PEDIATRIC PRACTICE

Sports Medicine

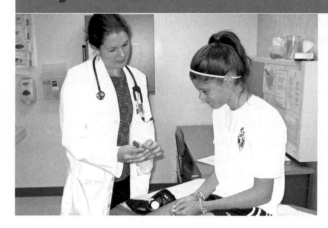

NOTICE

PEDIATRIC PRACTICE

Sports Medicine

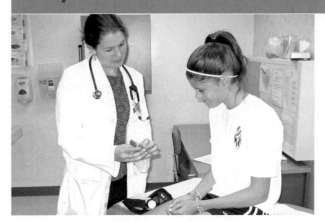

EDITORS

Dilip R. Patel, MD, FAAP, FSAM, FAACPDM, FACSM
Professor of Pediatrics and Human Development
Michigan State University College of Human Medicine
Primary Care Sports Medicine Fellowship Program
Kalamazoo Center for Medical Studies
Kalamazoo, Michigan

Donald E. Greydanus, MD, FAAP, FSAM, FIAP(H)
Professor of Pediatrics and Human Development
Pediatric Residency Program Director
Michigan State University College of Human Medicine
Kalamazoo Center for Medical Studies
Kalamazoo, Michigan

Robert J. Baker, MD, PhD, FACSM, ATC
Associate Professor of Family Medicine
Michigan State University College of Human Medicine
Program Director
 Family Medicine Primary Care Sports Medicine Fellowship
Kalamazoo Center for Medical Studies
Team Physician, Bronco Athletics, Western Michigan University
Family Medicine Residency Program
Kalamazoo, Michigan

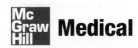 **Medical**

New York Chicago San Francisco Lisbon London Madrid Mexico City
Milan New Delhi San Juan Seoul Singapore Sydney Toronto

Pediatric Practice: Sports Medicine

Copyright © 2009 by The McGraw-Hill Companies, Inc. All rights reserved. Printed in China. Except as permitted under the United States Copyright Act of 1976, no part of this publication may be reproduced or distributed in any form or by any means, or stored in a data base or retrieval system, without the prior written permission of the publisher.

1 2 3 4 5 6 7 8 9 0   CTP/CTP   12 11 10 9 8

ISBN 978-0-07-149677-3
MHID 0-07-149677-7

This book was set in Minion by Aptara®, Inc.
The editors were Anne M. Sydor and Robert Pancotti.
The production supervisor was Sherri Souffrance.
The illustration manager was Armen Ovsepyan.
Project management was provided by Sumbul Jafri, Aptara®, Inc.
The designer was Janice Bielawa; the cover designer was David Dell'Accio.
Cover photographs:
Large image at right: Physician examining a boy. (Credit: Tetra Images/Getty)
Small image at left: Radiograph of a child's hand.
China Translation & Printing Services, Ltd., was printer and binder.

This book is printed on acid-free paper.

Library of Congress Cataloging-in-Publication Data

Pediatric practice. Sports medicine / editors, Dilip R. Patel, Donald E.
Greydanus, Robert J. Baker.
      p. ; cm.
   Includes bibliographical references and index.
   ISBN-13: 978-0-07-149677-3 (hardcover : alk. paper)
   ISBN-10: 0-07-149677-7 (hardcover : alk. paper)
   1.   Pediatric sports medicine.   I. Patel, Dilip R.   II. Greydanus,
Donald E.   III. Baker, Robert J. (Robert Jon), 1963– IV. Title: Sports
medicine.
   [DNLM: 1.   Athletic Injuries. 2.   Adolescent. 3.   Child. 4.   Health
Status. 5.   Sports—physiology. 6.   Sports Medicine—methods.   QT 261
P371 2009]
  RC1218.C45P45 2009
  617.1'027083—dc22
                                                          2008014397

Dilip R. Patel dedicates this work to his wife, Ranjan, and son, Neil, who once again endured and supported his crazy scholarly pursuits.

Donald E. Greydanus dedicates his efforts in this book to "my big brother, Robert John Greydanus, who introduced me to the wonderful world of sports as a child in the baseball fields and basketball courts of our hometown, Hawthorne, New Jersey. Thanks, Bob! I also dedicate my efforts to my daughters, Marissa, Elizabeth, Suzanne, and Megan—I watched the interplay of life and sports in your lives as you grew up. Thanks for the education and your enduring love!"

Robert J. Baker dedicates this work to his wife, Lynette, and children, Amanda, Katie, and Paul, who sacrificed their time for dad.

A Special Dedication

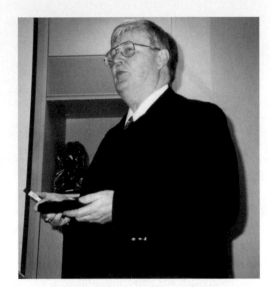

Eugene F. Luckstead, MD

Pediatric Practice: Sports Medicine is dedicated to Eugene F. Luckstead, MD, one of the pioneers and true giants of pediatric sports medicine. During the past 30 years, Dr. Luckstead ("Gene") has inspired, motivated, and taught so many of us in the field of pediatric sports medicine and continues to do so with the same zeal, passion, enthusiasm, and dedication. Over the years, he has guided hundreds of young athletes and their families through good times and bad times as they ventured into sports. Gene has taught us not only the science but more importantly the art of practicing pediatric sports medicine. One of his numerous contributions to the field is the book *Medical Care of the Adolescent Athlete.*

With great affection and admiration, we dedicate *Pediatric Practice: Sports Medicine* to Eugene F. Luckstead, MD.

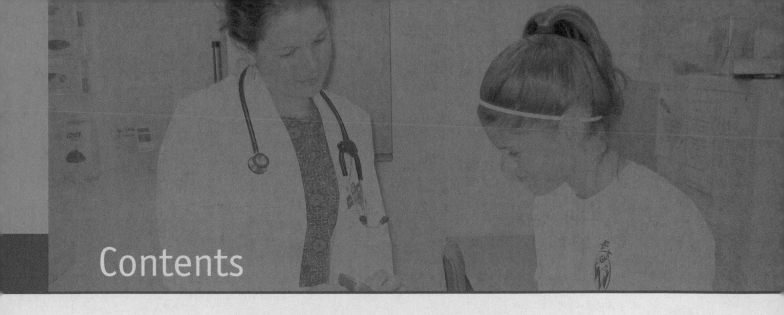

Contents

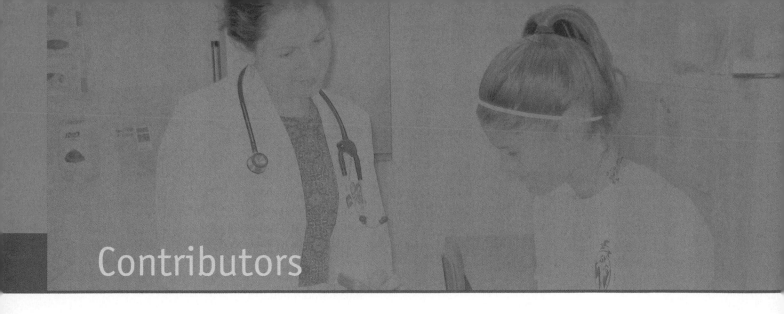

Contributors

General Pediatrician Reviewer

Arthur N. Feinberg, MD
Professor, Pediatrics and Human Development
Michigan State University College of Human Medicine
Pediatric Residency Program
Kalamazoo Center for Medical Studies
Kalamazoo, Michigan

Medical Illustrator

Megan M. Greydanus, BFA
Portage, Michigan

Medical Photography and Research Assistant

Neil D. Patel
Undergraduate Studies
University of Michigan
Ann Arbor, Michigan

Authors

Robert J. Baker, MD, PhD, FACSM, ATC
Associate Professor of Family Medicine
Michigan State University College of Human Medicine
Program Director
Family Medicine Primary Care Sports Medicine
  Fellowship
Kalamazoo Center for Medical Studies
Team Physician, Bronco Athletics, Western Michigan
  University
Family Medicine Residency Program
Kalamazoo, Michigan

Sarah Bancroft, DO
Kansas City University of Medicine and Biosciences
Kansas City, Kansas

Steven Cline, MD
Orthopedic Sports Medicine
Assistant Research Director for Orthopedic Residency
  Program
Michigan State University Kalamazoo Center for
  Medical Studies
Kalamazoo, Michigan

Daniel G. Constance, MD, MS, ATC
Primary Care Sports Medicine
Department of Family Medicine
Michigan State University Kalamazoo Center for
  Medical Studies
Kalamazoo, Michigan

Joseph D'Ambrosio, MD, DMD
Program Director, Internal Medicine-Pediatrics
  Combined Residency Program
Associate Professor
Michigan State University Kalamazoo Center for
  Medical Studies
Kalamazoo, Michigan

Eugene Diokno, MD, FAAP
Primary Care Sports Medicine
Arnold Palmer Sportshealth Center
Union Memorial Hospital
Baltimore, Maryland

Martin B. Draznin, MD, FAAP
Pediatric Endocrinology
Professor of Pediatrics and Human Development
Michigan State University College of Human Medicine
Kalamazoo Center for Medical Studies
Kalamazoo, Michigan

Cynthia Feucht, PharmD, BCPS
Assistant Professor
Ferris State University College of Pharmacy
Michigan State University, Kalamazoo Center for
  Medical Studies
Kalamazoo, Michigan

Donald E. Greydanus, MD, FAAP, FSAM, FIAP(H)
Professor of Pediatrics and Human Development
Pediatric Residency Program Director
Michigan State University College of Human Medicine
Kalamazoo Center for Medical Studies
Kalamazoo, Michigan

Douglas N. Homnick, MD, MPH, FAAP
Pediatric Pulmonology
Professor of Pediatrics and Human Development
Michigan State University College of Human Medicine
Kalamazoo Center for Medical Studies
Kalamazoo, Michigan

Manmohan K. Kamboj, MD, FAAP
Pediatric Endocrinology
Professor of Pediatrics and Human Development
Michigan State University College of Human Medicine
Kalamazoo Center for Medical Studies
Kalamazoo, Michigan

Ashir Kumar, MD
Pediatric Infectious Diseases
Professor, Department of Pediatrics and Human
  Development
Michigan State University College of Human Medicine
East Lansing, Michigan

E. Dennis Lyne, MD, FAAP
Pediatric Orthopaedic Surgery
Professor of Orthopaedic Surgery
Orthopaedic Residency Program
Michigan State University College of Human Medicine
Kalamazoo Center for Medical Studies
Kalamazoo, Michigan

Timothy J. Michael, PhD
Associate Professor of Exercise Science
Department of Health, Physical Education, and
  Recreation
Western Michigan University
Kalamazoo, Michigan

Michael G. Miller, EdD, ATC, CSCS
Associate Professor and Program Director
Graduate Athletic Training Education
Department of Health, Physical Education,
  and Recreation
Western Michigan University
Kalamazoo, Michigan

Dilip R. Patel, MD, FAAP, FSAM, FAACPDM, FACSM
Professor of Pediatrics and Human Development
Michigan State University College of Human Medicine
Primary Care Sports Medicine Fellowship Program
Kalamazoo Center for Medical Studies
Kalamazoo, Michigan

Helen D. Pratt, PhD
Clinical Psychology
Professor of Pediatrics and Human Development
Michigan State University College of Human Medicine
Director of Behavioral-Developmental Pediatrics
Kalamazoo Center for Medical Studies
Kalamazoo, Michigan

Dale Rowe, MD
Spine Surgery
Professor of Orthopaedic Surgery
Program Director
Orthopaedic Surgery Residency Program
Michigan State University College of Human Medicine
Kalamazoo Center for Medical Studies
Kalamazoo, Michigan

Alfonso Torres, MD
Director of Pediatric Nephrology
Assistant Professor of Pediatrics and Human
  Development
Michigan State University College of Human Medicine
Kalamazoo Center for Medical Studies
Kalamazoo, Michigan

Artemis K. Tsitsika, MD, PhD
Adolescent Medicine
Department of Pediatrics
P&A Kyriakou Children's Hospital
Athens, Greece

David H. Van Dyke, MD
Pediatric Neurology
Professor of Neurology and Pediatrics
Department of Pediatric and Human Development
Michigan State University College of Human Medicine
East Lansing, Michigan

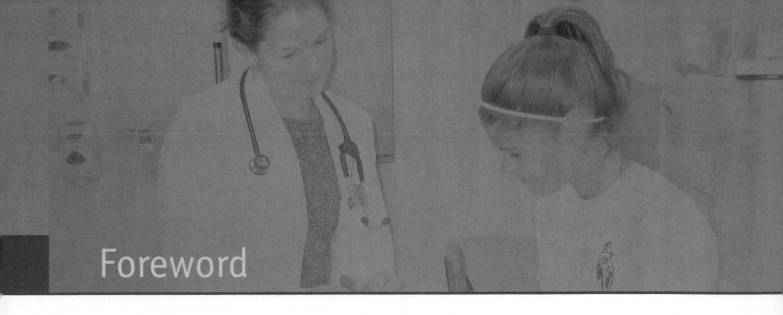

Foreword

"Children are not small adults." This phrase embodies the essential elements of pediatric practice and helps to remind practitioners that infants, children, and adolescents have unique developmental, physiologic, and psychosocial concerns.

Sport participation is an integral aspect for every child and adolescent growing up in a contemporary society. It is estimated that 30 million children and adolescents participate in organized sports and many more participate in recreational activities every year in the United States. They engage in sports for a variety of reasons ranging from fun to serious, intensive competition. Some young persons even take part in activities that push their physiologic and psychologic limits, such as climbing Mount Everest. Those practitioners who provide medical care to young athletes appreciate and understand that, compared with adults, the implications of such sport participation and physical activity are vastly different and often unique, physiologically, psychologically, and socially, for children and adolescents. An understanding of the interrelatedness between physical, cognitive, and psychosocial growth and development and sport participation by children and adolescents is fundamental to pediatric sports medicine.

Pediatricians and other health care practitioners who provide medical care to young athletes are at the front line to guide them appropriately as they engage in sports. Thus, pediatricians have the privilege and responsibility to influence positively and to promote a lifelong choice of regular physical activity.

The editors and authors of *Pediatric Practice: Sports Medicine* represent an integration of outstanding expertise and experience in various aspects of pediatrics as it applies to the practice of sports medicine. *Pediatric Practice: Sports Medicine* covers the following topics in a practical and concise manner: aspects of growth and development with implications for sport participation, a detailed review of major medical conditions, acute and overuse injuries of the musculoskeletal system, and aspects of the team physician and on-field emergencies. The information is organized in a consistent format with numerous tables and is profusely illustrated with numerous figures, including algorithms and hundreds of full-color photographs.

Pediatric Practice: Sports Medicine is a "must-have" book for every medical practitioner who provides care to children and adolescents.

Sandra J. Hoffmann, MD, MS, FACSM, FACP
Fellow of the American College of Sports Medicine,
Board of Trustees (2006–2009) of the American College
of Sports Medicine,
Associate Professor
Department of Family Medicine
Idaho State University School of Medicine

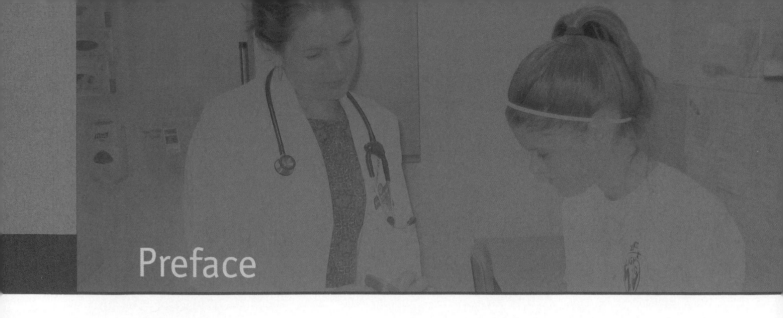

Preface

Providing medical care to children and adolescents engaged in sports and various recreational physical activities is truly a team effort. The field of sports medicine has evolved from the integration and application of the concepts derived from many different basic and clinical exercise science disciplines. The goals of primary care sports medicine are to apply these concepts and knowledge for lifelong health promotion, and to practice prevention and medical management of diseases in relation to physical activity, for those who engage in sports and other physical activities.

In sports medicine literature (including this book), the terms physical activity, exercise, and sports are often used interchangeably. *Physical fitness* is generally defined as a set of attributes that a person has regarding the ability to perform physical activities that require aerobic fitness, endurance, strength, or musculoskeletal flexibility. The degree of individual physical fitness is influenced by a combination of physical activity and genetic ability. *Physical activity* is defined as any bodily movement produced by skeletal muscles which results in an expenditure of energy. *Exercise* is a physical activity that is planned and structured. Physical activity is integral to sport participation but participation in *sports* occurs within a social context. For children and adolescents, physical, psychological, and social growth and development have direct implications for sport participation and vice versa.

Our goal is to provide a perspective of the child and adolescent athlete within the context of their growth and development. Young children engage in a wide range of play and physical activities that is spontaneous and fun and are able to stay within the limits of their abilities. As they get older and especially as they reach adolescence, sport participation takes on a new meaning: extrinsic influences from adult society tend to increase and sport participation changes from being simply fun to being a more organized, planned, and purpose-driven activity. In pediatric sports medicine, most patients seen by practitioners are in the adolescent age group; this group is the major focus of our book.

The main goal of *Pediatric Practice: Sports Medicine* is to provide guidance on a range of issues encountered by the pediatrician or other medical practitioner caring for children and adolescents in the office or clinic setting. Because it is impossible to cover every problem encountered in one's practice, we have included conditions that are commonly seen and can be managed in the primary care setting. Some topics are included because they have significant implications for the health and well-being of the athlete. Other topics, although considered uncommon in pediatric athletes, are included because we have encountered these problems often enough over the years. Many conditions that once were considered problems affecting only the adult athlete are being seen in adolescents because of the increasing trend of adolescents to participate in sports more intensely, more competitively, and at younger ages than before.

We would like to express our most sincere thanks to Anne M. Sydor, executive editor at McGraw-Hill, for her encouragement and professional guidance of this project from start to finish with great zeal. We also thank Robert Pancotti, project development editor at McGraw-Hill, for making sure, among other things, that all words and numbers match and for his incredible patience throughout this work. Thanks also to the other staff members at McGraw-Hill who diligently worked on this book. Dilip Patel would like to thank Donald Greydanus for introducing him to something called "sports medicine" in the early years of his training. Dilip Patel also expresses his heartfelt appreciation and thanks to Terry Nelson, MD, for his years of support, teaching, and wisdom in sports medicine, and all the staff at K Valley Orthopedics for their commitment to sports medicine. We are indebted to our medical students, residents, and sports medicine fellows over the years for keeping us on our toes and honest. Once again, special thanks to Megan Greydanus for her excellent drawings.

Special thanks and appreciation to Dr. Robert Carter, CEO and Assistant Dean at Michigan State University Kalamazoo Center for Medical Studies, for fostering an environment in which scholarly pursuits like this one are possible.

We sincerely hope that our readers will find this book useful in their daily practice and will be inspired and motivated to seek more knowledge and acquire more skills in pediatric sports medicine.

Dilip R. Patel
Donald E. Greydanus
Robert J. Baker

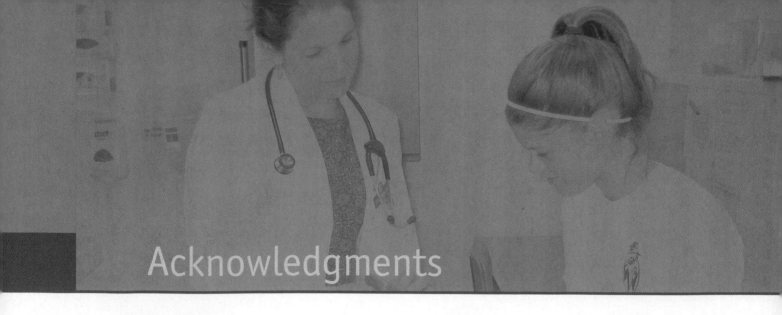

Acknowledgments

The editors wish to extend their sincere thanks to:

William Arbogast, Brenda Chapman, Teri Coburn, Daren Webb, Rainer Liebert, Matt Eberhardt, K. C. Zomer, April Eby, Tina Thompson, Mercedes Licavoli, and Jessica Groth, all from Western Michigan University, Sports Medicine Clinic, Kalamazoo, MI, for their active engagement and participation in various aspects during the development of this book.

Stu Myers, Human Resuscitation Learning Lab, Department of Emergency Medicine, Michigan State University, Kalamazoo Center for Medical Studies, Kalamazoo, MI, for help with the use of and providing the photographs for the "SimMAN" and the automated external defibrillator.

Amy Esman and Kim Douglas, Administrative Assistants, Department of Pediatrics, Michigan State University Kalamazoo Center for Medical Studies, for help with preparation of manuscripts.

Eugene Diokno, Kelsey Twist (Baltimore, MD); Matt Eberhardt, Mercedes Licavoli, Jennifer Groth, Jasmin Willis, Monica Lininger (Western Michigan University, Sports Medicine Clinic, Kalamazoo, MI); Kathleen Ryan, Rita Brust, Kristin Bayuk, Teresa Byrne, Erin Ruth, Elizabeth Mettler, and Elena Lewis (Pediatric Residency Program, Michigan State Kalamazoo Center for Medical Studies), Flora Bacopoulou (Athens, Greece), Molly Kooi, Alyssa Kooi (Portage, Michigan), for assistance with the photographs.

Sarah Bancroft, Kansas City University of Medicine and Biosciences, Kansas City, KA, for providing medical student review for the chapters on musculoskeletal injuries.

Neil D. Patel, of Portage, MI, for invaluable technical help with aspects of using information technology during the preparation of the manuscripts, artwork, and photographs.

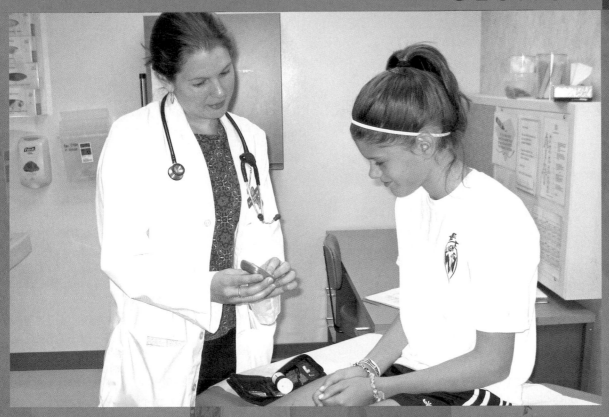

General and Basic Concepts

CHAPTER 1

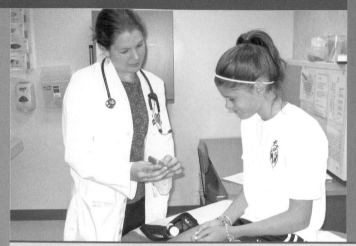

Child Neurodevelopment and Sport Participation

Dilip R. Patel and Helen D. Pratt

Stories of child prodigies, who began to learn a specific sport as early as age 3, may encourage parents to question whether or not they too should be enrolling their very young children in sport training programs. This raises the issue of neurodevelopmental maturation and readiness of the child to effectively and safely engage in sports, especially competitive sports. This chapter reviews the definition of neurodevelopment, normal child development as relevant to sport participation, and sport readiness. The discussion is limited to *typically developing children*.

Several broad fundamental principles underlie our understanding of child development (Table 1-1).[1-20] In order to effectively engage in and benefit from sport participation, all children and adolescents need to have mastered several fundamental skills.[21] Further refinement of skills is necessary for a child and adolescent to move from participation for *fun* to participation at a *competitive* level; at this level, skills must be highly developed to such a degree that it will limit who can play competitive sports. Children and adolescents who cannot master fundamental skills or who have other impediments to refining those skills can still be involved in sports activities, but may require special adaptations or equipment.[15,22,23]

DEFINITION OF NEURODEVELOPMENT

Neurodevelopment in a broad sense refers to the growth and maturation of the nervous system as well as the sensory and perceptual abilities of the child.[6,11,12,18,19,24,25] Normal growth and development is characterized by individual variations in the rate of progression and achievement of milestones, and the sequential nature of this progression. Although largely determined by genetic factors, environmental factors (such as opportunity, nutrition, and social context) also play a significant role in the overall development of a child or adolescent. Capute noted that motor milestones are mostly influenced by the maturation of the neurologic system, whereas social and adaptive skills are influenced largely by environmental factors, such as social expectations, education, and training.[18]

The term *neurodevelopment* encompasses various domains, which can be broadly categorized as physical or somatic, neurologic, sensory–perceptual, cognitive, and

Table 1-1.

Key Principles of Child Development

1. Growth and maturation is an on-going and continuous process.
2. Neurologic, somatic, cognitive, and social development of the child and adolescent progress at the same time as interdependent factors, and therefore must be considered together as one looks at development and sport participation.
3. Although different developmental milestones are recognized at specific ages, appearance of these milestones often varies considerably in between children.
4. The *sequential* nature of development remains the same in typically developing children (i.e., a child must first have neurologic maturity in order to stand and walk; no amount of training will make a child walk before a certain level of neurologic maturity is reached).
5. It is generally well recognized that there will always be children who will be at either end of the developmental spectrum.

psychosocial or emotional. Gesell described "streams" of development to include gross motor, fine motor, visual-motor problem solving, expressive language, receptive language, and social and adaptive skills.[9,26] Fagard notes that a "skill refers to the proficiency with which an integrated activity is carried out."[27] With increasing levels of maturity, there is an increasing level of integration and interaction among different domains. Although *quantitative* progress (i.e., number of milestones) in development is more apparent and often measured, *qualitative* progress (e.g., not only that the child is able to jump or throw, rather how well he or she is able to jump or throw) in motor and developmental skills is equally or more important to sport participation.[28–32] Developmental progression and refinement of certain fundamental sport-related tasks (such as catching, throwing, kicking, various other ball-handling skills, and others) naturally occurs over time with advancing age and overall neurodevelopmental maturation and is further enhanced by sports-specific skills training.[2,3,4,24,28,31,33–39] Malina refers to increase in size as *growth* and rate of progress toward a mature state as *maturation*.[20,40,41]

STAGES OF NEURODEVELOPMENT AND IMPLICATIONS FOR SPORT PARTICIPATION

The Infant and the Toddler

It is not unusual to see many infants and toddlers being initiated into sports programs as exemplified by swimming and gymnastics; a crawling race for infants has also been reported.[3,41,42] The American Academy of Pediatrics (AAP) recommends that children are not developmentally ready for swimming lessons until after 4 years of age.[3,42] Early participation in swimming programs has neither been shown to decrease the later risk of drowning nor does it increase the skill of swimming in children.[3,43]

Infants attain gross and fine motor skills along a predetermined and sequential path.[1,3,4,19,30,44] Attempts at acquisition of specific motor skills by early training usually are not successful.[41,45] For example, children must have neuromotor maturation before they can walk, and children who walk earlier than at an "average" age will not necessarily learn other motor skills earlier.

THE PRESCHOOL YEARS

Physical Growth and Motor Development

During the preschool years, from approximately 3 to 5 or 6 years of age, the physical growth slows down compared

to infancy and toddlers stages; however, acquisition of basic neuromotor, language, and cognitive skills increase rapidly.[25,46] The development of better postural and balance control allows preschoolers to learn how to ride a bicycle without training wheels, catch a small ball thrown from 10 ft away, and use their hands to manipulate objects (such as objects used for drawing and elementary writing skills).[4,7,14,19,25,27,39,43,46–48]

Children between ages 3 and 4 years can broad jump approximately 1 ft, hop up to six times, and catch a ball against their chest.[19] By the end of 4 years, a child can skip on one foot, climb up a jungle gym, throw overhand, and catch a large ball.[19] A child can also stand on one foot for up to 5 seconds, kick a ball forward, catch a bounced ball most of the times, and move backward as well as forward with agility.[4,7,24,25,43,47–49]

By age 5, children have better balance, coordination, body strength, and endurance, although still far less compared with adolescents and adults. By the end of age 5, children can run smoothly, gallop, do a one-foot skip, hop up to nine times on one foot, throw a ball with shift of their bodies, catch a ball with both hands, ride a tricycle well, swing, and do somersaults.[17,19,48] By age 6, most children can run, throw a small ball at a target, and hit the target; girls can skip but boys may not. Children by 6 years of age can jump up 1 ft and broad jump up to 3 ft.[19] Once children have learned these skills, their continued use results in further refinement.[7,50] Throughout childhood, the effects of training and skill development are directly related to age-specific changes in the neuromotor, metabolic, cardiopulmonary, and cognitive/integrative systems.[4,7,25,47] Muscular strength and muscular endurance can be improved during the childhood years with the use of higher repetition-moderate load resistance training programs during the initial adaptation period.[4,41,43,51,52]

Cognitive Development

During the preschool years, children can remember basic information, recall that information on demand, and answer simple "who" and "what" questions. Their memory is enhanced by visual aides, and they tend to learn from trial and error.[7,44] Preschool children generally have short attention spans (5–15 minutes) and poor selective attention; they can distinguish simple similarities and differences and can understand simple analogies; and they can identify the missing parts of familiar objects. Also, they can follow simple rules but will need visual cues and frequent reminders.

Language Development

Children by age 5 have a vocabulary of approximately 2500 words, and by age 6, it is approximately 5000 words.[19] Typically, the speech of a preschooler is 100% intelligible to strangers.[14,17,19,53] By age 5, the child can speak sentences of up to five words, use future tense, can name four colors, and count 10 or more objects.[19,53] They may still have difficulty understanding words that sound alike but have different or multiple meanings. At this age, the ability to comprehend complex or compound sentences is limited. Coaches and trainers who give multiple instructions may find that many of their young players become lost in the words or get distracted. Children will be better able to follow instructions given using simple sentences combined with visual cues (such as pictures), which demonstrates the expected action. Sentences should be clear, concise, and devoid of words that have multiple or complex meanings. Use of training tapes to teach a skill may be helpful, if the language used matches the words that will be used when directing a particular skill; it is also critical that the words and skills are shown in a way that depicts the actual intended situation or environment. Coaches and parents can begin to teach children how to communicate when the children are frustrated, tired, angry, happy, or excited. This will aid in their overall communication skills development.

Social and Emotional Development

Children between the ages 3 and 5 or 6 years are *egocentric,* and thus they have difficulty taking the view of another person or understanding why they cannot always be first.[44,46] They are learning to interact with their environment and engage in cooperative play with other children. By age 6, they play best with children of the same gender. Children learn autonomy and trust through their successes or failures.[44,46] Preschoolers are unable to compare their own abilities to that of other children.[7,14,19] They may become upset when they lose or may want others to focus only on their performance. They may not understand why one child is allowed more "play" or "demonstration" time, and they usually want their needs met immediately.

Visual Development

At this age children may not have a fully developed capacity for tracking objects or people and judging the velocity of moving objects.[7,8,18,19] Children younger than 6 or 7 years are farsighted, and their limited ability to track objects and judge the speed of moving objects is owing to their vision limitation and not owing to a lack of coordination.[7,11] In softball, for instance, a pitcher with limited ability to judge velocity might throw the ball too fast. The batter who is accustomed to a slow pitch, but also has a limited ability to track and judge velocity, may be hit in the head because he or she will not be able to determine the trajectory of the ball, process in time

this critical information, and then coordinate the movements to pull the body out of the ball's path.

Auditory Development

The ability to understand the sounds they hear is developing rapidly in children in this age range.[11,19,25,41] The multiple sounds that occur in most sport environments can be very confusing for a child at this level of development. In a typical setting, a coach or a trainer may be giving the child instructions, while the parent is yelling directions and various members of the audience are also offering advice. Children may have difficulty discriminating which words they should listen to and may become distracted or confused. Other sounds such as those of whistles and bells can simply add to this perceived cacophonous situation. The ability to listen *selectively* matures as the child grows. All sports require players to listen and comprehend spoken language as well as sounds and to coordinate that information with other events and actions in their *specific* sports environment.

Perceptual Motor Development

These children know their right from their left body parts and can locate the right and left of other people or objects.[46] They can also locate themselves in relation to other objects.[46] They have a better orientation of their bodies in space, but may not be able to control the intensity and trajectory of a gross motor action.[7,8] They may throw a ball to another child, but at a velocity that is too fast and results in the other child being hurt when the ball hits him. Or the child may kick at a soccer ball, but the aim is off and he or she kicks another child. A child who runs toward a base may trip and fall in an attempt to beat the ball to the baseman.

The act of catching a ball is an example of complex motor planning that involves temporal sequencing, body awareness, eye–hand coordination, and visual–spatial skills.[4,31,33,38,39] Children at this age will do better if they are told where the ball will be thrown (i.e., saying and demonstrating: "I am going to throw the ball to you; I will throw it to your chest area; hold your hands up to your chest.") The adult throws a medium-sized ball slowly using exaggerated movements to allow the child time to mentally process and coordinate visual, mental, and gross motor skills; the child also needs time to estimate the temporal sequence, judge the velocity of the ball, determine body position, move arms and hands to the chest, and grasp the ball as it reaches the appropriate distance to his or her body. By following these multiple tasks, the child has just performed the complex motor function of catching. With practice, the child can learn to catch a ball thrown toward other body parts from a distance of up to 10 ft.[2]

Implications for Sport Participation

By age 5 or 6, most children can remember simple rules and play games that require only simple decision-making skills.[7,8,44,46] Their ability to generalize rules to different aspects of a sport activity other than the context in which it was learned is limited or even nonexistent. Children at the *concrete-operational* stage of cognitive development only understand clear and concise information. Children younger than 6 to 8 years do not always understand the purpose or competitive nature of a game even though they know and understand the basic rules.[7,8,44,46]

For example, these children will all swarm around a soccer ball to kick it, because they know that is what you are suppose to do. However, they may not understand that they are to engage in a cooperative effort with their peers to move the ball down the field to score points by kicking the ball between their opponent team's goal posts. This form of "beehive" soccer is frustrating to coaches and parents, but it is actually normal behavior for children at this level of *cognitive development*.[8,26,41] All the physical skill and knowledge of the game can be thwarted by a player's stage of cognitive development. If one player kicks the ball in an unanticipated direction, another player may not be able to engage in rapid decision making needed to change his or her position or process a strategy to compensate for this unexpected event. Changes in the demands of the sport during a game or a season will most likely result in chaos; these children are less likely to be able to change their performance to meet the "new" competitive requirements of their game.[8] It is best to encourage participation in a variety of different activities that allow preschool age children to practice, refine skills, and have fun.[47] In order to establish the best learning environment for these children, it is important to focus on cooperation and socialization abilities as well as learn critical thinking and perceptual motor skills.[8,47]

Preschool children need to engage in activities that allow them to travel (i.e., hop, skip, run, slide, crawl, creep, slither, and climb) in different directions and on different surfaces (i.e., flat, inclined, wavy, wet, and dry).[47] They also need to exercise postural control and balance (i.e., head stands and hanging).[47] Preschool children should experience what it feels like to be out of balance and in balance, they need to move their bodies up and down in space while out of contact with the ground (i.e., jumping, hopping, skipping, bouncing, and leaping), and they need to experience different forms of contorting their bodies (i.e., turning, spinning, rolling, twisting, tumbling, gesturing, bending, stretching, and reaching).[47] It is important for them to learn about directionality (i.e., up, down, sideways, backward, and forward) and different temporal sequences (i.e., going quickly or slowly, fast or slow, and moving one's body in time to different forms of music as well as different rhythms or sound patterns).[44,46,47]

Children need to experience a variety of shapes of objects through the visual memory, symbolic memory, linguistic, kinesthetic, and proprioceptive properties of each shape (i.e., round, oval, square, thin, twisted, and straight).[47] Also, they should experience physical properties of objects (especially sports objects such as bats, ball, hockey sticks, or rackets) and experience a variety of concepts and actions (such as *strong* versus *weak*, *heavy* versus *light*, *smooth* versus *rough* or *bumpy*, *smoothly* verses *jerkily*, *push* verses *pull*, and *receive* versus *send*). Each of these repeated experiences will integrate over time and provide children with foundational skills that will allow them to overcome physical and mental challenges of various sports. These experiences will also help children develop confidence in their ability to perform skills necessary for most sport participation and possibly prevent the development of the fear of being struck by a ball.[7,8,47]

MIDDLE CHILDHOOD

Physical Growth and Motor Development

By the middle years (6–10 or 11years) most children have established adult walking patterns.[11,25,54] There is a synergistic cooperation of the physiologic, neurologic, and musculoskeletal systems that allows children at this level of development to adopt a walking frequency to optimize physiologic cost, symmetry, and stability.[54]

Physical growth is fairly steady during the elementary school years; gender differences in height and weight are less noticeable than in later developmental stages.[11,25] At this stage children also develop the initial awareness of more effectively and efficiently using their gross motor functions. Gender differences are noted in certain motor tasks during middle years.[2,7,28,30,31,36,37,55] As with most fundamental physical skills, boys at this age have a slight advantage in explosive power needed for actions such as vertical jump, long jump, running speed, and throwing for distance. Girls learn to strike objects, jump, kick, and throw later than boys; but they learn to hop, skip, and catch a little earlier than boys.[30,31] Girls have the advantage of having better balance than boys at this stage of development.[30,31] By age 7, children show interest in learning to bat and to pitch and can pedal a bicycle well.[19,48,53] By age 8, the motor movements are more graceful and rhythmic, and children begin to learn soccer or baseball.[17,53] By age 9, they can engage in vigorous physical activities, participate in team play, catch a fly ball, and can balance on one foot for at least 15 seconds; they like to wrestle, play ball, and be part of a team.[17,19,30,31,48,53]

By age 10 or 11, most children have mastered all fundamental motor skills.[4,7,8,19,25,41] Hitting a baseball or tennis ball and shooting a basketball are examples of skills that are easiest to learn at this age. Aerobic and anaerobic capacities increase steadily during middle childhood but are still quite limited compared to adolescents. Children now can perform other sophisticated motor functions such as overarm throwing and overhead striking as employed in tennis.[8,56]

As children mature, they will continue to experience improvement in their posture, balance, and reaction times with practice. The refinement of these skills may be influenced by many factors, including somatotype, gender, training, and motivation; this makes age predictions for a specific child as "ready" to participate in all sports a difficult task.[5,8,23,30,41,43,57,58]

Cognitive Development

Children at this age have considerable difficulty with futuristic thinking; they see things as here and now, right or wrong, and black or white.[17,19,44,46,59] Discussions about morality and future consequences of current behavior are useless. They engage in *magical thinking* and may believe they have unique powers that will protect them from harm.[46,53] These children cannot think through the consequences of their actions to know that jumping from a high place may result in serious injury, for example, mimicking wrestling stunts seen on television; thus, children believe they have same abilities as these highly trained athletes. Their attention spans are longer now, but they may still be easily distracted. They can plan and execute simple motors sequences.

There is further development of memory and rapid decision making; they can understand the intent of instructions given and can follow directions.[8,46] Critical thinking and problem-solving skills are further developed during the middle years.[19,44,46,53] They can apply factual knowledge to familiar situations but may not be able to extrapolate that knowledge to unique or new situations. They are beginning to understand the purpose of the rules they learned earlier. Judgment and decision making improve significantly by the end of the middle years.[26,60] They can adopt another person's spatial perspective much better. Children at this age clearly recognize differences between personal performance and the performance or skill of others.[23] They accurately discriminate between those children that are popular and those who are not. They begin to identify those children who are "smart" and those who are "dumb."[23] They are now very aware of their body image.[44,46,61]

Language Development

Use of complex language skills increases considerably during the middle years. By now children can give complex directions to others and have the cognitive ability to understand a broader range of words and their symbolic use.[19,23,48,53] They understand words with multiple, similar, and different meanings. Children who have mastered age-appropriate language skills will have a better chance of understanding and articulating sports instructions. Language is used as part of the socialization environment in sports to transmit rules or instructions, to praise, and to critisize.

Social and Emotional Development

At this stage children are developing a sense of right or wrong and usually like to play by the rules; they become upset with peers who do not follow the rules.[2,26,44,46,60] They are able to follow limits set by others. During these middle years, children enjoy playing organized games and delight in peer comparisons of athletic prowess. Children at this age generally know it is not okay to make fun of other players. They are now better able to control their anger or hurt feelings when they cannot get their own way. Those children with more advanced skills may not yet understand that their "gifts" may be time limited; some in fact become less motivated to learn and practice to refine those skills.[23]

Special attention from coaches, other players, and their parents (because of their athletic success) may facilitate positive social adaptation of these children. However, the less gifted or skilled child may become more withdrawn and less socially adept. It is important for adults in this environment to recognize these issues and build in confidence-enhancing activities for **all** children. The focus should be on practice, correcting weak areas, developing overall skills, engaging in multiple activities, and doing one's best. Such a foundation gives children a broader set of criteria on which they can base their self-esteem or belief in their own abilities. They should be involved in more than one sport (at least one *noncompetitive* type) and other activities that contribute to other aspects of their development (i.e., music, voice, singing, art, stamp collecting, reading, or debate). The more well-rounded the athlete, the easier it is to maintain a healthy balance.

Visual and Auditory Development

These children have improved visual acuity, tracking ability, and a more mature level of visual–perceptual motor integration; however, their sense of *directionality* may not yet be fully developed.[7,8,17,19] Auditory discrimination is now well developed, and children can begin to listen *selectively* and thus the confusion they might have experienced in the early childhood years becomes significantly less.[7,14,19] They can more clearly distinguish the directions and comments of coaches, trainer, and parents from other "noises" in the crowd.

Perceptual Motor Development

Balance is still somewhat limited because these children are just starting to integrate visual, vestibular, and proprioceptive cues at a more sophisticated level.[8,19] These children have the visual motor capacity, manual dexterity, basic analytical thinking, problem-solving skills, and motor-planning skills necessary for most sports.[7,8,14,17,19,41,53]

Children's ability to estimate the arrival of a simulated moving object on a target based on three different motions (constant *velocity*, constant *acceleration*, and constant *deceleration*) was analyzed by Benguigui and Ripoll.[62] Results showed that timing accuracy improved mainly between the age of 7 and 10 years, tennis practice accelerated the development of timing accuracy, and acceleration or deceleration of the moving object or target had no effect on the timing accuracy of any of the tested groups (ages 7, 10, 13, and 23 years). Additionally, they concluded that with practice, a 7-year-old could develop a level of performance very similar to that of the older participants. Tennis practice induced an acceleration of the development of the perceptual motor process involved in tennis that requires the player to engage in coincidence timing tasks necessary to target the trajectory of a specific moving object in order to intercept it. This study illustrates a child's ability to link sensory input and motor output even at an *early* age.[62]

Pienaar et al. found that they could develop the essential physical and motor skills in a 10-year-old rugby players in South Africa.[63] They successfully developed a practical method of selecting and developing the basic skills and abilities needed to play rugby: catching, passing, running, kicking, sprinting, passing for accuracy over a specific distance, two-handed lateral pass, pull-ups, zigzag run, 50-yard dash, ball-changing skills, strength and endurance training, vertical jumping, throwing a ball through a circle to hit a target, running and throwing at a specific target, making lateral passes, agility runs, sit and reach, flexed arm hang, speed, and endurance.[63]

Implications for Sport Participation

The reactions and feedback of coaches, trainers, parents, and other professionals to the behaviors, attitudes, beliefs, and actions of children at this developmental level are crucial to helping these children successfully transition from childhood to adolescence. Children during the middle years exhibit early levels of judgment, thinking, problem solving, and a variety of physical abilities and emotional reactions; however, they have little prior history and limited perspective to allow them to put their experiences in context.[8,19,46,59] They are still developing their *sense of self* in terms of confidence, esteem, consciousness, and body awareness.[26,44,46,60] Their abilities to handle the reactions of others to their words and behaviors are still limited. They do not have *abstract thought* yet and may not understand that their ability to hit a pitched ball during a baseball game is related to how much time they spend practicing hitting a ball between games.[15,23,44,46,59] They may incorrectly assume that being able to hit a ball is something you can either "do" or "not do." For example, a girl at age 10 may think she cannot throw a ball as well as her male peers because when she was 7 years old, she could not compete with the boys; she may then give up on trying to play ball because she thinks she is not "good" at that sport. She will need encouragement to continue to play and will need to be told her skills may develop more fully as she practices.

If sports activities are focused on skill development and incorporate problem solving, anger management, as well as cooperative play, children can learn to enjoy sport participation and develop appropriate skills to support competitive play that is both fun and instructive. Children at this age will often become confused and very emotional if they are criticized too severely or if adults (especially coaches and parents) scream, yell, use harsh tones of voice, and animated physical or facial gestures to give feedback. These children will attend only to the emotion of the message and not to the message itself. They will personalize the negative impact of the message and not be able to learn or gain an instructive quality of what the adult is saying or is trying to say. Children during these middle years can engage in more complex sport activities that enhances the refinement of the fundamental skills they acquired during preschool years. They should participate in activities that help them learn to use their skills in a variety of settings. Children should receive instructions in a "show and tell" format delivered in short intervals and intertwined with free play and drills.[8] As these children are just beginning to compare their performance with those of their peers, involvement in competitive sports should be minimal.[8] It is more important to work on the perceptual motor skills, decision-making skills, and problem-solving skills necessary for participation in a number of different sports, rather than prematurely specializing in one or two sports.[41,51,64] Entry-level soccer, baseball, tennis, track, swimming, tumbling, or gymnastics are all examples of appropriate activities.[7] By the end of middle childhood, the normally developing child has mastered the basic skills identified in the functional domains (e.g., language, auditory, perceptual motor). The focus shifts to highlight the importance of the adolescent growth spurt, higher order cognitive functions, and psychosocial development.

Many parents wonder whether their child's sports talent can be identified early and developed further to reach elite or Olympic level. Researchers have used complex measurements of physical, behavioral, and psychologic characteristics to identify talented child athletes; however, numerous interrelated variables (such as the continuous process of growth and development, varying selection processes at different levels, different sport-specific demands, and cultural factors) make it extremely difficult to identify and accurately predict athletic excellence at an early developmental stage.[2,5,6,8,15,26,41,51,65]

Although research is limited, some reports suggest that early intensive training and specialization in sport before a child is developmentally ready have neither shown enhancement in current performance nor guarantee future athletic success.[26,38,41,51,63,64,66] In fact, some athletes may develop stress-related physical as well as emotional problems stemming from intense early participation; these problems include overuse injuries (such as stress fractures), overtraining syndrome, menstrual disorders, stress injuries to growth plates, depression, anxiety, conversion reactions, and disordered eating behaviors.[26,32,41,50,51,58,64,67]

Regular training enhances neuromuscular adaptive responses and contributes to improved sports-specific skills and performance.[15,35,41,51,68–71] Somatotype, motor skills, age, nutritional status, physiologic as well as psychologic factors, perceived physical abilities, training level, genetic endowment, and injury risk are the major independent variables influencing performance.[41,43,50,51,58,70,72–75] Although, mesomorphy and to a lesser extent ectomorphy are positively associated with enhanced performance, successful athletes tend to have or acquire somatotypes characteristic of individuals already successful in a particular sport.[2,62] For the most part, motor skills are chronologic age and gender dependent; in general, the efficiency of such skills progressively improves throughout childhood and into early adolescence and is influenced by environmental factors.[4,28,33,37,39,40,43,55,72] Lower anaerobic and aerobic capacity to some extent may also reduce performance in the child. The relationship between endurance, performance, and aerobic capacity, however, is not strong at any age during childhood A number of mental factors such as motivation, aggression, spirit, and self-confidence are also related to sports performance; however, their specific correlation is unclear at present. Some of the factors that *negatively* impact on performance levels include inadequate nutrition, a history of previous injury, excessive training schedules, decreased fitness, decreased endurance, joint looseness, and certain personality traits.

NEURODEVELOPMENTAL READINESS FOR SPORTS

Sports readiness refers to a stage when the child has reached the necessary maturity to learn a given sport-related task.[5,6,8,26,32,41,51,57] In other words, it is a process in which the child acquires the motor, physical, cognitive, social, and adaptive abilities and is ready to meet the demands of a given sport. Readiness to play and to compete is influenced by biologic, physiologic, psychosocial, and environmental factors.[3,5,7,13,26,31,32,41,51,58]

Participation in sports requires that the child can coordinate certain motor, cognitive and physiologic functions, such as movements of the extremities, breathing, thinking, balancing, and many more. The ability to coordinate different actions is influenced by a child's level of thought processing ability, thinking speed, agility, flexibility, strength, and endurance.

Some researchers have proposed that there are certain critical periods when sport skills are learned best.[2,41] On the other hand, *not all* children must learn such skills during these periods. Because there are multiple factors influencing readiness and varying rates of growth and development progression, it is not possible to *reliably* identify athletic talent and predict future athletic excellence in children.[3,5,7,8,26,30,41,64] Seefeldt's classic study showed that by elementary school age, 60% of children were able to perform the following tasks at age-appropriate levels: throwing, kicking, running, jumping, catching, striking, hopping, and skipping[30,31] (Figure 1-1). Major cognitive milestones with implications for sport participation are summarized in Table 1-2.[1,4,5,7,8,23,25,26,31–33,41,51,57,76] The progression of motor and adaptive skills from immature to more mature stage is illustrated in Figures 1-2–1-4.

Table 1-2.

Major Sport Participation-Related Cognitive Milestones

Cognitive Maturiy	Age (yr)
To compare one's own abilities in sport to that of others	≥6
To understand the competitive nature of sport	≥9
To understand the complex tasks of a given sport	≥12

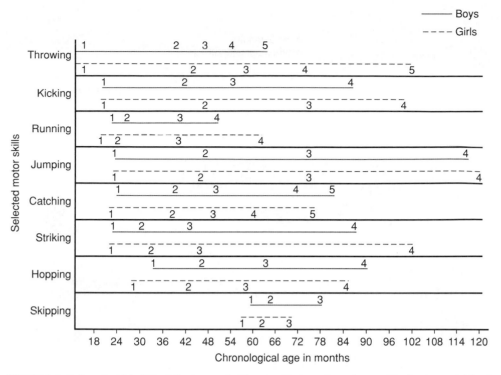

FIGURE 1-1 ■ Age at which 60% of the boys and girls were able to perform at a specific developmental level for selected fundamental motor skills. Numbers refer to the developmental stages of that motor skill.

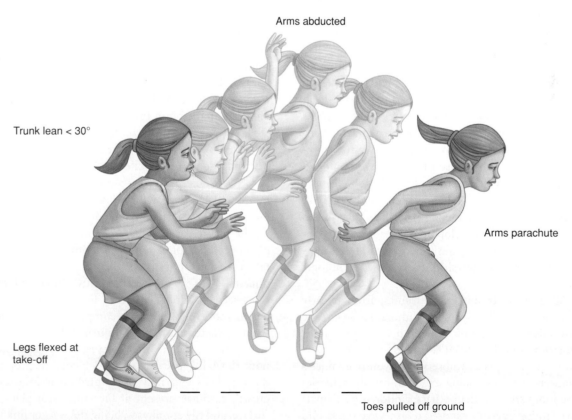

FIGURE 1-2 ■ Pattern of long jump in the beginner.

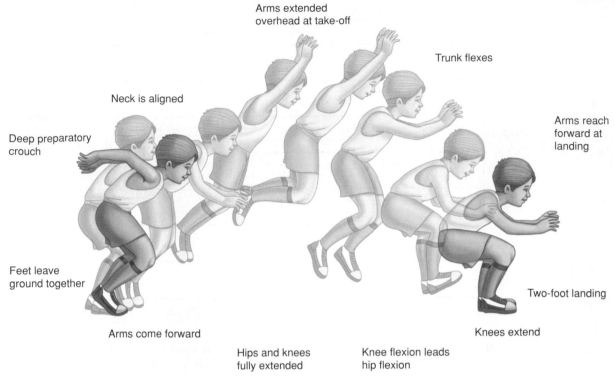

Arms extended
overhead at take-off

Trunk flexes

Neck is aligned

Arms reach
forward at
landing

Deep preparatory
crouch

Feet leave
ground together

Two-foot landing

Arms come forward

Knees extend

Hips and knees
fully extended

Knee flexion leads
hip flexion

FIGURE 1-3 ■ Pattern of long jump in an advanced jumper.

NEURODEVELOPMENT AND INJURIES

Numerous reports have discussed the implications of young athlete's growth and development for specific risks, unique characteristics, and short- and long-term complications of sport-related injuries; these reports have suggested appropriate precautionary and preventive measures.[42,45,66,73,77–91] Young children can be predisposed to injuries because of neurodevelopmental immaturity. They may lack the motor skills as well as the cognitive abilities to comprehend the demands and risks of a sport. Sometimes parents or coaches may fail to appreciate the *normal* developmental readiness of their children and unknowingly push them beyond their limits, resulting in both physical as well as psychologic injury.

Adverse effects of intensive training from an early age have been described by many authors. These include overuse injuries, effects on growth, delayed menarche, amenorrhea, and disordered eating; dysfunctional eating patterns are especially observed in young gymnasts and dancers. For developing children, certain activities may be more stressful than others. Children participating in triathlons may be exposed to excessive stress, and

the AAP recommends that they be specifically designed for children considering their developmental stage.[82] There is a significant risk of injury to young children from trampolines; the AAP recommends that trampolines not be used in home, in routine physical education classes, or in outdoor playgrounds.[42] Sports-related, mild, traumatic brain injuries in still developing young athletes can have significant long-term consequences as suggested by recent reports; including cognitive, memory, and fine motor functions.[21,90,91]

The adolescent years present with special risks for injuries related to growth and development.[86] The rapid increase in height and weight during adolescence also results in increased force and momentum when two players collide, for example, in football and other contact collision sports, this may increase the risk of injuries.[45,66,73,84,86,91] Paradoxically, enhanced motor skills seen in adolescents may lead the athlete into a higher, more intense level of competition, also exposing them to increased risk for injuries.[5,66,84,90] The motor awkwardness and relative decrease in musculotendinous flexibility because of myoosseous disproportion during adolescence may also contribute to injuries. The growth cartilage present at the epiphyseal plate, joint surface, and the apophyses, being the weaker link in the

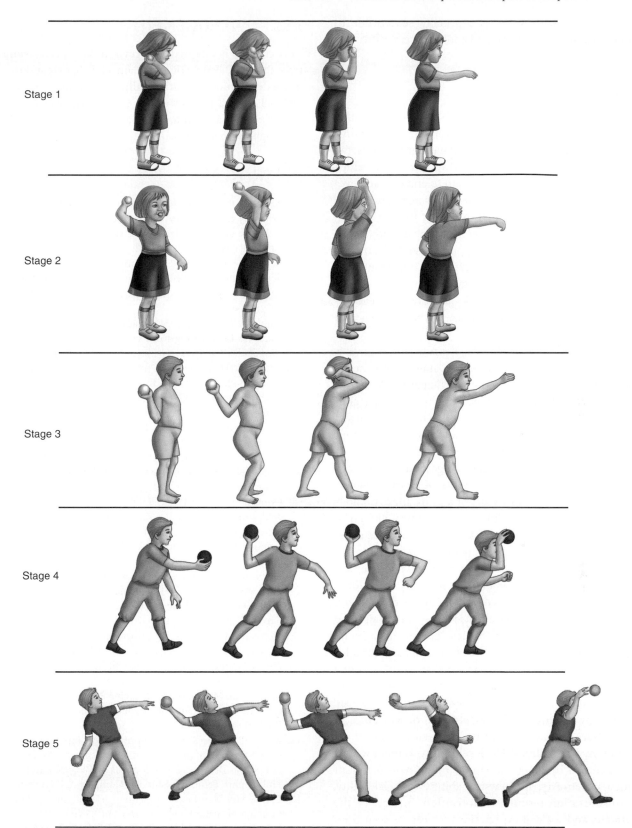

FIGURE 1-4 ■ Developmental sequence of throwing behavior.

musculoskeletal system, is especially susceptible to injuries during childhood and adolescence.[45,85,86,88]

SUMMARY

Neurodevelopmental maturation is a complex, continuous process, encompassing a number of domains. Although the rate of developmental progress varies, the *sequence* remains the same during normal development. Early training does *not* seem to enhance achievement of specific abilities at an earlier age; indeed, the neurologic system must first mature at its own normal pace. It is not possible to predict future athletic excellence. Different areas of development (somatic, neurologic, cognitive, and psychosocial) function in an integrated and interdependent fashion and should be considered together as one looks at the overall development of the child and the adolescent, when dealing with sport participation.

A child's level of physical, neuromotor, cognitive, perceptual–motor, and psychologic maturation should guide the level of specific sport participation. As shown by an earlier study, 60% of elementary school age children were able to perform the following tasks: throwing, kicking, running, jumping, catching, striking, hopping, and skipping.[30] The sense of social comparison is not achieved until after 6 years of age, and the ability to understand the competitive nature of sports is generally not achieved until 9 years of age. By approximately 12 years of age, most children are mature enough to comprehend the complex tasks of sports and are physically as well as cognitively ready to participate and compete in most sports. Sport participation is generally a *positive* experience for the vast majority of children and adolescents and should be encouraged for them. However, to avoid adverse consequences, participation should be appropriate to the developmental stage and personal interests and abilities of the child and the adolescent; it should neither be a reflection of parental "dreams" nor societal expectations. *All* children can participate in some level of physical activity; however, they may require special adaptations or assistance, if they have physical, cognitive, behavioral, social, or emotional disabilities. The level of involvement will be determined by many factors including neurodevelopmental maturity, age, physical ability, financial ability, transportation resources, motivation, interest of the athlete, and societal expectations. As can be seen from this overview, there are no sure answers to the question when is a particular child optimally ready to perform a given set of tasks required by a sport and common sense and clinical judgment should largely guide such decisions.[6]

ACKNOWLEDGEMENT

This chapter is adapted and revised with permission from Pratt HD, Patel DR, Greydanus DE. Sports and the neurodevelopment of the child and adolescent. In: DeLee JC, Drez D, Miller MD, eds. *Orthopaedic Sports Medicine*. Philadelphia, PA: Saunders; 2003:624-42. Copyright Elsevier 2003.

REFERENCES

1. Annett J. The acquisition of motor skills. In: Harries M, Williams C, Stanish W D, Micheli L J, eds. *The Oxford Textbook of Sports Medicine*. Oxford, England: Oxford University Press; 1994:136-148.
2. Beitel PA, Kuhlman JS. Relationships among age, sex, depth of sport experience with initial open-task performance by 4 to 9-year-old children. *Percept Mot Skills*. 1992;74:387-398.
3. Blanksby BA, Parker HE, Bradley S, Ong V. Childrens readiness for learning front crawl swimming. *Aust J Sci Med Sport*. 1995;27(2):34-37.
4. Branta C, Haubensticker J, Seefeldt V. Age changes in motor skills during childhood and adolescence. *Exerc Sport Sci Rev*. 1984;12:467-520.
5. Illingworth RS. *The Development of the Infant and Young Child*. 7th ed. London, UK: Churchill Livingstone; 1980.
6. Dyment PG. Sports and the neurodevelopment of the child. In: Stanitski CL, DeLee JC, Drez D, eds. *Pediatric and Adolescent Sports Medicine*. Philadelphia, PA: WB Saunders; 1994:12-15.
7. Gomez JE. Growth and maturation. In: Sullivan AJ, Anderson SJ. *Care of the Young Athlete*. Park Ridge, IL: American Academy of Orthopaedic Surgeons, and Elk Grove Village, IL: American Academy of Pediatrics; 2000: 25-32.
8. Harris SS. Readiness to participate in sports. In: Sullivan AJ, Anderson SJ, eds. *Care of the Young Athlete*. Park Ridge, IL: American Academy of Orthopaedic Surgeons, Elk Grove, IL: American Academy of Pediatrics; 2000:19-24.
9. Hofmann AD. Adolescent growth and development. In: Hofmann AD, Greydanus DE, eds. *Adolescent Medicine*. 3rd ed. Stamford, CT: Appleton and Lange; 1997:11-22.
10. Kreipe RE. Normal somatic adolescent growth and development. In: Mc Anarney ER, Kreipe RE, Orr DP, Comerci GD, eds. *Textbook of Adolescent Medicine*. Philadelphia, PA: WB Saunders; 1994:44-67.
11. Kelly DP. Patterns of development and function in the school-aged child. In: Behrman RE, Kliegman RM, Jenson HB, Staton BF, eds. *Nelson Textbook of Pediatrics*. 18th ed. Philadelphia, Penn: WB Saunders Company; 2007:139-145.
12. Levine MD. Neurodevelopmental variation and dysfunction among school-aged children. In: Levine MD, Carey WB, Crocker AC, eds. *Developmental-Behavioral Pediatrics*. 3rd ed. Philadelphia, PA: WB Saunders; 1999:520-535.
13. Patel DR. Principles of developmental diagnosis. In: Greydanus DE, Feinberg A, Patel DR, Homnick D, eds. *Pediatric Diagnostic Examination*. New York: McGraw Hill Medical; 2008.

14. Needleman RD. Growth and development. In: Behrman RE, Kliegman RM, Jenson HB, eds. *Nelson Textbook of Pediatrics.* 16th ed. Philadelphia, PA: WB Sanuders; 2000:23-65.

15. Patel DR, Pratt HD, Greydanus DE. Adolescent growth, development, and psychosocial aspects of sports participation: An overview. *Adolesc Med: State Art Rev.* 1998;9(3):425-440.

16. American Academy of Pediatrics. Participation in boxing by children, adolescents, and young adults. Committee on Sports Medicine and Fitness. *Pediatrics.* 1997;99(1):134-135.

17. American Academy of Pediatrics Committee on Psychosocial Aspects of Child and Family Health. *Guidelines for Health Supervision III.* Elk Grove Village, IL: American Academy of Pediatrics; 1997.

18. Accardo PJ, Accardo JA, Capute AJ. A neurodevelopmental perspective on the continuum of developmental disabilities. In: Accardo PJ, ed. *Developmental Disabilities in Infancy and Childhood.* 3rd ed. Baltimore, MD: Paul H. Brooks Publ; 2008:3-25.

19. Dixon SD, Stein MT, eds. *Encounters with Children: Pediatric Behavior and Developmen.* 4th ed. Philadelphia, PA: Mosby; 2006.

20. Malina RM, Bouchard C. Oded Bar-Or, eds. *Growth, Maturation, and Physical Activity.* 2nd ed. Champaign, IL: Human Kinetics; 2004.

21. American College of Sports Medicine. *Guidelines for Exercise Testing and Prescription.* 7th ed. Baltimore, MD: Williams and Wilkins; 2005.

22. Rowland T. *Children's Exercise Physiology.* 2nd ed. Champaign, IL: Human Kinetics; 2005.

23. Patel DR, Greydanus DE, Pratt HD. Youth sports: More than sprains and strains. *Contemp Pediatr.* 2001;18(3):45-76.

24. Caterino MC. Age differences in the performance of basketball dribbling by elementary school boys. *Percept Mot Skills.* 1991;73:253-254.

25. Feldman H. Developmental-behavioral pediatrics. In: Zitelli BJ, Davis HW, eds. *Atlas of Pediatric Physical Diagnosis.* 4th ed. ST Louis, MO: Mosby-Wolfe; 2002:58-86.

26. Erickson E. *Childhood and Society.* New York: WW Norton and Co., Inc; 1963.

27. Fagard J. Skill acquisition in children: A historical perspective. In: Bar Or O, ed. *The Child and Adolescent Athlete.* Oxford, England: Blackwell Science; 1996:74-91.

28. Butterfield SA, Loovis EM. Influence of age, sex, balance and sports participation on development of throwing by children in grades K-8. *Percept Mot Skills.* 1993;76:459-464.

29. Rieser JJ, Pick HL, Ashmead DH, Garing AE. Calibration of human locomotion and models of perceptual-motor organization. *J Exp Psychol Hum Percept Perform.* 1995;21(3):480-497.

30. Seefeldt V. The concept of readiness applied to motor skills acquisition. In: Magill RA, Ash MJ, Smoll FL, eds. *Children in Sports.* 2nd ed. Champaign, IL: Human Kinetics; 1982:31-37.

31. Seefeldt V, Haubenstricker J. Patterns, phases, or stages: An analytical model for the study of developmental move-

ment. In: Kelso JAS. Clark JE, eds. *The Development of Movement Control and Coordination.* New York: John Wiley and Sons; 1982:309-318.

32. Stryer BK, Tofler IR, Lapchick RA. Developmental overview of child and youth sports in society. *Child Adolesc Psychiatr Clin N Am.* 1998;7:697-724.

33. Bodie DA. Changes in lung function, ball-handling skills, and performance measures during adolescence in normal schoolboys. In: Binkhorst RA, et al. eds. *Children and Exercise XI.* Champaign, IL: Human Kinetics; 1985:260-268.

34. Dirix A, Knuttgen HG, Tittle K, eds. *The Olympic Book of Sports Medicine.* Melbourne, FL: Blackwell Scientific Publications; 1988:194-211.

35. Hermiston RT. Functional strength and skill development of young ice hockey players. *J Sports Med.* 1975;15:252-265.

36. Krombholz H. Physical performance in relation to age, sex, social class and sports activities in kindergarten and elementary school. *Percept Mot Skills.* 1997;84:1168-1170.

37. Loovis EM, Butterfield SA. Influence of age, sex, balance and sports participation on development of sidearm striking by children in grades K-8. *Percept Mot Skills.* 1993;76:459-464.

38. Oliver I, Ripoll H, Audiffren M. Age differences in using precued information to preprogram interception of a ball. *Percept Mot Skills.* 1997;85:123-127.

39. Strohmeyer HS, Williams K, Schaub-George D. Developmental sequence for catching a small ball: A prelongitudinal screening. *Res Q Exerc Sport.* 1991;62(3):257-266.

40. Malina RM. Physical growth and biologic maturation of young athletes. *Exerc Sport Sci Rev.* 1994;22:389-433.

41. Smoll FL, Smith RE, eds. *Children and Youth in Sport: A Biopsychosocial Perspective.* Madison, WI: Brown and Benchmark, Inc; 1996.

42. American Academy of Pediatrics Committee on Injury and Poison Prevention and Sports Medicine and Fitness. Swimming programs for infants and children. *Pediatrics.* 2000;105:868-870.

43. Birrer RB, Levine R. Performance Parameters in Children and Adolescent Athletes. *Sports Med.* 1987;4:211-227.

44. Piaget J. Intellectual Evaluation from Adolescence to Adulthood. *Hum Dev.* 1972;1-12.

45. Burgess-Milliron MJ, Murphy SB. Biomechanical considerations of youth sports injuries. In: Bar-or O, ed. *The Child and Adolescent Athlete.* Oxford, England: Blackwell Science; 1996:173-188.

46. Piaget J, Inhelder B. *The Psychology of the Child.* New York: Basic Books; 1969.

47. Lewis BJ. Structuring movement experiences for preschool children. *Child Care Health Dev.* 1978;4:385-395.

48. Shelov SP, ed. *American Academy of Pediatrics: Caring for Your Baby and Young Child Birth to Age 5.* Rev ed. New York: Bantam Books; 1998.

49. Bardy BG, Laurent M. How is body orientation controlled during somersaulting? *J Exp Psycholo: Hum Percept Perform.* 1998;24(3):963-977.

50. Yan JH, Thomas JR Thomas KT. Children?s age moderates the effect of practice variability: A Quantitative review. *Res Q Exerc Sport.* 1998;69(2):210-215.

51. Cahill BR Pearl AJ, eds. *Intensive Participation in Children?s Sports.* Champaign, IL: Human Kinetics; 1993.

52. American Academy of Pediatric Committee on Sports Medicine and Fitness and School Health. Organized sports for children and pre-adolescents. *Pediatrics.* 2001; 107:1459-1462.

53. Gesell A, Ilg FL, Ames LB. *The Child from Five to Ten.* New York: Harper and Row Publishers; 1946.

54. Jeng S, Liao H, Lai J, Hou J. Optimization of walking in children. *Med Sci Sports Exerc.* 1997;29(3):370-376.

55. Smoll FL Schultz RW. Quantifying gender differences in physical performance: A developmental perspective. *Dev Psychol.* 1990;26(3):360-369.

56. Messick JA. Prelongitudinal screening of hypothesized developmental sequences for the overhead tennis serve in experienced tennis players 9 to 19 years of age. *Res Q Exerc Sport* 1991;62(3):249-256.

57. Begel D. The psychologic development of the athlete. In: Begel D, Burton RW, eds. *Sport Psychiatry: Theory and Practice.* New York: WW Norton; 2000:3-21.

58. Smoll FL, ed. *Children and Sport.* 2nd ed. Champaign, IL: Human Kinetics; 1982:31-37.

59. Gemelli R. *Normal Child and Adolescent Development.* Washington, DC: American Psychiatric Press; 1996.

60. Erickson E. *Identity, Youth and Crisis.* New York: WW Norton and Co, Inc; 1968.

61. Abe JA, Izard CE. A Longitudinal study of emotion, expression and personality relations in early development. *J Pers Soc Psychol.* 1999;77(3):566-577.

62. Benguigui N, Ripoll H. Effects of tennis practice on the conincidence timing accuracy of adults and children. *Res Q Exerc Sport.* 1998;69(3):217-223.

63. Pienaar AE, Spamer MJ, Steyn HS. Identifying and developing rugby talent among 10-year-old boys: A practical model. *J Sports Sci.* 1998;16:691-699.

64. American Academy of Pediatrics Committee on Sports Medicine and Fitness. Intensive training and sports specialization in young athletes. *Pediatrics.* 2000;106(1):154-157.

65. Fagenbaum AD, Westcott WL, Loud RL Long C. The effects of different resistance training protocols on muscular strength and endurance development in children. *Pediatrics.* 1999;104(l):1-7.

66. Smith AM, Stuart MJ, Wiese-Bjornstal DM, Gunnon C. Predictors of injury in ice hockey players: A multivariate, multidisciplinary approach. *The American J Sports Med.* 1997;25(4):500-507.

67. Tofler IR, Stryer BK, Micheli LJ, et al. Physical and emotional problems of elite female gymnasts. *NEJM.* 1996; 335:281.

68. Hahn T, Foldspang A, Ingemann-Hansen T. Dynamic strength of the quadriceps muscle and sports activity. *Br J Sports Med.* 1999;33:117-20.

69. Lillegard WA, Brown EW, Wilson DJ, Henderson R, Lewis E. Efficacy of strength training in prepubescent to early postpubescent males and females: Effects of gender and maturity. *Pediatr Rehabil.* 1997;1(3):147-57.

70. Roemmich JN, Rogol AD. Physiology of growth and development: Its relationship to performance in the young athlete. *Clin Sports Med.* 1995;14(3):483.

71. Sharkey BJ. Neuromuscular training. In: Sullivan AJ, Grana WA, eds. *The Pediatric Athlete.* Park Ridge, IL: American Academy of Orthopaedic Surgeons; 1990:21-26.

72. Beunen G, Malina RM. Growth and physical performance relative to timing of the adolescent spurt. *Exerc Sport Sci Rev.* 1988;16:503-540.

73. Finch CF, Elliott BC, McGrath AC. Measures to prevent cricket injuries: An overview. *Sports Med.* 1999;28(4): 263-272.

74. Livingood AB, Goldwater C, Kurtz RB. Psychological aspects of sports participation in young children. In: Camp BW, ed. *Advances in Behavioral Pediatrics.* Greenwich, CT: Jai Press; 1981:141-169.

75. Ryckman RM, Hamel J. Perceived Physical Ability Differences in the Sport Participation Motives of Young Athletes. *Int J Sport Psychol.* 1993;24:270-283.

76. Nelson MA. Developmental skills and children's sports. *Physician Sports Med.* 1991;19:67-79.

77. American Academy of Pediatrics Committee on Injury and Poison Prevention Policy Statement. Skateboard and scooter injuries. *Pediatrics.* 2002;109:542-543.

78. Brenner JS; and American Academy of Pediatrics Council on Sports Medicine and Fitness. Overuse injuries, overtraining and burnout in child and adolescent athlete. *Pediatrics.* 2007;119:1242-1245.

79. American Academy of Pediatrics Committee on Sports Medicine. Strength training by children and adolescents. *Pediatrics.* 2001;107:1470-1472.

80. American Academy of Pediatrics Committee on Sports Medicine and Fitness. Injuries in youth soccer: A subject review. *Pediatrics.* 2000;105(30):659-661.

81. American Academy of Pediatrics Committee on Sports Medicine and Fitness. Risk of injury from baseball and softball in children 5 to 14 years of age. *Pediatrics.* 1994; 93(4): 690-692.

82. American Academy of Pediatrics Committee on Sports Medicine and Fitness. Triathlon participation by children and adolescents. *Pediatrics.* 1996;98(3):511-512.

83. American Academy of Pediatrics Policy Statement: Fitness, activity, and sports participation in the preschool child. *Pediatrics.* 1992;90(6):1002-1004.

84. Duggleby T, Kumar S. Epidemiology of juvenile low back pain: A review. *Disabil Rehabil.* 1997;19(12):505-512.

85. Hewett TE, Lindenfeld TN, Riccobene JV, Noyes FR. The effects of neuromuscular training on the incidence of knee injury in females athletes: A prospective study. *Am J Sports Med.* 1999;27(6):699-706.

86. Linder MM, Townsend DJ, Jones JC, et al. Incidence of adolescent injuries in junior high-school football and its relationship to sexual maturity. *Clin J Sports Med.* 1995;5:167-170.

87. Metzl JD, Micheli LJ. Youth Soccer: An epidemiologic perspective. *Clin Sports Med.* 1998;17(4):663-673.

88. Micheli LJ. Overuse injuries in children's sports: the growth factor. *Orthop Clin N Am.* 1983;14:337.

89. Patel DR, Baker RJ. Musculoskeletal injuries. *Prim Care Clin Off Pract.* 2006;33(2):545-580.

90. Pieter W, Zemper ED. Head and neck injuries in young taekwondo athletes. *J Sports Med Phys Fit.* 1999;39(2): 147-153.

91. Powell JW, Barber-Foss KD. Traumatic brain injury in high school athletes. *JAMA.* 1999;282(10):958-963.

CHAPTER 2

Adolescent Growth and Development, and Sport Participation

*Donald E. Greydanus and
Helen D. Pratt*

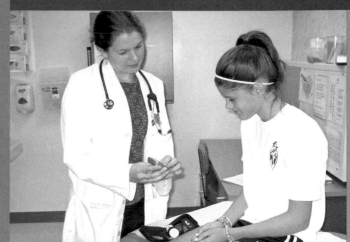

TRANSITION TO THE ADOLESCENT YEARS

During the preschool years, physical growth, neurologic growth, and maturation are quite rapid and apparent, with new skills being acquired at a rapid pace. This process continues throughout the middle years with a somewhat slower pace. As the child enters puberty, rapid development of physical and sexual characteristics becomes more apparent, accompanied by important psychosocial development. The onset and rate of progression of pubertal events vary considerably among adolescents; however, the changes occur in a *predetermined sequence*.[1,2] The adolescent may perceive sport experiences quite differently based on the influences of several variables: the differences in physical and psychosocial development, states of adolescent development (early: 10–13 years of age; middle: 14–16 years of age; and late: 16–20 years of age), as well as those who mature early or late.[3–8] Also, gender differences become more apparent and significant for sport participation during adolescence (Figure 2-1). Clinically, it is important to assess an adolescent's sexual maturity rating (SMR) or Tanner staging (Figures 2-2–2-4), because chronologic age does not necessarily correlate well with many physiologic and somatic changes. Skeletal maturity is best assessed by measurement of bone age.

Selected aspects of somatic, sexual, and skeletal growth and maturation during adolescence (especially relevant to sport participation and performance) and their developmental continuity and inter-relatedness have been the subject of extensive review in the literature.[1,2,4,9,10–22]

Weight

In males, the average weight gain during its peak is approximately 9 kg/y with a *range* of 6 to 12.5 kg/y; in females it is approximately 8 kg/y with a *range* of 5.5 to 10.5 kg/y.[1,19,21] In males, the peaks of growth spurts in height, weight, and muscle occur at the same time, while in females these occur in sequence in that order.[2,16]

Height

Peak height velocity (PHV) refers to the maximal rate of linear growth during adolescence. Females reach PHV by 12 years of age during SMR 3, usually 6 to 12 months before menarche (onset of menstruation); their average *gain* is 8 cm/y, while the *range* is 6 to 10.5 cm/y.[1,2,19] Males usually reach their peak height velocity by 14 years at SMR 4, with an average *gain* of 9 cm/y and a *range* of 7 to 12 cm/y.[1,2,19] During the early growth spurt, growth of the shoulders in males and that of hips and pelvis in females are the most noticeable changes. In general, linear growth first occurs in the lower extremities, followed by the torso and then the upper extremities.

Body Composition

There are significant gender differences in changes in body composition as described in terms of fat mass (FM), fat free mass (FFM), and body fat distribution.[8,9,13,17,20] In general, both males and females tend to increase both FM as well as FFM from the early to middle adolescent years.[6] However, males may show a transient decrease in fat accumulation in extremities during PHV; females continue to gain fat through late adolescence. By SMR 4 and 5, the fat mass in females can reach twice that of males. There is a relatively predominant deposition of fat in lower trunk and thighs in females. The pattern of growth of FFM is similar to that noted for growth in height and weight. *Body mass index* (BMI) (weight in kg/stature in meters squared)

has been shown to have a better correlation with FM than weight.[23] The calculated value is compared to the population norm tables. One limitation of BMI is the fact that factors other than FM, such as muscle mass and bone mass, affect the numerator and may incorrectly give a high value in someone with high-muscle mass and not FM.[17]

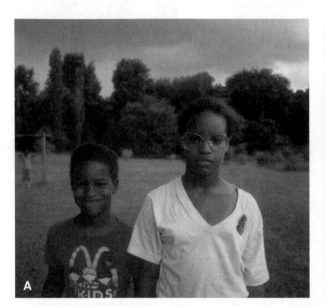

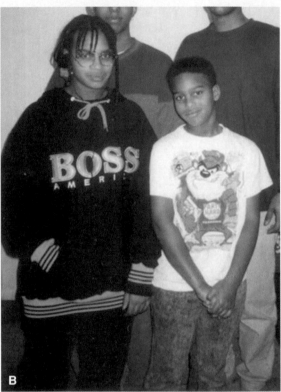

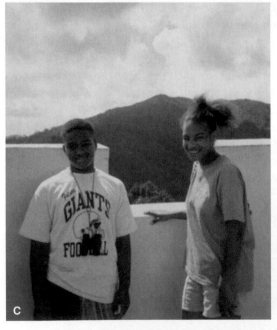

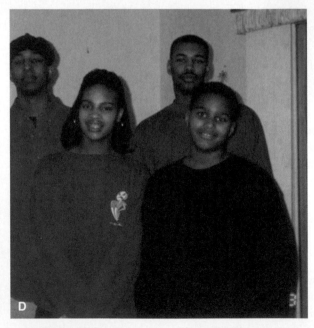

FIGURE 2-1 ■ Gender differences become more apparent and significant during progression from early to late adolescence and are most apparent in growth velocity and height as evident in these photographs of the brother and sister. *(continued)*

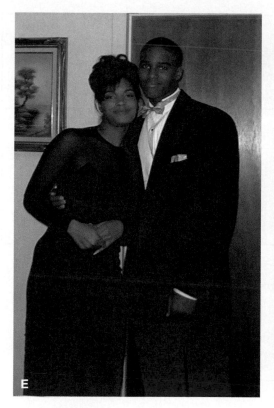
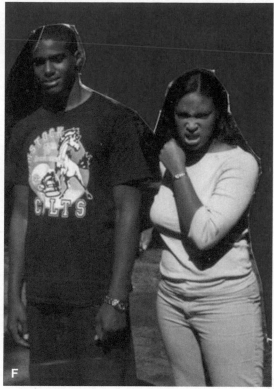

FIGURE 2-1 ■ *Continued.*

Application of BMI in sports classified by weight categories has been found useful in such sports as wrestling, bodybuilding, and weightlifting.

Flexibility

Typically, skeletal growth precedes that of *musculo-tendinous* growth during early to midadolescence; this partly contributes to a relative decrease in musculo-tendinous flexibility in some adolescents, especially males.[4,6,20] In general, females are more flexible compared with males. In males, overall flexibility tends to decrease from late childhood to midadolescence; in females, it tends to show a slight increase during early adolescence, plateauing by 14 or 15 years of age.[8,16,20,21] Decreased flexibility is particularly noticeable in hamstrings and ankle dorsiflexors, especially in dancers and gymnasts.[6,21] Flexibility is influenced by *internal factors* such as bone structure, muscle volume, and tissue elasticity (i.e., muscles, tendons, joint capsules, and ligaments). *External factors,* which influence flexibility include room temperature, warm-up time, and physical exercise.[24]

Muscle Growth and Strength

Growth in muscle mass is seen both in males and females during adolescence. Since androgens partly influence this growth, it is relatively more pronounced in males compared with females. There is also a linear increase in muscle strength in both males and females, with males showing a period of relative acceleration or spurt around age 13, females reach a plateau by age 15 with no apparent spurt.[4,2,14,20] The peak increase in muscle strength follows a peak in muscle mass by approximately 12 months.[2,8,20] The response to strength training is best seen during SMR 4 and 5 in both males and females.[2,4,6,14,25]

Bone Mass

Weight bearing and loading, along with proper diet, are essential to optimal bone growth. The largest percentage of lifetime acquisition of bone mineral density occurs during the second decade of life.[10,12,13] Peak bone mass during adolescence is determined by many factors, including genetic influences, exercise, calcium intake, and hormonal status.[10,13] Thus, lack of proper nutrition seen in some athletes who engage in drastic weight control measures may predispose them to *deficiencies* in bone mass accumulation.[8,13]

Implications of Early and Late Maturatizon

Early development is characterized by advanced bone age compared with chronologic age, and *late development* by

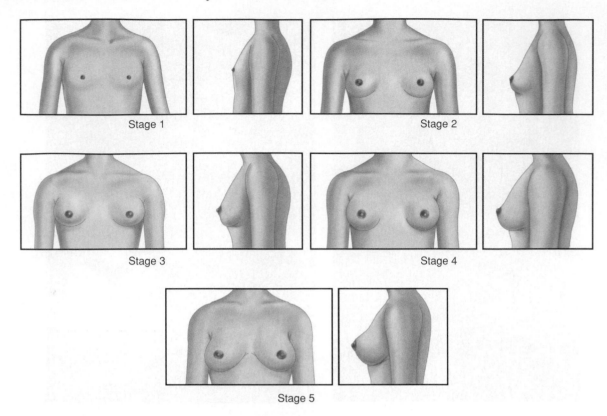

Stage 1   Preadolescent: juvenile breast with elevated papilla and small flat areola.

Stage 2   The breast bud forms under the influence of hormonal stimulation. The papilla and areola elevate as a small mound, and the areolar diameter increases.

Stage 3   Continued enlargement of the breast bud further elevates the papilla. The areola continues to enlarge; no separation of breast contours is noted.

Stage 4   The areola and papilla separate from the contour of the breast to form a secondary mound.

Stage 5   Mature: areolar mound recedes into the general contour of the breast; papilla continues to project.

FIGURE 2-2 ■ Maturational stages of female breast development.

delayed bone age compared with chronologic age.[1,2,19] Early developing males may have PHV before 13 years of age, while females may reach PHV before 11 years of age; late developing males may not reach PHV before 15 years of age, while females may not reach PHV before 13 years of age.[1,2,16,18,19,21,23,26]

Boys, who mature *early* tend to be taller and have greater muscle mass, fat mass, as well as strength (i.e., arm, grip, and explosive) compared with average or late maturing boys; jumping and sprinting are examples of explosive strength. Adolescent boys who are *late* maturers are relatively smaller in stature, weaker, and less coordinated; they may experience frustration, anxiety, and disappointment when not being able to meet performance expectations while playing sports. They may even be ignored by peers as well as coaching staff.

In comparison to average or late maturing female peers, early maturing girls tend to be taller, have greater fat mass and fat free mass, greater weight for height, relatively shorter legs, and broader hips; however, this only gives them a modest (if any) advantage in sports. In fact, early maturing girls may be at a disadvantage socially, as well as in certain motor tasks, and may not be considered ideal for such sports as gymnastics, dancing, diving, and figure skating.[21] On the other hand, girls who mature later are taller, have lower weight for height, less FM, relatively longer legs, and narrower hips; they may be at an advantage socially, perform better on tests of upper extremity strength, and are better suited for sports such as gymnastics and figure skating.[21]

EARLY ADOLESCENCE

Physical Growth and Development

Rapid changes in physical growth and motor skills characterize *early* adolescence. Many adolescents, especially males, begin to demonstrate special skills and talents during this time. Because, normally girls often experience the onset of puberty earlier than boys, they

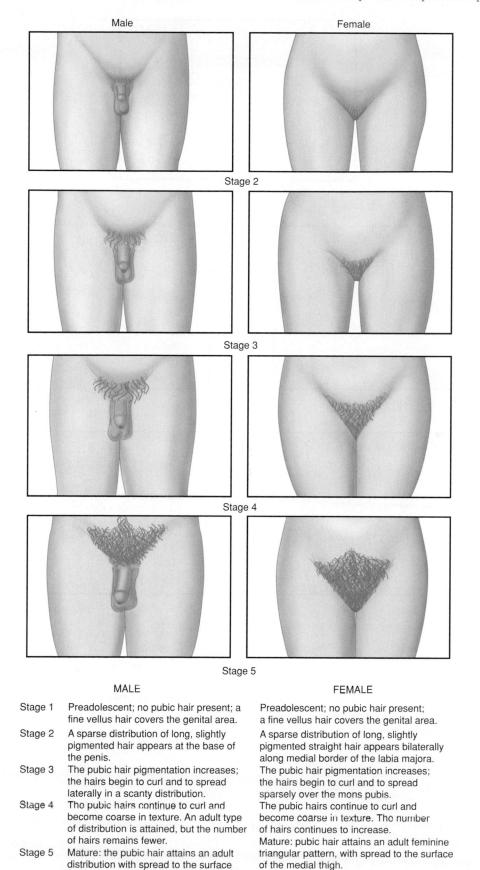

FIGURE 2-3 ■ Maturational stages of male and female pubic hair development.

	MALE	FEMALE
Stage 1	Preadolescent; no pubic hair present; a fine vellus hair covers the genital area.	Preadolescent; no pubic hair present; a fine vellus hair covers the genital area.
Stage 2	A sparse distribution of long, slightly pigmented hair appears at the base of the penis.	A sparse distribution of long, slightly pigmented straight hair appears bilaterally along medial border of the labia majora.
Stage 3	The pubic hair pigmentation increases; the hairs begin to curl and to spread laterally in a scanty distribution.	The pubic hair pigmentation increases; the hairs begin to curl and to spread sparsely over the mons pubis.
Stage 4	The pubic hairs continue to curl and become coarse in texture. An adult type of distribution is attained, but the number of hairs remains fewer.	The pubic hairs continue to curl and become coarse in texture. The number of hairs continues to increase.
Stage 5	Mature: the pubic hair attains an adult distribution with spread to the surface of the medial thigh. Pubic hair will grow along linea alba in 80% of males.	Mature: pubic hair attains an adult feminine triangular pattern, with spread to the surface of the medial thigh.

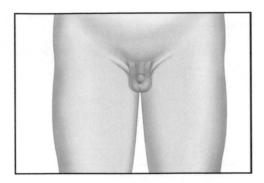

Stage 1

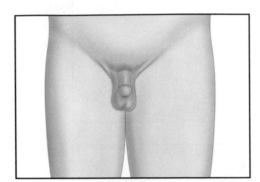

Stage 2

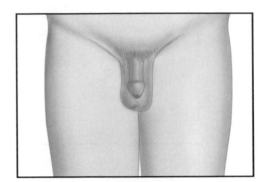

Stage 3

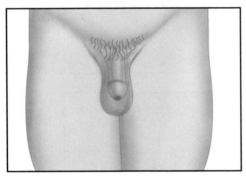

Stage 4

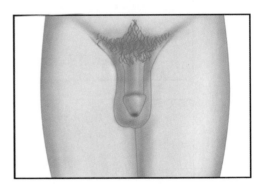

Stage 5

Stage 1   Preadolescent: testes, scrotum, and penis identical to early childhood.

Stage 2   Enlargement of testes as result of canalization of seminiferous tubules. The scrotum enlarges, developing a reddish hue and altering its skin texture. The penis enlarges slightly.

Stage 3   The testes and scrotum continue to grow. The length of the penis increases.

Stage 4   The testes and scrotum continues to grow; the scrotal skin darkens. The penis grows in width, and the glans penis develops.

Stage 5   Mature: adult size and shape of testes, scrotum and penis.

FIGURE 2-4 ■ Maturational stages of male genital development.

may become temporarily taller and heavier than boys of the same age. Differences in physical performance, early in adolescence are more strongly influenced by the age at the onset of puberty and environmental conditions than by the chronologic age.[4,8,18,21,27,28] As adolescents become older, gender differences become increasingly more a function of environmental factors.

Physical differences can be dramatic in some adolescents, especially boys. A wide variability in the rate of progression of growth, physical skills, and overall development may contribute to increased concerns about body image in some adolescents. Increases in muscle mass, strength, and cardiopulmonary endurance that occur during puberty are greater than at any other age.[2,6,20,21,29] Males show sharp increases in tasks that require muscle strength such as vertical or horizontal jumping, throwing, and sprinting; females show a gradual improvement or reach a plateau in their performance of these skills.[6,16,18,21]

Cognitive Development

Piaget contends that early adolescents are just beginning the *Formal Operational Stage* of cognitive development, with improved inductive and deductive reasoning abilities.[30–33] While they develop prepositional logic in which they can think about thinking itself, they may also note an awakening sense of morality and altruism. Also, future time perspective has not been fully developed during early adolescence, and they are still at a concrete level of cognitive functioning.[1,31,32,34] It should also be noted that some adolescents may never shift to this stage of thinking and remain at the *concrete* phase of thinking.

However, for many, there is a beginning of abstract thinking, analytical abilities, problem solving skills, and transitional skills.[30,32,33,35–37] Selective attention and memory are more mature; they now have a cognitive ability to understand and remember complex strategies for sports such as football and basketball. During adolescence, the focus shifts away from acquisition to the cognitive aspects of language development, such as the ability to understand the semantics of language and the ability to use language to convey the variety and quality of information. Adolescents, at this age can understand the basic theories and concepts behind how a sport is played.[38] They can use symbols, signs, and coded words to understand plays the coach or trainer is asking them to perform. They can use such language to communicate to others who understand the special language related to specific sport activities. They may still have some limitations, but with practice and patience will continue to grow in their use of this vital communication domain.

However, problems may arise as a result of this developing process.[39] Since behavior and consequences are processed on a "here and now" basis, they often fail to extrapolate general rules of the game from one situation to another. Early adolescents may attribute success or failure in athletics to their uniqueness and may fail to connect regular training or practice to future athletic success. Early adolescents are preoccupied with physical (bodily) concerns and may respond to minor injuries with out-of-proportion reactions. Normal comparisons (and finding differences or similarities) between self and peers may cause the adolescent to be either distressed or feel superior.

As reasoning abilities become more sophisticated, some adolescents may argue and disagree with adults; arguments with their coaches, trainers, or referees may result in penalties or ejections from games. Because, these adolescents lack life experience, their *magical thinking* tendency may be problematic for some. They still need approval from their peers and may go to great lengths, even get in trouble to gain their acceptance. They may impulsively engage in high-risk taking behaviors, much to the dismay of parents and coaches.

Psychosocial Development

From approximately 11 to 14 years of age, a convergence of body image and motor skills occurs.[38] Sport participation provides an early opportunity for independence and emancipation.[15,29] Comparison with peers, worry over perceived physical differences, and sexual relationships may occupy much of their time.[1,5,40,41] Peers and adults in the environment can independently weigh consequences of their decisions before taking action. Peer acceptance is important, but the approval and support from family are still *significant* guiding forces.[32,33] These adolescents are also able to enjoy and take pride in increasingly complex accomplishments in sports as well as academics and begin to improve their self-image. Some studies suggest that adolescents who experience consistent successes tend to develop a positive self-image, while those who experience repeated failures tend to develop a less healthy self-image.[3,5,21,36,42]

Implications for Sport Participation

Most early adolescents are ready for entry level competitive sports including football, basketball, baseball, or tennis.[38] However, these young adolescents continue to require a great deal of demonstrations along with verbal instructions. Although continued participation in different activities is generally preferable, depending on innate abilities and talent, they may begin to specialize in their favorite sport, if *they* choose this type of concentrated effort.

The behavior of adolescents is influenced by the behavior of the adults and peers in their environment. Bullying and teasing may be seen at this developmental stage with potentially negative effects. Early adolescents cannot often depersonalize criticism, and they may even believe the coach or trainer hates them. These adolescents have limited life experiences and may be highly sensitive to negative comments from others (i.e., "You are a lousy hitter! You hit like a girl! You shouldn't be in this sport because girls don't belong here! You don't have any talent and should drop out!"). At the other end of this continuum, adults might say things that are meant to be positive, but may cause problems when the *precocious* athlete is no longer bigger, stronger, or better than his peers (i.e., "You don't need to practice, you are a gifted player! You are better than the other kids! You are going to be a superstar!").

MIDDLE ADOLESCENCE

Physical Growth and Development

Specialization of gross motor skills continues during middle adolescence.[6,38] Most adolescents experience continued increase in muscle mass, strength, and cardiopulmonary endurance that began during early adolescent years. In a study by Hahn et al. of competitive athletes aged between 14 and 24 years, dynamic strength of the quadriceps muscle was significantly higher in males than in females and positively associated with body weight, years of jogging, years of soccer, and weekly hours of basketball.[43] Sport-specific adaptation may reflect high levels of running and jumping activity that occurs in sports such as soccer, European team handball, basketball, badminton, tennis, competitive gymnastics, swimming, and jogging.[24,43]

There is also continued gain in agility, motor coordination, power, and speed.[4,16,20] Females generally perform better than males in tasks which require balance as a main component. Females generally do not improve in motor performance after age 14, while males continue to improve throughout adolescence.[4,16,20,21] In males, maximal speed peak occurs *before* peak height velocity, while strength and power peaks *follow* peak height velocity; no such clear pattern is observed in females.[4,16,17,20,21]

Between 12 and 14 years of age, a transient period of *motor incoordination* may occur during the adolescent growth spurt, primarily in boys.[4,8,16,21] It typically lasts only for approximately 6 months and is believed to be because of a temporary disturbance of performance tasks that require balance. However, some experts doubt its clinical significance as well as its existence. Multiple factors may account for the differences in motor coordination seen in these adolescents; however, no unique sociocultural, anthropometric, or physical activity characteristics have been identified in these adolescents. If such a period of motor incoordination is bothersome to the adolescents or their family, reassurance is all that is needed in the absence of a specific neuromuscular disorder.

Cognitive Development

During middle adolescence, there is improved abstract thinking and an increasing ability to understand consequences of behavior.[1,6,30,32,44] With increased ability to understand their sport, creative use of helpful strategies and techniques along with their execution is now possible.[45,46] The athletes can now observe their own behavior in a match, analyze what they did correctly, and what they did not do well; they can also compare and contrast that behavior to their personal best and other training data, evaluate strengths and weaknesses, determine what needs to change, modify action plan, design and formulate a new approach, implement that approach, and begin the process again.[45–47] They can now perform these functions with or without the aid of a coach or trainer; however, their input or feedback is still often valued.

Psychosocial Development

During middle adolescence, there is an increased level of independence from parents and authority figures.[32,33] They are capable of multiple relationships, and improved critical thinking skills help expand their roles and options.[1,41] Adolescents, now begin to rely more and more on peers as their frames of reference versus parents. They use peer feedback to set personal goals and rules of conduct. They identify with nonparental adults; the coach can become a very influential role model at this stage.[8] During middle adolescence, feelings are very intense and risk taking behavior can cause conflicts with parents and authority figures. Sport participation is often used to impress others and to achieve social status while risk taking in sports occurs with increasing frequency.[8,42] Media images of professional athletes exert greater influence at this stage of development, and can potentially foster unrealistic expectations of fame and fortune from sports.[3,7,8,21,36,42]

Implications for Sport Participation

During middle adolescence, some adolescents may find it difficult to adjust to the somatic growth spurt. Adolescents, who wrestle may find it difficult to maintain a personally desired lower weight in spite of pathogenic weight control measures. They often refuse to move to a higher weight class for fear of losing in a category where they would be at the lower end of weight limits. Female athletes may also find they are now heavier and then engage in as many high-calorie-burning sport activities as much as possible to keep their weight down. Female adolescents, who dance may also engage in various excessive weight control measures to keep their ultra thin figures.

Other adaptations to sports include the need for some to increase bulk, weight, strength, and endurance. The more competitive the sport, the more pressure is on athletes to meet a specific standard and body type. For example, regardless of how talented they may be, adolescents who play defensive tackle in football may not be considered competitive by their coaches and trainers. If they want to be selected for high school varsity or college teams, they are encouraged to gain weight, lift weights, run, engage in multiple activities, and increase their flexibility and agility. Because, these adolescents are still at a developmental stage where peer pressure and the need to please significant adult figures is important, they may engage in unhealthy practices, such as using anabolic steroids or other drugs, in an attempt to achieve weight gain or bulk.[6,15,42] These adolescents may understand the consequences of taking steroids, but their caution may be overridden by their stronger need for popularity and peer recognition. Such negative adaptations to sport participation may present significant problems for some adolescents.

Adolescents at this stage of development have the requisite skills to recognize and understand the demands of a particular sport and can decide if they want to engage in the necessary behaviors to meet those requirements. Competitive sports are appropriate and can be a rewarding experience; however, it is essential to recognize the emotional needs and personal limitations of each athlete and provide him or her with *multiple* avenues to access peer approval and acceptance.

LATE ADOLESCENCE

Physical Growth and Development

Most adolescents reach full physical maturity by the end of this stage of development, although, they will continue to develop specialization of gross motor skills. Males continue to gain in strength, speed, and size during late adolescence at a slower rate compared to earlier years; females continue to accumulate fat mass that may negatively impact performance. Muscular strength and aerobic capacity continue to increase into adulthood, but at slower rate than during early puberty.

Cognitive Development

Late adolescent years are characterized by more realistic goals about one's sport abilities and participation. Other issues, such as dating and future career plans, become more important than sports. Intellectual and functional capacities as well as abstract thought processes are now well developed, while decision making becomes future oriented and personal values are now clearer and well defined.[1,30–33] Late adolescents have the cognitive ability to understand and remember complex strategies for sports; their perceptual motor abilities are fully developed.[6] Adolescents are now fully capable of competitive

sports and specialization; however, most of them still prefer sports for fun.

Psychosocial Development

By late adolescence, most issues of emancipation should be essentially resolved and final pubertal changes have been completed.[32,33] At this stage, the adolescent is better able to deal with pressures from parents, coaches and society, as well as handle personal failures. The well-adjusted adolescent, who is mentally and physically healthy has developed a secure, acceptable body image, and gender role. The adolescent athlete now has a more realistic view of the role of sports in the overall scheme of his or her life.[3,5,7,8]

Visual and Perceptual Motor Development

Perceptual-motor and visual-motor abilities are now well developed and highly sophisticated . Bardy and Laurent studied how body orientation is controlled during somersaulting in male gymnasts (ages 23–26 years) by looking at the kinematics of backward standing somersaults.[48] They found that vision plays a significant role in increasing the athlete's ability to successfully complete trials over a *no-vision* condition. Expert gymnasts were able to use their vestibular and somatosensory systems to control their body orientation in the air, help them balance their bodies, control the angle of their jumps, and temporarily stabilize their bodies when landing from a jump. During a no-vision condition, subjects were still able to successfully execute many somersaults, but the authors could not fully explain this ability. They speculated that the gymnasts may have used stored visual representations to control their body orientations in the absence of actual visual cues. The authors concluded that the vestibular and somatosensory systems need the input of vision to be fully operational in these athletes.[48]

Implications for Sport Participation

Late adolescents have the physical, cognitive, social, emotional, visual-motor capabilities, and perceptual-motor capabilities to adapt their skills to meet the demands of most sports. The adolescent may or may not necessarily achieve the elite skills and psychologic motivation to engage in professional or Olympic sports. Adolescents at this stage can participate in any sports for fun, recreation, fitness, and exercise; those who are able to qualify for competitive sports can also make independent determinations as to whether or not they wish to participate in *any* sport activity.

GROWTH, DEVELOPMENT, AND TRAINING

Studies show that regular training or sport participation does *not* affect the timing, rate, or magnitude of peak height velocity.[4,8,11,14,16,17,20,21,49] Regular weight training may contribute to an increase in FFM and favorably alter the FM to FFM ratio. Endurance training also may result in improved aerobic capacity; however, the effects of growth itself and of training may be difficult to differentiate, especially in adolescents. Resistance training results in improvement in muscular strength in preadolescents as well as adolescents.[14,20,21,25,49,50–52] The strength gain in prepubescent children may be more a reflection of improved neuromuscular adaptation, than actual muscle hypertrophy.

ACKNOWLEDGMENT

This chapter is partly adapted and revised with permission from Pratt HD, Patel DR, Greydanus DE. Sports and the neurodevelopment of the child and adolescent. In: DeLee JC, Drez D, Miller MD, eds. *Orhopaedic Sports Medicine.* Philadelphia, PA: Saunders; 2003:624-642. Copyright Elsevier 2003.

REFERENCES

1. Hofmann AD. Adolescent growth and development. In: Hofmann AD, Greydanus DE, eds. *Adolescent Medicine.* 3rd ed. Stamford, CT: Appleton and Lange; 1997:11-22.
2. Kreipe RE. Normal somatic adolescent growth and development. In: McAnarney ER, Kreipe RE, Orr DP, Comerci GD, eds. *Textbook of Adolescent Medicine.* Philadelphia, PA: WB Saunders; 1994:44-67.
3. Begel D. The psychologic development of the athlete. In: Begel D, Burton RW, eds. *Sport Psychiatry: Theory and Practice.* New York: WW Norton; 2000:3-21.
4. Beunen G, Malina RM. Growth and physical performance relative to timing of the adolescent spurt. *Exerc Sport Sci Rev.* 1998;16:503-540.
5. Farrell EG. Sports medicine: psychologic aspects. In: Greydanus DE, Wolraich ML, eds. *Behavioral Pediatrics.* New York: Springer-Verlag; 1992:425-434.
6. Gomez JE. Growth and maturation. In: Sullivan AJ, Anderson SJ, eds. *Care of the Young Athlete.* Park Ridge, IL: American Academy of Orthopaedic Surgeons, and Elk Grove Village, IL: American Academy of Pediatrics; 2000:25-32.
7. Patel DR, Greydanus DE, Pratt HD. Youth sports: more than sprains and strains. *Contemp Pediatr.* 2001;18(3):45-74.
8. Patel DR, Pratt HD, Greydanus DE. Adolescent growth, development, and psychosocial aspects of sports participation: an overview. *Adolesc Med State Art Rev.* 1998;9(3):425-440.
9. American College of Sports Medicine. *Guidelines for Exercise Testing and Prescription.* 7th ed. Baltimore, MD: Williams and Wilkins; 2006.
10. Bailey DA, Faulker RA, McKay HA. Growth, physical activity, and bone mineral acquisition. *Exerc Sport Sci Rev.* 1994;24:233-266.
11. Cahill BR, Pearl AJ, eds. *Intensive Participation in Children's Sports.* Champaign, IL: Human Kinetics; 1993.
12. Hergenroeder AC. Bone mineralization, hypothalamic amenorrhea, and sex steroid therapy in female adolescents. *J Pediatr.* 1995;126:683-689.
13. Hergenroeder AC, Klish WJ. Body composition in adolescents athletes. *Pediatr Clin N Am.* 1990;37:1057-1084.
14. Lillegard WA, Brown EW, Wilson DJ, Henderson R, Lewis E. Efficacy of strength training in prepubescent to early postpubescent males and females: effects of gender and maturity. *Pediatr Rehabil.* 1997;1(3):147-157.
15. Luckstead EF, Greydanus DE. *Medical Care of the Adolescent Athlete.* Los Angeles, CA: PMIC; 1993.
16. Malina RM. Physical growth and biologic maturation of young athletes. *ExercSport Sci Rev.* 1994;22:389-433.
17. Malina RM, Bouchard C, eds. *Growth, Maturation, and Physical Activity.* Champaign, IL, Human Kinetics; 1991.
18. Marshall WA, Tanner JM. Variation in the pattern of pubertal changes in girls. *Arch Dis Child.* 1969;44:291-303.
19. Needleman RD. Growth and development. In: Behrman RE, Kliegman RM, Jenson HB, eds. *Nelson Textbook of Pediatrics.*16th ed. Philadelphia, PA: W B Sanuders; 2000: 23-65.
20. Roemmich JN, Rogol AD. Physiology of growth and development: its relationship to performance in the young athlete. *Clin Sports Med.* 1995;14(3):483.
21. Smoll FL, Smith RE, eds. *Children and Youth in Sport: A Biopsychosocial Perspective.* Madison, WI: Brown and Benchmark, Inc; 1996.
22. Levine MD. Neurodevelopmental dysfunction in the school age child. In: Behrman RE, Kliegman RM, Jenson HB, eds. *Nelson Textbook of Pediatrics.* 16th ed. Philadelphia, Penn: WB Saunders Company; 2000:94-100.
23. McArdle WD, Katch FI, Katch VL. Body composition assessment and sport-specific observations. In: McArdle WD, Katch FI, Katch VL, eds. *Sports and Exercise Nutrition.* Baltimore, MD: Williams and Wilkins, ; 1999:374-425.
24. Hahn T, Foldspang A, Vestergaard E, Ingemann-Hansen T. One-leg standing balance and sports activity. *Scand J Med Sci Sports.* 1999;9:15-18.
25. Purcell JS, Hergenroeder AC. Physical conditioning in adolescents. *Curr Opin Pediatr.* 1994;6:373-378.
26. Marshall WA, Tanner JM. Variation in the pattern of pubertal changes in boys. *Arch Dis Child.* 1970;45:13-24.
27. Bodie DA. Changes in lung function, ball-handling skills, and performance measures during adolescence in normal schoolboys. In: Binkhorst RA, et al, eds. *Children and Exercise XI.* Champaign, IL: Human Kinetics; 1985:260-268.
28. Branta C, Haubensticker J, Seefeldt V. Age changes in motor skills during childhood and adolescence. *Exerc Sport Sci Rev.* 1984;12:467-520.
29. Nelson MA. Developmental skills and children's sports. *Physician Sports Med.* 1991;19:67-79.
30. Abe JA, Izard CE. A Longitudinal study of emotion, expression and personality relations in early development. *J Pers Soc Psychol.* 1999;77(3):566-577.
31. Gemelli R. *Normal Child and Adolescent Development.* Washington, DC: American Psychiatric Press; 1996.

32. Piaget J. Intellectual evaluation from adolescence to adulthood. *Hum Dev.* 1972;1-12.

33. Piaget J, Inhelder B. *The Psychology of the Child.* New York: Basic Books; 1969.

34. Greydanus DE, Pratt HD. Psychosocial considerations for the adolescent athlete: lessons learned from the US. *Asian J Pediatr Pract.* 2000;3(3):19-29.

35. American Academy of Pediatrics. Participation in boxing by children, adolescents, and young adults. Committee on Sports Medicine and Fitness. *Pediatrics.* 1997;99(1): 134-135.

36. Erickson E. *Childhood and Society.* New York: WW Norton and Co, Inc; 1963.

37. Ewing MW, Seefeldt VS, Brown TP. Role of organized sport in the education and health of American children and youth. *Institute for the Study of Youth Sports.* East Lansing, MI: Michigan State University; 1996.

38. Harris SS. Readiness to participate in sports. In: Sullivan AJ, Anderson SJ, eds. *Care of the Young Athlete.* Park Ridge, IL: American Academy of Orthopaedic Surgeons, and Elk Grove, IL: American Academy of Pediatrics; 2000:19-24.

39. Elkind D. *The Hurried Child: Growing Up Too Fast, Too Soon.* Reading, MA: Addison-Wesley; 1988.

40. Gesell A, Ilg FL, Ames LB. *The Child from Five to Ten.* New York: Harper and Row Publishers; 1946.

41. Greydanus DE, ed. *American Academy of Pediatrics: Caring for Your Adolescent.* New York: Bantam Books; 1991.

42. Patel DR, Luckstead EF. Sport participation, risk taking, and health risk behaviors. *Adolesc Med State art rev.* 2000;11(1):141-155.

43. Hahn T, Foldspang A, Ingemann-Hansen T. Dynamic strength of the quadriceps muscle and sports activity. *Br J Sports Med.* 1999;33:117-120.

44. Metfessel N.S, Michael WB, Kirsner DA. Instrumentation of Bloom's & Krathwol's taxonomies for writing of educational objectives. *Psychol Sch.* 1969;6:227-231.

45. Ryckman RM, Hamel J. Perceived physical ability differences in the sport participation motives of young athletes. *Int. J. Sport Psychol.* 1993;24:270-283.

46. Zimmerman BJ, Kitsantas A. Developmental phases in self-regulation shifting from process goals to outcome goals. *J Educ Psychol.* 1997;89(1):29-36.

47. Tofler IR, Stryer BK, Micheli LJ, et al. Physical and emotional problems of elite female gymnasts. *NEJM.* 1996;335:281.

48. Bardy BG, Laurent M. How is body orientation controlled during somersaulting? *J Exp Psychol Hum Percept Perform.* 1998;24(3):963-977.

49. Sharkey BJ. Neuromuscular training, In: Sullivan AJ, Grana WA, eds. *The Pediatric Athlete.* Park Ridge, IL: American Academy of Orthopaedic Surgeons; 1990:21-6.

50. American Academy of Pediatrics Committee on Sports Medicine. Strength training, weight and power lifting, and body building by children and adolescents. *Pediatrics.* 1990;86(5):801-803.

51. Erickson E. *Identity, Youth and Crisis,* New York: WW Norton and Co, Inc; 1968.

52. Fagenbaum AD, Westcott WL, Loud RL, Long C. The effects of different resistance training protocols on muscular strength and endurance development in children. *Pediatrics.* 1999;104(l):1-7.

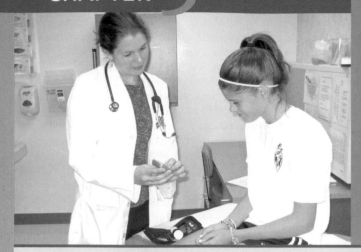

CHAPTER 3

Psychosocial Aspects of Youth Sports

Dilip R. Patel, Donald E. Greydanus, and Helen D. Pratt

INTRODUCTION

In contemporary American society, participation in sports is considered a rite of passage for children and adolescents. Over the past five decades there has been a fundamental shift in the context in which children become involved in sports. Prior to the 1950s sports were largely a matter for local communities to organize for their youth; since the early 1950s, however, sports have shifted from being youth-organized activities to adult-organized activities for the youth and from being fun oriented, spontaneous activity to highly organized competitions.[1–3] Today's youth have little say in the conduct of the organized sports, which largely reflect adult perspectives. At the same time, one must acknowledge the tireless efforts of thousands of well-meaning adult volunteers making such sport experiences possible for youth.

At the outset, we should draw a distinction between professional and youth sports. In the professional athletics, sport is athlete's full-time occupation and he or she makes a living from sport. On the other hand for children and adolescents, sport is one of many activities they do as part of growing up. Within the context of American culture, the term youth sports refers to "any of the organized sports programs that provide a systematic sequence of practices and contests for children and youth."[1] Approximately 20 to 35 million children and adolescents participate annually in organized sport programs (Table 3-1).[1–4] The most popular sports include football, basketball, track and field, baseball, softball, wrestling, tennis, swimming, volleyball, cross-country running, and golf. Approximately 80% of total participants are involved in nonschool programs, and 20% in school-based programs.[1] There is a significant trend toward increasing participation in nonschool programs and decreasing participation in school programs. There is none to minimal research or published information on the youth who are not part of the organized sports and those who quit. Many children take part in other valuable alternative activities such as recreational sports, music, and various other arts. Many more enjoy walking, hiking, camping, and other equally healthy activities.

Table 3-1.

Organized Youth Sports Programs

School sponsored

Intramural—Competition is between teams within a school

Interscholastic—Competition is between teams from different schools. These are governed by National Federation of State High School Associations.

Nonschool sponsored

Agency sponsored—These are local sports programs with national affiliation; usually limited to one sport, for example, Little League Baseball.

Club sports—Participants in these programs pay for services. Programs are conducted year round; competitive; and located in special facilities. For example, ice skating, gymnastic clubs.

National youth service organizations—Sport is just one of many youth activities; for example, YMCA.

Recreational programs—These programs emphasize fun and skill development, are noncompetitive, and all participate. For example National Recreation and Park Association programs.

Based on data from Ewing MW, Seefeldt VD, Brown TP. Role of Organized Sport in the Education and Health of American Children and Youth. East Lansing, MI: Institute for the Study of Youth Sports, Michigan State University; 1996.

A basic understanding of the psychosocial dynamics of youth sports by the pediatrician will help facilitate early recognition and effective management of potential problems. We review the salient aspects of organized youth sports in the United States, such as developmental issues, factors influencing participation or attrition, the psychology of injury, violence in sports, use of performance-enhancing substances, eating disorders, competitive stress, health risk behaviors, and effects of intensive participation. We seek to delineate the critical role of the pediatrician in this context and suggest a clinical approach. Pediatricians provide medical care to athletes on a regular basis in their practice. Because of their knowledge of growth and development of the children and adolescents, pediatricians are in a unique position to apply this knowledge and in guiding the athlete and his or her family through the ups and downs of many wonderful years of sport participation.

SPORTS AND PSYCHOSOCIAL DEVELOPMENT

In spite of the perceptions held on both sides of the arguments regarding the benefits and risks associated with organized youth sports programs in the United States, evidence suggest that sport participation is inherently neither a "good" nor a "bad" experience for children.[1,5–9] The most crucial factor determining whether children and adolescents will have a positive or negative experience from sports is neither the sport participation itself nor in what form; rather it is how adults impart or chose to impart this experience to the participants. The overall outcome from sport participation is the result of interplay among multiple mediating factors: the athlete, family, peers, coach, and societal attitudes as well as expectations. In fact, the vast majority of youth like sports and have a positive experience from "normal" level of participation; some children who engage in "intensive" participation may be more likely to experience problems associated with sports.

Many lifelong benefits from regular physical activity, either in the form of exercise or sport, have been well documented. Although, physical exercise and sports are inherently related and the terms are often used interchangeably, sport has a distinct social dimension.[10] Many potential contributions of sport to psychological and social development of a child are enumerated in Table 3-2.[1,8,11,12]

Sports provide a setting for the child to test personal abilities. Self-perception is influenced by feedback from peers, coach, parents, and spectators. Behavior of adults and peers also influence self-perception. Positive feedback, encouragement, and focus on fun and participation rather than the outcome—a win or a loss—will contribute to

Table 3-2.
Potential Contributions of Sports to a Child's Psychosocial Development

Psychologic development
Improved self-esteem, self-perception, self-confidence
Enhanced personal coping abilities
Increased motivation

Social development
Provides opportunity for self-evaluation and social comparison
Enhances social competence
Provides socialization experiences for the athlete and family
Teaches personal responsibility
Provides experience in dealing with authority
Fosters competitiveness, teamwork

Moral Development
Fosters independence and builds character
Teaches sportsmanship and fair play

increased self-esteem. Sports experience provides the opportunity for learning how to handle success or failure, and to realize that the most important thing is the effort rather then the result. Many physical as well psychosocial benefits from sport participation by children and youth with chronic disease and physically and mentally challenging conditions have been well documented.[13]

Children learn to compare their own abilities and skills with those of peers and assess their own level of competence. They learn the value of practice and preparation resulting in better performance. Many facets of social competence can be enhanced through sport, such as teamwork, cooperation, interpersonal skills, leadership skills, and self-discipline.[1,14] Sport provides a setting in which appropriate physical aggressiveness can be learned and taught under supervised and controlled circumstances.[1,8] Within the context of athletics, many friendships are made between athletes and between families, across racial and ethnic groups, and across socioeconomic groups.[14] For older children and adolescents, sport participation provides opportunity for learning how to appropriately interact with adult authority figures other than their parents. Many children learn the value of fairness and the concept of right and wrong from their sport experience.

Sometimes sport can have negative influence also.[7,8] If the child is pressured to compete, this can contribute to stress and decreased motivation to continue in sports. A perception of failure and criticisms from adults and peers can lead to decreased self-esteem. Sports can also expose children to negative adult behaviors.

Some researchers have noted that sport participants are less likely to engage in delinquent behaviors and suggested sport as alternative to gangs for youth.[1]

However, the contribution of sports to decreased health risk behaviors, decreased teenage pregnancy rate, decreased truancy, improved grades, decreased smoking, and decreased depression remains controversial and subject of on going research and debate.

FACTORS MEDIATING SPORT PARTICIPATION EXPERIENCE

Sport experience occurs within the larger sociocultural context and is, therefore, influenced by many factors, most significantly peers, parents, and coaches.[10,11,15-19] The place of sports in contemporary society, societal attitudes on success and failure, media portrayal of sports, and societal expectations of young athletes also play influencing role.

Peers

As children grow older, they spend increasingly more time with peers. Athletic ability is considered to be an important characteristic of social status by boys while physical appearance is considered more important by girls, especially by older children and adolescents.[1,7] Peer approval of athletic performance and abilities is highly valued by athletes and their families. They also begin to compare their own abilities with those of peers. Thus, peers become the most significant source of information for appraisal of personal abilities and self-worth as well as a most important socializing influence, especially for adolescents.[8-10,15] Athletic ability, an important marker for social status, is most highly valued by high school students; they would rather succeed in athletics than in academics.[1] Participation in team sports is believed to greatly increase the teenager's popularity and peer acceptance. Sport participation becomes the sole motivation for some students to stay in school.[1]

Athletes enjoy more peer acceptance when the team is successful; on the other hand, a loss may result in rejection and intense criticism.[10,15] The athlete has to be a team player and needs to be cooperative with teammates; at the same time, he or she must compete with friends. Pursuit of athletic excellence and success may potentially lead to alienation from peers, because of jealousy. Whether to continue high level athletics or not depends upon the athlete's need for peer acceptance or need for personal achievement.[8,12] Memories of success or failure in athletics and with peers remain with individuals throughout their lives.

Family

The family is the most important support system for an athlete. Parents have the greatest influence on children younger than 10 to 12 years.[10,15] Parental attitudes and feedback affect a child's self-perception of his or her own capabilities, and emotional outcomes from sports involvement. Whether sport participation is a positive or a negative experience is greatly dependent upon parental influence. Parents can provide positive evaluations, encouragement for their efforts, support for sport participation, realistic expectations of winning or losing, and involve the children in decisions about participation; these factors all contribute to an overall positive sport experience.[7,8] Some children are more likely to enjoy and do well in sport. For the vast majority of athletes parental influence leads to a positive sport experience. However, for other athletes, parents can be a source of negative influence.

Some parents may have unresolved needs of their own (such as unfulfilled athletic wishes from childhood), and identify their self-esteem with athletic success of their children.[9,16,20-22] This creates undue pressure on children to perform and excel in sports. Some parents consider sport participation by their child as an investment for future rewards such as athletic scholarship or financial success.[7,14] In other instances a child's success in athletics may become a symbol of social status for parents, and parents may enter into unhealthy competition to push their children to perform.[7] A child's success in sport becomes the sole focus at the expense of development in other psychological and social aspects. In few instances parental over involvement, e.g., yelling at children or other parents or fighting with coaches, can lead to aggressive behaviors at the game or practice, with negative influence on social and psychological development of the child athlete. Parent may become angry at the child who loses, makes mistakes, or wants to drop out of one or more sports.[14] Children may be pushed to continue to participate despite injury; parents may shop physicians for favorable opinion and may even request surgical or hormonal treatments to enhance athletic abilities of their children.[7,14,16,22] For the athletes who want to pursue competitive athletics, parents have to invest considerable energy, time, and financial resources, often stressing the family system.[7,8] The balance between appropriate positive encouragement and over involvement can be difficult to achieve by all family members.

Coach

The influence of a coach on the child and adolescent athlete's life in and out of sports has been well recognized.[1,7,11,15,20,23,24] The coach's role, interactions, and influence changes over time for the young child playing sports for fun to that of the child or adolescent engaged in intense participation for competitive athletics. The coach becomes increasingly more important for the adolescent.

The coach is involved in player selection, recruitment, determining the role of the athlete in the team, training, game plan preparation, and foster team cohesion.[12] The child's behaviors, self-perceptions, and self-esteem are greatly influenced by a coach's interpersonal behaviors, values, goals, and priorities that are set.[12,16] Casual remarks by a coach can have significant effects on an athlete, as for example in dieting behaviors or use of performance-enhancing substances. For most youth sports, the coach's priority is mainly to ensure enjoyment of the participants; for more competitive settings and those potentially leading to a life in professional sports, the goal becomes winning at all costs. A vast majority of coaches are volunteer coaches with no formal training in coaching or child development, and thus, may not have a developmentally appropriate coaching style.[8] In fact one study notes that many coaches at the junior high level tend to have an aggressive behavior, and tend to have inappropriately high expectations for performance and behavior for their athletes.[14]

Not unlike parents, some coaches may have their own unmet needs and may be living them through their athletes. On the other hand, the adolescent may also have unmet dependency needs and become dependent on the coach as an adult figure or fatherly figure (surrogate parent) in a so-called dependency relationship. Also incidences of sexual exploitation of athletes by coaches have been reported.[5,7,25,26] Thus, parents walk a fine line between giving total control of the child to the coach and being over involved themselves.

Coaches can have a great positive influence on the moral and social development of a child and an adolescent. This influence involves setting good examples by their own behaviors and attitudes; coaches can act as advisors and help adolescents in trouble as well as teach them prosocial values, teamwork, and cooperation. A philosophy of winning which has been developed for coaches of youth sports is outlined in Table 3-3.[8]

Table 3-3.

Philosophy of Winning: Coaching Effectiveness Training Program of Smoll and Smith

Winning is not everything, nor is it the only thing
Failure is not the same thing as losing
Success is not synonymous with winning
Children should be taught that success is found in striving for victory (i.e., success is related to effort)

Based on Smoll FL, Smith RE, eds. Children and Youth in Sport: A Biopsychosocial Perspective. Madison, WI: Brown and Benchmark; 1996.

Society and Media

Sports have become a major economic factor in society. It is estimated that the sport industry ranks tenth with revenues of $120 billion in the United States.[7] Media portrayal of professional athletics can be highly influential in shaping young athlete's perceptions of athletics, with potential fame and success.[27] Many professional athletes are heroes and role models for children and adolescents. The importance of winning reinforces the message that winning at all costs is success in life! However, only a very handful of youth may ever be fortunate enough to reach the glory and fame of elite and professional athletics. For the many that are left behind, the unrealistic expectations can be detrimental. More importantly youth must understand that success in professional athletics does not necessarily translate into success in overall life.

Many elite and professional athletes and their media exposure can also be a positive influence. Athletes can serve as positive role models by contributing to youth programs back into their schools and communities. Some athletes show self-determination and value of hard work by succeeding in spite of physical handicap or socioeconomic barriers. Also coverage of local youth sports can potentially be quite positive.

REASONS TO PARTICIPATE IN SPORTS

An athlete's attitudes, personality, and personal motivation play central roles in sports participation. Many individual factors (cognitive and physical maturity, importance of success in sports) and environmental factors (rewards from sports, type of sport, sociocultural factors, coaching style) influence individual motivation.[28–30] Some athletes are primarily motivated to improve personal sport skills and to do their personal best (intrinsically or mastery-oriented); others are motivated to excel in comparison to peers (extrinsically or outcome-oriented).[31] Mastery-oriented athletes enjoy playing the sport, and for them, success is personal improvement and the effort itself. For outcome-oriented athletes, success mean winning the game, and thus, a loss can be difficult to tolerate.

Many youth have unrealistic expectations from sports. Studies suggest that in middle and high school years 40% to 50 % of students, especially boys, intend (dream) to become professional athletes.[32] Their reasons to pursue professional athletics in the future were the "rewards" of athletic participation such as money, social status, praise from others, independence, and the admiration of women. It was not for the "fun" of sports.

Table 3-4.		
Reasons to Play, to Quit, and To Be Left Out of Sports		
Reasons to Play	**Reasons to Quit**	**Reasons To Be Left Out**
Fun. *The most common reason.*	Injury *The most common reason*	Exclusionary selection process
Personal motivation	Being cut from the team	Low priority on physical education in
Physical fitness	Needing job	school curricula
Socialization	Inconvenient schedule	Lack of skilled coaches
Way out of limited socioeconomic	Conflicts with nonsports activities	Fear of injury
situations	Lack of playing time	Low socioeconomic status
Status symbol	Overemphasis on competition	Lack of local community based programs
Rewards	Overzealous coach	Overemphasis on winning
Family/parental wish	Dislike for coach	Low cultural priority
Societal expectations	Competitive stress	Adverse parental attitudes
Media influence	Lack of fun	Lack of female coaches
	Peer disapproval	Being female
	Personal sense of failure	
	Depression	
	Burnout	
	Failure to meet other's expectations	

However, for the vast majority of children and youth, the most common reason to participate in sport is to have fun and be with friends. Motivation and reasons to be involved in sport also vary depending upon the age and developmental stage of the child. Young children tend to focus on having fun and being with friends, while adolescents may want to achieve status among peers, or "impress" others. Many other reasons are enumerated in Table 3-4.[8,12,30,33]

REASONS TO QUIT SPORTS

Attrition refers to those who drop out of a sport before the season officially ends.[1,34] Studies suggest that attrition from youth sports generally begin by age 10 years and peak at 14 to 15 years.[1] Highest rates of early dropout are noted in gymnastics and the least in football. Fifty percent of sports participants may drop out by the time they reach early adolescence.[1] One study of high school students noted that 26% dropped out from one sport; this increases to 29.8% when attrition from more than one sport was considered.[34] Injury was cited as the most frequent reason for quitting sports. Intensive participation in organized sports beginning at an early age has been noted to be an important contributing factor to early attrition; one study noted 75% dropout rate by age 15 years among those who began participating in organized sports by age 7.[14]

Dropout may be either athlete-initiated or because of reasons not under an athlete's control. Some authors consider dropping out to be a normal process in which the athlete is trying out different activities.[35] There is very little information on the relationship between developmental stage and reasons to quit sports. It is noted that reasons to quit are different at different ages and developmental level. In one study, elementary school students cited overemphasis on winning as a main reason; while high school students cited conflicts of interest as a main reason.[35]

Contrary to popular belief, burnout is just one of many reasons to drop out from sports. Burnout is a response to chronic stress from intense sport participation and the athlete no longer enjoys the sport.[17] The athlete perceives that he or she is not able to meet the demands of the sport and perform adequately. Table 3-4 outlines a number of other reasons for quitting sports.

REASONS TO BE LEFT OUT OF SPORTS

It can be difficult to imagine that there are children and adolescents not in the "game" with so many youth apparently participating in sports at all levels, and with daily mass media exposure to sport. However, a recent report on youth sports noted that "sports in America represent a highly exclusionary process, with only the elite performers accorded a share of the spotlight."[1] A closer scrutiny of youth sports scene indicates that a large number of children and adolescents do not participate in organized sports because of many perceived or real barriers in adult-organized competitive sports.[1,7,8,34]

In addition to sports being a highly selective process, other important considerations include female gender, low socioeconomic status, and cultural influence as barriers for sport participation.[8,11] Because of social bias, boys tend to be encouraged more for sports than are girls. Also, girls who do participate do so at a relatively later age than do boys, and then tend to drop out early.[1] Importantly, there are very few female role models, and only 1 out of 10 coaches is a female.[1] Low socioeconomic conditions are especially important consideration for the inner city urban youth; as more programs move away from local schools and communities to suburbs, they become less affordable. In many cultures, sports are a low priority compared to academic achievement and children are not particularly encouraged to be actively involved in sports. Table 3-4 lists some of the various barriers for sports participation by youth. Research is limited on those who are left out.

PSYCHOLOGY OF THE INJURED ATHLETE

The psychological response to injury depends on many factors such as the emotional maturity of the child or adolescent, severity and type of injury, the extent to which it will limit participation at present or in the future, individual pain tolerance, ability to cope, personal motivation, one's place in the team, seasonal timing, context of the injury, and support from family and others.[9,36–39]

The vast majority of young children and adolescents cope well with injury and the inability to play, since they hope that their injury will heal and they will be able to resume sport participation.[38] Some athletes may cherish the special attention given to them during rehabilitation. They may take pride in having a cast signed by friends. A few will find it difficult to adjust and may manifest anger, frustration, and a depressed mood following injury. Late adolescent athletes in highly competitive or elite-level sports may go thorough emotional stages similar to other loss, beginning with disbelief, denial, and isolation and followed in succession by anger, bargaining, depression, and acceptance and resignation.[10,19,37] Fortunately, for most children and adolescents the progression from denial to recovery is of short duration. A few athletes may manifest multiple somatic symptoms and do not recover as expected. In these athletes, further assessment is indicated to find complicating factors such as underlying depression, fear and anxiety, secondary gain, or conflicts with parents.

Management of parental anxiety can be even more challenging. Parents should be helped to understand the implications of injury on future sport participation and the emotional reactions of the athlete. Pediatricians play an important role in helping an athlete and parents during this period by recognizing potential problems, having realistic expectations, and not yielding to external pressures to return athlete prematurely to sports, in the best interests of an athlete. A pediatrician may also consult a psychologist who can help the athlete with a number of cognitive-behavioral techniques during the rehabilitation process.[40]

THE TALENTED ATHLETE

Some children naturally excel in certain sports. Knowing this many parents wonder whether these talented children can be identified early and their talent developed further to reach elite or Olympic level. Researchers have used complex measurements of physical, behavioral, and psychological characteristics to identify talented child athletes.[8,12] Numerous interrelated variables (such as continuous process of growth and development, varying selection process at different levels, different sport-specific demands, and cultural factors) make it extremely difficult to identify and predict athletic excellence at an early developmental stage.[8]

The main goal of some high performance youth sports programs is to identify athletes who will succeed at state, national, or Olympic levels.[12] Athletes in such programs may start intensive training as early as age 3, with the intention to perfecting the sport-specific skills.[8] Such parents are advised to involve the child in this process, allow the child to participate in important decisions, be careful of over involvement and respect the child's aspirations, and consider potential negative effects on other critical aspects of development and on family life.

HIGH-RISK HEALTH BEHAVIORS

The issue of certain high-risk health behaviors (such as aggressive and violent acts, use of performance-enhancing substances, substance abuse, weight control and dieting behaviors) by adolescents in the context of athletics has been a subject of debate.[41–45] Whether adolescent athletes are more or less likely to engage in such behaviors is not clear. Studies comparing adolescent athletes and nonathletes are limited and do not allow any definite generalizations or conclusions. From limited data, it seems that while the vast majority of adolescent athletes engage in a healthy lifestyle a subset may be at higher risk of engaging in dangerous behaviors. On the other hand some researchers suggest that youth sports are a deterrent to negative behaviors and may lead to less aggression, less involvement in gang activities, and less delinquency.

Aggression and Violence

Many reports in the scientific as well as lay press have looked at sports-associated aggressive and violent behaviors among athletes and spectators, however a clear link between sports and aggressive behaviors cannot be established conclusively.[30,46–50] Some researchers have theorized that sport may be a venue for youth to engage in aggressive acts in a socially acceptable manner.[21] Aggression in sport is considered to be a learned behavior. It is relatively more common in team and contact sports (such as ice hockey, football), and among male athletes.[8,10] Athletes may react aggressively because of pressure to compete and win with no intention to harm others. On the other hand violent behaviors with intent to harm opponents to gain unfair advantage are not only unethical but also highly dangerous. Coaches and parents can help young athletes to express their frustrations and anger in an appropriate, socially acceptable manner. Media portrayal of aggression and violence in professional sports may also influence youth, though such behavior is not necessarily representative of most youth sports.[27] In fact acts of violence in youth sports are not common.

Use of Performance-Enhancing Substances

There has been an increased use of drugs and nutritional supplements by adolescents in order to enhance sports performance.[30,51] The pressure to excel and meet social and individual expectations; advice from a coach, parents, or peers; use by peers; youth-targeted marketing; and lack or misinformation on risks all may contribute to such use of performance-enhancing substances.[5,52,53] Use of such substances by adolescents should be considered within the broader context of adolescent risk taking and substance abuse behaviors. See Chapter 7 for further discussion of this topic.

Weight Control and Eating Disorders

There is a wide spectrum of eating and dieting behaviors seen in adolescent athletes ranging from seasonal weight control to full syndromes of anorexia or bulimia nervosa.[54–59] Such disordered eating behaviors are more common in athletes participating in weight class sports (e.g., wrestling, weight lifting), aesthetic sports (e.g., gymnastics, figure skating, diving), and endurance sports (e.g., long-distance running, cycling, swimming).[59,60] In weight class sports, the athlete must meet a specific weight in order to compete in a particular category; in the aesthetic sports, the athlete is judged subjectively based on lean appearance; and in endurance sports, a lean body type and low weight are considered important to enhance performance. There are numerous cultural and societal attitudes toward weight and appearance contributing to dieting and disordered eating behaviors in adolescents.[61] With the exception of weight control by some male athletes (such as wrestlers, football players, jockeys, and long distance runners) disordered eating and pathogenic weight control behaviors are most common among female athletes who constitute almost 95% of this total.[61] Studies suggest that the prevalence of disordered eating behaviors in athletes range from 5% to 33% or more (compared to 1%–3% in general population).[57,58,61] Numerous acute and long-term medical complications associated with pathogenic weight control practices including premature osteoporosis and death should be of great concern and have been well documented.[61,62]

PSYCHIATRIC CONDITIONS

Some mental health conditions can have special significance for athletes. Eating disorders and substance abuse have been alluded to previously. Salient aspects of depression, attention deficit hyperactivity disorder, competitive stress, and anxiety as these relate to athletics are considered below.

Depression

Depression in an adolescent athlete may be owing to an injury resulting in an inability to return to sport, failure to meet others expectations, substance abuse, or underlying overt depressive disorder. The athlete who suddenly loses interest and drops out from team should be evaluated further. Athletes can also effectively mask depression. Prevalence of depression is not necessarily higher in athletes and in fact some studies suggest less depression and suicidal ideation in athletes than in youth who do not participate in sports.[63–65]

Attention Deficit Hyperactivity Disorder

Athletes with attention deficit hyperactivity disorder (ADHD) may perceive that they are better at sports and other physical activity than academics.[41] Thus they may have a tendency to be more involved in sports compared to those who do not have ADHD. These athletes may need more attention and guidance from coaches and other adults to make their sport experience a positive one. Stimulant medications (methylphenidate, amphetamines) commonly used in the treatment of ADHD are banned from athletics by the United States and International Olympic Committees because of the concern over abuse and unfair advantage by athletes who use them.[66] Researchers have noted that fine motor coordination, balance, attention, and concentration all improved in sports played when athletes with ADHD are on stimulants.[66] Also there is a high degree of individual differences in response to different stimulants and effects on sport performance vary depending upon the tasks involved in particular sport.

Competitive Stress and Anxiety

Children and adolescents experience different levels of stress from competitive sports. This depends upon the specific situation, an athlete's perception of the situation, and his or her ability to cope.[17,67] The stress of competition can result in symptoms of anxiety. A number of factors may contribute to anxiety, such as type of sport (individual more than team), level of competition, underlying anxiety traits, fear of failure, fear of not meeting adult expectations, reactions of peers and adults, pressure from coach and parents, significance of winning, and outcome of the competition (loss).[8,17] Research indicates that for most children, sport participation is no more stressful than many other childhood activities where competition is involved and performance is measured.[8]

It is important for the pediatrician to recognize that athletic stress can present as any number of psychosomatic complaints including, chest pain, abdominal pain, headaches, fatigue, shortness of breath, and hyperventilation. This understanding will facilitate early recognition of such problems.

Stress can also manifest as sudden inability to perform (choking) when least expected during the competition.[5] The athlete may not be able to move his or her body and there may or may not be associated anxiety. In addition stress can manifest as prolonged deterioration of performance (slump) lasting for many weeks to months.[5]

INTENSIVE SPORT PARTICIPATION

Some athletes engage in intense sport participation because of their own love for sports, personal motivation (dream), because of parental pressure or societal influences. These athletes begin training as early as 5 or 6 years of age and continue training through-

out the year; they generally specialize in a single sport, and may spend as much as 4 hours every day involved in practice or game.[12,14] These athletes often travel away from home for games or special training. Some researchers contend that such time commitment to sports may take time away from normal social and developmental activities, possibly leading to isolation.[7,12,30] The athlete and the family must carefully weigh the long-term priorities (namely academic versus athletic) and consider the fact that only a few will be fortunate enough to reach professional or Olympic levels. It is estimated that out of two million children participating each year in competitive gymnastics only seven or eight make it to Olympic games; also only 1 in 2300 high school senior basketball players will be skilled enough to play at the NBA (National Basketball Association) level.[14]

Some athletes may develop stress-related problems stemming from intense participation. These include depression, stress-related anxiety, conversion reactions, and disordered eating behaviors. A few will develop overtraining syndrome and may drop out completely from all sports. An athlete who is too embarrassed to quit, or is pressured to continue, may cause sports-related self-injury in order to drop out gracefully. In addition to many psychological concerns, intense training has been associated with menstrual disorders, and overuse injuries of the musculoskeletal system. Also, the emotional, financial, and time commitment on the part of the family can stress the family system, leading to diverse family problems.[28]

A CLINICAL APPROACH TO PSYCHOSOCIAL ISSUES

The pediatrician has many opportunities to intervene with the athlete and his or her family. The athlete may present with a specific sports-related concern such as minor musculoskeletal injury, questions regarding the safety of supplement use, or requesting to learn how to lose weight. Parents may be concerned that their son or daughter suddenly quit the team. Each well or health maintenance visit presents an opportunity to discuss many sport-related issues on a routine basis as part of anticipatory guidance (Table 3-5). Other scenarios in which a pediatrician has the opportunity to see athletes include when an athlete presents with a sport-related concern, a nonsport-related concern within the context of sport participation or at the sideline or in office with an injury.

After the pediatrician has obtained routine psychosocial history, focused questions related to sport participation can be used (Table 3-6). The examination

Table 3-5.

Anticipatory Guidance

Developmental readiness

Readiness for competitive sports depends on child's developmental stage, sociocultural environment, parental attitudes, as well as skills and demands required of a particular sport.

Desire to compare skills to others develops by age 6–7 y; cognitive understanding of social and competitive nature of sports is developed by age 8–9 y.

All psychological skills needed for competitive sports may not be achieved before age 11 or 12 y.

During elementary school years expose the child to different activities; emphasis should be on participation and fun rather then outcome.

Talent identification

It is very difficult to identify specific athletic talent in a child with any certainty. Because of many variables (genetics, effects of growth and development) involved, it is not possible to reliably predict future athletic excellence.

Academics and athletics

Those students who are involved in cocurricular activities including sports (and others such as debate, music, voluntary activities, student governing) also generally do well in academics. Academic failure should not be the sole reasons to not allow athlete to continue participation.

Gender and sports

Girls can participate in all sports and should be encouraged and allowed to do so.

Program philosophy

Know the primary goal of the youth sport program before enrolling. Be sure it matches with child's readiness as well as purpose of participation.

Coaching philosophy

Be aware of the coaching style and philosophy. Win at all cost attitudes may not lead to best outcome from sports. Be involved and do not abandon your parental role nor abdicate all control to the coach.

Odds of success

Only a handful of children and adolescents will ever make it to the elite or professional level. Nurture realistic expectations. Avoid the temptation of using sports to achieve other goals (for example scholarships, financial gain, fame, social status).

Chronic disease

Children and adolescents with chronic disease, and physically or mentally challenging conditions should be appropriately matched to sports activities they can participate in. This will have great physical and psychological benefits.

Benefits versus risks

Sports participation can be beneficial or detrimental depending upon the child's experience. Whether the experience is a positive or negative one depends on involved adults and societal attitudes and goals.

Intensive participation

Intensive and early participation in sports does not necessarily lead to future athletic success. In fact it may result in detrimental effects.

---

should include a mental status examination. The overall goal of this assessment is to determine whether the problem is really related to sport participation or there is an underlying medical disorder presenting in the context of athletic activity. A number of indicators of potential problems associated with sport participation are listed in Table 3-7.

The vast majority of problems can be successfully managed by the pediatrician. In some instances, further consultation with a sport psychologist or other professional with expertise in sports may be needed who can offer further assessment, counseling (individual and family), and cognitive-behavioral sports performance enhancement interventions. The pediatrician can get involved with local community sport programs to influence their philosophy, and act as a helpful

resource, educator, and advisor to parents, athletes, and officials.

Organized sport is an exclusionary process, leaving many children and adolescents out of such activities. These youth who feel left- out and discouraged, and their families should be counseled that not being in organized sport activities is not the "end of the world." All children and adolescents can benefit from informal play activities. Some children may be in sports that they are not suited for and may well benefit from a different sport or other activity of their own choosing. Many extracurricular activities can be as enjoyable and worthy as organized sport. These include art, music, and dance, individual sports that one likes (such as swimming, tennis, and martial arts), walking, jogging, camping, hiking, and many more.

Table 3-6.

Sport-Related Psychosocial Screening

1. Does the athlete or parents have a specific sport-related concern?
2. Does the athlete participate in organized sports or plays recreationally?
3. What is the level of participation? How many hours per week? Does the athlete often travel away from home for games or special training?
4. How is the athlete doing in school? Does he or she participate in any nonsports activities?
5. Does the athlete have any professional sport hero? Does the athlete aspire to be like him or her?
6. Do the parents or coaches exert undue pressure on the athlete to participate or perform?
7. Who wants the athlete to participate and why?
8. Is sport the sole focus to the exclusion of other activities? Do parents or the athlete perceive he or she is overinvovled or underinvolved in sports?
9. Why does the athlete want to participate in sports?
10. Why do parents want the athlete to participate in sports?
11. How important is winning to the athlete, the parents, the coach?
12. How do athlete and parents handle a win or a loss?
13. What do the athlete and parents know about the philosophy of the coach, team or the program in which the athlete participates?
14. Is the athlete exempted from other responsibilities because of his or her status as an athlete? Is he or she asked to share the expenses of sport participation?
15. Is the athlete compared to athletic siblings? Or is he or she the last hope for the family to achieve athletic success?
16. Do parents like to participate in sports? Were they involved as children? Have they expressed any unfulfilled wishes for athletic achievement?
17. What do parents think of opposing team's coach? Parents? Fans?
18. Has a parent (or parents) been barred from attending game ? Have there been involved in fights with other parents or a coach?
19. Have parents made excessive financial commitment for sports ? Have they moved to new location, or the athlete moved, to participate in sports?

Partly based on data from Begel D, Bruton B, eds. Sport Phychiatry: Theory and Practice. New York: Norton Professional Books; 2000; Stryer BK, Tofler IR, Lapchick R. A developmental overview of child and youth sports in society. Child Adolesc Psychiatr Clin N Am. 1998;7:697; Murphy SM. The Cheers and the Tears: Healthy Alternative to the Dark Side of Youth Sports Today. San Francisco: Jossey-Bass, Inc.; 1994.

Table 3-7.

Indicators of Potential Problems

Athlete centered
Failure to recover from injury as expected
Recurrent injuries
Sudden withdrawal from sports
Noncompliance with medical treatment or recommendations
Use of performance-enhancing substances
Undue focus on weight control; pathogenic weight control behaviors
Thrill seeking behaviors from high-risk sports
Unrealistic personal expectations of rewards from sport participation
Deteriorating performance
Aggressive and violent behavior on and off the field
Increased interpersonal conflict with teammates or coaches
Focus on athletics at the expense of other activities
Signs of posttraumatic stress disorder following major injury
Signs of adjustment disorder, depression, anxiety
Psychosomatic symptoms
Signs of sexual exploitation

Family/parent centered
Parental overinvolvement or lack of involvement
Out of control parental behaviors (yelling, fights with coach or other parents)
Competition between parents with respect to their child's athletic success
Parental view of sports as a means to an end (rewards such as scholarship)
Vicarious living through a child's sport participation
Repeated reminders to the athlete about time, money, emotional commitment
Ignoring injuries, pushing athlete to continue participation despite injury

Coach centered
Exploitation of athletes to fulfill personal unmet athletic needs
Excessive control over athlete
Win at all cost philosophy
Preferential selection, favoritism
Encouraging aggression/ violence
Repeated criticisms of athlete
Excessive punitive actions for mistakes

Organization centered
Focus on few talented athletes, exclusionary process
Winning at all costs philosophy

ACKNOWLEDGMENT

This chapter is adapted, with permission, from Patel DR, Greydanus DE, Pratt HD. Youth sports: more than sprains and strains. *Contemp Pediatr.* 2001;18(3): 45-72.

REFERENCES

1. Ewing MW, Seefeldt VD, Brown TP. *Role of Organized Sport in the Education and Health of American Children and Youth.* East Lansing, MI: Institute for the Study of Youth Sports, Michigan State University; 1996.
2. Federation of Sports Medicine and World Health Organization. Sports and children: consensus statement on organized sports for children. *Bull World Health Organ.* 1998;76(5):445.

3. Luckstead EF, Greydanus DE. Psychology and physiology of adolescence. In: *Medical Care of the Adolescent Athlete.* Los Angeles, CA: PMIC; 1993:3-16.

4. Sullivan AJ, Anderson ST, eds. *Health Care of the Young Athlete.* Elk Grove Village, IL: American Academy of Pediatrics and American Academy of Orthopaedic Surgeons; 2000.

5. Begel D, Bruton B, eds. *Sport Phychiatry: Theory and Practice.* New York: Norton Professional Books; 2000.

6. Micheli LJ, Jenkins MD. *Sportswise: An Essential Guide for Young Athletes, Parents, and Coaches.* Boston, MA: Houghton Mifflin Co; 1990.

7. Murphy SM. *The Cheers and the Tears: Healthy Alternative to the Dark Side of Youth Sports Today.* San Francisco: Jossey-Bass, Inc.; 1994.

8. Smoll FL, Smith RE, eds. *Children and Youth in Sport: A Biopsychosocial Perspective.* Madison, WI: Brown and Benchmark; 1996.

9. Singer RN, Murphey M, Tennant LK, eds. *Handbook of Research on Sport Psychology.* New York: Mcmillan; 1993.

10. Patel DR, Pratt HD, Greydanus DE. Adolescent growth, development and psychosocial aspects of sports participation: an overview. *Adolesc Med.* 1998;9:425.

11. Coakley JJ. *Sport in Society: Issues and Controversies.* St. Louis, MO: Mosby-Year Book Publishers; 1998.

12. Cahill BR, Pearl AJ, eds. *Intensive Participation in Children's Sports.* Champaign, IL: Human Kinetics; 1993.

13. Dykens EM, Rosner BA, Butterbaugh G. Exercise and sports in children and adolescents with developmental disabilities: Positive physical and psychosocial effects. *Child Adolesc Psychiatr Clin N Am.* 1998;7:757.

14. Stryer BK, Tofler IR, Lapchick R. A developmental overview of child and youth sports in society. *Child Adolesc Psychiatr Clin N Am.* 1998;7:697.

15. Geigle-Bentz FL, Bentz BG. Psychological aspects of sport. In: Stanitski CL, DeLee JC, Drez D, eds. *Pediatric and Adolescent Sports Medicine.* Philadelphia, PA: WB Saunders; 1994:77-93.

16. Libman S. Adult participation in youth: a developmental perspective. *Child Adolesc Psychiatr Clin N Am.* 1998;7:725.

17. Gould D. Intensive sport participation and the prepubescent athlete: competitive stress and burnout. In: Cahill BR, Pearl A, eds. *Intensive Participation in Children's Sport.* Champaign, IL: Human Kinetics; 1993:19-38.

18. Farrell EG. Sports medicine: psychological aspects. In: Greydanus DE, Wolraich ML, eds. *Behavioral Pediatrics.* New York: Springer-Verlag; 1992:425-434.

19. Greydanus DE, Pratt HD. Psychological considerations for the adolescent athlete: lessons learned from the United States experience. *Asian J Pediatr Prac.* 2000;3(3):19.

20. Arnstein RL. Emotional problems of adolescent athletes. In: Gallagher JR, Heald FP, Gavell DC, eds. *Medical Care of the Adolescent.* New York: Appleton-Century-Crofts; 1976:272-278.

21. Thornton JS. Springing young athletes from the parental pressure cooker. *Phys Sportsmed.* 1991;7:92.

22. Tofler IR, Knapp PK, Drell MJ. The "achievement by proxy" spectrum: recognition and clinical response to pressured and high-achieving children and adolescents. *J Am Acad Child Adolesc Psychiatry.* 1999;38:213.

23. Brown BR, Butterfield SA. Coaches: a missing link in the health care system. *Am J Dis Child.* 1992;146:211.

24. Dishman RK. Exercise and sport psychology in youth 6 to 18 years of age. In: Gisolfi CV, Lamb DR, eds. *Youth, Exercise, and Sports.* Indianapolis, IN: Benchmark Press; 1993:47-98.

25. Brackenridge CH, Kirby S. Playing it safe: assessing the risk of sexual abuse to elite child athletes. *Int Rev Sociol Sport.* 1997;32:407.

26. Jaques R, Brackenridge C. Child abuse and the sports medicine consultation. *Br J Sport Med.* 1999; 33(4):229-230.

27. Kinkema KM, Harris JC. Sport and the mass media. *Exerc Sport Sci Rev.* 1992;20:127-159.

28. Hellstedt JC. Invisible players: a family systems model. In: Murphy SM, ed. *Sport Psychology Interventions.* Champaign, IL: Human Kinetics; 1995:117-146.

29. Lindquist CH, Reynolds KD, Goran MI. Sociocultural eterminants of physical activity among children. *Prev Med.* 1999;29:305.

30. Patel DR, Luckstead EF. Sport participation, risk taking, and health risk behaviors. *Adolesc Med.* 2000;11(1):141-155.

31. Weiss MR, Chaumenton N. Motivational orientations in sport. In: Horn TS, ed. *Advances in Sport Psychology.* Champaign, IL: Human Kinetics; 1994:61-100.

32. Stiles DA, Gibbons JL, Sebben DJ, Wiley DC. Why adolescent boys dream of becoming professional athletes. *Psychol Rep.* 1999;84:1075.

33. Weiss MR. Children in sport: an educational model. In: Murphy SM, ed. *Sport Psychology Interventions.* Champaign, IL: Human Kinetics; 1995:39-70.

34. DuRant RH, Pendergrast RA, Donner J, et al. Adolescents' attrition from school sponsored sports. *Am J Dis Child.* 1991;145:1119.

35. Petlichkoff LM. The drop-out dilemma in youth sports. In: Oded Bar-Or, ed. *The Child and Adolescent Athlete.* London, England: Blackwell Science; 1996: 418-432.

36. Ahren DK, Lohr BA. Psychosocial factors in sports injury rehabilitation. *Clin Sports Med.* 1997;16:755.

37. Heil J. *Psychology of sport injury.* Champaign, IL: Human Kinetics; 1993.

38. Smith AD. Rehabilitation of children following sport and activity-related injuries. In: Oded Bar-Or, ed. *The Child and Adolescent Athlete.* Cambridge, MA: Blackwell Science; 1996:224-242.

39. Smith AM. Psychological impact of injuries in athletes. *Sports Med.* 1996;22(6):391.

40. Weinberg RS, Comar W. The effectiveness of psychological interventions in competitive sport. *Sports Med.* 1994;18(6):406.

41. Aaron DJ, Dearwater SR, Anderson R, et al. Physical activity and initiation of high-risk health behavior in adolescents. *Med Sci Sports exerc.* 1995;27:1639.

42. Baumert PW, Henderson JM, Thompson NJ. Health risk behaviors of adolescent participants in organized athletics. *J Adolesc Health.* 1998;22:460.

43. Ferron C, Narring F, Cauderay M, et al. Sport activity in adolescence: associations with health perceptions and experimental behaviours. *Health Educ Res.* 1999;14(2): 225.

44. Forman ES, Dekker AH, Javors JR, et al. High-risk behaviors in teenage male athletes. *Clin J Sports Med.* 1995;5:36.

45. Nattiv A, Puffer JC, Green GA. Lifestyles and health risks of collegiate athletes: a multi-center study. *Clin J Sports Med.* 1997;7:262.

46. Levin DS, Smith EA, Cladwell LL, Kimbrough J. Violence and high school sports participation. *Pediatr Exer Sci.* 1995;7(4):379-388.

47. Pipe AL. Sport, science, and society: ethics in sports medicine. *Med Sci Sport Exerc.* 1993;25:888.

48. Pratt HD, Greydanus DE. Adolescent violence: concepts for a new millennium. *Adolesc Med.* 2000;11(1):103.

49. Young K: Sport and collective violence. *Exerc Sport Sci Rev.* 1991;19:539.

50. Russell GW, Arms RL, Mustonen A. When cooler heads prevail: peacemakers in sports riot. *Scand J Psychol.* 1999;40:153.

51. Catlin DH, Murray TH. Performance enhancing drugs, fair competition, and Olympic sport. *JAMA.* 1996;276:231.

52. DuRant RH, Rickert VI, Ashworth CS, et al. Use of multiple drugs among adolescents who use anabolic steroids. *N Engl J Med.* 1993;328:922.

54. American Academy of Pediatrics Policy Statement. Adolescents and anabolic steroids: a subject review. *Pediatrics.* 1997;99(6):904-908.

55. Epps RP, Lynn WR, Manley MW. Tobacco, youth, and sports. *Adolesc Med.* 1998;9:483.

56. American Academy of Pediatrics Policy Statement. Promotion of healthy weight control practices in young athletes. *Pediatrics.* 1997;97:752.

57. Brownell KD, Rodin J, Wilmore JH. *Eating, Body Weight and Performance in Athletes: Disorders of Modern Society.* Philadelphia, PA: Lea and Febiger; 1992.

58. Garner DM, Rosen LW, Barry D. Eating disorders among athletes: research and recommendations. *Child Adolesc Psychiatr Clin N Am.* 1998;7:839.

59. Sundgot-Borgen J. Eating disorders among male and female elite athletes. *Br J Sports Med.* 1999;33:434.

60. Tofler IR, Stryer BK, Micheli LJ, et al. Physical and emotional problems of elite female gymnasts. *N Engl J Med.* 1996;335:281.

61. Comerci GD, Greydanus DE. Eating disorders: anorexia nervosa and bulimia. In: Hofmann AD, Greydanus DE, eds. *Adolescent Medicine..* Stamford, CT: Appleton & Lange; 1997:683-702.

62. American College of Sports Medicine Position Stand. the female athlete triad. *Med Sci Sport Exerc.* 2007;39(10): 1867-1882.

63. Lidstone JE, Amundson ML, Amundson LH. Depression and chronic fatigue in the high school student and athlete. *Prim Care.* 1991;18:283.

64. Older MJ, Mainous AG, Martin CA, et al. Depression, suicidal ideation, and substance use among adolescents. Are athletes at less risk? *Arch Fam med.* 1994;3:781.

65. Puffer JC, McShane JM. Depression and chronic fatigue in athlete. *Clin Sports Med.* 1992;11:327.

66. Hickey G, Fricker P. Attention deficit hyperactivity disorder, CNS stimulants and sport. *Sports Med.* 1999;27(1): 11.

67. Raglin JS. Anxiety and sport performance. *Exerc Sport Sci Rev.* 1992;20:243.

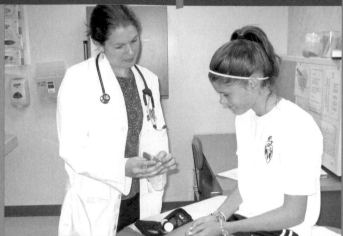

CHAPTER 4

Introduction to Pediatric Exercise Physiology

Robert J. Baker

INTRODUCTION

The field of pediatric exercise physiology is still an emerging science. Biological maturation and large variations in morphology of this group raise challenges in studying and describing physiologic responses in children and adolescents. Because of this variability, chronologic age is not a reliable means of comparison. Tanner staging has merit clinically, but not shown to be as reliable in exercise physiology. There is a lack of means to standardize measures for size and development. There are ethical aspects, which makes research in this population more challenging than its adult counterpart. Studies need to be appropriately designed with clear benefit outweighing risk in this vulnerable population. In fact, actual long-term risk of type of exercise may not be completely known.

The adolescent period appears to be unique because of the impact of the changing hormone milieu which is occurring. Prior to this period, the child's growth is largely driven by growth hormones. During pubertal growth, reproductive hormones come into play. This change affects not only growth and development, but physiologic responses as well (Figure 4-1).

GROWTH AND DEVELOPMENT

A clear understanding of factors that promote growth itself is lacking. However, physical development of organ systems such as the cardiac, ventilatory, and musculoskeletal are considered the driving force of physiologic improvement of performance and capacity in children. Acute and chronic exercise may stimulate growth factors by impacting binding proteins and

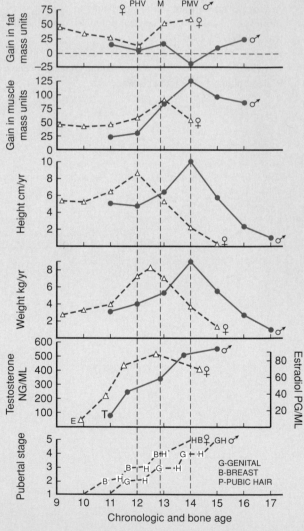

FIGURE 4-1 ■ Relationship between spurt in height, weight, muscle mass (fat free mass), fat (fat mass), testosterone levels, sexual maturity rating, and chronologic age.

receptor sites. Growth factor variations with exercise may be associated with nutritional variation resulting in biological markers of overuse.

Increased sex hormones present in puberty leads to a variety of changes in physiologic functioning that impact exercise performance. Exercise training has been associated with an inhibition of hypothalamic–pituitary–gonadal axis. This impact of regular exercise on reproductive functioning may be mediated by nutritional state, caloric balance, body composition, or some combination of these. Regular vigorous exercise has been shown to slow linear growth in gymnasts only. While the significance of this inhibition of hormones is not completely understood, low estrogen levels may have a long-term effect on bone development.

Metabolic pathways in response to activity are thought to vary with development of children. Anaerobic glycolysis progressively rises as children age, whereas aerobic metabolic capacity declines. These changes progress steadily throughout childhood without significant influence of puberty. The relationship of this phenomenon to body size mimics the pattern seen in adults.[1]

RESPONSES TO EXERCISE

Exercise responses in children are often compared to adults based on current understanding of adult exercise physiology. There are variations in responses between these two groups. Some of this variation is present despite normalization for size. A summary of physiologic responses for children is listed in Table 4-1.

In spite of challenges in testing physiologic factors, studies have monitored responses to acute exercise. Many protocols exist for testing aerobic and anaerobic fitness. No single method is considered best.

Exercise testing is limited by heterogeneity of techniques. Variations in physiologic responses to treadmill activity versus cycle ergometer have been described. Further, minute oxygen consumption (VO_2) is not directly related to treadmill grade and speed in children as is the case in adults.[2] Lack of biomechanical familiarity with the treadmill may lead to metabolic inefficiencies. Also, relative perceived exertion scales do not correlate with exercise intensity in children, as they do in adults. Children do appear to recover faster from physical activity compared to adults. This faster recovery for children may be related to lower power generation.

Cardiovascular Responses

Maximal oxygen uptake (VO_{2max}) is a function of several body systems. VO_{2max} increases concomitantly with growth in children until age 18 in boys and age 14 in girls (Figure 4-2). Until age 12, absolute VO_{2max} values increase at the same rate in both genders, although boys have higher values as early as age 5. These values were significantly in excess of those recorded for average adult population. Bar-Or found that values in boys remained stable for ages 6 to 17, values in girls were less than those in boys and remain stable until age 11 or 12, then decline each year thereafter.[1] Children between ages 6 and 17 showed a mean anaerobic threshold of 58% VO_{2max}. For college age males, the mean was 58.6% VO_{2max}. Adult males had a mean of 49% to 63% VO_{2max}, and adult women had a mean of 50% to 60%.

The pattern of relative magnitude of cardiovascular response to progressive and sustained dynamic exercise appears to be qualitatively similar between adults and children. With VO_{2max} and anaerobic threshold as indicators of cardiovascular potential in childhood,

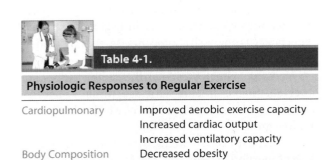

Table 4-1.

Physiologic Responses to Regular Exercise	
Cardiopulmonary	Improved aerobic exercise capacity
	Increased cardiac output
	Increased ventilatory capacity
Body Composition	Decreased obesity
	Decreased body fatness
	Increased lean body mass
Muscle strength and endurance	Improved musculoskeletal function
	Prevention of muscle atrophy and injury
	Increased strength
	Increased oxidative capacity
Flexibility	Improved musculoskeletal function
	Prevention of joint contractures

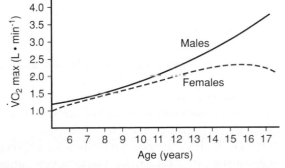

FIGURE 4-2 ■ Development of absolute VO_2 max with age in boys and girls.

these appear equal to that of adults. Stroke volume is increased in exercising children to match cardiac output to size and meet metabolic demands. At rest, heart rate accounts for matching metabolic demands. Heart rate response to maximal exercise is protocol dependent.

Resting heart rate declines during the course of childhood. Stroke volume increases in proportion to left ventricular size. While maximum heart rate remains constant during childhood, stoke volume during maximal exercise increases in proportion to body size and left ventricle size. Therefore, stoke volume serves as the determinant of increase in maximal cardiac output in the growing child.

Maximal cardiac output increases in proportion to VO_2 in absolute values. VO_{2max} remains stable during childhood. In females, maximal cardiac output may decline in relation to weight. Cardiac output in children is dependent on cardiac function. Circulatory adaptations to increased work are not affected by maturation. Myocardial oxygen uptake relative to heart mass at rest remains constant. Myocardial contractility is independent of age and maturation. Myocardial oxygen uptake during maximal exercise increases, as children grow, because of a rise in systolic blood pressure. Maximal oxygen consumption may be moderately heredity related, but left ventricle size is minimally influenced by genetics. No maturational changes occur in exercise myocardial function during childhood.

Maturational changes do not appear to affect myocardial performance or cardiac loading. Maximal stroke volume changes with age are a direct result of increased left ventricular chamber size. These changes are in direct relationship to body dimension. With aging, heart rate decreases because of intrinsic sinus node maturation. Resting cardiac output and VO_{2max} increase in absolute values but decline relative to body mass. Peripheral factors also play a role in meeting the demands of exercise. Arteriolar dilation in active muscle tissues will deliver increased blood flow to active muscle. The pumping action of the skeletal muscle will also augment the flow as well.

During submaximal activity, walking or running economy improves throughout childhood. Though the cause is unclear, this relationship holds for scaling for size. Improved coordination, substrate utilization, or elastic recoil forces may play a role. With increasing age in childhood, VO_{2max} at a given work intensity will decline. Endurance performance also improves with aging.

Cardiovascular responses to resistance exercise in children are similar to those in adults. Both systolic and diastolic blood pressures rise. Heart rate and cardiac output show limited changes. While the acute response to high-intensity physical activity is qualitatively similar to adults, there are quantitative differences. Children and adolescents have higher heart rates, a higher arterial-venous oxygen (a-vO_2) difference, lower diastolic and systolic blood pressures, lower stroke volume, and lower cardiac output for any given level of VO_{2max}.

Ventilatory Responses

Much as there are similar qualitative responses of the cardiovascular system to exercise between children and adults, there are likewise similar patterns of responses in the ventilatory system. In response to the acute exercise bout, ventilation increases in children as in adults, however prepubertal children demonstrate certain anatomic and functional characteristics.

Childhood ventilatory responses to exercise include lower relative tidal volumes, higher breathing rates, higher ventilation rates (V_e), and higher ventilatory equivalents (V_e/VO_2) compared to adults. Thus, children have relative inefficiency in breathing compared to adults. However, children demonstrate more than adequate VO_{2max} and anaerobic threshold levels relative to body size, and qualitatively similar hemodynamic and ventilatory responses to acute exercise.

Children hyperventilate during exercise resulting in an increased ratio of minute ventilation to oxygen consumption at all intensities. Arterial concentration of carbon dioxide (PCO_2) is lower. This results in greater pH at maximal exercise in children. Thus, ventilatory compensation appears exaggerated in the face of less lactate production. There is no understanding of these variations in children. This hyperventilatory response is less obvious as children grow, possibly owing to hormonal influence of puberty. Children breathe more rapidly and with greater frequency in relation to a given tidal volume. Less lung compliance and greater airway resistance in children may explain this response. In spite of this, normal arterial oxygenation is maintained at maximal exercise.

Resting metabolic rate increases with age. Resting tidal volumes (V_t) increase as the lung grows. Breathing frequency (f_b) progressively declines. Minute ventilation expressed relative to body weight decreases with age. At a given submaximal workload the same changes are observed: that is f_b falls with age while V_t and V_e increase. Submaximal V_e per body weight declines as children grow.

Maximal exercise ventilation rises with age in close proportion to body size. Maximal ventilation relative to body size remains stable throughout childhood. While frequency of breathing decreases progressively, maximal ventilation relative to body size decreases with aging. Males typically demonstrate greater volumes compared to females. Children typically have a greater ventilation rate relative to intensity of exercise. Training will improve ventilation rate, as VO_{2max} improves, as a result of improved tidal volume. Resting tidal volumes increase with aging while breathing rate decreases. Overall, resting ventilation related to body size decrease with age. Children breathe more rapidly than adults in response to submaximal work.

Peripheral Blood Flow Responses to Exercise

Total oxygen uptake relative to body size decreases with aging. Activity of aerobic enzymes is greater in children than in adults. Slow twitch oxidative muscle fibers are larger in children than in adults. The a-vO$_2$ difference at rest and with maximal exercise appears to be independent of age. Peripheral blood flow is improved by an increase in hemoglobin. Blood hemoglobin concentration rises slowly during childhood, without gender differences. At puberty, significant increases are observed in males secondary to bone marrow stimulation by testosterone. Training does not influence hemoglobin concentration in children. A blood volume relative to body mass does not change during childhood. Other factors, such as increased capillarization and increased density of capillaries in muscle also improve peripheral blood flow to active tissue. Children may demonstrate a smaller decline in plasma volume during acute exercise compared to adults.

Metabolic Responses

Children are metabolically inefficient at similar workloads compared to adults. This metabolic inefficiency does not necessarily occur during all types of activity. Research is conflicting as to the extent that children metabolize fatty acids compared to adults. In children, electrolyte movement from muscle to blood stream does not appear to be significantly different from adults. However, because of improved muscle blood flow, acid base balance and lactic acid mobilization may be improved. Muscle breakdown products such as creatine kinase do not rise to the same extent as in adults. This may reflect a lesser force per muscle fiber in children, or simply shorter circulation time.

Children rely more on oxidative rather than anaerobic metabolism compared to adults. Children demonstrate not only lower intramuscular glycogen and CrP stores, compared with adults, but also utilize them to a lesser extent during exercise. Children have a lower phosphofructokinase and lactate dehydrogenase activities and demonstrate a faster CrP resynthesis. Therefore, children demonstrate a lesser glycolytic capacity.[3]

Muscular Responses to Exercise

Children anatomically show smaller muscle fibers with greater density of blood capillaries, which results in shorter distance of blood diffusion with muscle tissue. Young children possess muscle fiber numbers, types, and distribution similar to that of adults. Increased strength during maturation is almost entirely owing to increase in muscle tissue growth. Males tend to be stronger than females at any age, especially in muscle groups of the upper body. This difference in muscle strength by gender and age can be eliminated if strength is expressed per unit cross-sectional muscle area. Males show greater muscle endurance compared to females. Compared to adults, children demonstrate lower anaerobic power production.[4] Boys are capable of producing more anaerobic power compared to girls.

Children demonstrate greater energy expenditure during weight bearing activities such as running and walking compared to adults. This exercise inefficiency does improve throughout childhood. Factors such as deceased stride length, greater stride frequency, and faster rate relative to body size compared to adults contribute to greater relative exercise intensity.

Neurologic Responses to Exercise

Children have a limited use of higher-hierarchy motor units. This leads to a higher relative reliance on lower-hierarchy motor units. Electromyography (EMG) data suggest a faster recovery of neuromotor function. The neuromotor system determines magnitude of power production and affects the extent of fatigue.

RESPONSES TO TRAINING

Speed, endurance, and strength normally improve as a result of natural growth and development. There is evidence that in certain areas, specifically in aerobic training, prepubertal children may differ from adults in their adaptation to training. Training effects are seen in several body organs. Although young swimmers have shown enlarged left ventricular dimensions, the cardiovascular response to endurance training in children does not increase myocardium size as is seen in adults with "athlete's heart." However, children will improve maximal cardiac output with endurance training. Myocardial hypertrophy is seen in children. There is an increase in glycogen stores and oxidative enzyme activity as well as increased left ventricular mass.

Young athletes do not demonstrate significant changes in pulmonary functioning with endurance training. As with VO$_{2max}$, maximal ventilation does not typically change significantly with training. There is an increase in efficiency and endurance of accessory ventilator muscles. Intensive training for young girls has been associated with later onset of menarche. Numerous factors including low body fat, energy deficit, psychological stress, and nutritional deficiencies may play a role. The immune system may be compromised by heavy training. Studies have suggested a greater incidence of viral infections in adult athletes compared to nonathletes. Training in children has been associated with leukocytosis, elevation of B and T cell, as well as a higher count of natural killer cells. While heavy intensity training may compromise the immune system, moderate intensity training may lead to either no change or improve immune functioning. This is similar to the adult response.

Many biochemical changes occur in response to training. Oxidative function improves with an increase in number and volume of mitochondria, and increased glycogen storage. Peripheral blood flow improves with an increase in blood volume, circulating hemoglobin, and increased cellular myoglobin content.

Musculoskeletal function and morphological changes are minimal in response to training. Increased oxidative fibers normally seen in adults are not seen in children. Muscle hypertrophy is significantly less in females and immature males compared to adolescent males. Flexibility in children is affected to a greater extent by growth than training. However, static stretching can be demonstrated to increase static flexibility in children and adults.

In general, both aerobic and anaerobic training has only a modest effect on children. Young children can benefit significantly from strength training though by different mechanism from adults and adolescents. Significant alterations in heart and lung function that are described in adults have not been seen in children. Weight bearing exercises may have benefit on bone mineralization, however, females with amenorrhea could be at risk for osteoporosis. There are benefits of physical fitness described in Table 4-1.

Aerobic Fitness

With training, children can increase VO_{2max}. This increase however may be one-third of what is seen in adults. With similar program design, the rise in VO_{2max} for children was 5% to 10% compared to 15% to 30% in adults.[5] Some children demonstrated no increase in VO_{2max}. Possibly a ceiling exists for children before puberty. High daily level of physical activity seen in children compared to adults may have a training effect. This may explain this ceiling phenomenon. Maximal oxygen consumption may to be proportionally lower because of the relatively high starting values. Further, structured programs may not significantly increase activity levels.

Usual daily activity is not likely to impact fitness. Spontaneous activity typical for children tends to be short-burst, without significant endurance. If children are deprived of daily activity, there is not a measurable decrease in VO_{2max}. There does not appear to be a strong relationship between VO_{2max} and habitual physical activity. Habitual physical activity is not a useful predictor of VO_{2max}, as daily variation in physical activity may not substantially alter maximal oxygen utilization. Therefore, possibly biological differences are responsible for the blunted response.[6]

Maximal stroke volume is increased by increased plasma volume and improved oxygen extraction in muscles. This effect is even greater after puberty. However, improvement in actual performance in endurance events is limited compared to this improvement in oxygen consumption.

Maximal oxygen consumption that occurs with aging is determined by increasing active muscle tissue. These changes are accompanied by an increase in functional capacity of aerobic enzyme system with age. During this period cardiac size also increases in concert to match oxygen delivery and cellular consumption. With age maximal stroke volume, maximal cardiac output increase with increasing ventricular size. Plasma volume, vagal tone, and hormonal changes affect left ventricular size of the heart. A lower heart rate at rest and submaximal workloads results as stroke volumes increase.

Increases in endurance performance with age are independent of VO_{2max}, rather submaximal exercise economy. It is the balance of aerobic and anaerobic enzyme function that defines performance during growth. Controlling for body size, there is little difference in maximum aerobic power between boys and girls.

Maturation is associated with an increase in resting metabolic rate. Relative to body size and surface area, the metabolic expenditure decreases. VO_{2max} increases with age associated with increase in size of the active muscle tissue. Before puberty, differences based on gender are minimal, although male values tend to be consistently higher. Endurance performance does improve dramatically through childhood.

Anaerobic Fitness

Children commonly engage in play activity that is of short-burst. These activities would appear anaerobic in nature. Anaerobic performance is generally difficult to measure. There is no established standard regimen of activity intensity and duration for anaerobic training and there is no simple laboratory marker for anaerobic fitness. Therefore, most data is focused in evaluating aerobic fitness and capacity. Aerobic capacity is better defined and easier to measure. Further, aerobic fitness is more directly related to health outcomes. Although the evaluation of anaerobic performance is limited, factors relating to maturation, growth, and anaerobic performance will be considered.

Children have long been shown to possess anaerobic power capacity that is lower compared with adults. For children, peak torque and peak power output reach only approximately 60% to 80% that of adults. Children recover faster from high-intensity exercise. There was a faster recovery of ventilatory rate, heart rate, and $\dot{V}O_2$ in prepubertal boys compare to men. The relative faster recovery time may be multifactorial. Children have lower maximal speed, maximal force, maximal power, which may allow for rapid recovery in children. . Qualitatively, there is also shorter delay between the onset of exercise and the peaking of metabolites in the blood. This would allow the recovery process to commence earlier.

Performance on the cycle ergometer, Wingate test is most often used to evaluate anaerobic performance. Studies indicate children's performance on this test can be improved with anaerobic training, but such training fails to improve sprint time. Peak and mean anaerobic power rise with chronologic age, both absolute and in proportion to size. Further, both maximal and submaximal exercise lactate levels increase with age.

Ventilation in relation to oxygen consumption falls as children grow. Anaerobic threshold is greater in trained versus untrained children. Thus, while ventilatory efficiency is present, there may be some training effect.

The amount of habitual short-burst activity declines as children grow. Glycolytic activity and production of lactic acid increase during this period. In fact, because of a limit in activity of phosphofructokinase, which plays an important role in the anaerobic glycolitic process, children appear to be inefficient in anaerobic metabolism. Children's ability to engage in short-burst activity may not be related to anaerobic metabolic capacity as much as other factors such as biomechanical, neuromuscular, or morphological factors. Development of anaerobic fitness improves with increasing age, but improvements are greater than can be accounted for by changes in body size alone. There is an observed rise in lactate and catecholamines during progressive exercise testing with age.[7] Although testosterone does not appear to play a role, there is evidence for age-related difference in epinephrine and norepinephrine.

Strength Training

Relative strength gains in children and adults are the same. Prepubertal strength improves by mechanisms other than size. Neurologic adaptations are considered the main explanation. Studies show that strength training can result in substantial and significant increases in strength even in preadolescents. Strength gains occur even if the confounding effects of growth and motor skill are controlled. This increase in strength during the preadolescent period is similar to the adult response.

Strength gains are dependent on sufficient training intensity and volume as well as the duration of such training. While the optimal combination of these factors is not known, improvements were seen for isometric, isotonic, and isokinetic training. The magnitude of increased strength observed was equivalent to that seen in adults. These strength improvements are similar in boys and girls. Clearly, increased strength in prepubertal children is not accompanied by an increase in muscle size. Therefore, factors such as neural adaptations or enhanced intrinsic force-producing capacity of muscle play some role.

Studies across childhood, including adolescents, have consistently reported comparable and some times greater relative strength trainability in preadolescents, compared to adolescents and adults. Preadolescents are probably less trainable in terms of absolute strength gains, but equally, if not more trainable in terms of relative strength compared to young adults.

Any loss in strength because of a reduction in training may be possibly at least partially offset by a concomitant growth-related increase in strength. Whether the strength gains will revert fully to growth-adjusted control levels will depend upon the magnitude of the initial strength gains and the duration of the detraining period. Training-induced strength gains during preadolescents are probably impermanent. A single weekly training session did not maintain strength gains compared to the growth-adjusted control level. Therefore, training-induced strength gains are probably impermanent, and that one high-intensity training session per week is probably insufficient for maintenance training at least during preadolescents.

Muscle power and muscle endurance may also be trainable in children, though there is less information. Power is difficult to measure. Programs with repetition of short-burst 5 to 30 seconds (i.e., cycling, or running near maximum) have been evaluated. There appears to be higher muscle power among trained individuals. Greater intensity is associated with greater training effect. Fitness level prior to training program is important in determining training response. The mechanism for trainability of muscle power and endurance may include neurologic changes, increase in diameter type I and type II fibers, increase in proportion of type I fibers, increase in glycogen content, increase in glycolytic and oxidative enzymes, and increased glycolytic flux.[3]

An appropriate strength training program should include: proper technique, strict supervision, and proper design for children. Weight-bearing activity may protect future osteoporosis. A health care practitioner should conduct an initial examination. The program design should be "conservative" relative to adult criteria. Finally, the program should include warm-up and cool down.

Strength training is associated with morphological adaptation. Muscle hypertrophy has not been reported in preadolescents, in spite of significant strength gains; this appears to be the same for boys and girls. Preadolescent strength gains are associated with anabolic hormones and growth factor. Size-independent strength gains in prepubertal children result from changes in neural mechanisms, motor unit firing, recruitment, or conduction velocity.

In adolescent boys, strength training increases muscle size, and this has been found from indirect and direct anthropometric measures of increased arm and thigh girth. Thus, hypertrophy appears to be more consistent outcome of strength or resistance training during adolescence. At puberty increases in muscle size and strength accelerate in males because of testosterone.

Increased strength during maturation is almost entirely owing to an increase in muscle tissue growth. Males tend to be stronger than females at any age in muscle groups of upper body. Differences in muscle strength by gender and age can be eliminated if strength expressed per unit cross-sectional muscle area. Muscle endurance is greater in males.

Childhood muscle tissue is similar to that of adults with respect to number, types, and distribution. Strength continues to increase with growth to early adulthood. Males tend to be stronger than females at any age, particularly in the upper body.

Flexibility varies in childhood. Children become less flexible as they age until it bottoms out between 10 and 12 years. In the early adolescent growth spurt there may be a short-term "tightness" in the joints, as a result of increased tension in connective tissue. Girls have been shown to be more flexible than boys. Static flexibility tends to decrease progressively after early adulthood. Dynamic flexibility decreases with age from childhood.

Neurologic

Muscular strength improves throughout childhood, a reflection of neural adaptations and increase in muscle size. Children are more limited in their ability to recruit and use higher-hierarchy motor units. This, most likely, is owing to neuromuscular immaturity in either neuromotor control or incomplete motor-unit differentiation. Children have increased resting vagal parasympathetic drive than adults. The central nervous system (CNS) plays a role in physical performance. Maturation of central neurologic factors play a role in improvements in motor performance. Perceptions of central fatigue by the brain may limit physiologic capacity. Possible intrinsic CNS influence on energy hemostasis may contribute to obesity in some children. Relative perceived exertion levels are variable in children.

Training-induced strength increases in preadolescent boys and girls have been attributed to undefined neurologic and neuromotor adaptations.[1] Resistance training-induced preadolescent and adolescent appear to be achieved in part by increase voluntary neuromuscular activation. Magnitude of changes in neuromuscular activation is generally smaller than observed increases in strength gain during preadolescence. In fact, the changes are more proportional to strength gains in males during adolescence.

Intrinsic adaptations during training indicate an improvement in twitch-specific tension.

Metabolic

There is a qualitative difference in intramuscular and circulatory transit times between children and adults. Children demonstrate a faster initial diffusion and initiation of metabolites breakdown. Lactic acid clearance rate is faster. Energy substrate replenishment and electrolyte and acid-base rebalance are faster in children. Though children may be less efficient metabolically, recovery is more rapid.

SUMMARY

Relative training responses include an absolute strength, which is greater in adolescents compared to preadolescents and equal relative strength gains in preadolescent and adolescent children. Muscle hypertrophy shows small gains in muscle size in preadolescent compared to adolescent children. Neuromuscular activation has greater potential for increased activation in preadolescent children. Motor skills of children show a greater potential for improvement because of lower lifetime exposure to these skills.

Potential benefits of strength training are improved sports performance and enhance body composition. Strength training may also reduce sports injuries, improve rehabilitation from injury, but this is still unproven.

For safety concerns competitive weight lifting, Olympic weight lifting, powerlifting, and bodybuilding are not recommended in children and adolescents. The American Orthopedic Society for Sports Medicine recommends a frequency of two to three 20- to 30-minute sessions per week. In the beginning, no resistance should be used until proper form is achieved (Table 4-2).[4] One set of 6 to 15 repetition should be the next step. The goal is three sets per session. Maximum lifts are not recommended.

DETRAINING

In adults neural drive decays at approximately the same rate as training. Since there is little, if any, effect

Table 4-2.

General Guidelines for Resistance Training

1. Screen for medical contraindications
2. Provide instruction and proper technique
3. Warm-up
4. Start light relative to body weight
5. Individualize
6. Train all major muscles both flexors extensors for balance
7. Full range of motion to maintain flexibility
8. Do not train more than 3 d/wk
9. Progress gradually
10. Cooldown
11. Select stable, sturdy, safe equipment
12. Stop with sharp pain or persistent pain

on muscle size in preadolescents, detraining may occur more quickly in preadolescents. Thus, loss of strength gains during detraining is owing to a reduction in neuromuscular activation and loss of motor coordination.

REFERENCES

1. Rowland TW. *Children's Exercise Physiology.* 2nd ed. Champaign, IL: Human Kinetics; 2005.
2. Stephens P, Paridon SM. Exercise testing in pediatrics. *Pediatr Clin North Am.* 2004;51(6):1569-1587.
3. Falk B, Dotal R. Child-adult differences in the recovery from high-intensity exercise. *Exerc Sport Sci Rev.* 2006;34(3): 107-112.
4. Blimkie CJR, Bar-Or O. Trainability of muscle strength, power and endurance during childhood. In: Bar-Or O, ed. *The Child and Adolescent Athlete.* Champaign, IL: Human Kinetics; 1996:113-122.
5. Paridon SM, Alpert BS, Boas SR, et al. American Heart Association Scientific Statement: clinical stress testing in the pediatric age group. *Circulation.* 2006;113:1905-1920.
6. Nelson MA, SS Harris. The benefits and risks of sports and exercise for children with chronic health conditions. In: Goldberg B, ed. *Sports and Exercise for Children with Chronic Health Conditions.* Champaign, IL: Human kinetics; 1995:13-30.
7. American College of Sports Medicine. *Guidelines for Exercise Testing and Prescription.* 6th ed. Baltimore, MD: Lippincott Williams Wilkins; 2000.

CHAPTER 5

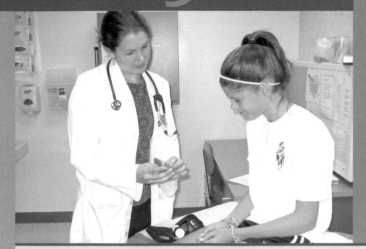

Strength Training and Conditioning

Michael G. Miller and
Timothy J. Michael

The idea of weight training for children (preadolescent and adolescent) has always raised questions. The concern most often raised is whether or not weight training puts children at an increased risk for injury. A secondary question that is raised is whether children would benefit from weight training, if they are not physiologically mature (e.g., low androgen levels). This chapter will review these issues and offer guidance to the proper (safe) training techniques and programs, followed by a review of the expected training responses and outcomes as characterized in the research literature.

Often the risk of the epiphyseal growth plate injuries is mentioned; however, to date there have only been a few published papers that document such injuries and often these injuries are owing to lack of adequate education (training) and supervision of the children. Often injuries are owing to improper lifting techniques or the participant's workloads are progressed to quickly. However, injuries may increase for the child athlete, who has inadequate strength for his or her chosen sport and in these cases weight training offers protection from potential injuries.

Children have been shown to increase their strength from participating in weight training programs. Two separate meta-analytic reviews[1,2] showed that children increased their strength with resistance training by 13% to 30%. These analyses also determined that there was a greater effect size seen in isotonic training, followed by isometric exercise and finally by isokinetic training. However, the reviews could not determine the optimal training program because the studies were limited by gender (mostly males), age range, differences in intensity, duration, and frequency. It is well documented that the strength (force) of a muscle is directly related to its cross-sectional area. Increase in muscle size is related to the androgen hormone. Because prepubertal children lack adequate androgen hormone, the strength gains at this age are largely believed to be because of neuronal adaptations. Various aspects of muscle strength testing, strength training, growth and maturation, metabolism, and muscle fiber types have been the subject of extensive body of published literature.[1-20]

DEFINITIONS

Concentric Muscle Action

When muscles respond in the manner for which they are activated, a specific motion either lengthening or shortening or no movement occurs. A concentric muscle action refers to a shortening of the muscle fibers accompanied by movement of the respective joint. The muscle is shortening because the actions of the muscle fibers are greater than the external resistance and the muscle shortens (Figure 5-1). Since the internal muscular forces are greater than the external resistance, it has also been described as performing "positive" work.

Eccentric Muscle Action

An eccentric muscle action results in a lengthening of the muscle accompanied by joint motion because the resistive forces are greater than the concentric forces of the muscle fibers. An example of an eccentric muscular action is the lowering of weight during a bicep curl (Figure 5-2). The weight is lowered in a slow and controlled manner resulting in the term "negative" work.

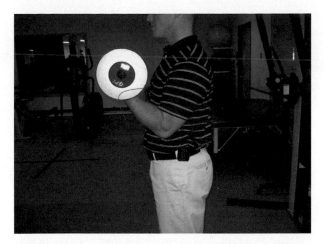

FIGURE 5-1 ■ Lifting a weight during biceps curl is an example of concentric muscle action in which the muscle shortens while performing positive work.

Isometric Muscle Action

An isometric muscle action has no change in length of the muscle, and is not accompanied by joint motion, because the external forces equal the contractile forces of the muscle. Because the total length of the muscle/tendon unit does not change, the work is said to be "zero."

Isotonic Exercise

Both concentric and eccentric muscle actions comprise the type of exercise called isotonic. Isotonic means same tension or same mass. In weight training, isotonic exercises include moving a person's body weight during an exercise or lifting free weights. While the mass of a weight being lifted during an exercise does not change, the external force will vary depending upon the joint

angle and joint angular velocity. The muscle tension during isotonic exercise will vary based upon the weight, joint velocity, muscle length, and type of muscle contraction (eccentric or concentric).

Isometric Exercise

Isometric exercise places tension or resistance on the muscle or muscle group without the joint movement. Isometric exercises are well suited for individuals beginning an exercise regimen or for individuals who have sustained an injury and have limited range of motion or strength[21]; however, the strength gained is usually limited by the specific joint angle when performing the exercise.

Isokinetic Exercise

Isokinetic exercises are those in which the movements occur at a constant angular velocity resulting in the same speed of movement. The speed at the joint angle is controlled via a machine called an isokinetic device with a constant resistance (Figure 5-3). Isokinetic

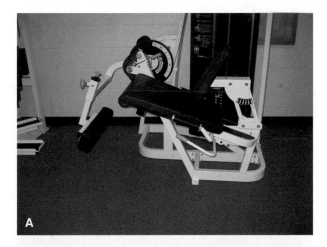

A

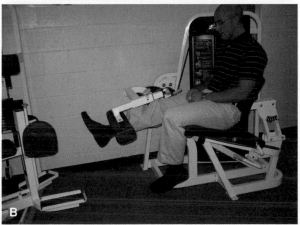

B

FIGURE 5-3 ■ During isokinetic exercise, the speed at the joint angle is controlled via the isokinetic machine or device.

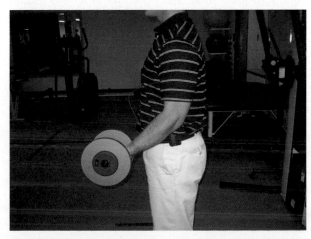

FIGURE 5-2 ■ Lowering the weight during a biceps curl is an example of eccentric muscle action in which the muscle lengthens while performing negative work.

devices are frequently used in rehabilitation and testing of muscular strength and power because of the reliability and safety of the devices. A drawback of using isokinetic devices is that the speed controlled by the devices seldom mimics the speed produced in natural movements.

Strength

Although, strength usually refers to the weight a person can lift, it is more appropriately defined as the maximal force that a muscle or a muscle group generates at a specific velocity.

Power

Power is defined as the time rate of performing work (Power = work/time) and work is defined as the product of force on an object and the distance the object moves (Work = force × distance over which the force is applied). These formulas are used in designing, implementing, and testing a strength-training program.

Plyometrics

Another type of exercise that combines power and strength is plyometrics. Plyometrics involves an eccentric loading of a muscle or a muscle group followed immediately by a concentric muscle action. The eccentric/concentric actions utilize the stretch reflex or stretch-shortening cycle in which the muscle is pre-loaded with energy during the eccentric phase (much like stretching a rubber bad apart) and the release of that stored energy for subsequent muscular actions (letting go of the rubber band). The stored elastic energy within the muscle is used to produce more force than can be provided by a concentric action alone.[22–24] Researchers have shown that plyometric training can contribute to improvements in vertical jump performance, acceleration, leg strength, and muscular power.[25–32] Most plyometric exercises include activities such as hops, depth jumps, bounds, skipping, jumps for the lower extremities, medicine ball drills, throwing, and other activities for the upper extremity.

Plyometric training program must follow recommended intensities and volumes and progress over time to avoid injury.[33] Training volume are usually categorized according to the number of foot contacts per training session, starting from a low number of foot contacts and progressing upward over several weeks. In addition, it is recommended that plyometric activities be incorporated no more than two to three times per week to prevent undue muscular injury or soreness.

PROGRAM DESIGN

Maturity

When beginning a strength-training program, the first factor to consider is the physical maturity of the individual. The physical maturity may prevent a child who is too small from properly being fitted to a machine when strength training or not coordinated in completing an exercise with the proper form. Alternate exercises are recommended for the safety of the children to prevent injuries. In addition to physical maturity, mental maturity should also be considered when developing an exercise program. Mental maturity may limit participation when the children cannot adequately follow directions or conduct themselves in an appropriate manner in the weight room to avoid risk of injury. Injuries occur less frequently during resistive training compared to actual athletic participation in children and maturity may be a predominate factor.[34]

Supervision

When conducting a strength-training program, adequate supervision and teaching the proper use of weight training equipment is imperative to decrease the likelihood of accidental injuries in the weight room facility.[35] Improper form, even at low intensity or resistance levels can lead to the risk of injuries when the intensity and resistance increases. Supervision should include not only verbal feedback about the proper form, movement, and breathing but also visual feedback where the athlete can see his or her movements using mirrors to be aware of poor biomechanics.[36] Research has shown that a properly supervised strength-training program can improve strength gains and exercise adherence versus unsupervised strength-training programs.[37,38] Children who participate in strength-training programs should also be taught the correct form and sound lifting techniques regardless of an equipment or body weight. Proper form and techniques will help the adolescents develop appropriate muscle strength and muscle balances and limits the potential for injury. This can be better accomplished with a lower athlete to supervisor ratio, especially in the early developmental phases of the strength-training program. It has been recommended that ratios of 1:10 up to 1:25 are adequate, depending upon the maturity and complexity of exercises performed.

Needs Analysis

Before initiating the strength-training program, it is imperative that the strength-training professional conducts a needs analysis to evaluate the physical requirements of a sport or athletic endeavor and evaluate the physical attributes of the children. Evaluation of the sport or athletic endeavor includes determining movement patterns, the physiologic requirements needed to participate in the sport (power, strength, or hypertrophy of the muscle), and an assessment of common injuries sites or potential for injuries.[39,40] Assessment of the children includes previous training background, training experience, age, maturity, and experience.

Determining the selection of exercise is dependent upon the goals and objectifies and the needs analysis. Most exercises can be classified as they relate to the body. *Core exercises* mean using large muscle groups that involve two or more joint movements (multijoint exercises). These include the muscles of the back, shoulders, chest, thigh, and hip. Smaller muscle groups that usually involve one joint (single-joint exercises) such as the biceps, forearm, calf, neck are called *assistance exercises*.

Training Frequency

Training frequency refers to the number of times strength-training sessions are completed in a given period. The training frequency is dependent upon many factors such as experience, training status, and other physical and sport requirements. Individuals who are inexperienced should begin a training program with relatively fewer sessions per week then increase as the training level of the individual progresses. In most cases, training sessions of one to two times per week is sufficient to begin stressing the body's systems to adapt to the strength-training programs. As with training sessions, it is recommended that at least 1 day but not more than 3 days of rest should be taken before the next session begins, but it is also dependent upon the child. As the children become more advanced, training sessions can increase up to three times per week.

More training sessions can be accomplished and provide adequate rest, if a *split routine* is used. A split routine divides the training session into groupings, split between the upper body and lower body exercises. For example, a 4d/wk training session can occur by exercising the lower body on Tuesdays and Fridays and the upper body on Mondays and Thursdays. This type of program allows enough rest and recovery for the muscle group before the next session.[41] Another alternative is to perform a "push" and "pull" exercise, where the strength-training program is divided into exercises in which the individual pushes weight (bench press, triceps extension) then pulls the weight (latissimus dorsi pull down or bicep curl). If the training loads are near the maximum capacity, more time for recovery will be required to minimize soreness and provide adequate rest. Some evidence exists that in previously trained individuals, recovery is quicker for training upper body muscles than lower body muscles when training with heavy loads.[42]

Training Load

In a strength-training program, the term *load* refers to the amount of weight used in that specific exercise. As the load becomes heavier, the number of times an individual can lift (repetitions or reps) the load decreases, whereas the load becomes lighters, more reps can be accomplished. Load is often described as a percentage of what a person can lift. Most strength and conditioning specialists describe the load as a percentage of a repetition maximum (RM). The RM can be expressed as the greatest amount of load lifted 1 time (1 RM) or as the amount of load lifted for a specified number of reps, usually expressed as a 5 RM or up to 10 RM when lifting with proper form.

Training load is useful to establish the baseline or estimated amount of load to lift per session. Usually, the training load is based upon the percentage of the 1 RM. It has been suggested that 1 RM be used for testing strength with core exercises and use multiple RM testing for the assistance exercises.[43] Determining the RM is dependent upon the goals of the individual and the demands of the sport. Heavy loads are useful for strength or power, moderate loads for hypertrophy, and light loads for muscular endurance. If an individual has strength-training experience, a 1 RM testing method can be used (Table 5-1).

If the individual has limited or no experience or he or she is an adolescent, estimating a 1 RM by using a multiple RM testing method is better suited. A 10 RM testing load is often recommended to estimate the 1 RM. The testing procedures are similar to the 1 RM procedures except for the number of reps lifted. Follow the steps for the 1 RM but use 10 reps for each set. Increase the weight for each set by half of the recommended loads for the 1 RM. As with the 1 RM testing protocol, determine the 10 RM within 5 total sets. After the 10 RM is found the individual estimated 1 RM can be calculated based on standard RM table while working with trainer or strength and conditioning specialist.

Although the RM testing has some flaws, it is still one of the best methods to determine loads used for resistance training exercises.[44,45] Another method that is not commonly used but can be a good indicator of strength and power is a 1 RM equivalent. The 1 RM equivalent is a formula that takes into account the weight lifted and reps multiplied by an numeric equivalent.[46]

$$1 \text{ RM equivalent} = (\text{Weight lifted} \times \text{Number of reps} \times .03) + \text{weight lifted}$$

Table 5-1.

One RM Testing Method

1	Warm up	Before initiation of RM testing, have the individual perform general warm-up for 5–10 minutes with 1 set of 10 reps using weight that can be easily lifted. Performing too may warm-up sets can fatigue muscles and decrease the accuracy of the testing
2	Rest	1 min
3	Lift	Use a load that can be lifted between three and five times by adding weight to the warm-up set. Add 10–20 lbs to, or 5%–10% of, the weight lifted in the warm-up
4	Rest	2 min
5	Lift	Use a load estimated to be near maximum load that can be lifted for 2–3 reps. Find load by adding increasing the weight lifted in step 3. Add 10–20 lb to, or 5%–10% of, the weight lifted, for upper body exercises; 30–40 lbs or 10%–20% for the lower body exercises
6	Rest	2–4 min
7	Lift	Increase the load (weight lifted) by following weight recommendations in step 5 and have the individual attempt 1 RM
8	Rest	2–4 min
9	Lift	If step 7 attempt was successful repeat the step. If step 7 failed, decrease the weight to be lifted as follows: subtract 5–10 lbs from, or 2.5%–5% of weight attempted in step 7 for upper body; 15–20 lb or 5%–10% for lower body. With the new weight attempt 1 RM
10	Repeat	Repeat the steps as necessary to find the 1 RM. 1 RM should be determined within five lifting attempts or sets

(Adapted from Baechle and Earle, 2000 (43))

For example, suppose you have a soccer player who lifted 100 pounds for incline bench press a total of 14 times, his or her 1 RM equivalent will be equal to $(100 \times 14 \times .03) + 100 = 142$. Although not as accurate as the 1 RM procedure, it can be used for inexperienced athletes and for any athlete where safety is a concern.

The RM that will be used for determining resistance during a strength-training program, however, will need to be adjusted as the children learn the technique and become more experienced and as the muscles adapt to the stimulus. Many individuals just add weight randomly without determining the best resistance for overloading the muscles to increase gains. One method used that is relatively conservative and perhaps beneficial for children who are strength training is the "2 for 2 rule."[47] This particular method increases the load for the individual when the load becomes too easy. The rule states that the load should increase, if the individual can perform 2 or more reps over the assigned reps for that particular exercise over two consecutive workouts (Table 5-2).

A set is defined as the number of reps performed before a rest period. For example, if an athlete is to perform three sets of 10 reps, he or she would be lifting the weight 10 times in one set followed by a rest period and repeat the process another two more times for a total of 3 sets. When describing the volume, the sets and reps are written in a format that is easy to decipher. In the above example, the training program would be written as 3×10, where 3 represents the sets and 10 represents the reps lifted per set. Begin the training load by performing one set of six to eight exercises with 10 to 15 reps per exercise of all major muscle groups, then progress anywhere from one to three sets with 6 to 15 reps.[35]

Training Volume

The training volume describes the total amount of load lifted during a strength-training session. The volume is

Table 5-2.

2 for 2 Rule Protocol

Exercise	Lat pull down
Goal reps	10
Goal sets	3
Load	Increase if, on the last set, the individual can perform 12 reps for two sessions
If past training experinece increase load by	5–10 lb for upper body exercises 10–15 lb for lower body exercises
If limited or no past training increase load by	2.4–5 lb for upper body exercises 5–10 lb for lower body exercises

(Adapted from Baechle and Earle, 2000 (43))Tab

dependent upon the weight lifted, the reps, and sets. The total volume during a strength-training session is dependent upon the goals of the session, training focus, and time of year as reviewed in the section of periodization. Volume is calculated by multiplying the sets times the reps times the weight lifted per rep. For example, suppose an individual is slated to perform 3 × 10 reps with 20 pounds for the biceps curl, the formula would be written as 3 × 10 × 20, with the first number representing the sets, the second number representing the reps, and the third number represents the weight lifted per rep. By multiplying the numbers together, the training volume for that particular exercise would be 600 lbs. If each set has a different weight associated with it, the volume is calculated per each set and then all sets are added together. For example, the scenario above may be assigned as 1 × 10 × 15, 1 × 10, × 20, 1 × 10 × 25, the volume for each set is calculated then all sets added together to find a 600 lb training volume.

Warm-Up and Cool Down

Research suggests that any exercise program should have components that assist with flexibility and movements that prepare the body for the activity. Before conducting an exercise program, some type of warm-up protocol is recommended to increase the flexibility and raise the body's temperature. The warm-up period usually has two distinct phases: general and specific. The general warm-up consists of 5 to 10 minutes of a slow jog, stationary bicycling, or other general activity to increase the heart rate, muscle temperature, respiration rate, and decrease joint viscosity.[48] The specific warm-up consists of activities that are similar to the tasks or movements that the individual will perform in his or her sporting activity and usually lasts for 8 to12 minutes in total time. The cool down is usually a light exercise, similar to the general warm-up, for the purpose of eliminating waste products from the muscles and to help decrease heart

rate and respirations. The cool down is performed after the activity and lasts for approximately 5 minutes.

Flexibility

After the general warm-up, it is recommended that a flexibility program be incorporated to increase joint movement and muscle extensibility. There are several types of flexibility techniques that are used (Table 5-3). Static flexibility is classified as the range of motion about a joint during passive motion without external force, gravity, partner, or machine to apply the stretch that does not elicit the stretch reflex.[49] It is a slow stretch that is held in position for approximately 30 seconds. Ballistic stretching involves a bouncing type of movements in which the end position is not held. A dynamic stretch is similar to a ballistic stretch except that the bouncing movements are avoided and that the specific movements often mimic the type of activity that the individual will perform during his or her activity. Proprioceptive neuromuscular facilitation (PNF) is another type of stretching technique that uses both concentric and isometric actions to facilitate muscular inhibition that usually need to be done with a knowledgeable partner.

Resistance Training Intensity and Goals

The selected sets, reps, weight lifted, and total volume of the training sessions are all focused on the specific goals and objectives of the individual and any sport or activity requirement. The training program should focus on key elements to ensure individual safety, attainable goals, proper form, and technique. An analysis of the individual and sport is required before developing and implementing a strength-training program. Athletes, who are relatively untrained or inexperienced should begin their resistive training session with lightweight

Table 5-3.

Stretching Techniques

Type of Stretch	Static	Ballistic	Dynamic
Definition	Movements that are held at the end range of motion for up to 30 s	A movement in which a bouncing motion is used and the end position is not held	Similar to ballistic stretching and sport-specific warm-up, but eliminates the bouncing movement
Example	Touching the toes	Reaches for the toes, bounces at the end, and quickly goes back up. The activity is repeated with each stretch preceding the last session	Runner, who takes long strides to increase leg motion similar to the running pattern

Table 5-4.

Example of a Beginner Strength-Training Program

Sets	1
Reps	10–15
Load	Use a load that the adolescent can lift for the desired number of reps
Muscle groups Exercised	Abdominals, quadriceps, hamstrings, lower back, shoulder, chest, middle back

Table 5-6.

Resistance Training Goals and Intensity

Goal of Training	Sets	Reps	Load or Weight
Muscle strength	2–6	Less than 10	Moderate
Muscle power	2–5	Less than 8	Moderate
Muscle hypertrophy	3–6	12	Heavy
Muscle endurance	6–8	More than 12	Light

and multiple reps (Table 5-4). It has been recommended that these athletes begin with low resistance and reps between 13 and 15 until they become more experienced in technique and develop muscular strength.[50] For more experienced athletes, reps between 8 and 12 are recommended (Table 5-5). As the athletes become acclimated and adapt to the exercise, loads can increase by following the 2 for 2 rule.

Adolescent athletes can safely participate in two to three resistive training session per week.[35,50] It has been recommended that young athletes begin by performing one to three sets of 8 to 12 reps on all major muscle groups.[51–53] All reps should be with weight that can be lifted with proper technique and form to prevent injury or developing faulty body mechanics. After several training sessions and resistive training experience, athletes can progress to specific weight training goals to develop strength, power, hypertrophy, and muscular endurance (Table 5-6).

Rest Periods

The time between sets and exercise is called a rest period. Rest period length vary according to the specific type of training being performed (i.e., strength, power, and endurance), load lifted, and athletes' training status.[43] The heavier the loads lifted, the longer the rest period between sets. If training for strength and power,

rest periods between sets range form 2 minutes up to 5 minutes, with a longer rest period for power exercises since the loads and intensity is much heavier. Hypertrophy training has shorter rest periods of 30 seconds to 90 seconds to stress the muscle before adequate recovery time. Endurance training has the shortest rest periods, usually less than 30 seconds between the sets (Table 5-7).

PERIODIZATION

The term periodization refers to the overall training program throughout the year. It is divided into sections or cycles in order to maximize gains by altering the volume and intensities of exercise to help increase performance, minimize overtraining, or decrease the frequency of chances of training plateaus. Usually, the volume is high with lower intensity of work and as the time progresses to a competition period, the volume decreases and intensity and sport-specific techniques increase. The periodization model can be incorporated with athletes/ teams where the individual has previous strength-training experience and is often used at the high school level and beyond.

The periodization model is divided into specific time periods. The overall time period or division is called the *macrocycle*. The macrocycle comprises the

Table 5-5.

Example of an Intermediate to Advanced Strength-Training Program

Sets	1–3
Reps	8–15
Load	Dependent upon the individual goals
Exercises	Squat, dead lift, chin-ups, bench press, power clean (advanced movement), lat pulldown, abdominal crunches, biceps and triceps curls, calf raises, stability, or ball exercises

Table 5-7.

Guideline for Rest Periods

Strength-Training Goal	Rest Period Time
Muscular endurance	Less than 30 s
Muscular hypertrophy	30–90 s
Muscular strength	2–5 min
Muscle power	2–5 min

entire training year. Within the macrocycle, smaller sub-cycles called mesocycles are incorporated. A *mesocycle* is a training period that lasts anywhere from weeks to month, dependent upon the goals and objectives of the training plan and athlete. In most training plans, there are four mesocycles: off-season, preseason, in-season, and postseason. Within a mescocycle are shorter training periods designed specifically based on the training variations that can last from 1 to several weeks called a *microcycle*. It has been suggested[54] that a transition period, or a period of specific technique training be placed between the preparatory period and the competition period and ending transition period for active rest, thus changing the overall macrocycle into four distinct periods, preparatory, transition (used for technique training), competition, and transition period (used for active rest after the competition period). This model is useful for novice or inexperienced athletes.

The Preparatory Period

The preparatory period is usually divided into several mesocycles and encompasses the longest training time of all the periods. The purpose of the preparatory period is to develop conditioning beginning at low intensities and high volumes and minimize actual sport-specific technique training. Within the preparatory period are three microcycles that are focused on particular types of training volume and intensities, the hypertrophy/endurance phase, basic strength, and the strength/power phases.

Hypertrophy/endurance phase

The hypertrophy/endurance phase takes place in the beginning phases of the preparatory phase and lasts approximately up to 6 to 8 weeks. The overall purpose of this phase is to increase lean body mass and metabolic and muscular endurance for later periods. The volume remains high while the intensity is low, using higher reps per set. Intensities range from 50% to 75% of the athlete's 1 RM with three to six sets of 10 to 20 reps.

Basic strength phase

The basic strength phase follows the hypertrophy/endurance phase and is geared toward strengthening the muscles that will be specifically used in the sport's primary movements. Strength-training activities begin to target the types of movements required for the sport and the loads become heavier and the reps become fewer. The intensities are usually around 80% to 90% of the athlete's 1 RM, with three to five sets of four to eight reps per exercise.

Strength/power phase

The strength/power phase is the last phase in the preparatory period and focuses on the developing power exercises using higher loads and lower volumes. Typically, the intensity is around 75% to 95% of the athlete's 1 RM, with three to five sets and two to five rep per exercise.

First Transition Period

Before the next mesocycle, the first transition period is used to provide a break from the training and focuses on technique and skill for the sport. This microcycle is relatively short in duration, usually 1 to 2 weeks. After the completion of the first transition period, the competition period beings.

Competition Period

The competition period focuses on developing the peak power and strength training while decreasing the overall training volume. In this period, sport-specific techniques and skills training increase for the athletes. Usually, the competition periods lasts for the entire sporting season, anywhere from several weeks to several months in duration, depending upon the type of sport. The longer the duration of the competition period, the harder it is to maintain peak performance. The goals of a longer competition phase are to have the athletes maintain strength and power while training at moderate intensities and volumes. For a short competition period, the training intensity should be high (>90% of the athletes 1 RM) with minimal number of sets and reps (1–3). If training for a longer competition period, the intensity is approximately 80% to 85% of the athlete's 1 RM with two to three sets of six to eight reps.

The Second Transition Period

The second transition period, or active rest period, follows the competition period. This period lasts approximately several weeks and is geared to nonsporting activities at low intensities and volumes. This period is meant to allow the athlete to rest, relax, and rehabilitate injuries.

TYPES OF EXERCISES

General guidelines for strength training are summarized in Table 5-8. Adolescents can use a variety of training exercises (modalities) to improve their strength and power. These include weight machines, free weights, or their own body weight. While children may be a little small for adult weight machines found in most gyms, using extra padding for support will allow children to use them properly. Children, who are just beginning a structured weight training program benefit from using weight machines since they are easy to learn and easy to perform.[55] However, if training for a sporting event,

Table 5-8.

General Guidelines for a Strength-Training a Program

1. Establish a strength-training program that is both challenging and exciting for children to participate.
2. Qualified strength and conditioning professions such as those certified by the *National Strength and Conditioning Association* should be used for developing strength-training programs for children. Coaches must have the scientific and clinical background in adolescent development to create and develop adequate strength-training programs.
3. Make sure all children have a preparticipation screening prior to any strength-training program by qualified physicians or allied health professionals to examine for preexisting conditions or injuries. A standard health history questionnaire followed by a physical examination that includes flexibility, strength testing for weakness, muscle imbalances, and reflexes will help detect potential risks for strength training.
4. If the preparticipation screening detects physical limitations or strength deficits, a comprehensive program to correct these deficiencies should be addressed as a priority when beginning a strength-training program.
5. Strength-training programs for adolescents should emphasize submaximal efforts, using their body weight or bars with no added weights and concentration on muscular strength and endurance instead of power exercises. The strength-training program should first focus on mastery of technique and motor skills with lightweight before progressing to heavier resistance training and more complex multijoint exercises.
6. Avoid 1 RM lifts.
7. Perform all exercises through a full range of motion and with proper form.
8. Instruct children on the proper methods to breath during exercise and make sure they do not hold their breath.
9. Have an adequate supervision in the strength training facility that includes the use of spotters, if necessary.
10. Make sure the facility is safe, well ventilated, and illuminated properly.
11. Strength training should be performed only two to three times a week with an adequate rest and recovery between sessions. Each session should comprise a general warm-up period, flexibility, resistance training and workout program, specific tasks, and a cool down period.

incorporating more complex exercise, such as in free weights, is recommended only after mastering the technique of all introductory exercises. Advanced multijoint exercises, such as the Olympic lifts, can be introduced after mastery of preparatory or introductory exercises upon the direct supervision and guidance of a strength and condition specialists.

Focus on core musculature, such as abdominals, low back, and hips. Keep the load relatively light when beginning a strength-training program for adolescents, since the majority of gains are attributed to the increase coordination of the neuromuscular patterns versus actual muscle size increases.[56] After an acclimation period to strength training and mastery of introductory exercises, focus on large multijoint exercises that incorporate the major muscle groups. These include exercises such as chin-ups, squats, and military press for adolescents with an emphasis on correct supervision and form/technique while performing these exercises. Exercises that involve a combination of strength, power, and dynamic movements, such as with therapeutic balls or medicine balls should be incorporated into the strength-training program to develop balance, stability, and coordination.

REFERENCES

1. Falk B, Tenenbaum G. The effectiveness of resistance training in children. A meta-analysis. *Sport Med.* 1996; 22(3):176-186.

2. Payne VG, Morrow JR Jr., Johnson L, Dalton SN. Resistance training in children and youth: a meta-analysis. *Res Q Exerc Sport.* 1997;68(1):80-88.
3. Sunnegardh J, Bratteby LE, Nordesjo LO, Nordgren B. Isometrics and isokinetic muscle strength, anthropometry and physical activity in 8 and 13 years old Swedish children. *Eur J Appl Physiol.* 1988;58:291-297.
4. Ramsay JA, Blimkie CJR, Smith K, Garner S, MacDougall JD, Sale DG. Strength training effects in prepubescent males. *Med Sci Sports Exerc.* 1990;22(5):605-614.
5. Weltman A, Janney C, Rians CB, et al. The effects of hydraulic resistance strength training in prepubertal males. *Med Sci Sports Exerc.* 1986;18(6):629-638.
6. Ozmun JC, Mikesy AE, Surburg PR. Neuromuscular adaptations following prepubescent strength training. *Med Sci Sports Exerc.* 1994;26:510-514.
7. Faigenbaum AD, Zaichkowsky LD, Wescott WL, Micheli LJ, Fehlandt AF. The effects of a twice-a-week strength training program on children. *Pediatr Exerc Sci.* 1993;5: 339-346.
8. Falk B, Eliakin A. Resistance training, skeletal muscle and growth. *Pediatr Endocrinol Rev.* 2003;1(2):120-127.
9. Cooper DM. Evidence for and mechanisms of exercise modulation of growth. *Med Sci Sports Exerc.* 1994;26:733-740.
10. Saavedra C, Lagasse' Bouchard C, Simoneau JA. Maximal anaerobic performance of the knee extensor muscles during growth. *Med Sci Sports Exerc.* 1991;23:1083-1089.
11. Inbar O, Bar-Or O. Anaerobic characteristics in male children and adolescents. *Med Sci Sports Exerc.* 1986;18:264-269.
12. Blimkie CJR, Roche P, Hay JT, Bar-Or O. Anaerobic power of arms in teenage boys and girls: relationship to lean tissue. *Eur J Appl Physiol.* 1988;57:677-683.

13. Eriksson BO, Gollnick PD, Saltin B. *Muscle metabolism and enzyme activities after training in boys 11-13 years old. Acta Physiol Scand.* 1973;87:485-497.

14. Falgairette G, Duche P, Bedu M, Fellman N, Coudert J. Bioenergetic characteristics in prepubertal swimmers. *Int J Sports Med.* 1993;14:444-448.

15. Bell RD, Macdougall JD, Billeter R, Howald H. Muscle fiber types and morphometric analysis of skeletal muscle in 6-year-old children. *Med Sci Sports Exerc.* 1980;12:28-31.

16. Fournier M, Ricci J, Taylor AW, Ferguson R, Monpetit R, Chaitman B. Skeletal muscle adaptation in adolescent boys: sprint and endurance training and detraining. *Med Sci Sports Exerc.* 1982;14:453-456.

17. Belanger AY, McComas AJ. Contractile properties of human skeletal muscle in childhood and adolescence. *Eur J Appl Physiol.* 1989;58:563-567.

18. Mero A. Blood lactate production and recovery from anaerobic exercise in trained and untrained boys. *Eur J Appl Physiol.* 1988;57:660-666.

19. Falgairette G, Bedu M, Fellmann N, Van Praagh E, Coudert J. Bio-energetic profile in 144 boys aged 6 to 15 years with special reference to sexual maturation. *Eur J Appl Physiol.* 1991;62:151-156.

20. Kuno S, Takahashi H, Fujimoto K, et al. Muscle metabolism during exercise using phophorus-31 nuclear magnetic resonance spectroscopy in adolescents. *Eur J Appl Physiol.* 1994;70:301-304.

21. Garrick JG, Webb DR. *Sports Injuries: Diagnosis and Management.* Philadelphia, PA: WB Saunders; 1990.

22. Asmussen E, Bonde-Peterson F. Apparent efficiency and storage of elastic energy in human muscles during exercise. *Acta Physiol Scand.* 1974;92:537-545.

23. Pfeiffer R. Plyometrics in sports injury rehabilitation. *Athletic Ther Today.* 1999;4(3):5.

24. Wathen D. Literature review: explosive/plyometric exercises. *Strength Cond.* 1993;15(3):17-19.

25. Adams K, O'Shea JP, O'Shea KL, Climstein M. The effects of six weeks of squat, plyometrics, and squat plyometric training on power production. *J Appl Sports Sci Res.* 1992;6:36-41.

26. Anderst WJ, Eksten F, Koceja DM. Effects of plyometric and explosive resistance training on lower body power. *Med Sci Sports Exerc.* 1994;26:31.

27. Brown ME, Mayhew JL, Boleach LW. Effects of plyometric training on vertical jump performance in high school basketball players. *J Sports Med Phys Fitness.* 1986;26:1-4.

28. Clutch D, Wilton B, McGown M, Byrce GR. The effect of depth jumps and weight training on leg strength and vertical jump. *Res Q Exerc Sport* 1983;54:5-10.

29. Crowder V, Jolly SW, Collins B, Johnson J. The effects of plyometric push-up on upper body power. *Track Techn.* 1990;39:59-67.

30. Hennessy L, Kilty J. Relationship of the stretch-shortening cycle to spring performance in trained female athletes. *J Strength Cond Res.* 2001;15(3):326-331.

31. Miller MG, Berry DC, Bullard S, Gilders R. Comparisons of land-based and aquatic-based plyometric programs during an 8-week training period. *J Sport Rehab.* 2002;11:269-283.

32. Paasuke M, Ereline J, Gapeyeva H. Knee extensor muscle strength and vertical jumping performance characteristics in pre and post-pubertal boys. *Pediatr Exer Sci.* 2001;13:60-69.

33. Piper TJ, Erdmann LD. A 4-step plyometric program. *Strgth Cond.* 1998;20(6):72-73.

34. Hamill BP. Relative safety of weightlifting and weight training. *J Strength Cond Res.* 1994;8:53-57.

35. Faigenbaum AD, Kraemer WJ, Cahill B, et al. Youth resistance training: position statement paper and literature review. *Strength Cond.* 1996;18:62-75.

36. Myer GD, Ford KR, Hewett HE. Rationale and clinical techniques for anterior cruciate ligament injury prevention among female athletes. *J Athl Train.* 2004;39:352-364.

37. Coutts AJ, Murphy AJ, Dascombe BJ. Effect of direct supervision of a strength coach on measures of muscular strength and power in young rugby league players. *J Strength Cond Res.* 2004;18:316-323.

38. Mazzetti SA, Kraemer WJ, Volek JS, et al. The influence of direct supervision of resistance training on strength performance. *Med Sci Sports Exerc.* 2000;32:1175-1184.

39. Fleck SJ, Kraemer WJ. *Designing Resistance Training Programs.* 2nd ed. Champaign, IL: Human Kinetics; 1997.

40. Kraemer WJ. Exercise prescription in weight training. A needs analysis. *NSCA J.* 1983;5(1):64-65.

41. Hunter GR. Changes in body composition, body build, and performance associated with different weight training frequencies in males and females. *NSCA J.* 1985;7(1):26-28.

42. Hoffman JR, Kraemer WJ, Fry AC, Deschenes M, Kemp M. The effects of self-selection for frequency of training in a winter conditioning program for football. *J Appl Sport Sci Res.* 1990;4:76-82.

43. Baechle TR, Earle RW. *Essentials of Strength Training and Conditioning. National Strength and Conditioning Association.* 2nd ed. Champaign, IL: Human Kinetics; 2000.

44. Hoeger W, Barette SL, Hale DF, Hopkins DR. Relationship between repetitions and selected percentages of one repetition maximum. *J Appl Sport Sci Res.* 1987;1(1):11-13.

45. Hoeger W, Hopkins DR, Barette SL, Hale DF. Relationship between repetitions and selected percentages of one repetition maximum. A comparison between untrained and trained males and females. *J Appl Sport Sci Res.* 1990;4:47-54.

46. Landers J. Maximum based on reps. *J Strength Cond Res.* 1985;6:60-1.

47. Baechle TR, Groves BR. *Weight Training: Steps to Success.* 2nd ed. Champaign, IL: Human Kinetics; 1998.

48. deVries HA. *Physiology of Exercise for Physical Education and Athletics.* Dubuque, IA: Brown; 1974.

49. Corbin CB, Dowell LJ, Lindsey R, Tolson H. *Concepts in Physical Education. Dubuque.* IA: Brown; 1978.

50. Faigenbaum AD, Loud RL, O'Connell J, et al. Effects of different resistance training protocols on upper body strength and endurance development in children. *J Strength Cond Res.* 2001;15:459-465.

51. Rhea MR, Alvar BA, Burkett LN. Single versus multiple sets for strength: a meta-analysis to address the controversy. *Res Q Exerc Sport Dec.* 2002;73:485-488.

52. Rhea MR, Alvar BA, Burkett LN, et al. A meta-analysis to determine the dose response for strength development. *Med Sci Sports Exerc.* 2003;35:456-464.

53. Hedrick A. Training for hypertrophy. *Strength Cond.* 1995;17(3):22-29.

54. Matveyev LP. *Periodization of Sports Training.* Moscow: Fiscultura I Sport; 1966.

55. Faigenbaum AD. Resistance training for adolescent athletes. *Athletic Therapy Today.* 2002;7(6):30-35.

56. Haff GG. Roundtable Discussion: youth resistance training. *Sand C Journal.* 2003;25(1):49-64.

CHAPTER 6

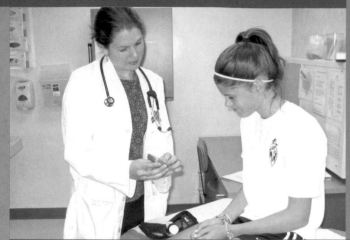

Sports Nutrition
Robert J. Baker

There appears to be a dichotomy among children and adolescents. On the one hand is a population of youth with increasing obesity, on the other hand, active youth are involved in several sports or extensively in a single sport. Access to electronic equipments such as computers, video games, and television has lead to a more sedentary lifestyle. At the same time, ready access to high-energy food has resulted in excess caloric consumption and weight gain, whereas, athletes who train intensely may have a difficult time consuming adequate calories. More youth are participating in intense training and sports such as football, soccer, swimming, tennis, distance running, even triathlons, and marathons. These athletes may need to consume a rather large number of calories to meet the needs for intense activity on top of growth and development.

DAILY CALORIE NEEDS

Baseline caloric demands are determined by the weight. Factors such as growth, age, and physical activity will increase metabolic demand. In children and adolescents, this can increase caloric demand greatly over the basal metabolism. Growth alone can increase basal metabolism significantly. Weight and more specifically body composition can affect metabolism. As lean body mass increases, so do energy requirements increase. Because children and adolescents are less efficient compared to adults when physically active, their energy requirements may be increased 20% to 30% for given level of activity.

Based on the length of physical activity, three different metabolic pathways may serve as the primary metabolic pathways (Figure 6-1).[1] In very short burst of activity, the phosphagen pathway provides the main source of energy. And the athlete performs an activity such as an Olympic lift or 1 repetition maximal lift, phosphocreatine, a chemical present in muscles of the body, can be broken down to immediately release energy for activity. As a readily available energy source, lasting only a few seconds, this source is depleted very early in activity.

As longer physical activity is performed, the anaerobic glycolysis pathway meets the body's energy demands. This pathway provides energy by the breakdown of glycogen. In this metabolic pathway, the energy is regenerated faster without breaking down glucose completely. Longer activities such as sprints, short-distance swimming, and short bouts of weightlifting would be associated with anaerobic glycolysis.

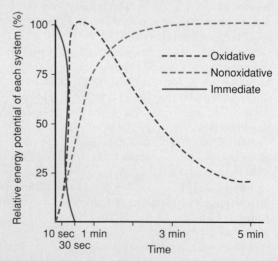

FIGURE 6-1 ■ Energy sources for muscle as a function of activity duration. Schematic presentation showing how long each of the major energy systems can endure in supporting all-out-work. (*From Brooks GA, Fahey TD, White TP. Exercise Physiology. New York: McGraw Hill Medical; 2005.*)

Long-duration endurance physical activity is associated with the aerobic glycolysis pathway. Ultimately, the glucose metabolized by this pathway is broken down completely to water and carbon dioxide. In the process, significantly more energy is released. Aerobic glycolysis pathway being a more complicated pathway, more metabolic resources are invested in it to supply a greater release of energy from each molecule. Also, fats may be metabolized to a greater extent during longer aerobic activity. During constant or intermittent running activities over longer periods of time aerobic glycolysis would contribute most significantly to energy production. Athletes playing soccer, basketball, hockey, and distance runners would be the examples.

BASIC NUTRITION SOURCES

Carbohydrates, proteins, and fats are the three basic sources of calories in the human diet (Figure 6-2).[2] Carbohydrates represent a readily usable energy source. Fats represent a calorie dense source of energy. A significant number of calories are released in the body as these longer chain molecules are broken down. As carbohydrates and fats as energy sources in the body are fully consumed, proteins within the body will be metabolized as a final source of energy. Children and adolescents may have an increased requirement for calorie intake compared to adults. Increased calories are required for growth and development. Since children and adolescents have increased energy consumption for physical activity compared to adults, the young athletes may have a slightly greater calorie requirement.[3]

Carbohydrates

Carbohydrates are the primary energy source for physical activity of the body. For this reason, 50% to 60% of the calories in the athlete's diet should be carbohydrates. Consumed carbohydrates may be broken down into glucose circulating in the blood. Blood glucose serves as a ready source of energy in the cells. Consumed carbohydrates may be mobilized to the liver for glycogen storage or finally mobilized in the muscle for storage as muscle glycogen. Liver glycogen can be mobilized to maintain blood glucose to other tissue. Muscle glycogen stores can be metabolized within the muscle during prolonged physical activity as an energy source.

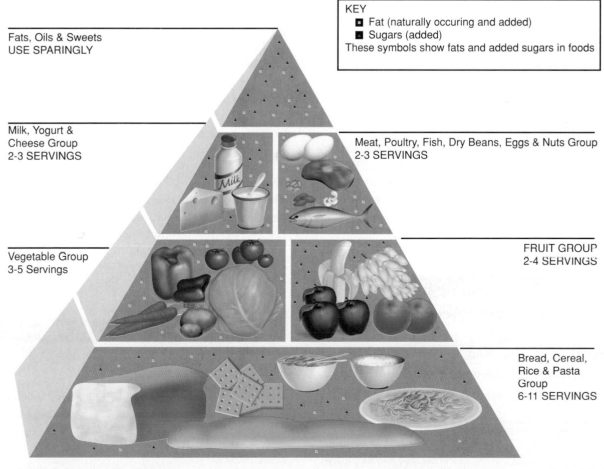

KEY
■ Fat (naturally occuring and added)
■ Sugars (added)
These symbols show fats and added sugars in foods

Fats, Oils & Sweets
USE SPARINGLY

Milk, Yogurt &
Cheese Group
2-3 SERVINGS

Meat, Poultry, Fish, Dry Beans, Eggs & Nuts Group
2-3 SERVINGS

Vegetable Group
3-5 Servings

FRUIT GROUP
2-4 SERVINGS

Bread, Cereal,
Rice & Pasta
Group
6-11 SERVINGS

FIGURE 6-2 ■ The food pyramid.

Blood glucose is regulated by insulin and exercise. In the resting state, insulin facilitates the uptake of glucose by the cell. Exercise is associated with an upregulation of membrane bound glucose receptors, which results in an increase uptake of glucose by the active cell. Thus, exercise will increase the effect of insulin.

Carbohydrates can be classified based on a glycemic index. Carbohydrate rich foods will affect blood sugars based on the complexity of the carbohydrate. Foods with a higher percentage of complex sugars will be digested and absorbed more slowly. These foods will have a low-glycemic index and contribute to less elevation in blood glucose. Examples would be dairy foods, fruits, pasta, dried beans, and nuts. Foods with a higher percentage of simple sugars would be digested and absorbed more rapidly and result in greater increase in blood sugars. Examples of these high-glycemic index foods would be carrots, white potatoes, honey, white bread, corn chips, and sports drinks. Other foods such as rice cakes, crackers, soda, wheat bread, ice cream, sweet potatoes, and potato chips would have a moderate glycemic index and a mix of complex and simple sugars.

Athletes competing in endurance activity may experience an increase in blood glucose by consuming high-glycemic index foods just prior to activity. Some athletes, who consume high-glycemic index foods may experience hypoglycemia because of overproduction and effect of insulin. This may actually decrease performance because of rebound insulin overload. Consumption of low-glycemic index foods several hours before exercise for some athletes can help to maintain a more even blood glucose level.

Timing of the carbohydrate consumption in relationship to exercise may affect performance. Generally, the pre-event consumption of carbohydrate should satisfy hunger and elevate blood glucose without causing insulin rebound phenomenon. This may be achieved by consuming most carbohydrates several hours prior to the event (Table 6-1).[4]

Carbohydrate loading may improve performance in long-endurance events. This technique should only be repeated twice during a season. Loading begins 1 week prior to the event with the depletion of glycogen stores. During the first 3 days, the athlete increases activity while decreasing the percentage of carbohydrate consumed at each meal. After the glycogen depletion phase, the athlete replenishes glycogen stores slowly by gradually decreasing workout bouts and increasing the percentage of carbohydrates consumed on the days leading up to the event. While this technique is effective in adults, it has not been studied in children.[5]

Protein

Proteins are an alternate energy source when stored glycogen and fat are depleted during endurance exercise. More importantly, proteins provide the building blocks for muscle development and repair. Increased protein intake has been suggested for active individuals as well children and adolescents who are experiencing growth and development (Table 6-2).[6]

Not meeting the body's protein requirements can result in muscle mass wasting, lowered immunity, decreased injury repair, and fatigue. This is common in athletes who are attempting to lose weight by restricting calories. Repeated injury with poor recovery can be the hallmark of protein deficiency in athletes. Exceeding the protein requirements can result in increased body fat, dehydration by nitrogen loss, and calcium loss. Increased protein consumption is often associated with carbohydrate deficiency. The end result is poor athletic performance.

Fats

The final energy substrate macronutrient in the body is fat. Fats serve as a high-caloric storage source of energy. Not more than 30% of dietary calories should be from fats. Limiting fat intake can limit energy storage as well as essential fat deficiencies. Significantly, limiting fat intake can

Table 6-1.

Suggested Carbohydrate Intake for Physical Activity

When	How Much (g)	How
Before activity	300	Several hours before the activity
During activity	30	Every hour during the activity
After activity	75	Within 30 min after cessation of activity
	100	Every 60 min for 2 h after cessation of activity

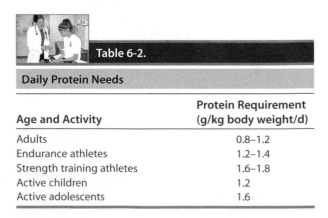

Table 6-2.

Daily Protein Needs

Age and Activity	Protein Requirement (g/kg body weight/d)
Adults	0.8–1.2
Endurance athletes	1.2–1.4
Strength training athletes	1.6–1.8
Active children	1.2
Active adolescents	1.6

result in deficiencies in the fat-soluble vitamins A, D, E, and K. Children with developing nervous tissue are at risk with fat deficiency. Fat consumption should be evenly divided between saturated, polyunsaturated, and monounsaturated fat sources. Saturated fats should not account for greater than 10% of total dietary caloric intake.

WEIGHT CONTROL

Nutrition and Weight Control

Weight gain or weight loss is based on caloric balance. Simply put, if the athlete consumes more calories than are expended, he or she will gain weight as do football players. If the athletes consume less calories than are expended, they will loose weight as sportspersons in figure skating, gymnastic, wrestling, who are seeking to loose weight.

Weight Loss

Obesity among children is on the raise. This most likely is related to an increasing sedentary life style as well as poor dietary habits. Time spent in sedentary activities such as computer games and television viewing is on the rise. To make matters worse, these activities are associated with the consumption of high-caloric snacks. Over the last 30 years, obesity among children has increased 106%. In adolescent boys (12–17), obesity has increased by 146% and 69% in females.[7]

Favorable changes in body composition may occur with regular physical activity. Studies show a decrease in visceral fat. Body mass and percent body fat may also decrease with an increase in fat-free mass. Exercise can decrease insulin resistance in juvenile obesity associated with type 2 diabetes.

The activity program should include adequate intensity to result in body composition changes. While exercise modality is not as important, it should include a component to increase aerobic fitness. Children will be motivated by enjoyable activity and rewards for attainable goals. Parents should be involved in the program to serve as role models.

Athletes in sports such as gymnastics and figure skating may be motivated to loose weight to improve performance. Wrestlers are motivated to loose weight to compete in lower weight classes. Any weight loss program for children and adolescents should be professionally supervised.[8] Restricting caloric intake can interfere with growth and development. Protein deficiencies as well as micronutrient deficiencies may occur, if a balanced diet is not followed. A multivitamin may be beneficial, if there is a specific concern, however, a good balanced diet is best.[1]

Weight Gain

In sports such as football, where size may be an advantage for certain positions, young athletes may seek to gain weight. Other young athletes, who are generally underweight may seek to gain weight as well. Simply increasing caloric intake will increase weight. However, without proper training this weight gain will primarily be fat. This added weight will result in decreased efficiency of the young athlete and decreased performance. Long-term effects of weight gain in young athletes are unknown. In light of increasing obesity and chronic diseases such as diabetes, hypertension, cardiovascular disease, and arthritis, these athletes may be at increased health risk in later life. As with weight lose, body composition should be monitored in any young athlete wishing to gain weight.

Eating Disorders

Females in sports with an emphasis on slender appearance are at greatest risk for eating disorders. Males involved in a sport with weight requirements may also be at risk. The physician should be aware of athlete with bulimia that may be involved in unsafe practices of self-induced vomiting, use of diuretics, use of cathartics, or overexercising. Athletes will often minimize or deny these behaviors. Anorexic athletes will often have a distorted body image. Valid diagnostic survey instruments are available for eating disorders.[9] Athletes, male, and female with suspected eating disorder should be managed with the team approach consisting of nutritionist, counselor, and physician.

BODY COMPOSITION

Weight alone is probably not an accurate reflection of body fat especially in athletes. Body mass index (BMI) is easily calculated from weight and height. Young athletes may have a higher weight and BMI because of increase larger muscle mass as opposed to fat. There are several methods to estimate body composition. Each method has its advantages and disadvantages. Hydration status can affect all body composition measurements. Young athletes seeking to lose weight should be evaluated based on body composition rather than weight alone. Athletes may consider themselves overweight, yet actually have a lower percent body fat. While there is no ideal body composition for individual athlete by sport, most would recommend maintaining 5% or greater body fat.

Underwater Weighing

This method of estimating body composition is based on the concept that muscle is denser in water and sinks, whereas fat is less dense and floats. This method is considered the gold standard of body composition estimation; however, error in measurement can result from inaccurate estimation of lung volume.[1] This error can be significant, if the subject is unable to empty lungs underwater because of fear. While measurements can be very accurate, athletes with a fear of water should not be evaluated by this method.

Skin-Folds Measurement

Subcutaneous fat can be estimated by skin-fold thickness. Skin-fold measurements taken from various body areas, often chest, biceps, abdomen, and thigh can be placed in a valid equation which will estimate percent body fat. This method can be very accurate for average athletes. Muscular athletes with very low body fat may be underestimated. Those with extra body fat may be overestimated. Other factors such as technical skill, quality of calipers, and equation can also affect accuracy.

Bioelectrical Impedance

The bioelectrical impedance method estimates the body fat based on the body's resistance to electrical current. Tissue with less water content will have greater impedance. Hydration status significantly affects the accuracy of this method. Impedance devices are relatively small and affordable and require little skill on the part of the technician. Reproducibility can be quite good, if hydration is controlled.[1] Validation studies are lacking.

Dual Energy X-Ray Absorptiometry (DEXA)

Body composition can be estimated based on x-ray attenuation of tissue in two planes. This method can accurately estimate whole body or regional body fat. The equipment is expensive and does result in radiation exposure. The most common clinical application is to estimate bone density.

MICRONUTRIENTS

The daily requirements for major micronutrients are summarized in Table 6-3.

Iron

Iron plays a role in hemoglobin and myoglobin synthesis. Deficiencies may lead to a decrease in the oxygen carrying capacity of blood and oxygen delivery in the muscles. Iron is usually adequately stored in the body. Iron deficiency may occur in very active athletes in

Table 6-3.

Daily Recommended Intake for Micronutrients

Nutrient	Males (y)		Females (y)	
	9–13	14–18	9–13	14–18
Calcium (mg)	1300	1300	1300	1300
Iron (mg)	8	11	8	15
Zinc (mg)	8	11	8	9
Energy (kcal)	2279	3152	2071	2368

warm environment where iron is lost through sweat. For females, heavy menses, which may be experience at menarche, may result in iron deficiency. Other diseases associated with blood loss of cell degradation can be associated with a decrease in iron stores and anemia.

Mild anemia has been recognized in girl distance runners.[9] Low levels of ferritin and hemoglobin in these athletes is associated with decreased performance. For this reason, some recommend screening of these athletes and iron supplementation, with or without vitamin C.

Iron can be increased in the diet by consuming lean meat, cooking with iron skillet, cooking vegetables a shorter period of time with less water, or using iron-fortified breads and cereals. Supplementing with a vitamin C source, such as orange juice, can improve iron uptake from the gastrointestinal tract. The recommended dietary allowance for iron is 8 mg for 9- to 13-year-old and 11 to 15 mg for 14 year to 18-year-old adolescents.

Vegetarian athletes are reliant upon nonhaeme iron source from plants as opposed to haeme iron of animal products.[10] Decreased bioavailability of iron in these plant sources raises concern for iron deficiency in the vegetarian. Consumption of soy product along with vitamin C from fruits and vegetables partially offsets the lower absorption and results in adequate iron stores in these athletes.

Calcium

Calcium plays a role in bone density. Calcium supplementation is recommended for individuals with osteopenia. Females with disordered eating and amenorrhea are at increased risk of osteopenia. These three together in a female athlete is referred to as the female athlete triad. A young female with a low bone density is a concern because maximum bone density is achieved by age 25 to 30 years. Low bone density at an early age can place the individual at serious risk of fracture at an even earlier age. Early diagnosis and treatment of amenorrhea may reverse some bone lose.

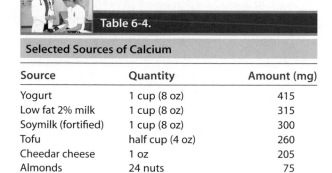

Table 6-4.

Selected Sources of Calcium

Source	Quantity	Amount (mg)
Yogurt	1 cup (8 oz)	415
Low fat 2% milk	1 cup (8 oz)	315
Soymilk (fortified)	1 cup (8 oz)	300
Tofu	half cup (4 oz)	260
Cheedar cheese	1 oz	205
Almonds	24 nuts	75

Table 6-5.

Daily Vitamin Needs During Adolescence

Vitamin	Daily Need
Vitamin D	5 μg
Thiamin	0.9–1.2 mg
Riboflavin	0.9–1.3 mg
Niacin	12–16 mg
Vitamin B-12	1.8–2.4 μg
Vitamin C	45–75 mg
Folate	300–400 μg

A calcium intake of 1300 mg/d is recommended. Dairy products and dark green leafy vegetables are the best dietary sources (Table 6-4). Calcium supplements are available as well. Because vitamin D plays a role in the absorption of calcium, some recommend supplementation with 5 μg/d of this vitamin.[11]

Zinc

Zinc plays a role in immune function and protein synthesis as well as blood formation. Because animal products are the best sources of zinc, the vegetarian athlete is at risk of zinc deficiency. Athletes who participate in hot humid environment may loose substantial zinc in sweat. Legumes, whole grains, cereals, nuts, seeds soy, and dairy products are good sources of zinc.

Chromium

Chromium is a trace element, which is a cofactor for insulin receptor binding. It thus enhances insulin's effect on glucose uptake. As a trace element, there is no recommended daily allowance of chromium. Chromium picolinate is often advertised as a fat burner. Because of its action, it could theoretically mobilized fat and enhance fat metabolism. However, this has not been clearly demonstrated. Thus, its safety and efficacy in young athletes is not known.

Vitamins

A healthy, balanced diet is the best source of vitamins. Mega doses of any vitamin have not been shown to be beneficial. The fat-soluble vitamins, A, D, K, and possibly E, may be toxic in large doses. Most of the water-soluble vitamins, B-complex and C, are not absorbed in excess and do not necessarily pose the same risk. Because vitamin C does play a role as a cofactor in tissue healing and growth, some may recommend this vitamin for athletes with illness or injury. It is unclear, if

mega doses improve healing over adequate amounts of intake. Vitamin C does enhance iron absorption and can be recommended along with iron supplementation for athletes with anemia. Many B-complex vitamins play a role as cofactors in energy metabolism. Mega doses of these vitamins do not seem to enhance metabolism significantly unless a deficiency is identified.

Vitamins A, C, and E are known as antioxidants because they do play a role scavenging free radials. A free radical is the chemical substance produce as a byproduct during exercise. The free radical can cause significant cell damage, if not metabolized. Studies have not clearly shown whether supplementation with these antioxidants is beneficial.[3] The daily needs for vitamins during adolescence are listed in Table 6-5.

Fluids

Fluid balance in young athletes can be a challenge because of several risk factors. Young athletes have greater surface area to mass ratio, greater metabolic heat production, and lower sweat rate. All of which can contribute to greater thermoregulatory stress in the hot humid environment. Thus, because of a smaller physical size, limited cardiac capacity, and metabolic inefficiency, young athletes may be more susceptible to thermoregulatory stress, heat exhaustion, and heat stoke.

There are no studies that have examined core temperature changes in children. However, like adults, children are thought to voluntarily dehydrate during long-endurance activities.[6] Young athletes should be encouraged to consume fluids during prolonged activity in a hot humid environment. With acclimatization, sweat production increases and can cause greater fluid and electrolyte loss.

There is currently controversy regarding fluid replacement recommendations for athletes. Young athletes may be at risk of hyponatremia as are their adult counterparts. Certainly, young athletes may have inexperience of sport, lower body weight, slow pace of activity, excessive drinking, and free accessibility of fluids. These, along with female sex and activity lasting longer than 4 hours, are risk factors for hyponatremia. Fluids with lower concentration of electrolytes, sodium, potassium, and chloride may be beneficial. In addition, a small concentration of carbohydrates may provide energy replacement as well as encourage intake by improving taste. Heat-related illness and fluid replacement are reviewed in Chapter 30.

REFERENCES

1. Bonci L. Nutrition. In: McKeag DB, Moeller J, eds. *ACSM Primary Care Sports Medicine*. Philadelphia, PA: Lippincott, Williams and Wilkins; 2007:37-49.

2. US Department of Health and Human Services & USDA. *Dietary Guidelines for Americans*. 2005. Available at www.healthierus.gov/dietaryquidelines. Accessed September 17, 2007.

3. Bar-Or O, Barr S, Bergeron M, et al. Youth in Sport: nutritional needs. *Sports Sci Exch*. 1997;8(4):1-4.

4. American College of Sports Medicine, American Dietetic Association & Dietitians of Canada. Joint Position Statement: nutrition and athletic performance. *Med Sci Sports Exerc*. 2000;32(12):2130-2145.

5. Conrad E. Preventing nutritional disorders in athletes: Focus on the basics. *Curr Sports Med Rep*. 2002;1:172-178.

6. Bar-Or O. Nutrition for child and adolescent athletes. *Sports Sci Exch*. 2000;13(2):1-5.

7. Bar-Or O. Childhood obesity: A world-wide epidemic. Gatorade Sport Science Institute. Available at www.gssi-web.com/hottopicarticle/july2001:2001. Accessed September 15, 2007.

8. Manore MM. Exercise and the institute of medicine recommendations for nutrition. *Curr Sports Med Rep*. 2005;4:193-198.

9. Gabel KA. Special nutritional concerns for the female athlete. *Curr Sports Med Rep*. 2006;5:187-191.

10. Venderley AM, Campbell WW. Vegetarian diets: Nutritional considerations for athletes. *Sports Med*. 2006;36(4):293-305.

11. Unnithan VB, Goulopoulou S. Nutrition for the pediatric athlete. *Curr Sports Med Rep*. 2004;3:206-211.

Suggested Further Reading

American Dietetic Association. Adolescent Nutrition: special issue. *J Am Diet Assoc*. 2002;102(3).

Bar-Or O. The juvenile obesity epidemic: strike back with physical activity. *Sport Sci Exch*. 2003;16(2):1-6.

Habash DL. Child and adolescent athletes. In: *American Dietetic Association Sports Nutrition*. 4th ed. New York: American Dietetic Association; 2006:229-252.

Landry GL, Bernhardt DT. Nutrition. *Essentials of Primary Care Sports Medicine*. Champaign, IL: Human Kinetics; 2003:167-183.

Petersons M, Bruss MB, Bruss JB. Adolescent nutrition. In: Greydanus DE, Patel DR, Pratt HD, eds. *Essential Adolescent Medicine*. New York: McGraw Hill; 2006:615-634.

Rowland TW. Iron deficiency in the adolescent athlete. In: Bar-OrO, ed. *The Child and Adolescent Athlete*. Cambridge, MA: Blackwell Science; 1996:274-286.

Steen SN. Nutrition for the school age child athlete. In: Bar-Or O, ed. *The Child and Adolescent Athlete*. Cambridge, MA: Blackwell Science ;1996:260-273.

Steen SN, Bernhardt DT. Nutrition and weight control. In: Anderson SJ, Sullivan JA, eds. *Care of the Young Athlete*. Chicago, IL: American Academy Orthopedic Surgeons; 2000:81-94.

Williams MH. Exercise effects on children's health. *Sports Sci Exch*. 1993;4:1-2.

CHAPTER 7

Performance-Enhancing Drugs and Supplements

Donald E. Greydanus and Cynthia Feucht

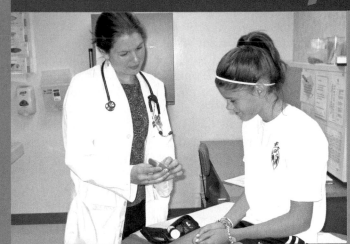

> *"He cures most successfully in whom the people have the greatest confidence."*
>
> Galen, 180 AD

INTRODUCTION

Western history first records myriad medical treatments in 1550 BC in the *Ebers Papyrus,* which is a 110-page scroll containing 700 formulas and remedies (animal, vegetable, and mineral) used by ancient Egyptian healers.[1,2] Historical records from ancient China and India also reveal extensive herbal and plant-based pharmacopoeias.[3] The attempt by athletes to improve their sports performance by taking various remedies and drugs has been observed for thousands of years. For example, athletes taking part in the ancient Greek and Roman games consumed various mixtures of mushrooms, figs, and opioids that contained stimulants such as strychnine, and other substances in attempts to seek victory over opponents in sports competition.[4,5]

Athletes in the 20th-century Olympics events also used strychnine to gain a competitive edge, even though it was known as a potential poison. Indeed, part of the 20th-century Olympic history is the discovery of various substances taken by some athletes in attempts to win and attempts by the Olympics Committees to find and stop these attempts.[5] Athletes of all ages in the 21st century are willing to take a wide variety of drugs, concoctions, herbals, "health" foods, and others if they feel it will help "win" the game and sometimes even if they know deleterious effects may occur. Many athletes take various chemicals even without any evidence of their benefit or lack of safety. Very few of the thousands of herbal remedies now

available have been shown to improve health or even sports performance. Despite this, billions of dollars are spent by athletes hoping for an edge in their sports competition.[4–7]

The United States Pure Food and Drug Act of 1906 was passed by the US Congress, which prevented adulterated or misbranded food and drugs from being manufactured, sold, or transported across the state lines.[4] The 1938 Federal Food, Drug, and Cosmetic Act (FFDCA) then made it law that medications be tested for *safety*; however, it was not until 1962 that the Harris-Kefauver Amendment of the FFDCA was passed making it law that these drugs must be proven *effective* for their intended use prior to marketing.[4]

In order to avoid the close supervision provided to medications, intense lobbying convinced the US Congress to pass the 1994 Dietary Supplement Health and Education Act (DSHEA) in which "dietary supplements" were placed in a *separate* category. These chemicals were legally defined as substances that were mineral, vitamin, herb, other botanical substances, amino acid, or constituents of these products, metabolites, or even related concentrations, extractions, or combinations of these substances.[8] The result is that makers of these products do not need to prove the safety or efficacy of their products. While they cannot claim to prevent, treat, or cure a specific disease, they can denote that the product will "maintain health or normal structure and function."[8]

The unfortunate result of this 1994 law is that the public is inundated with a wide variety of products with a dietary supplement label and producing all types of claims for improved health. Athletes are also overwhelmed with a plethora of products claiming to help them become more successful sports participants who will perform better and be in improved health. In 1999, more than $12 billion was spent on "dietary supplements" and the public was bombarded with more than 89 supplement brands and 300 products competing for the attention of the public, including athletes, with unproven claims of improved health and improved sports performance.[9] Since the implementation of the DSHEA in 1994, several ingredients have been found to be harmful by the FDA, and thus removed from the market.[10] The first such agent to be removed was ephedrine alkaloids, in 2004, because of the cardiovascular effects it had.[10] The most recent act is the 2006 Dietary Supplement and Nonprescription Drug Consumer Protection Act, which mandates that supplement and OTC manufacturers report serious adverse effects to the FDA within 2 weeks of the claim.[10] While additional measures have been enacted to help protect athletes from adverse consequences, there is still the need of clinicians to educate athletes and their parents to what is known and not known about these substances.[11]

DEFINITIONS

An *ergogenic* drug is one that presents with claims of improved sports performance, whether allowing one to run faster, jump higher, or whatever it takes to perform better in one's chosen sports.[4] "Ergogenic" comes from the Greek word, *érgon* (to work) and *gennan* (to produce) and when applied to a chemical or drug, implies that the consumer will be able to "work" better. If applied to sports, the claim will be the athlete can "work better" at his or her chosen sport.[5] Substance-induced *enhanced* sports performance refers to improved sports results in the athlete. Reasons to use these products are listed in Table 7-1.

In 1963, the Council of Europe developed a definition of *sports doping* as "the administration or use of substances in any form alien to the body or of physio-

Table 7-1.

Claims of Ergogenic Agents

1. Serve as an energy source
2. Decrease fatigue in sports events
3. Increase lean body mass and strength
4. Decrease adipose tissue
5. Alter weight in desirable directions
6. Improve aerobic capacity
7. Enhance motor capacity
8. Enhance overall sports performance

Table 7-2.

Drugs and Supplements Misused by Adolescent Athletes [4,7]

1. Anabolic steroids, dehydroepiandrosterone
2. Antioxidants
3. Amphetamines
4. Beta-hydroxy-beta-methylbutyrate (HMB)
5. Blood
6. Caffeine
7. Calcium
8. Carnitine
9. Chromium
10. Creatine
11. Dimethyl sulfoxide (DSMO)
12. Diuretics
13. Ephedrine
14. Iron
15. Nonsteroidal anti-inflammatory drugs (ibuprofen, mefenamic acid, naproxen, etc.)
16. Oxygen
17. Pangamic acid ("Vitamin B15")
18. Protein and amino acids
19. Sodium bicarbonate.
20. Vitamins
21. Minerals:
    Boron
    Chromium
    Vanadium
    Iron
    Selenium
22. Erythropoietin (EPO)
23. Inosine
24. Gamma oryzanol (ferulic acid, FRAC)
    Ginkgo biloba
    Ginseng
    Yohimbine (Yohimbe)
25. Illicit drugs (alcohol, marijuana, tobacco, methamphetamine, cocaine, methcathinone, etc.)

logical substances in abnormal amounts and with abnormal methods by healthy persons with the exclusive aim of attaining an artificial and unfair increase in performance in competition."[12] The word "doping" comes from the Dutch word, *dop*, referring to a mixture of opium given to stimulate racing horses.[5] Agents that have been used in attempts to improve sports performance include anabolic steroids, testosterone, creatinine, oxygen, amphetamines, ephedrine, iron, blood, and others as listed in Table 7-2.[4–7,9,12–20]

EPIDEMIOLOGY

The claims listed in Table 7-1, as outrageous as they seem, are powerful enough to entice thousands of athletes to try them. Encouragement to buy these agents can come from coaches, trainers, fellow athletes, "nutrition" store employees, magazine advertisements, professional athletes, and others. Since much of the known research has been performed on adult males involved in competitive sports, the actual short-term and long-term effects on children and adolescents are practically unknown. Even though the purity and even actual chemical that are found in these products is not clear, sports doping remains a very popular phenomenon among all ages of athletes. Anabolic steroids and creatine are among the most popular sports doping agents.[4–7,9,12–20]

Prevalence rates vary among studies and depend on several demographic factors including age, athlete or nonathlete, and the type of sports participation. Studies have noted that 5% to 11% of high school males and 0.5% to 2.5% of high school females experiment with *anabolic steroids* (see next section).[4] Approximately half of those who use anabolic steroids start are younger than 16 years and approximately one-third are not athletes. The Monitoring the Future Study has assessed the annual prevalence rates of anabolic steroid use among the US high school students from 1989 to 2006. In the 2006 Monitoring the Future Study, the annual prevalence rates for steroid use were 1.2%, 1.9%, and 2.7% among males and 0.6%, 0.5%, and 0.7% in females in the 8th, 10th, and 12th grades, respectively.[21] The Centers for Disease Control and Prevention's 2005 Youth Risk Behavioral Surveillance (YRBS) examined the annual prevalence rates of anabolic steroid use among the US high school students from 1991 through 2005. This study noted a lifetime steroid prevalence use of 4.8% among high school males and 3.2% among high school females.[22] The rates were consistently higher in males than females throughout the study period but the gender gap has narrowed in recent years. More than 300,000 high school students have used anabolic steroids and it is estimated that 3% to 7% of adolescents use these drugs.[6] Studies indicate that anabolic steroid use is more common in athletes than in nonathletes.[23–25] Among athletes, football players are commonly implicated but use has also been demonstrated in other sports such as gymnastics, weight training, basketball and baseball.[23,24] Reasons cited for steroid use include improving athletic capability and increasing strength among athletes to improving appearance and enhancing overall well-being in nonathletes.[23,25]

Creatine has gained popularity as a performance-enhancing substance among adolescents. Creatine is an essential amino acid that helps supply energy to muscles and has been touted to decrease muscle fatigue and improve muscle performance. One study by Smith and Dahm surveyed 328 high school athletes between the ages of 14 and 18 years and found that 8.2% of male athletes used *creatine* as a supplement and the use increased with age.[26] Most of those who used creatine learned of its use from a friend and purchased it in a health food store.[26] In another study, more than 1000 middle and high school athletes were surveyed with 5.6% of respondents reporting use of creatine and use also increased with age.[27] Studies continue to support the widespread use of supplements by athletes of all ages.[28–30]

SPECIFIC DRUGS AND SUPPLEMENTS

Anabolic Androgenic Steroids

Anabolic steroids or androgenic anabolic steroids, listed by the FDA since 1990 as Schedule III controlled drugs, are synthetic testosterone derivatives that are well-known in the athletic community.[4–6,31,32] Testosterone was isolated in 1935 as a chemical to provide a positive effect on overall metabolism. Anabolic steroids interact with a wide variety of receptors, including glucocorticoid, progestin, estrogen, and androgen. Anabolic steroids have been used since the 1940s to improve strength in body builders and others. "Anabolic" refers to its ability to stimulate protein synthesis and "androgenic" refers to its stimulation of male secondary sex characteristics. The term "steroid hormones" or "steroids" refers to the fact that these chemicals are derived from cholesterol and are in a class that includes corticosteroids and sex hormones (i.e., progesterone, estrogen, and testosterone). Table 7-3 lists various

Table 7-3.

Anabolic Steroids

A. Injectable steroids
   1. Testosterone cypionate (Testim®)
   2. Testosterone enanthate (Depo-Testosterone®)
   3. Nandrolone phenpropionate (Durabolin®)
   4. Nandrolone decanoate (Deca-Durabolin®)
B. Oral steroids
   1. Oxandrolone (Oxandrin®)
   2. Oxymetholone (Anadrol®)
   3. Stanozolol (Winstrol®)
C. Topical steroids
   1. Testosterone transdermal (Androderm®)
   2. Testosterone gel (Androgel®)

anabolic steroids. *Dianabol®* was removed from the official market because of the high level of abuse associated with it.

Use and effectiveness

Anabolic steroids are taken in various regimens, typically in prolonged and very high (*supraphysiologic*) doses in attempts to achieve optimal pharmacologic effects. One method is called "stacking" that involves cycles of 6 to 12 weeks of high dose use and then no use, followed by more cycles of heavy use.[4,7] Many use a "pyramiding" plan in which oral and injectable doses are increased over time from 10 to 100 times a physiologic or therapeutic dose and typically obtained from veterinary supplies.[31] A therapeutic oral dose is one used for management of various medical illnesses, and is often 2 to 20 mg, depending on the specific steroid being prescribed. Athletes often take several agents together with doses up to 200 mg/d.

The intended purpose is to increase lean body mass and strength while some only want to improve overall appearance. Research does show that high doses of anabolic and androgenic steroids in association with adequate training and protein intake does lead to an increase in water retention, lean body mass, muscle mass, and overall body weight.[4–7] These effects may be very beneficial to some athletes and are noted only if involved in intensive training regimens; otherwise the athlete may gain weight but not increase overall strength. The exact impact on the athlete's performance based on doping with anabolic steroids is controversial and not predictable. However, the publicized use by some professional and college athletes has led many adolescents to conclude they should take them, especially those involved in wrestling, football, body building, sprinting, shot putting, discus throwing, and weight lifting.

Side effects

Side effects of anabolic steroids are complex, numerous, and potentially very serious, as noted in Table 7-4.[4–6,31–33] Female athletes seek to take doses of steroids that will increase muscle mass and strength but not cause masculinization. These include hirsutism and clitoromegaly that may be permanent and deepening of the voice that is permanent. Female athletes may also develop amenorrhea, skin coarseness, and male-pattern baldness. Severe acne and hair loss can be seen in both males and females.

Gynecomastia may be seen in some males and is partly irreversible. Prostate hyperplasia can occur with possible heightened risk for the development of prostate cancer. Also noted in males are reduced

Table 7-4.

Anabolic Steroids Side Effects

1. Masculinization of females
   a) Hirsutism
   b) Clitoromegaly
   c) Deepening of voice
   d) Alopecia (males also)
2. Fluid retention and hypertension
3. Growing athletes:
   a) Acceleration of maturation
   b) Early epiphyseal closure
   c) Shortened ultimate adult height
4. Psychological changes with rise in:
   a) Aggressiveness
   b) Irritability
   c) Depression
5. GI irritation
6. Hyperglycemia
7. Acne vulgaris (can be severe)
8. Decrease in glycoproteins (FSH and LH) with:
   a) Decreased sperm
   b) Decreased testosterone levels
   c) Reduction in testicular size
9. Increase in tendon injuries
10. Increase in liver function tests and liver failure
11. Heptic neoplasms (including a hepatocellular carcinoma)—peliosis hepatitis
12. Prostatic enlargement
13. Gynecomastia
14. Hyperlipidemia
15. Potential rise in cardiovascular disorders
16. Wilm's tumor (at least one case report)

Reprinted from: Greydanus DE, Patel DR. Sports doping in the adolescent athlete: the hope, hype, and hyperbole. Pediatric Clin North Am. 2002; 49(4): 829-55, with permission from Elsevier.

levels of FSH and LH, testosterone levels, and testicular size. The reduction in testicular size is reversible, though abnormalities in germinal elements can continue for several months after stopping anabolic steroid use.

Of particular concern in the adolescent is the effect of anabolic steroids on bone growth. Early in puberty, androgens are responsible for bone growth and towards the end of puberty they are responsible for epiphyseal closure.[34] As a result of the premature closure, a reduction can be observed in adult height.[34] Adolescents are also at an increased risk for muscle strains or ruptures with more intense training.[34]

Adverse events associated with anabolic steroids include effects on the liver and range from mild to severe with the incidence varying with dosage, length of use, and agent chosen.[34] The oral 17-alpha alkyated anabolic steroids have been associated with much of the hepatoxicity as noted in Table 7-4.[35] Injectable anabolic steroids increase the risk for hepatitis (B and C), HIV/AIDS, and other complications from the use of nonsterile needles. There may be increased platelet aggregation, cardiac hypertrophy, myocardial infarction, and sudden death with anabolic steroid use.

Clinician response

The response of physicians who care for young athletes should be to educate them to the real and unacceptable dangers that anabolic steroids present, dangers that far outweigh any potential benefit to weight or strength gain.[36] Anabolic steroids have been banned by the National Collegiate Athletic Association (NCAA), International Olympic Committee, and various professional sporting associations. Young adolescents who are still developing cognitive skills may not be able to appreciate the dangers of drugs taken now that will cause serious medical damage later in life. Even older athletes with "adult" thinking skills may choose the risks of such drugs for the potential of "winning at any cost" philosophy. Even coaches and trainers may be drawn into allowing harm to their athletes if it leads to a winning season while some parents may condone use of these drugs if parents conclude it will lead to a college sports scholarship or a "successful" professional sports career. Thus, society must be clearly educated to these dangers and though some of these steroids are used to treat management of wasting caused by HIV/AIDS or chronic renal failure, these drugs should not be used by athletes to improve sports performance.

Use of concomitant agents

Athletes who take anabolic steroids may take additional drugs to boost the anabolic effects of steroids, including androstenedione, human growth hormone (hGH), DHEA (dehydroepiandrosterone), methamphetamine, and clenbuterol.[4–6] Diuretics are taken to reduce fluid retention or dilute urine in attempts to prevent a positive sports doping test. These diuretics include spironolactone, furosemide, and hydrochlorothiazide. Tamoxifen is an antiestrogen taken by athletes abusing anabolic steroids in attempts to avoid feminization effects. hCG and clomiphene are taken after the end of an anabolic steroid cycle to reduce hypogonadotrophic hypogonadism and to reduce testicular atrophy and infertility.[34] ACTH (corticotrophin) is taken to increase endogenous corticosteroids to induce euphoria, while various narcotics and other illicit drugs are also abused for their euphoric effects. Additional drugs abused include stimulants, analgesics

(such as oxycodone, meperidine, morphine, hydrocodone, others), antibiotics, and corticosteroids.

DHEA (dehydroepiandrosterone)

DHEA is a hormone produced in the adrenal glands and testicles and is converted to androstenedione or androstenediol. These are subsequently converted to testosterone and testosterone and androstenedione can further be aromatized to estrone and estradiol.[37] DHEA became available in 1996 as an OTC nutritional supplement and is used by some athletes as an alternative to anabolic steroids.[38] It is proposed that DHEA can increase testosterone and insulinlike growth factor (IGF-1) which have anabolic properties. DHEA has been touted to reduce fat, promote muscle mass, increase strength, and improve sexual performance, and a wide range of doses have been used, from 50 to 100 mg/d up to 1600 mg a day.[4,38] Studies have not supported these claims including a study by Broeder and colleagues deemed the "Andro Project."[39] Patients took androstenedione, androstenediol (200 mg daily), or placebo along with a high-intensity resistance-training program for 12 weeks.[39] The authors found that testosterone levels increased transiently but returned to baseline by 12 weeks and neither agent improved lean body mass or increased muscle strength when compared to placebo.[39] They also noted that estrone and estradiol levels were significantly elevated.[39] Side effects are not well known owing to few long-term studies. DHEA has been associated with irreversible virilization in women and gynecomastia in men.[38] Theoretically, high doses could lead to excessive androgen levels and produce the same side effects as anabolic-androgenic steroids.[38] DHEA is banned by many sporting organizations.

Androstenedione

Androstenedione is an androgen that is a precursor of testosterone, dihydrotestosterone, estrone, and estradiol and is produced in the adrenal glands and testes.[4,7] It was legally available until 2004 when the Anabolic Steroid Control Act was enacted. Because of the potential for serious health adverse events of androstenedione that were similar to anabolic-androgenic steroids, androstenedione was placed into scheduled III controlled substance.[38–40] DHEA was not added because of claims by the lobbyists that it was effective as an antiaging substance and had minimal risks.[38–40] Androstenedione is taken as a "T-booster" and used to raise testosterone ("T") levels and increase muscle mass using high doses such as 100 to 300 mg/d and also used 60 minutes before a sports event.

Androstenedione is taken in a pill form in the US and nasal form in Europe, often in combination with different anabolic steroids in various cycling patterns. As with DHEA, androstenedione does not effectively raise testosterone levels nor increase lean body mass, muscle strength or improve performance.[38] Androstenedione has a similar side effect profile compared to anabolic steroids. It is banned by most sporting organizations and should not be taken by growing individuals or those at risk for breast cancer and prostate cancer.[4,7] Despite the fact that androstenedione can no longer be produced as a dietary supplement, it remains a popular sports doping drug, though use among high school students in the United States has dropped since 2001.1[21]

Human Growth Hormone

Growth hormone is secreted from the pituitary gland in a pulsatile fashion that varies with gender and age.[40,41] Concentrations are higher in neonates and during puberty and are positively influenced during slow wave sleep, exercise, hypoglycemia, amino acid intake (leucine and arginine), increased temperature, and stress.[40,42] Growth hormone leads to the production of IGF-1, which mediates the anabolic actions of growth hormone.[40] This results in increased total body protein turnover and muscle mass.[40] Despite a lack of evidence to support, hGH is claimed to have anabolic effects that increase lean body mass and decrease fat mass.[40] It is also purported to enhance performance within endurance and power sports.[40,43] As a doping agent, hGH is often used in combination with anabolic steroids in power sports or with erythropoietin in endurance sports because of their theoretical synergistic effect.[44] The use of chronic, high doses by athletes has the potential to lead to significant side effects ranging from infection (caused by nonsterile needles) to hypertension, insulin resistance, osteoarthritis, and visceromegaly to name a few.[40,45,46] hGH is difficult to detect in those using it, and hGH bought from the black market may contain growth hormone obtained from human pituitary glands and increases the risk for disease transmission.[40] Its exorbitant cost, at $3000 or more per month, still does not prevent its widespread illegal use.[4,7]

Gamma-hydroxybutyrate (GHB)

GHB (*"Liquid Ecstasy," "G," "Georgia home boy"*) is a central nervous system depressant that reduces inhibition and induces euphoria.[4,47] It has been used medically to treat cataplexy. However, GHB is taken by various athletes such as body builders who hope that growth hormone will be increased during sleep resulting in increased muscle growth. It has also become a popular date rape pill since GHB is a tasteless, odorless, and colorless chemical that can be placed in a liquid to induce sedation and amnesia lasting for several hours. Subsequently, a sexual assault can take place and the victim has no memory of this event or the perpetrator. GHB is quickly cleared from the body and difficult to detect. An overdose of this chemical leads to severe respiratory depression, coma, and death.

GHB is produced as a clear liquid or white powder and can be made by local, clandestine laboratories with ingredients and instructions easily found on the Internet. The production of GHB and its use as a sports doping agent is now illegal owing to its toxicity. Therefore, some athletes are using precursors or metabolites of this chemical, such as GBL (gamma-butyro-lactone) or 1-4 butanediol (BD), an industrial solvent. Some nutritional supplement manufacturers are now using BD (instead of GHB) and one can find various combinations of these drugs in "health food" stores where it is marketed as a muscle builder, sleep-inducing drug, or sexual performance enhancer. BD can be found in floor stripper and paint thinner products and its ingestion can induce emesis, coma, seizures, and death.

Ephedrine

Ephedrine is the primary alkaloid derived from *Ephedra sinica* which is also known as ma huang.[48] Other alkaloids include pseudoephedrine, norephedrine and norpseudoephedrine.[48] Traditionally ephedrine has been used to relieve cold symptoms but the purpose within sports-related events include weight loss, enhance alertness, and lessen feelings of fatigue to improve performance.[48–51] Ephedrine is a sympathomimetic and exerts a variety of CNS, cardiovascular, and metabolic effects.[48] Numerous adverse effects are noted with these products, including elevated blood pressure, seizures, insomnia, tremors, arrhythmias, anxiety, cerebrovascular accidents, myocardial infarctions, paranoid psychosis, and death. Ephedra was banned by the FDA in 2004 because of serious adverse events including death and is banned by numerous amateur and professional sport organizations.[48,52] Because of the ban on ephedra, supplement manufacturers have turned to *Citrus aurantium* (also known as bitter orange, sour orange, Zhi shi) which contains synephrine.[53,54] Synephrine is a milder sympathomimetic with a similar action and side effect profile to ephedrine.[50] *Citrus aurantium* has been banned by some sports organizations and athletes should be cautioned to avoid these products.

Clenbuterol (Clensasma; Broncoterol)

Clenbuterol is a beta-agonist (substituted phenylethanolamine) available in Europe, Central America, and South America.[4,7] Traditionally it is used to manage asthma at a dose of 0.02 to 0.04 mg/d. It has also been used with anabolic steroids in unproven hopes of reducing adipose tissue and augmenting lean body mass at doses up to 0.16 mg/d. It is given orally for full absorption and has a long half-life of 34 hours. Clenbuterol is used as an ergogenic agent in a 2-day-on and 2-day-off pattern with complete discontinuation of the drug before the sports event, since it can be detected up to 4 days after the use.

Side effects include headaches, anxiety, dizziness, tremor, nausea, tachycardia, and insomnia. It has also been implicated in inducing myocardial infarction, cardiac arrhythmias, cardiac muscle hypertrophy, and cerebrovascular accidents. Use of this product is banned by various sporting organizations (Table 7-5).

Creatine

Creatine is a nonessential amino acid synthesized in the liver, kidneys, and pancreas from glycine, arginine, and methionine.[4,7,55] It is found in fish, meat, milk, and other foods. Meat and fish are key food sources and provide more than half of the daily requirement. The typical diet provides 1 to 2 grams a day of creatine. Creatine supplement (creatine monohydrate or with phosphorus) is available as a crystalline powder that is tasteless and dissolves in liquids and it has become the most popular "nutritional" supplement among athletes.[4–7,12,26,27,56]

Ninety-five percent of creatine is stored in skeletal muscle and the remaining 5% is found in the heart, brain and testes.[55] Within the skeletal muscle, one-third of creatine is stored as free creatine and two-thirds is stored in a phosphorylated form. Creatine is an energy substrate for skeletal muscle contraction and cells with high energy requirements utilize creatine as phosphocreatine, functioning as a donor of phosphate to produce adenosine triphosphate (ATP) from adenosine diphosphate (ADP). Skeletal muscle cells store sufficient phosphocreatine and ATP for approximately 10 seconds of high-intensity exercise. Creatine supplementation is provided with the purpose of augmenting resting phosphocreatine levels in muscles and also free creatine to delay fatigue for a brief time and allow sustained sports performance. Phosphocreatine maintains increased energy ATP levels, provides action as a proton buffer, and its use can lead to reduced glycolysis. As the phosphocreatine levels drop, glycolysis

Table 7-5.

Drugs Banned from Various Sports Competitions (Partial List)

A. Anbaolic steroids (see Table 7-3)
B. Beta blockers
  1. Atenolol
  2. Metoprolol
  3. Propanolol
C. Diuretics
  1. Furosemide
  2. Hydrochlorothiazide
  3. Spironolactone
D. Narcotics
  1. Dextropropoxyphene (Darvon)
  2. Morphine
  3 Meperidine (Demerol)
E. Peptide hormones
  1. ACTH (Corticotropin)
  2. EPO (Erythropoietin)
  3. hCG (human chorionic gonadotropin)
  4. hGH (human growth hormone)
F. Stimulants
  1. Amphetamines
  2. Caffeine
  3. Ephedrine
G. Others
  1. Local anesthetics
  2. Corticosteroids
  3. Alcohol
  4. Illicit drugs, including marijuana, cocaine, amphetamines

Reprinted from Greydanus DE, Patel DR. Sports doping in the adolescent athlete. Asian J Paediatr Pract. 2000;4:9-14.

increases. The optimal amount of exercise eventually ceases because of muscle fatigue as a result of an increase in hydrogen ions, lactate accumulation, and a reduction in ATP.

Controversy still surrounds creatine as to whether it is an ergogenic agent. Differences in study methodology and potential bias in results make it difficult to draw sound conclusions regarding its efficacy.[48,55] Multiple reviews have concluded that creatine does improve muscle power with short bouts of near-maximal to maximal exertion and improve performance with repeated bouts of maximal exertion.[48,57–59] Some athletes may have a low intracellular concentration of creatine and not respond to supplementation; others may have a high level at baseline and may also not respond. There are no studies that note any improvement in long-term endurance sports and most *in vivo* studies with creatine supplementation show no ergogenic effects at all.[4,7]

Table 7-6.

Side Effects of Creatine Supplementation[4–7,26,27,56]

Common
Weight gain owing to fluid (water) retention
Abdominal pain
Nausea, emesis
Diarrhea
Dyspepsia
Anxiety
Fatigue
Headaches
Rash
Dyspnea
Elevation in serum creatinine

Less Common
Muscle cramps
Muscle strain
Dehydration in hot/humid weather
Suppression of endogenous synthesis of creatine
Renal dysfunction
Atrial fibrillation
Rhabdomyolysis

Table 7-7.

Claims of Manufacturers of Amino Acids as Ergogenic Agents

1. Antioxidant effects
2. Reduce lactate accumulation
3. Ammonia detoxification
4. Various anticatabolic and anabolic effects
5. Augmented lean muscle mass
6. Augmented production of growth hormone
7. Augmented levels of serotonin and somatotropin
8. Muscle glycogen sparing
9. Sports performance enhancement

Athletes typically take a loading dose of 20 g/d (5 g four times a day) for 5 to 7 days followed by a maintenance dose of 2 to 5 g each day. The aim of this or other supplement schedules is to optimize phosphocreatine levels in muscle. Because of a decrease in muscle creatine over time despite supplementation, cycling has been suggested to counteract this phenomenon.[48,60] Cycling consist of three phases: a loading phase of 1 week, a maintenance phase of 5 to 8 weeks and an off-cycle phase of 2 to 4 weeks.[48] Increased muscle mass may occur (0.5–2 kg in 1 month), especially if the supplementation occurs with exercise. However, the increased muscle mass is owing to water retention and not increased protein synthesis. Because of the possibility for dehydration and heat illness, it is recommended to stay well hydrated with six to eight glasses of water per day while taking creatine.[48]

One of the first large-scale studies to document creatine use was conducted by the NCAA in 1997.[48,54] More than 14,000 athletes from Division I–III sports were surveyed and results indicated a 32% use of creatine in the previous 12 months.[48,54] Since then, additional studies continue to document the widespread use from adolescent to professional athletes. Annual sales of more than $200 million are noted and its popularity continues despite the mixed results of studies evaluating its ergogenic effects. Although creatine is generally regarded as safe, a number of side effects are noted (Table 7-6). There are no long-term studies available and it is not banned by the major sports organizations. However, the American College of Sports Medicine recommends that athletes younger than 18 years do not use creatine supplement.[42]

Protein and Amino Acid Supplements

Protein and amino acid supplements are a popular group of nutritional supplements long advocated as sports-enhancing agents.[4,7,9,15–17] Nutritionally adequate amounts of these substances are important for the health of humans and active athletes may need more protein than inactive individuals (see Chapter 6-5). Protein and amino acid supplements may help someone who has a deficient diet for a variety of reasons.

Protein and amino acid supplements have been used by athletes to speed recovery from exercise and increase body mass and strength.[48] The debate has continued over any potential sports performance effects when taking excessive amounts by someone who has a normal nutritional intake.[9] Table 7-7 lists some of the unproven claims made by manufacturers of these products. Side effects of amino acid supplementation include metabolic imbalance, diarrhea at high doses, and adverse reactions to various impurities found in these products. Table 7-8 reviews some of these chemicals, while Table 7-9 reviews sports doping claims in regard to mineral supplementation.

Antioxidants

Antioxidants include *ascorbic acid (vitamin C), beta carotene (precursor of vitamin A),* and *alpha tocopherol*

Table 7-8.

Amino Acid Supplements[4,7]

Amino Acid		Manufacturer Claims
Arginine	Semiessential amino acid; stimulates human growth hormone and insulin secretion; increases creatine stores; stimulates protein synthesis	Increases muscle mass and strength if takingl 2–10 g/d along with resistance training
Aspartates	Salts of aspartic acid (nonessential AA)	Spares muscle glycogen stores, serve as a substrate for energy production, enhance exercise performance
Branched-chain amino acids (BCAAs)	Leucine (essential AA); Isoleucine (essential AA); Valine (essential AA)	Aid in endurance exercise by decreasing fatigue. Wide variety of health benefits including sports doping effects.
L-Carnitine	Essential AA found in meat and dairy products; synthesized from lysine and methionine in the liver and kidneys; all but 5% found in muscle and heart tissue	Improve the oxidation of fatty acid; decrease the accumulation of lactate and spare muscle glycogen
Glutamine	Nonessential amino acid; most abundant AA in human muscle and plasma; found in almonds, soybeans, and peanuts	Induces release of human growth hormone and ACTH; linked to overall enhanced high intensity resistance training effects; optimizes immune function.
Glycine	Nonessential amino acid; important for the synthesis of proteins, ATP, creatine, glycogen, and others	Overall health enhancement; precursor to creatine but lack of ergogenic effect
HMB (beta-hydroxy-beta-methylbutyrate)	Metabolite of leucine; non essential nutrient; found in breast milk, catfish, citrus fruits	Proposed to increase lean body mass and strength; also may decrease protein breakdown and enhance repair mechanisms; provided as an "anabolic" supplement during strength training, sometimes with creatine; also used in hopes of preventing weakened immune responses after intensive physical activity
Linoleic acid (Conjugated linoleic acid [CLA])	Linoleic acid is a nonessential AA found in heat-treated cheese, milk, yogurt, beef, and venison; CLA is derived from linoleic acid isomers	CLA is given in hopes of increasing lean body mass and decrease body fat; proposed to enhance the immune and bone mineral status of the consumer
Lysine	Essential AA; L-lysine is a necessary building block for protein synthesis; found in meat, poultry, dairy food and wheat germ; stimulates growth hormone secretion.	Involved in glycogen synthesis and energy production; wide variety of health benefits are proposed when taken as a supplement
Ornithine	Nonprotein amino acid; used for the production of L-arginine, L-proline, and polyamines; stimulates growth hormone secretion (high dose)	Anabolic effects, improves athletic performance, enhances immune system, and aids In wound healing; may be used in conjunction with arginine for ergogenic effects
L-tryptophan	Essential AA	Overall health enhancement; in 1980s, was linked to eosinophilia-myalgia syndrome (EMS) and deaths due to impurities found in the product; purported to aid sleep, enhance mood and decrease carbohydrate cravings; L-tryptophan still consumed today by athletes

Table 7-9.

Mineral Supplements[4,7]

Mineral		Manufacturer Claims
Boron	Substance that is essential for plants, not humans; found in foods of plant origin: noncitrus fruits, nuts, legumes, leafy vegetables	Increase muscle mass by augmenting testosterone; increase lean body mass and strength
Calcium	Mineral and metallic bivalent element that is found in dairy products; daily intake should be 1000–1300 mg/d for 11–24 y olds; supplement if athlete is on a low calcium diet; yogurt and skim milk may be acceptable to athletes concerned with consuming fat in dairy products	Supplementing will improve bone health. Beneficial if on a low calcium diet.
Chromium	Essential trace element; found in prunes, meats, nuts, mushrooms, apples, raisins, whole grain breads, broccoli, wine, beer, brewer's yeast; intake is often poor in the general population; lost in the urine during exercise, though not as much for those with regular exercise; chromium picolinate is the most common chromium supplement	Help in glucose metabolism, regulate insulin , levels improve body composition and aid in weight loss.
Iron	Metallic element that occurs in heme (i.e., hemoglobin, myoglobin, others); sources include red meats, fish, poultry, lentils, and beans; essential component of proteins involved in oxygen transport and regulation of cell differentiation and growth	Supplementation will enhance performance in those who are deficient
Magnesium	Alkaline earth element involved in various physiologic functions, including energy metabolism and muscle contraction; sources include green vegetables, nuts, and seeds and whole unrefined grains	Improved muscle efficiency, raise lactate synthesis, raise oxygen consumption, increase strength
Vanadium; Vandyl Sulfate	Vanadium is an essential trace mineral; found in mushrooms, soybeans, shellfish; no known deficiency state described in humans	Increase muscle mass, lower blood glucose, increase glycogen synthesis and storage, insulin-like action

(vitamin E).[4,17] Various products containing these and other antioxidants are marketed as sports doping agents by lessening injury from free radicals and other "reactive oxygen" chemicals that are produced during exercise. Lipid peroxidation affects oxidative stress and is one of the mechanisms related to injury. Antioxidants may decrease injury by reducing lipid peroxidation. Antioxidants may be particularly useful for smokers, mountain climbers, those with diabetes mellitus, situations in which one is chronically exposed to air pollution, and those (including athletes) with a limited antioxidant diet.

The benefit of antioxidant supplementation in athletes with normal diets remains unproven. Adverse events may result from taking very high doses of vitamin C and beta carotene. Guidelines for those wishing to take antioxidant supplementation include 10,000 to 30,000 IU of beta-carotene, 250 to 1000 mg of vitamin

C, and 400 IU of vitamin E daily.[4,17] The recommended daily allowance (RDA) of vitamin E is 22.5 IU/d and 75mg/d (females) to 90mg/d (males) for vitamin C. No RDA has been established for beta-carotene.

Miscellaneous Agents

Table 7-10 reviews a variety of other agents with proposed sports performance enhancements. These include alpha-lipoic acid, beta-blockers, blood doping, caffeine, carbohydrates, choline, chrysin, DMSO (dimethyl sulfoxide), erythropoietin (EPO), illicit drugs, inosine, nonsteroidal anti-inflammatory agents, probiotics, sodium bicarbonate, *Tribulus terrestris*, and other miscellaneous agents (gamma oryzanol, Ginkgo biloba, Ginseng, Yohimbine, and others).[4,7,47,56,61–73]

Table 7–10. (Continued)

Miscellaneous Agents[48,60]

Agent		Claims of Benefit and Adverse Effects	Effect on Performance
Probiotics	Ingestion of live food ingredients (*i.e., Lactobacillus species, Bifidobacterium species, and yeast*); can be found naturally in fermented foods such as yogurt, sauerkraut, others.	Various overall health benefits proposed, such as improvement in immune function, gastrointestinal function, others; proposed sports doping effect based on reduction in exercise-induced fatigue	Not proven; under current research
Sodium bicarbonate	Alkaline salt	Used to delay fatigue during bouts of exercise that are limited by acidosis; may be helpful where blood flow can increase to accommodate an increase in by-products due to muscles at work Adverse effects: nausea, cramps, diarrhea, severe metabolic alkalosis with excessive doses	Yes
Tribulus terrestris	Medicinal herb; active ingredients are steroidal glycoside (saponins); often used for infertility, erectile dysfunction, and low libido	Proposed that it increases tesosterone by ↑ LH levels as well as DHEA and estrogen; leads to improvement in sports performance; may enhance mood and libido Adverse effects: cytotoxic, hepatotoxic, phototoxic, and neurotoxic	Not proven
Water	Essential liquid needed for life; necessary for hemodynamic balance and avoidance of heat-related disorders.	Excessive water intake can lead to water intoxication and severe electrolyte dysfunction and death.	Excessive intake not ergogenic and must be avoided.
Yohimbine (Yohimbe)	Yohimbe is an evergreen tree found in Western Africa; Yohimbine is an alkaloid found in the inner bark of the tree; primarily used to treat impotence	Promoted as an ergogenic substance by enhancing testosterone and aiding fat loss	Not proven; *Caveat emptor!*

REFERENCES

1. Porter R. *The Greatest Benefit to Mankind: A Medical History of Humanity.* New York, NY: WW Norton & Co.; 1998.
2. Scholl R. Der Papyrus Ebers. Die grösste Buchrolle zur Heilkunde Altägyptens (Schriften aus der Universitätsbibliothek 7), Leipzig, Germany, 2002.
3. Grollman AP. Alternative medicine: the importance of evidence in medicine and medical evidence. *Acad Med.* 2001;76 (3): 221-223.
4. Greydanus DE, Patel DR. Sports doping in the adolescent athlete: the hope, hype, and hyperbole. *Pediatr Clin N Am.* 2002;49(4);829-855.
5. McDevitt ER. Ergogenic drugs in sports. In: DeLee JC, Drez D Jr, Miller MD, eds. *DeLee & Drez's Orthopaedic Sports Medicine: Principles and Practice.* Philadelphia, PA: Saunders/Elsevier; 2003:471-483.
6. Laos C, Metzl JD. Performing-enhancing drug use in young athletes. *Adolesc Med.* 2006;17:719-731.
7. Greydanus DE, Patel DR. Sports doping in the adolescent athlete. *Asian J Paediatr Prac.,* 2000;4(1):9-14.
8. Talalay P, Talalay P. The importance of using scientific principles in the development of medicinal agents from plants. *Acad Med.* 2001;76 (3):175-184.
9. Chorley JN. Dietary supplements as ergogenic agents. *Adolesc Health Update.* 2000;13(1):1-7.
10. Gregory A, Fitch R. Sports medicine; performance-enhancing drugs. *Pediatr Clin N Am* 2007;54:797-806.
11. Sampson W. The need for educational reform in teaching about alternative therapies. *Acad Med.* 2001;76(3): 248-250.

12. American Academy of Pediatrics Committee on Sports Medicine and Fitness. Policy statement: use of performance-enhancing substances. *Pediatrics.* 2005;118:1151-1158.

13. Koch J. Performance enhancing substances and their use among adolescent athletes. *Pediatr Rev.* 2002;23:310-317.

14. Metz J. Performance-enhancing drug use in the young athlete. *Pediatr Ann.* 2002;31:27-32.

15. Armsey TD, Green GA. Nutrition supplements. Science vs. hype. *Phys Sportsmed.* 1997;25:77-92.

16. Blazevich AJ, Giorgi A. Effect of testosterone administration and weight training on muscle architecture. *Med Sci Sports Exerc.* 2001;33:1688-1693.

17. Powers SK, Hamilton K. Antioxidants and exercise. *Clin Sport Med.* 1999;18:525-536.

18. Silver MD. Use of ergogenic aids by athletes. *J Am Acad Orthop Surg.* 2001;9:61-70.

19. Yesalis C, Bahrke M. Doping among adolescent athletes. *Clin Endocrinol Metab.* 2000;14:25-35.

20. Tokish JM, Kocher MS, Hawkins RJ. Ergogenic aids: a review of basic science, performance, side effects, and status in sports. *Am J Sports Med.* 2004;32:1543-1553.

21. Johnston LD, O'Malley PM, Bachman JG, Schulenberg JE. *Monitoring the Future National Results on Adolescent Drug Use; Overview of Key Findings, 2006.* Bethesda, MD: National Institute on Drug Abuse; 2007. NIH Publication 04-5506.

22. Eaton DK, Kann L, Kinchen S, et al. Youth risk behavior surveillance-United States. 2005. *MMWR.* 2006;55(SS-5):1-108.

23. Castillo E, Comstock R. Prevalence of use of performance-enhancing substances among United States adolescents. *Pediatr Clin North Am.* 2007;54:663-675.

24. Whitehead R, Chillag S. Elliott D. Anabolic steroid use among adolescents in a rural state. *J Fam Pract.* 1992;35(4):401-405.

25. Scott DM, Wagner JC, Barlow TW. Anabolic steroid use among adolescents in Nebraska schools. *Am J Health Syst Pharm.* 1996;53(17):2068-2072.

26. Smith J, Dahm D. Creatine use among a select population of high school athletes. *Mayo Clin Proc.* 2000;75:1257-1263.

27. Metzl JD, Levine SR, Gershel JC. Creatine use among young athletes. *Pediatrics.* 2001;108: 421-425.

28. Berning JM, Adams KJ, Bryant SA, et al. Prevalence and perceived prevalence of anabolic steroid use among college-aged students. *Med Sci Sports Exerc.* 2004;36:S350.

29. Reeder BM, Patel DR. The prevalence of nutritional supplement use among high school students: a pilot study. *Med Sci Sports Exerc.* 2002;34(Suppl 1):S193.

30. Kayton S, Cullen RW, Memken JA, Rutter R. Supplement and ergogenic aid use by competitive male and female high school athletes. *Med Sci Sports Exerc.* 2002;33:S193.

31. American Academy of Pediatrics. Adolescents and anabolic steroids: a subject review. Committee on Sports Medicine and Fitness. *Pediatrics.* 1997;99:1-7.

32. Evans N, Parkinson A. Steroid use and the young athlete. *ACSM Fit Society Page.* 2005;(Fall):5-8.

33. Avary D, Pope HG Jr. Anabolic-androgenic steroids as a gateway to opioid dependence. *N Engl J Med.* 2000;342:1532.

34. Casavant M, Blake K, Griffith J, et al. Consequences of use of anabolic androgenic steroids. *Pediatr Clin North Am.* 2007;54:677-690.

35. Hall RCW, Hall RCW. Abuse of supraphysiologic doses of anabolic steroids. *South Med J.* 2005;98:550-555.

36. Goldberg L, MacKinnon D, Elliot D, et al. The adolescent training and learning to avoid steroids program: preventing drug use and promoting health behavors. *Arch Pediatr Adolesc Med.* 2000;154:332-338.

37. Labrie F, Luu-The V, Lin S, et al. The key role of 17beta-hydroxysteroid dehydrogenase in sex steroid biochemistry. *Steroids* 1997;62:148-158.

38. Smurawa T, Congeni J. Testosterone precursors: use and abuse in pediatric athletes. *Pediatr Clin North Am.* 2007;54: 787-796.

39. Broeder CE, Quindry J, Brittingham K, et al. The andro project. *Arch Intern Med.* 2000;160:3093-3104.

40. Buzzini S. Abuse of growth hormone among young athletes. *Pediatr Clin North Am.* 2007;54:823-843.

41. Ho K, Evans W, Blizzard R, et al. Effects of sex and age on the 24-hour profile of growth hormone secretion in man: importance of endogenous estradiol concentrations. *J Clin Endocrinol Metab.* 1987;64(1):51-58.

42. Muller E, Locatelli V, Cocchi D. Neuroendocrine control of growth hormone secretion. *Physiol Rev.* 1999;79(2):511-607.

43. Jenkins P. Growth hormone and exercise: Physiology, use and abuse. *Growth Horm IGF Res.* 2001;11(Suppl A):S71-S77.

44. Schnirring L. Growth hormone doping: the search for a test. *Phys Sportsmed.* 2000;28(4):16-18.

45. Cittadini A, Berggren A, Longobardi S, et al. Supraphysiological doses of GH induce rapid changes in cardiac morphology and function. *J Clin Endocrinol Metab.* 2002;87(4):1654-1659.

46. Melmed S. Medical progress: acromegaly. *N Engl J Med.* 2006;355(24):2558-2573.

47. Greydanus DE, Patel DR. The adolescent and substance abuse: current concepts. *Dis Mon.* 2005;51(7):387-432.

48. Lattavo A, Kopperus A, Rogers P. Creatine and other supplements. *Pediatr Clin North Am.* 2007;54:735-760.

49. Tokish J, Kocher M, Hawkins R. Ergogenic aids; a review of basic science, performance, side effects, and status in sports. *Am J Sports Med.* 2004;32(6):1543-1553.

50. Lombardo J. Supplements and athletes. *South Med J.* 2004;97(9):877-879.

51. DesJardins M. Supplement use in the adolescent athlete. *Curr Sports Med Rep.* 2002;1:369-373.

52. Keisler B, Hosey R. Ergogenic aids: an update on ephedra. *Curr Sports Med Rep.* 2005;4:231-235.

53. Fugh-Berman A, Myers A. Citrus aurantium, an ingredient of dietary supplements marketed for weight loss: current status of clinical and basic research. *Exp Biol Med.* 2004;229:698-704.

54. The National Collegiate Athletic Association. NCAA study of substance use and abuse habits of college student-athletes. http://www.ncaa.org/sports_sciences/education/199709abuse.pdf. Accessed June 20, 2008.

55. Gosa B, Walker P. Common nutritional supplements used to enhance athletic performance. US Pharmacist. http://www.uspharmacist.com/print.asp?page=ce/10555 3.default.htm. Accessed September 7, 2007.

56. Terjung RL, Clarkson P, Eichner ER, et al. American College of Sports Medicine Roundtable: The physiological and health effects of oral creatine supplementation. *Med Sci Sport Exerc.* 2000;32(3):706-717.

57. Terjung R, Clarkson P, Eichner R, et al. The American College of Sports Medicine roundtable on the physiological and health effects of oral creatine supplementation. *Med Sci Sports Exerc.* 2000;32(3):706-717.

58. Hespel P, Maughan R, Greenhaff P. Dietary supplements for football. *J Sports Sci.* 2006;24(7):746-761.

59. Ciocca M. Medication and supplement use by athletes. *Clin Sports Med.* 2005;24:719-738.

60. Derave W, Eiginde B, Hespel P. Creatine supplementation in health and disease: what is the evidence for long term efficacy? *Mol Cell Biochem.* 2003;244:49-55.

61. Bent S, Tiedt TN, Odden MC, Shlipak MG. The relative safety of ephedra compared to other herbal products. *Ann Intern Med.* 2003;138:468-471.

62. Green BA. Recreational drug use in athletes. In: DeLee JC, Drez D Jr, Miller MD, eds. *DeLee & Drez's Orthopaedic Sports Medicine: Principles and Practice.* Philadelphia, PA: Saunders/Elsevier; 2003:483-492.

63. Greyanus DE, Patel DR. Attention deficit hyperactivity disorder across the lifespan. *Dis Mon.* 2007;53(2):65-132.

64. Petersons M, Bruss MB, Bruss JB. Adolescent nutrition. In: Greydanus DE, Patel DR , Pratt HD, eds. *Essential Adolescent Medicine.*New York, NY: McGraw-Hill Medical Publishers;2006:615-634.

65. Panel on Macronutrients, Standing Committee on the Scientific Evaluation of Dietary Reference Intakes. *Dietary Reference Intakes for Energy, Carbohydrate, Fiber, Fat, Fatty Acids, Cholesterol, Protein, and Amino Acids (Macronutrients).* Washington, DC: National Academy Press; 2002.

66. Nichols AW. Probiotics and athletic performance: a systemic review. *Curr Sports Med Rep.* 2007;6:269-273.

67. Clancy RL, Gleeson M, Cox A, et al. Reversal in fatigued athletes of a defect in interferon γ secretion after administration of *Lactobacillus acidophilus. Br J Sports Med.* 2006;40:351-354.

68. Cogeni J, Miller S. Supplements and drugs used to enhance athletic performance. *Pediatr Clin North Am.* 2002;49:435-461.

69. Burns RD, Schiller MR, Merrick MA, Wolf KN. Intercollegiate student athlete use of nutritional supplements and the role of athletic trainers and dieticians in nutritional counseling. *J Am Diet Assoc.* 2004;104: 246-249.

70. Green GA, Catlin DH, Starcevic B. Analysis of over-the-counter dietary supplements. *Clin J Sports Med.* 2001;11: 254-259.

71. Elliott DL, Goldberg L, Moe EL, et al. Preventing substance use and disordered eating: Initial outcomes of the ATHENA (athletes targeting healthy exercise and nutrition alternatives) program. *Arch Pediatr Adolesc Med.* 2004;158:1043-1049.

72. Hampton T. More scrutiny for dietary supplements? *JAMA.* 2005;293:27-28.

73. Patel DR, Greydanus DE. Nutritional supplement use by young athletes: an update. *Int Pediatr.* 2005;29(1):15-21.

CHAPTER 8

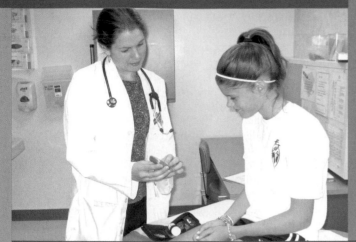

Preparticipation Evaluation

Donald E. Greydanus and
Dilip R. Patel

A careful medical history and physical examination are the cornerstones of effective clinical practice when caring for children and adolescents.[1] The frequency, format, contents, and usefulness of a sports preparticipation evaluation (SPPE) in predicting and preventing morbidity and mortality related to sport participation have not been validated by any long-term systematic research. Studies suggest that between 0.3% and 1.3% of the athletes are disqualified from participation based on SPPE findings and between 3.2% and 13.9% of the athletes require further evaluation.[2] In the United States all high school athletes are required to have an annual SPPE.

The athlete should receive an SPPE at least annually, preferably 6 to 8 weeks before the season or event to allow for adequate rehabilitation of most injuries that may be found and to allow for further medical evaluation of any other health problems identified.[2–6] SPPE is not meant to replace an annual comprehensive evaluation by the athlete's primary care pediatrician.[7] The main goals of the SPPE are to assess the general health of the athlete, to identify any health condition that may predispose the athlete to increased risk for injury or illness, and to match the athlete with the sport best suited for him or her depending on physical health, cognitive abilities, and athletic abilities.[8–10]

SPPE is best done in an office setting by the athlete's primary care physician. This will allow for continuity of care and exploration of a wider range of health-related issues in a confidential manner. SPPE is not a substitute for recommended health maintenance or preventive health visits. However, for some athletes SPPE may be the only health care visit. These athletes must be strongly recommended to establish care with a primary care physician. It is also suggested that SPPE should be integrated into the regular well child or preventive health care visits after 6 years of age thus avoiding the need for a separate visit for SPPE.

SPPE MEDICAL HISTORY

A comprehensive SPPE medical history as obtained from the athlete and parents is the most important aspect of the SPPE and can identify about three-quarters of important issues associated with sports participation. Youth are more comfortable fully clothed while the medical history is obtained. Data can be obtained from various sources, including the athlete, parents or guardians, previous medical records, and even school records. Standard questionnaires may be used for initial screening. Key elements to be explored in the history are summarized in Table 8-1.

History of Medical Conditions

The medical history should identify any known medical conditions (i.e., asthma, epilepsy, diabetes mellitus, hepatitis, high blood pressure, coagulation disorders, one functional kidney, one functional or anatomical eye, juvenile rheumatoid arthritis, spondylolysis, anorexia nervosa, pregnancy, depression, attention-deficit/hyperactivity disorder, and others).[2–4,7] Such knowledge will allow for proper management of these conditions in the athlete to ensure safe and continued sport participation.

History of Heat Disorders

A past history of heat-related illness is a risk factor for recurrent heat-related illness and this will allow for appropriate preventive measures to be implemented for the athlete.

Table 8-1.

Key Elements of SPPE History

Past history
Major trauma (musculoskeletal, head and neck, chest, abdomen)
Major surgeries (spine, cardiac, abdomen, genitourinary)
Chronic disease
Heat-related illness

Medications
Therapeutic medications
Nutritional supplements
Over-the-counter medications

Allergies
Environmental
Drug allergy
Food allergy
History of anaphylactic reactions
Exercise-induced allergic or anaphylactic reactions

Nutritional
Dietary habits
Attempts to manipulate weight
Recent weight loss or gain

Neurologic
Details of head and neck trauma
Symptoms of concussion (see Chapter 11)
History of seizures
Exercise-related headaches

Pulmonary
Exercise-related difficulty breathing
Chronic-exercise related cough
Persistent wheezing
Cardiovascular screening (see Chapter 14)

Health risk behaviors
Pathogenic weight control
High-risk sexual practices
Abuse of illicit drugs
Use of performance-enhancing agents

Other
Recent febrile illness
Undue fatigue
Hearing problems
Vision problems
Eye trauma and surgery
Missing paired organ
Musculoskeletal injuries
Immunization status
Menstrual history in females

History of Musculoskeletal Conditions

Ask about previous or current musculoskeletal problems so that they can be clearly identified and treated, resulting in minimal interference with the athlete's sports performance.[5,11] If there is a positive history for previous musculoskeletal injury, further inquiry is important regarding the nature of this injury, what treatment

Table 8-2.

Factors Influencing Eligibility for Sports Participation

1. What is the overall health status and fitness level of the athlete?
2. Is the desired activity a contact or noncontact sport?
3. What are the static or dynamic demands of the chosen sport?
4. What is the competition level of the athlete and his or her position?
5. What is the SMR or Tanner stage of the teen athlete?
6. Do the athlete and the parents/guardians understand the risks involved based on the desired sport and identified conditions of the athlete (e.g., epilepsy, diabetes mellitus, single kidney, and single eye)?
7. Are the athlete and family willing to change the sport if necessary based on results of the SPPE?
8. Does the athlete's medical condition, if any, place him or her or others at an increased risk for injury or illness?
9. Is it possible to allow limited participation?
10. Is it possible to modify the rules and conduct of the sport to accommodate the special needs of the athlete?

occurred, if there was full recovery from the injury or injuries, and if the athlete is engaged in overtraining.[12,13] If the athlete is allowed to return to sports without full rehabilitation, risks for additional injury are increased. It is important to rule out other causes of musculoskeletal pain or injury, such as neoplasm or infection.

History of Head and Neck Injuries

Minor head trauma is not uncommon in youth sports; it is important to evaluate for this possibility.[14] Thus a detailed history is taken regarding head and neck injury, as outlined in Table 8-2. Sport-related concussion may result in acute and chronic sequelae (see Chapter 11).[15–17]

History of Breathing Problems

Asthma is the most common chronic disease of children and adolescents and is diagnosed in approximately five million individuals younger than 18 years in the United States.[18–21] Asthma can have direct effects on the quality of life and if not adequately treated can adversely impact the athlete's sports performance. Pulmonary problems in athletes are discussed in Chapter 12.

History of Cardiovascular Disorders

A careful cardiovascular disorders assessment is critical to look for previously not recognized conditions while allowing an athlete to participate in sports at varying levels.[22–27] Cardiovascular screening (see Chapter 14 for detailed discussion) seeks to find those at increased risk for exercise-induced sudden cardiac death. A cardiac cause represents 95% of sudden death in adolescent and young adult athletes, while sudden cardiac death occurs in one to two per 200,000 athletes per year in the United States.[21,27]

Menstrual and Gynecologic History

The gynecologic history should seek information about menarche (age of menses onset), date of the last menstrual period, and the presence of menstrual problems such as amenorrhea (primary or secondary), dysfunctional uterine bleeding, or dysmenorrhea.[28,29] Female athletes involved in highly competitive sports may be at risk for the female athlete triad characterized by menstrual abnormality (such as amenorrhea), disordered eating behaviors, and osteopenia. [28–31]

The athlete should be screened for the possibility of sexual abuse and harassment.[32,33] Sexual harassment of female athletes can occur in a variety of ways, including salacious comments or suggestions, ridiculing of ability, sex-based comments, written threats with or without lewd jokes, unsolicited attention, sexual bullying, and others.[32,33] Specific issues of female athletes are further explored in Chapter 9.

Medication History

The SPPE should ask about what medication(s) the athlete is taking, and the athlete as well as the parents should understand potential adverse effects of these drugs.[3,4] Sometimes, sports officials should know about these medications as determined by the physician and the family (athlete as well as the parents or guardians). For example, the athlete should understand if the drug has a negative effect on sports performance, for example, beta blockers prevent optimal heart rate increase in response to physical activity. If the athlete is not in compliance with recommended medication, sports performance may be reduced, such as in the individual with poorly controlled diabetes mellitus who experiences diabetic reactions.[3,4,34]

Nonprescription drugs can lead to problems, as noted in the increased risks for heat illness if taking antihistamine medication, increased risk for trauma-induced bleeding in the athlete taking aspirin (acetyl salicylic acid) or increased risk for abdominal pain and bleeding from nonsteroidal anti-inflammatory drugs (NSAIDs). Performance-enhancing drugs and supplements are reviewed in Chapter 7.[35–37]

Presence of allergies

Ask about allergies including both environmental and drug allergies that may interfere with sports perform-

ance. The athlete should have appropriate medication for treating acute allergic reactions. An epinephrine injection kit should always be available for emergency treatment of anaphylactic reactions.

History of a Recent Febrile Illness

The athlete may be concerned about an upper respiratory tract infection or febrile illness that may interfere with optimal performance. However, a more serious threat is the uncommon development of myocarditis that may be the result of a viral illness leading to potentially lethal cardiac arrhythmias and sudden death (see Chapter 18).

History of Ophthalmologic Conditions

The SPPE should ensure that the athlete has proper vision and thus one should ask about visual acuity, eye symptoms, and history of eye surgery (Chapter 36).[3,4] Clearance for sports is dependent on normal or corrected normal visual acuity. Complex eye conditions will require evaluation and clearance by an ophthalmologist. Some eye conditions including retinal disorders can limit participation in certain sports.

History of Major Surgery

The SPPE should also ask about a history of major surgery, such as surgery of spine, chest, and abdomen. If there is a history of cardiac surgery for congenital heart disease, the current cardiac health should be understood as well as what risks continue for physical activity at all levels. This is true for any major surgery and the physician, athlete, and family need to know if the athlete has fully recovered and is cleared by the surgeon for some or all levels of exertion.

Diet and Weight Control Practices

Competitive athletes may use a variety of weight control and dietary methods in futile attempts to allow improved sports performance sometimes because of sport-required weight categories.[28–31] These measures may not only fail to aid the athlete's performance but may be harmful as well. Thus, it is important to ask about these practices that may include irregular nutrition intake, fad diets, ignoring overall nutrition, or symptoms of eating disorders. It is also important to ask about recent changes in weight, whether gains or losses.

History of Immunizations

Any time the child or adolescent is seen by the physician, one should ask about the patient's immunization status.[7] It is not just important to check on the status of the athlete's tetanus booster or Hepatitis B immunization, but look at all the needed immunizations. Thus, the SPPE is an excellent time to look at and offer recommended immunizations. This will help to prevent or control a variety of outbreaks with vaccine preventable diseases, such as influenza, Hepatitis A, and measles (see Chapter 18). The SPPE is the main or only time that some children or adolescents see a primary care physician and thus, provision of immunizations is a very critical part of the SPPE.

SPPE PHYSICAL EXAMINATION

A thorough physical examination is part of the SPPE with special focus on cardiovascular (see Chapter 14), neurologic, and musculoskeletal components.[1,3,4,38] The physical examination of athletes for preparticipation evaluation is conducted in the same manner as any complete head-to-toe physical examination.

The sexual maturity rating (SMR) or Tanner stage of the athlete should also be assessed to help identify those with delayed, normal, or precocious puberty. (see Figures 2-1 and 2-2 in Chapter 2). It should be noted that athletes of the same weight but different SMR maturity are not of equal strength, since muscle is stronger than adipose tissue. Thus, an individual with an SMR of 4 to 5 is typically stronger than the obese individual with an SMR of 2 to 3. A young adolescent who is tall and has an SMR of 2 to 3 will not be as strong as an older youth who is short and has an SMR of 4 to 5, since it takes this younger adolescent some time to gain optimal muscle strength as he eventually matures to an SMR of 4 and 5.

Laboratory and Imaging Studies

There are no screening laboratory tests or imaging studies that are routinely recommended as part of the SPPE. A careful medical history and focused physical examination determines if specific testing is needed for sports clearance or for evaluation of identified potential problems.

QUALIFYING ATHLETES FOR SPORT PARTICIPATION

The results of the SPPE determine the status of sports participation eligibility of the athlete based on factors noted in Table 8-2. The athlete is matched with appropriate sport based on the classification of the sport. Sports are classified either based on the likelihood of bodily contact and collision or the degree of cardiovascular stress that a particular sport activity will induce. Therefore it is essential to understand the basic concepts of classification of sports.

Table 8-3.

Classification of Selected Sports Based on Potential for Bodily Contact

Contact/Collision	LimitedContact	Noncontact
Basketball	Baseball	Badminton
Field hockey	Cheerleading	Body
Football	Fencing	building
Ice hockey	Gymnastics	Bowling
Lacrosse	High jump	Discus
Martial arts	Racquetball	Golf
Rugby	Skating	Running
Wrestling	Skiing	Swimming
	Softball	Tennis
	Volleyball	

Classification of Sports

One of the factors determining the relative frequency and type of injuries in sports is the likelihood of bodily contact or collision. It is therefore useful to classify sports based on the likelihood of bodily contact (Table 8-3) so that the athlete and sport can be appropriately matched.[2] This type of classification, however, does not help assess the cardiovascular stress of a given sport and therefore classification of sports based on cardiovascular stress (Figure 8-1) is found to be more useful in determining participation eligibility for athletes with cardiovascular risk factors.[24,39] In this type of classification, sports are categorized based on exercise type and intensity.

Exercise types

The two types of exercises based on the mechanical action of the muscles involved are dynamic (isotonic) and static (isometric).[24,39] Dynamic exercise is characterized by rhythmic contractions of muscles accompanied by change in muscle length (shortening or lengthening), with movement of the joint over which the muscles act, and minimal intramuscular force. Static exercise on the other hand is characterized by contractions of muscles not accompanied by change in muscle length or joint movement and generation of large intramuscular force.

Based on the muscle metabolism or the energy system used, exercise can also be categorized as either predominantly aerobic or predominantly anaerobic types.[40] Aerobic exercise is oxygen-dependent long-term energy system with unlimited time to fatigue. Anaerobic exercise that uses the phosphocreatine-ATP pathway provides immediate energy for muscle action with a time to fatigue from 5 to 10 seconds, whereas anaerobic exercise that uses the glycogen-lactic acid (glycolytic) pathway provides energy for short-term action with time to fatigue from 60 to 90 seconds.

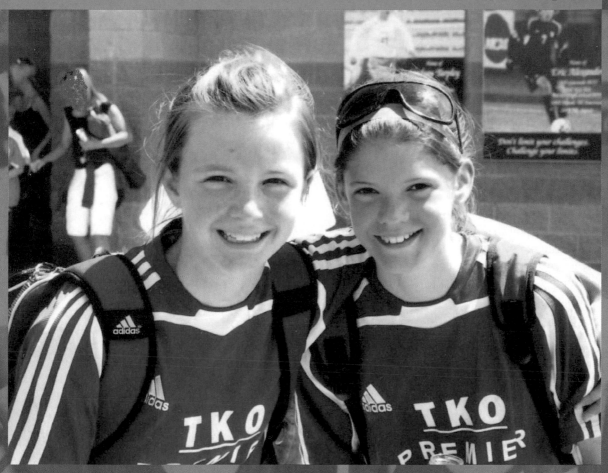

Medical Conditions and Sport Participation

CHAPTER 9

Special Considerations for the Female Athlete

Donald E. Greydanus and Artemis K. Tsitsika

Over the course of the 20th century, the adolescent female athletes became an important participant in the sports environment around the world.[1] Women were banned from the first Modern Olympics in 1896, but now make up a significant part of the Olympic games and not infrequently outshine the men. Beyond athletic competition and sporting events, the proven benefits of physical exercise on somatic and mental health are numerous; thus, adolescent females should be encouraged to participate in sport activities. This chapter reviews selected aspects of the adolescent female athletes that include stress urinary incontinence, breast injuries, pregnancy and exercise, menstrual dysfunction, and the female athlete triad Box 9-1. Iron deficiency anemia is increased in female athletes versus males and is discussed in the hematology chapter. An overview of the physiology of the female athletes is considered at this time.

PHYSIOLOGY

Both male and female children are basically equal in physical condition and have equal parameters as noted in Table 9-1. Male and female children have the same strength before puberty but these changes with the event of puberty. After puberty, females aged 11 to 12 years are 90% as strong as their male counterparts versus 85% as strong at ages 13 to 14 years and 75% at ages 15 to 16 years.[1] The specific responses to exercise training do vary from person to person based on willingness to train and genetic factors; however, being a female child or a male child does not influence these responses. There are, of course, individuals in general society who predict that female children are "poor" athletes in contrast to the males, resulting in a cultural attitude that can limit or even exclude the female athlete from training, often compounded by providing her with inferior sports equipment.

The consequences of puberty include an increase in body fat percentages, particularly in females, with an

---

Box 9-1 Referral to a Specialist

1. Stress urinary incontinence not improving with basic management (Table 9-4)
2. Chronic Jogger's nipple not responding to general care (Table 9-5)
3. Breast hematoma requiring drainage (Table 9-6)
4. Extensive breast laceration (s)
5. Breast pain preventing sports participation
6. Breast asymmetry
7. Breast lesion (s) of unknown etiology (Table 9-7)
8. Precocious puberty
9. Eating Disorder (Anorexia nervosa or bulimia nervosa)
10. Stress fracture (s)
11. Osteopenia or osteoporosis
12. Athletes with amenorrhea or oligomenorrha over 6 months (Tables 9-10 and 9-14)

Table 9-1.

Equal Parameters in Children (Prepuberty) of Both Sexes

Height
Weight
Strength
Endurance
Motor skills
Percent body fat
Hemoglobin levels
Risks of injury

Table 9-2.

Differences in Adolescent Females Compared to Males

Physiologic
Increased percentage of body fat
Skeletal maturation occurs earlier
Heart size and volume are smaller
Aerobic capacity is lower
Reduced testosterone levels
Basal metabolic rate is relatively lower
Lung volume is smaller and vital capacity is less

Anatomic
Shorter height
Wide hips with narrower shoulders
Relatively smaller total articular surface area
Relatively more fat around thighs and hips
Reduced muscle fibre size

eventual average body fat percentage of 23% to 27% in adult females versus 13% to 15% in adult males.[1] Intensive training in adolescent athletes can reduce these body fat percentages to 8% to 10% in female sprinters or 12% to 16% for distance female runners in contrast to 4% to 8% in highly trained male gymnasts. Table 9-2 notes other puberty-induced differences in females and males, as a result of changes induced by puberty.[1-3] There are fewer sweat glands in the female; however, her thermoregulatory capacity is similar to the male because she has less muscle bulk that produces less heat, less overall body mass, and a relatively larger surface area. However, there is an increased heatstroke risk in both genders, if they are obese, late in pubertal maturation, and exercise in hot environments.

The muscle fiber type proportion is similar in adolescent females and males; however, the muscle fiber size is reduced in females.[3] Females show a small increase in muscle strength once menstruation begins (menarche), while males show muscle strength gains throughout puberty (especially the 6–12 months following their growth spurt).[3] Females can never reach the muscle capacity of males, because of their lower testosterone levels. Testosterone like doping agents have been used in order to improve the athletic performance of females (see Chapter 6). Appropriate training can result in the adolescent female having upper body strength that is 30% to 50% that of male counterparts while the lower body strength an approximate 70% of males.[4,5] Females can benefit from age-appropriate weightlifting programs, maximizing muscle strength, and endurance. Such programs may help these athletes improve their performance and limit sport-induced injuries.

In the adolescent male athlete, his maximal speed peak occurs before his peak height velocity (PHV) while peaks in strength and power occur after PHV; this same pattern is not noted in the female. The adolescent female typically has her most rapid rate of weight gain in 12 to 14 months after her maximum growth velocity (sexually maturity rating [SMR] of 2 or 3). Also, she has a relatively small increase in muscle mass in contrast to a larger increase in body fat. There is an increased result in endurance and strength training in the female that is seen 12 to 24 months after her PHV (SMR of 4–5). Weight training produces only a small increase in muscle mass that can be seen, though some strength increase can be noted. There can be loss of subcutaneous adipose tissue and more muscle definition with extensive training.

Puberty allows males to grow into their sport because they are brought closer to their physical optimum that maximizes their sports performance. In contrast, adolescent females tend to grow out of their sport as these maturing athletes move away from their physical optimum for reduced sports performance.[1,6] Early adolescent females have better flexibility and balancing skills than early adolescent males, an advantage that begins in childhood and peaks at 14 or 15 years of age; males typically improve in flexibility from midadolescence until final puberty. The height and growth changes from childhood to adolescence allows the female to become competitive in various sports (i.e., basketball, volleyball, swimming, and others) as determined by her genetic potential and quality of sports training. The adolescent female has some advantage over the male in gymnastics and other sports that require excellent balancing proclivities because of her shorter extremities and lower center of gravity. Some research concludes that the center of gravity is not influenced by gender per se but more by the actual height and weight of the athlete.[1,6] The late maturing female may be more interested than her peers in sports that require a thin or lean body type, such as synchronized swimming, gymnastics, dance, and figure skating; these late maturing athletes may excel at these sports. Some female athletes deliberately attempt to delay their puberty and maintain a girlish figure by significantly reducing food consumption. Such abnormal eating patterns can lead to overt eating disorders and the female athlete triad, as reviewed later in this chapter.

STRESS URINARY INCONTINENCE (SUI)

Definitions and Epidemiology

The involuntary loss of urine during exercise or during sneezing or coughing is called SUI and it is described in 28% of nulliparous female sports participants with a mean age of 20 years.[7] SUI has prevalence rates that range from 10% to 55% in 15- to 64-year-old females.[8]

Table 9-3.
Exercise-Induced SUI Risk Factors

1. ↑ age
2. Female gender
3. ↑ parity
4. Strenuous or heavy exercising or physical activity
5. Sports that are high-impact
6. Hypoestrogenic amenorrhea
7. Obesity

Table 9-4.
Management Options for SUI

Basic education
Avoid pre-exercise overhydration (while avoiding dehydration)
Sanitary napkins
Pharmacologic therapy
Behavioral therapy
Kegal exercises (pelvic floor muscle strengthening)
Vaginal tampons or pessaries (cones)
Electrical stimulation
Biofeedback instructions

Pathogenesis

SUI is particularly noted in "high impact" sports that involve running and jumping found in track and field, gymnastics, and basketball; it is described much less often in females participating in sports such as skiing, jogging, skating, and tennis.[3,7–10] SUI risk factors are listed in Table 9-3 and the etiology is linked to an increase in intra-abdominal pressures because of exercise, resulting in urethral sphincteric unit changes.

Clinical Presentation

The athlete may be embarrassed by the incontinence and not voluntarily mention this event unless directly asked by the clinician. The history should point out if this occurs only during sports activity or is part of a picture of enuresis (daytime and/or nighttime) that has continued since childhood. The history can also note if risk factors are present, as indicated in Table 9-3. SUI describes a pattern of frequent or infrequent urinary incontinence that is only exercise-related. A general physical examination is done that may include a pelvic examination assessing pelvic floor anatomic integrity and abnormality of the posterior urethrovesical angle.[1,3] If the SUI is part of a larger incontinent pattern, laboratory testing can include a urinalysis, urine cultures, renal sonogram, voiding cystourethrogram, and others.[11,12]

Management

In most situations, the athlete can be educated that SUI is typically a benign, self-limited phenomenon that simply requires basic understanding of this condition along with such measures as prevention of pre-exercise excessive fluid intake and possibly the use of sanitary napkins placed prior to the exercise. The athlete, however, needs to avoid dehydration as well. Table 9-4 lists additional management options that are available in selected situations. The use of anticholinergic medications is not recommended, since these drugs can induce sweating dysfunction and heat disorders. Phenylpropolamine was removed from the US market because of reports of increased cerebrovascular accidents in females younger than 50 years of age. However, imipramine and pseudoephedrine hydrochloride are used by some clinicians to reduce the incidence of exercise-induced SUI.[1]

BREASTS AND SPORTS

Introduction

Breasts are modified, milk-producing apocrine glands anatomically situated within superficial thoracic fascial layers that are suspended from the anterior chest wall by fibrous septae called *Cooper's ligaments* and extend from the second to the sixth intercostal space (Figure 9-1).[13,14] The breast contains 15 to 20 lobes and excretory ducts opening into the nipple while the lobes contain alveoli (10–100). The breast contour is formed by connective tissue that is dense and fatty while

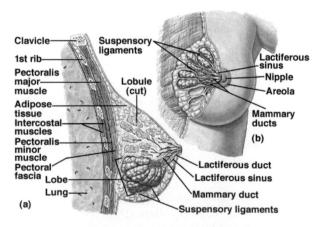

FIGURE 9-1 ■ Normal breast anatomy. *(Reproduced from Greydanus DE, Tsitsika AK, Gaines MJ. The gynecology system and the adolescent. In: Greydanus DE, Feinberg AN, Patel DR, Homnick DN, eds. The Pediatric Diagnostic Examination. New York: McGraw-Hill Medical; 2008:703. Copyright © The McGraw-Hill Companies, Inc.)*

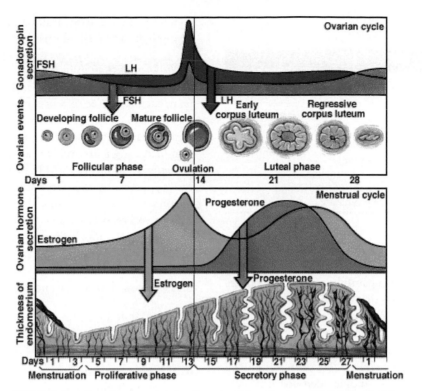

FIGURE 9-2 ■ Normal menstrual cycle. *(Reproduced from Greydanus DE, Tsitsika AK, Gaines MJ. The gynecology system and the adolescent. In: Greydanus DE, Feinberg AN, Patel DR, Homnick DN, eds. The Pediatric Diagnostic Examination. New York, McGraw-Hill Medical; 2008:719. Copyright © The McGraw-Hill Companies, Inc.)*

Cooper's ligaments provide some support to the breasts as they reach from the skin to the pectoralis muscle that is underneath the breasts (Figure 9-2). The areola is a darkened structure in the breast center that contains the nipple and also sebaceous glands called *Montgomery tubercules.*

Thelarche (breast bud stage or SMR 2) is the first clinical sign of puberty and normally occurs between 8 and 14 years of age, with a mean age of 9 to 11 years of age. Thelarche begins the process of clinical puberty with further breast development over the next few years and menarche (onset of menstruation) 2 to 5 years later.[13,14] An SMR 1 or Tanner stage 1 is defined by no breast development, 2 is the breast bud stage, 3 is further breast development, 4 is a doubled-contoured appearance with the areola and nipple separated from the breast in a secondary mound, and 5 is further breast enlargement with a single contour appearance (nipple separated from the rest of breast). A number of normal females never actually reach SMR breast stage 5 and stop their breast development at stage 4.

Effect of Exercise and Breast Size

There is only a small amount of muscle in breast tissue in the areola and thus, exercise does not affect breast size by impact on muscle tissue. There may be an appearance of exercise-increase in breast size, if the underlying pectoralis muscle is increased by intense physical activity.[15] Intense exercise can reduce the adipose tissue in the mammary gland leading to a smaller breast. Dieting can also change the breast size by increasing or decreasing breast adipose tissue. Also, exercise, even when very strenuous does not increase the athlete's risk for breast cancer.[16]

Nipple Injuries

Pathogenesis

The nipple is the most prominent part of the breast and thus can be injured in the course of sports activity. Jogging or other physical activity can injure nipple tissue by frequent nipple rubbing caused by friction between the nipple and cloth that covers the breast and nipple. This is called "jogger's nipple" or "bicyclist's nipple" and can be an acute or chronic injury worsened by a tight-fitting shirt, bra, or other irritating material rubbing against a nipple.[5,6,15, 17] Direct stimulation and exercise in cold weather that leads to nipple prominence by areolar muscle effects can lead to nipple irritation and trauma as well. It is more common in males than females and one classic reports notes a 20:1 male to female ratio of jogger's nipple in marathon runners.[18]

Table 9-5.

Prevention of Exercise-Induced Injury to Nipples

1. Place a plastic covering as a Band Aid or petroleum jelly over the nipples.
2. Always use a sports bra that fits well.
3. Try to avoid cold weather exposure.
4. Place wind breaking cloth over the chest.
5. Be very careful with trauma to the nipples during pregnancy when nipples are prominent.

Clinical presentation

Athletes can present with a painful, raw, and sometimes bleeding nipple or nipples that can be acute or chronic. If there is an accompanying unilateral pain mass under the areola often in association with a sanguineous or dark-brown nipple discharge, the differential diagnosis includes nonexercise-related disorders as an intraductal papilloma (papillomatosis), nipple adenoma, cystosarcoma phyllodes, papillary carcinoma, mammary duct ectasia, ductal hyperplasia, or infiltrating ductal adenocarcinoma.[19] If a mass is present, breast ultrasonography and fine needle aspiration are needed to study this condition further. However, most will present with a raw, bleeding nipple in association with exercise and no other findings on breast examination.

Management

Table 9-5 lists methods to prevent nipple trauma caused by exercise that includes a well-fitting sports bra. Management of overt nipple damage include using a proper sports bra, good hygiene, avoidance of ongoing nipple trauma, and antibiotic treatment of any secondary nipple infection.

Breast injuries

Pathogenesis

Besides injury to the nipple, sports activity may cause trauma to the breast tissue, in which direct trauma can cause breast contusions, abrasions, hematomas, or lacerations.[5,6,19] The injury may be from falls, seat belt injuries, sports equipment, elbows, kicks, or other trauma to the breast tissue. The sports bra itself may contribute to injury from bra clips, straps, hooks, or underwire metal. A breast contusion represents superficial rupture of capillaries, while a hematoma results from hemorrhage of deep blood vessel (s). Although a history of direct breast trauma is not always present, *Mondor's disease* may present as thrombophlebitis of superficial breast veins. If a female athlete has had sili-

cone-implanted breasts, trauma may lead to rupture of an implant in rare situations.

Clinical presentation

A breast *contusion* is typically mild with variable breast pain, edema, and ecchymoses over the injury. An *abrasion* presents as an excoriation or removal of superficial skin because of trauma; there may be secondary infection increasing pain over this abraded wound. A breast *hematoma* may be deep within mammary tissue and not easily appreciated as a localized collection of blood in the breast tissue because of a known or unknown breast trauma. A breast *laceration* is a variable sized cut in the breast skin. Mondor's disease presents as tenderness, redness, and swelling over superficial breast veins. Trauma-induced rupture of a silicone-implant leads to breast pain with bleeding and breast deformity.

Management

Table 9-6 reviews management of breast tissue injuries. Breast *contusions* are typically mild and resolved over 15 to 21 days. A *hematoma* usually resolves by itself with no need for aspiration; however, this resolution may take months to years and result in the development of fat necrosis and secondary induration, scarring, and calcification that may be mistaken for breast carcinoma.[1,15,19] Surgical closure of a breast *laceration* should occur with careful observation for the potential development of a painful breast abscess. Spontaneous resolution of Mondor's disease occurs usually over 1 to 2 weeks. An athlete

Table 9-6.

Management of Breast Tissue Injuries*

1. **Contusion**
   a. Application of cold every 15–20 min—several hours
   b. Appropriate analgesia
   c. Firm support
2. **Abrasion**
   a. Direct pressure to control bleeding
   b. Suturing may be necessary
3. **Laceration**
   a. Close with steri-strips or sutures
   b. Use good hygiene principles
   c. Apply a firm postclosure dressing
   d. She should wear a supportive bra (even at night)
   e. Pain and swelling can be reduced with a cold pack
   f. Provide a tetanus toxoid, if warranted
   g. Antibiotics may be needed, depending on the situation
4. **Hematoma**
   a. Most resolve without treatment
   b. Surgical aspiration may be necessary

*(Reprinted from: Greydanus DE, Patel DR. The female athlete: before and beyond. Pediatric Clin No Amer. 2002;49:553–580, with permission from Elsevier.)

with silicone implant rupture should be referred for removal of the implant.

Breast Pain

Pathogenesis

Breast discomfort or overt pain is not an uncommon event in female athletes involved in exercise and sports play. It is a concern often not mentioned by the adolescents unless directly asked by the clinician. It can prevent many females from taking part in sports activities. Breast soreness or tenderness caused by physical activity was reported in 31% of female athletes and 52% of this group also noted breast injury while involved in sports participation.[20] Considerable breast movement can occur in exercise such as noted with volleyball, basketball, running, gymnastics, and others. This pain or discomfort can be intensified with increase fluid retention in the breasts, noted during the premenstrual phase and other parts of the menstrual cycle as well as those with premenstrual syndrome. Excessive breast motion can lead to pectoralis muscle strain of fascial attachments and shoulder discomfort, especially in female athletes with large breasts. Breast pain can also be caused by various breast masses, as noted in Table 9-7.

Management

A well-fitted sports brassiere will prevent much of the pain and discomfort experienced by the female athlete by providing maximum breast support and reducing painful breast movement.[21,22] The sports bra should minimize breast motion by being well-fitted and able to lift as well as separate the breasts. It is important that the bra be made of material that is nonabrasive and "breathable" (in order to reduce sweating). It should not be old or worn-out and usually needs to be replaced on a regular basis, after every 6 months. The bra should have soft, firm cups, very few seams, and limited hooks that are padded. Some athletes will also benefit from padding of the bra and shoulder straps. Guidelines for sport bras have been published.[1,15,21,22] Excessive sweating may cause excoriation, development of abscesses, and cellulitis in the breast folds.

Breast Asymmetry

Pathogenesis

Breast asymmetry is a common event in adolescent females as they mature. By the time puberty is completed, one in four adult females still have visible breast asymmetry.[1,15] It is usually a normal variant, but a careful evaluation is needed for any female athlete who presents with breast asymmetry, especially looking for a mass in the larger breast (Table 9-7).

Management

Trauma may lead to breast injury, if proper protection is not provided and thus, a padded sports bra is recommended for these athletes. Foam inserts can be useful to the female with considerable breast asymmetry,

Table 9-7.

Causes of Breast Masses*

Fibroadenoma	Miscellaneous
Juvenile (giant) fibroadenoma	Nipple adenoma
Other fibroadenoma variants	Papillomatosis
Virginal hyperplasia	Ductal adenocarcinoma
Cystosarcoma phylloids	Mammary duct ectasia
Breast abscess	Intraductal granuloma
Breast cyst (including fibrocystic Breast disease and other breast mastopathies)	Sclerosing adenosis
	Keratoma of the nipple
	Interstitial fibrosis
Breast carcinoma	Granular cell myoblastoma
Intraductal papilloma	Angiosarcoma of the breast
Fat necrosis	Metastatic disease (e.g., leukemia, malignant lymphoma, ovarian malignancy, others)
Lipoma	Neurofibromatosis
Lymphangioma	Dermatofibromatosis
Hemangioma	Tuberous mastitis
	Papilloma sarcoidosis
	Hematoma
	Others

*(With permission from: Greydanus DE. Breast and gynecologic disorders. In: Hofmann, AD, Greydanus DE, eds. Adolescent Medicine. 3rd ed. Stamford, CT: Appleton and Lange; 1997:524.

sometimes found in stores catering to adults who underwent mastectomy. Swimmers may receive benefit from a bathing suit with breast supports.

Galactorrhea

Pathogenesis

There are many causes for an adolescent female who develops galactorrhea or nipple discharge not because of pregnancy. Etiology includes pituitary neoplasms, injury to the hypothalamus (i.e., infection, surgery, other), medications (i.e., phenothiazines, oral contraceptives, others), hypothyroidism, anxiety, depression, self-manipulation, and many others.[19]

Management

Management depends on the underlying etiology and includes stopping of the implicated medications or self-manipulation, correction of thyroid abnormality, if present, or treatment of a pituitary neoplasm, if present.[1,13,14, 15,19]

EXERCISE AND PREGNANCY

Pathogenesis

A dedicated female athlete or the one who is physically active may desire to remain exercising even if she is pregnant.[1,2] Concern has been raised that strenuous exercise would lead to fetal hypoxia by diverting blood from the fetus to the mother's muscles that are exercising or that exercise would cause fetal hyperthermia because of an increase in the mother's core temperature. However, there is no research supporting fetal damage while the mother is exercising and in general, such physical activity is considered good for the mother and safe for her fetus who is well-insulated from the effects of maternal exercise.

Management

The mother should be educated that her overall sports performance will be impaired because of the pregnancy (Table 9-8) and that there are contraindications to exercising during pregnancy (Table 9-9).[1,23–25] Guidelines to emphasize sensible exercising patterns have been developed.[23–25] An exercise plan can be developed for the pregnant athlete that is specific for her and based on common sense. This plan should take into account the exercise level before pregnancy occurred, but should in any case limit the physical activity to 15 minutes and avoid strenuous anaerobic activity. Activities and workouts not included in prepregnancy regimens or events should be avoided

Table 9-8.

Factors Impairing Sports Performance During Pregnancy

1. ↑ed Adipose tissue
2. Altered center of gravity
3. ↑ed Fluid retention
4. ↑ed Maternal blood volume
5. ↑ed Cardiac output
6. ↑ed Overall expenditure of energy
7. ↑ed Breast ducts
8. ↑ed Abdominal growth
9. ↑ed ligamentous laxity from ↑ed levels of estrogen and relaxin

while pregnant. Diabetes mellitus is not a contraindication to exercise while pregnant, if permitted by the athlete's clinician, and along with careful self-monitoring of the metabolic status in order to maintain physiologic stability.[26]

Pregnancy induces breast congestion and nipple prominence and thus, a well-fitting, supportive bra is recommended. Swimming is probably the best exercise for the pregnant individual and swimming is also an ideal form of physical activity for others, when increased weight is a factor.[1] Walking and bicycle riding are also safe for the fetus, though the mother should wear a helmet while biking and take care to avoid accidents. Activity that involves jumping should be discouraged because relaxin induces stretching of pelvic ligaments and

Table 9-9.

Contraindications to Exercise in Pregnancy

1. Preterm rupture of membranes
2. Prior and/or current preterm labor
3. Persistent bleeding (second or third trimester)
4. Intrauterine growth retardation
5. Pregnancy-induced hypertension
6. Incompetent cervix or cerclage
7. Development of dehydration
8. Vaginal bleeding
9. Muscle weakness
10. Calf pain (check for thrombophlebitis)
11. Dizziness
12. Tachycardia (heart rate over 180 beats/min)
13. Shortness of breath
14. Severe headache
15. Pain in the chest, hip, or back
16. Others as per the clinician's assessment in chronic illness; see guidelines[24,25]

potential injury. Exercise in the supine position is often avoided during the first trimester even if done with previous pregnancies. Physical activity that involves the upper body is fine unless the upper torso is subjected to mechanical stress. She should be instructed to avoid excessive physical activity, avoid work-outs in very hot weather, and avoid or stop the exercise, if febrile (i.e., over 38°C) or other conditions develop as noted in Table 9-9.

This athlete should not take part in sports such as weightlifting, horseback riding, scuba diving, and other water sports except, as noted, for basic swimming. It is best for her to avoid competitive events, especially if the risk of injury is high and/or it is a contact or collision sport. High-altitude exercising may increase obstetric risks while scuba diving can increase risk to the fetus from decompression injury and embolism.[25] Finally, the athlete may start back on her sports exercising regimen at approximately 4 to 6 weeks after a vaginal delivery and 6 to 8 weeks after a cesarean section.[5] Lactation is not a contraindication to having the mother resume her exercise patterns.[27]

MENSTRUATION AND SPORTS

Menstrual Physiology

Normal menstrual cycles are defined by three phases: *follicular, ovulatory,* and *luteal* and are governed by alterations in blood levels of estrogen and progesterone under the overall control of a responsive hypothalamic-pituitary-ovarian-uterine axis (Figure 9-2).[1,14,28] During the follicular phase, ovarian-produced estrogen is increased that results in endometrial growth character-

ized by a compact, proliferative stroma, and endometrial gland increase in number and length. Ovulation produces the corpus luteum that leads to production of estrogen and progesterone with progesterone-stimulated production of a secretory endometrium. As the luteal phases develops, this endometrium acquires an edematous stroma with glands that are tortuous and dilated. In the absence of pregnancy, the corpus luteum becomes atretic with resultant sudden drop in hormonal steroids (i.e., estrogen and progesterone) and then menstruation.

Menarche or the onset of menstrual periods normally develops between ages 9 and 16 years in the US with 12.4 years as the mean age for menarche.[29] Menarche usually develops 1 to 3 years after thelarche and this event is under many influences, including nutritional status, intensity of exercise patterns, weight, race, genetic factors, and others. An adolescent or adult with mature menstrual patterns will have menstruation with a mean interval of 28 days (±7 days) and a median loss of blood of 30 mL/mo (with an upper limit of 60–80 ml/mo).[28,29] A variety of abnormal menstrual patterns are noted in adolescent females, including those involved in sports (Table 9-10). Table 9-11 provides questions one can ask in taking a history of menstrual patterns in adolescent females.

Influence of menstrual cycles on athletic performance

Research generally does not demonstrate that the phase of the menstrual cycle negatively influences sports performance, though more research clearly is needed.[1,15,30-31] Anecdotal reports can be found that note dysmenorrhea or menstrual bleeding is worsened by exercise, while others conclude that these events are improved by

Table 9-10.

Abnormal Menstrual Patterns*

Condition	Comments
Amenorrhea	Absence of menses; can be *Primary* or *Secondary*
Oligomenorrhea	Infrequent, irregular bleeding at >45-day intervals
Menorrhagia	Prolonged (>7 d) or excessive (>80 mL) uterine bleeding occurring at regular intervals
Metrorrhagia	Uterine bleeding occurring at irregular but frequent intervals, the amount being variable
Menometrorrhagia	Prolonged uterine bleeding occurring at irregular intervals
Hypermenorrhea	Synonymous with menorrhagia
Polymenorrhea	Uterine bleeding occurring at regular intervals of <21 d
Breakthrough bleeding	Small amounts of bleeding between normal menstrual flows
Dysfunctional uterine bleeding	Abnormal (different from that patient's normal) uterine bleeding that is unrelated to an anatomic lesion

*(Reprinted with permission from: Greydanus DE, Tsitsika AK, Gains MJ. The gynecology system and the adolescent. In: Greydanus DE, Feinberg AN, Patel DR, Homnick DN, eds. The Pediatric Diagnostic Examination. New York: McGraw-Hill Medical; 2008:725.)

Table 9-11.

Menstrual History Questions*

1. Age when monthly/menstrual periods/cycle began (menarche)?
2. When was your last menstrual period?
3. How frequent are your periods?
4. Are the cycles regular (i.e., a defined number of days between the onset of 1 cycle and the onset of the next)?
5. What is the length (interval) between cycles?
6. How many days does the blood flow (or bleeding occurs)?
7. How much is the flow? Heavy? Medium? or Light? How many tampons or pads do you use per day?
8. How saturated are the pads/tampons?
9. Are there any clots?
10. Generally, what color is the blood?
11. Any bleeding between periods? How much?
12. Any bleeding with intercourse?
13. Any pain with menstrual periods?
14. Does the pain interfere with your school or other activities?

(Reprinted with permission from: Greydanus DE, Tsitsika AK, Gains MJ. The gynecology system and the adolescent. In: Greydanus DE, Feinberg AN, Patel DR, Homnick DN, eds. The Pediatric Diagnostic Examination. New York: McGraw-Hill Medical; 2008:724.)

physical activity.[1] For example, one report of 86 female soccer players concluded that female athletes with premenstrual symptoms identified more sports-related injuries during this time than in other menstrual phases; the athletes without premenstrual symptoms did not report any phase when injuries were more prevalent.[31] Athletes with dysmenorrhea or premenstrual syndrome may experience a limitation of their optimal sports performance because of interference from menstrual pain, edema, bloating, and other symptoms.

Influence of oral contraceptives on athletic performance

Sexually active adolescents, whether active athletes or not can be offered effective contraception, if they wish to avoid unwanted pregnancy.[32–36] Some athletes may refuse oral contraceptive pills (OCPs), fearing that reduction in sports performance may result. Some will not take OCPs because of fear of potential side effects or experience of such side effects as nausea, headaches, breast congestion, breast tenderness, and others. Research, however, generally concludes that no such impairment occurs when on oral contraception, and positive results may occur because of beneficial aspects of OCPs (Table 9-12).[31–37] OCPs can be taken on a longer basis to produce fewer menstrual cycles and improve the timing of menstruation (i.e., not during an important sporting event) by staying on active hormone pills. There are OCP formulations available to allow the female to prolong the time between cycles or the athletes can simply use the 21-day packs or the 28-day packs (minus the inactive pills) to achieve the same result.

Table 9-12.

Beneficial Effects of Oral Contraceptive Pills

↓ed dysmenorrhea
↓ed dysfunctional uterine bleeding (DUB)
↓ed anemia secondary to DUB
Timing of menstruation at times more convenient for the athlete
↓ed premenstrual syndrome (PMS)
Possibly less injuries for athletes with dysmenorrhea or PMS
Absence of unwanted pregnancy
Reduced bone mineral density loss
Possibly reduced stress fractures

FEMALE ATHLETE TRIAD

Female athletes may develop one or more **of a constellation** of problems that have been called the *female athlete triad*, consisting of *menstrual dysfunction* (as amenorrhea or oligomenorrhea), *dysfunctional eating patterns*, and *osteopenia* or *osteoporosis*. Much of these phenomena stem from the emphasis that different sports place on female athlete with regard to a lean body, a lean appearance, a prepubertal physique, and/or various weight levels (Table 9-13). These athletes may feel under immense pressure to obtain an "ideal" body for their sport leading them to wrestle with resultant menstrual/nutrition/exercise schemes.[38–42]

Table 9-13.

Sports Increasing Risks for Female Athlete Triad

1. **Prepubertal Appearance Emphasis**
   a. Figure skating
   b. Ballet
   c. Gymnastics
2. **Lean Appearance Emphasis**
   a. Dance
   b. Figure Skating
   c. Synchronized swimming
   d. Gymnastics
   e. Diving
3. **Lean Body Emphasis**
   a. Long-distance running
   b. Swimming
   c. Cross-country skiing
4. **Miscellaneous Weight Categories Emphasis**
   a. Rowing
   b. Judo
   c. Taekwondo
   d. Wrestling
   e. Weightlifting

Menstrual Dysfunction

Definitions and epidemiology

The absence of menstruation or amenorrhea can be primary or secondary (Table 9-10). *Primary* amenorrhea refers to absence of any menstruation by age 14 with a SMR of 1 or by age 16 regardless of the SMR. The cessation of menses after menarche for a total of 3 cycles or a total of 6 months without menses after menarche is called *secondary* amenorrhea.

Menstrual dysfunction is commonly seen in adolescent female athletes, whether amenorrhea (primary or secondary), oligomenorrhea (Table 9-10), or luteal phase disorders.[1,38–43] Secondary amenorrhea can be normal for 3 to 6 months during the first 2 years after menarche as it takes some time for menstrual maturity with regular cycles to develop. Also, the young adolescent female can delay the onset of menses by approximately 5 months for each year of strenuous exercise that develops before the onset of puberty, resulting in a 1- to 2-year or more delay in menarche.[1] Menstrual dysfunction is noted in 12% of swimmers and cyclists, 44% of ballet dancers, 50% of female triathletes, and 51% of endurance runners.[1] Secondary amenorrhea is noted in 10% to 20% of female athletes who are intensively exercising and up to two-thirds of "elite" athletes.[6] These sports include ballet, distance running, cycling, and gymnastics.

Pathogenesis

The menstrual dysfunction noted in female athletes involves a number of etiologic factors that can lead to amenorrhea or oligomenorrhea. These factors include pubertal level, age, weight, nutritional health or dysfunction, body fat percentage, level or intensity of exercise, stress (including pressure of the specific sport selected), genetic factors, and others. Sports such as gymnastics or dance encourage a thin body physique, though a low weight per se does not necessarily induce amenorrhea; athletes of the same weight can have differing menstrual patterns. The role of leptin in menstrual dysfunction in female athletes is not yet clear. Some have suggested that the intense level of physical activity can lead to an energy drain that the eating dysfunction noted in some athletes cannot correct, leading to hypothalamic amenorrhea with dysfunction of GnRH and LH pulsivity.[1,6,44] Also complicating and worsening this complex phenomenon is the potential presence of factors such as chronic illness, menstrual disorders in other family members, and a history of menstrual abnormality that predates the intense exercise patterns.

Clinical presentation

The athlete will present with a variety of menstrual dysfunction, whether primary or secondary amenorrhea, oligomenorrhea, or dysfunctional uterine bleeding patterns (Table 9-10).

Differential diagnosis

A careful assessment is necessary for the athlete who presents with amenorrhea or oligomenorrhea. The diagnosis of sports-related menstrual dysfunction is a diagnosis of exclusion after a careful search for other causes.[43] The evaluation should look for congenital anomalies, short stature, hypoestrogenemia, virilization, galactorrhea, and other conditions.[1,14,15] Table 9-14 lists a differential diagnosis for various menstrual dysfunctions along with suggested laboratory testing for each category. Figure 9-3 provides an algorithm for the evaluation of an adolescent with secondary amenorrhea and oligomenorrhea, while Figure 9-4 provides an algorithm for evaluation of an adolescent with dysfunctional uterine bleeding.

Management

Management of the female adolescent athlete with menstrual dysfunction depends on the underlying etiologic factors (Table 9-14). If her amenorrhea or oligomenorrhea is owing to physiologic immaturity, reassurance and the tincture of time should resolve this situation. It may take 1 to 5 years from menarche for ovulatory cycles to occur on a regular basis, with resultant normal menstrual patterns. The lack of ovulation prevents the development of a corpus luteum with the development of a luteal cycle. A trial of medoxyprogesterone acetate (10 mg orally for 5–10 days) will result in a withdrawal bleeding and reassure the clinician and patient of normal pelvic anatomy and physiology.[29] Primary dysmenorrhea is usually relieved to a major extent with the use of nonsteroidal anti-inflammatory agents and/or oral contraceptives.[29,33–36]

Management of the female athlete with exercise-induced menstrual dysfunction can be a challenging experience for both clinician and patient. If this athlete with delayed or absent menses reduces her level of training and increases her nutritional intake (including calcium intake), menarche or resumption of her menses usually results. If she is very thin, an increase in body weight of 10% or more would also resolve the abnormal menstrual pattern to a variable extent, if there are no other compounding factors. This athlete can be advised that her menstrual problems may be part of a chronic hypoestrogenic pattern that favors reduced bone marrow density (BMD), osteopenia, and eventually, osteoporosis. A bone density measurement is recommended in order to access current bone status. However, this athlete may be very dedicated to her sport and intense exercise patterns with low body fat status and not willing to change her life style.

Some clinicians adopt a "watch and wait" attitude to avoid alienating this young patient who is dedicated to her sport. Supplementation with daily calcium (1200–1500 mg) and vitamin D (400–800 IU) is advised for this athlete, if she has menstrual

Table 9-14.

Menstrual Disorders of Adolescent Females*

Gynecologic Disorder	Special Comments	Differential Diagnosis	Laboratory Testing
Amenorrhea (Primary)	Physiologic is the main cause; MRKH syndrome assoc. with renal abnormalities and spinal malformations Short stature with delayed sexual maturation: Turner syndrome; delayed sexual maturation + hypertension seen in 17-α-hydroxylase deficiency; Swyer syndrome; absence of smell sense suggests Kallmann syndrome; visual field deficits suggests brain tumor.	Physiologic Imperforate hymen Mayer-Rokitansky-Kuster-Hauser (MRKH) Syndrome; Turner syndrome (45,XO and mosaicism) Chronic illness Hypothalamic: Stress, eating disorders, exercise, depression; Androgen insensitivity syndrome (46 XY); Swyer syndrome; others: See the text.	Serum gonodotropins(FSH, LH), prolactin, TSH; Pelvic Ultrasound MRI Head CT scan/MRI Renal ultrasound/IVP(intravenous pyelogram; Karyotype Laparoscopy
Amenorrhea (secondary)	Pregnancy is the main cause: history of sexual activity—may present with a midline "pelvic mass"; causes of oligomenorrhea and secondary amenorrhea are essentially the same. Also important is history of dietary habits, exercise, stress; acne and hirsutism suggest elevated androgen levels; Athlete Triad Syndrome: amenorrhea, dysfunctional eating patterns, osteopenia-porosis.	Pregnancy; lactation; Stress, eating disorders, Chronic illness, Exercise-induced, prolactinoma (headaches visual field deficits, galactorrhea) PCOS (polycystic ovary Syndrome); See text.	Pregnancy Test (β-hCG) Progesterone challenge Serum estrogen, FSH, LH; bone mineral densitometry; Serum prolactin Thyroid screen; Head CT scan
Dysmenorrhea (Primary)	Pelvic pain during normal ovulatory menstruation; no underlying pelvic pathology. May also see gastrointestinal symptoms, headache, myalgia, sweating.	Physiologic	
Dysmenorrhea (Secondary)	May be seen at menarche or 3+ years postmenarche.	Endometriosis Pelvic inflammatory disease Reproductive tract anomalies Pelvic adhesions Cervical stenosis Ovarian masses Pelvic congestion syndrome Rule out urinary tract or Gastrointestinal causes	Laparoscopy STD screen Pelvic Ultrasound; MRI
Dysfunctional Uterine Bleeding (DUB)	Menstrual calendar useful to get accurate history of menstrual pattern; get sexual activity history; Establish presence/absence of ovulation: basal body temperature charts, serum	Anovulatory bleeding; Pregnancy, ectopic pregnancy; coagulation disorders (as von Willebrand disease, others), anatomic lesions, endometrial pathology;	CBC, platelets, **beta-HCG**, Pap smear, PT, aPTT, PFA, other coagulation disorders screening; D-21 progesterone; thyroid screen; STD screen; ultrasound

(continued)

Table 9-14. (Continued)

Menstrual Disorders of Adolescent Females*

Gynecologic Disorder	Special Comments	Differential Diagnosis	Laboratory Testing
	progesterone, urinary luteinizing hormone (LH) and possibly endometrial biopsy. rule out an STD; virilization evaluation necessary, if hirsutism present.	cervicitis or cervical dysplasia; pelvic inflammatory disease; ovarian cysts; polycystic ovary syndrome; severe stress, rapid or severe weight gain or loss, drug abuse; see text.	(transvaginal; pelvic), MRI; hysteroscopy.
Premenstrual Syndrome (PMS)	Variety of symptoms start before and end with menses	Premenstrual dysphoric disorder (PMDD); depression; anxiety; others, depending on the presenting symptoms	DSM-IV (2000) criteria for PMDD

Abbreviations: CBC: complete blood count; Pap: Papanicolaou smear; STD: sexually transmitted disease; MRI: magnetic resonance imaging; GI: gastrointestinal; ESR: erythrocyte sedimentation rate; F; Fahrenheit; C: Centigrade; HAIR-AN: hyperandrogenism, hirsutism, insulin resistance, acanthosis nigricans; DSM-IV: Diagnostic Statistical Manual-4th Edition (American Psychiatric Association); PT: prothrombin time; aPTT: activated partial thromboplastin time; PFA: platelet function analysis.
*(Used with permission from: Greydanus DE, Tsitsika AK, Gains MJ. The gynecology system and the adolescent. In: Greydanus DE, Feinberg AN, Patel DR, Homnick DN, eds. The Pediatric Diagnostic Examination. New York: McGraw-Hill Medical; 2008:743–748.)

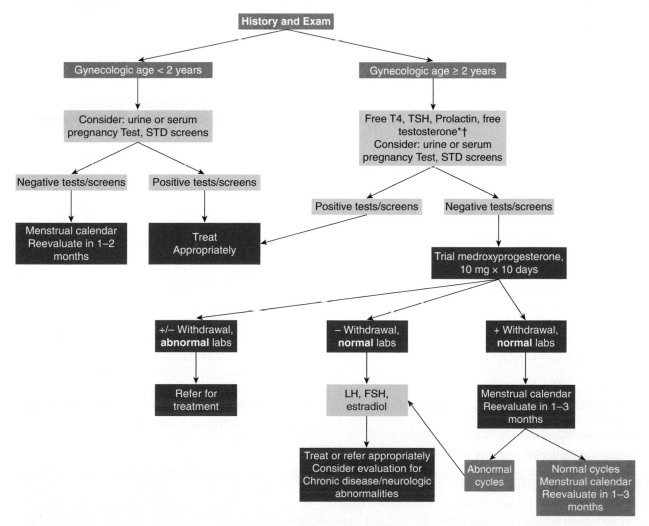

FIGURE 9-3 ■ Evaluation of secondary amenorrhea and oligomenorrhea in the adolescent. *Used with permission from reference #29.*

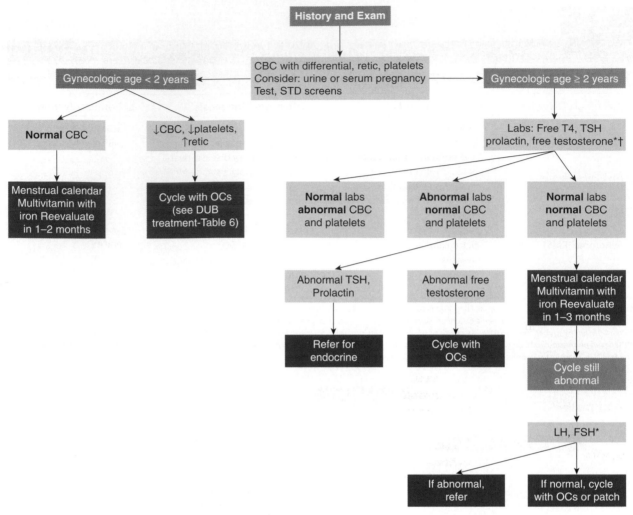

FIGURE 9-4 ■ Evaluation of dysfunctional uterine bleeding in the adolescent. *Used with permission from reference #29.*

dysfunction and/or abnormal eating patterns.[6] If low BMD is present, estrogen supplementation (conjugated estrogen or OCPs) has been suggested by some in efforts to preserve bone loss.[1] If she is amenorrheic and over past 3 years of her menarche, OCP prescription is suggested along with advise to reduce exercise levels and improve nutrition.[1] Some clinicians may provide estrogen supplementation earlier than age 16 or less than 3 years after menarche, especially with a history of a stress fracture.

However, such use of supplemental estrogen is controversial and of unproven benefit for this adolescent athlete to improve a low BMD status with or without weight gain. The estrogen does not resolve the underlying pathophysiology of the menstrual dysfunction or correct the low BMD. The athlete with chronic amenorrhea and low BMD may never develop a normal BMD even if the menstrual periods are normalized. One can provide a menstrual event with the OCP, but the abnormal menstrual pattern typically resumes once the

OCP is withdrawn. Side effects of the OCP may be distressing to the athlete, especially since OCPs under 50 mcg of ethinyl estrodiol may not positively effect bone mineral density.

Causes of a low BMD are complex, as reviewed in the osteoporosis section. The lowest BMD status are usually found in females who are thin and inactive, while thin female gymnasts who are amenorrheic usually have normal or increased bone density probably because of the high-mechanical forces developed by intense exercise with weight bearing leading to increased accretion of bone; this may offset the low BMD effects of a thin body habitus.[1] This effect can also be seen in ice skaters, tennis players, runners, and others. The overt implications of chronic amenorrhea and a possible hypoestrogenic status in this female teen athlete remain unclear at present for her immediate situation and long-term future. However, some of these athletes appear to be at increased risk for the development of osteoporosis as adults.

Disordered Eating

Definitions and epidemiology

Dysfunctional eating patterns are observed and self-recorded in 15% to 75% of adolescent female athletes often as a result of seeking optimal sports performance.[1,38–46] These abnormal patterns include fasting, self-induced vomiting, skipping meals, and/or use of drugs such as diet pills, laxatives, or diuretics. Many will not meet overt criteria for an eating disorder (i.e., anorexia nervosa or bulimia nervosa) as defined by the American Psychiatric Association's *Diagnostic and Statistical Manual of Mental Disorders*.[47] However, overt anorexia or bulimia nervosa is noted in athletes, as for example incidence reports of 5% to 20% of ballet dancers developing anorexia nervosa with the incidence dependent on the level of competition.[1]

Pathogenesis

There are times of increased vulnerability for this youth that increase the likelihood of acquiring abnormal eating patterns, as noted in Table 9-15. Athletes may become involved in sports that demand a thinner body than they have or can maintain without using ways to lose weight (Table 9-13). They are unable to keep up with the energy demands of their growing bodies and the intense exercise demanded by sports such as running, swimming, track, diving, gymnastics, ballet, and others (Table 9-13). They may develop hypothalamic amenorrhea that leads to low bone density at a time when they should rapidly be accumulating bone density and certainly not losing it.

Clinical presentation

The abnormal eating patterns of this athlete may not be easily detected, since she is not often willing to provide details of her diet. However, she may present with hypothalamic menstrual dysfunction with or without an evidence of osteopenia or osteoporosis. A variety of medical disorders can mimic an eating disorder, such as inflammatory bowel disease, substance abuse disorder,

Table 9-15.

Risk Factors for Abnormal Eating Pattern Acquisition

Growth spurt (with increased energy needs to sustain growth and exercise)
Loss of a loved one (such as family members, friends, coaches, trainers)
Educational transitions (such college or university entrance)
Cessation of competitive sports
Postpartum depression

diabetes mellitus, depression, and others. A careful history and physical examination with selected laboratory testing will eliminate these disorders as causative of the menstrual and nutritional dysfunction.

Management

Prevention is the best management tool for abnormal eating patterns or overt eating disorders. If she presents with hypothalamic amenorrhea or oligomenorrhea, the best management option is normalization of her weight, correcting her eating dysfunction, and improving any nutritional deficiencies.[1,38–46] The use of OCPs or other conjugated estrogens may improve low BMD in females with overt anorexia nervosa and severe malnutrition. However, the use of such agents is not proven to restore normal bone health and these females may never have a normal BMD. In some cases, the use of OCPs may lead to the development of a false perception of "normal" menstruation and limit the athlete's motivation to regain her weight. Developing a normal body weight seems critical to improving low BMD.

Osteoporosis

Pathogenesis

Research reveals that 50% to 63% of peak bone mass, or the amount of BMD accumulated in growth, develops in childhood while 37% to 50% occurs during the adolescent years through late adolescence.[1] Normal bone mass is acquired in the female adolescent who is of normal weight and normal estrogen status along with an adequate intake of calcium. The development of low BMD leads to the development of osteopenia and eventually osteoporosis, a condition that occurs with an increased frequency in female athletes with the female athlete triad.[1,48,49]

Table 9-16 lists factors that are important in the development of osteopenia/osteoporosis, including genetics (70%), estrogen status, body weight, intensity of exercise patterns, calcium intake, and others. Thus, the female athlete with a thin body habitus, hypothalamic amenorrhea, and abnormal eating patterns is at increased risk for low bone mineral density and stress fractures. This pattern can be seen in some runners and dancers, for example, if there is a hypoestrogenic state.

Management

As previously noted, the best option is *prevention* of osteopenia and osteoporosis, based on the risk factors listed in Table 9-16. An important factor in prevention is adequate calcium intake in childhood and adolescence. Daily calcium requirements for adolescents are 1200 to 1500 mg/d with an additional 400 mg/d for the female, who is pregnant or lactating. Calcium absorption is inhibited by oxalates, phytates, and iron, while absorption is enhanced by taking vitamin D, citric acid,

Table 9-16.

Risk Factors for Osteoporosis*

1. Limited calcium intake in childhood/adolescence
2. Positive family history (first-degree relatives) for osteoporosis
3. Low levels of physical (weight-bearing) activity
4. History of amenorrhea/irregular menses
5. Thin habitus (anorexia nervosa, others)
6. Alcoholism (toxic to bone-building cells and possibly induces decreased calcium absorption
7. Cigarette smoking (decreases estrogen effectiveness)
8. Medications (glucocorticoids, phenytoin, others)
9. Various chronic diseases (primary hyperparathyroidism, Cushing's syndrome, Addison's disease, leukemia, celiac disease, Crohn's disease, others)
10. Others[1,103]

(Reprinted from: Greydanus DE, Patel DR: The female athlete: before and beyond puberty. Pediatric Clin No Amer. 2002;49:553–580, with permission from Elsevier.)

and phosporus. Foods rich in calcium include skim milk, canned sardines, salmon with bones, plain or non-fat yoghurt, and others.

Prevention of osteoporosis also includes avoidance of estrogen deficiency, physical inactivity, and drug abuse (particularly cigarette addiction). Measures to correct hypothalamic amenorrhea or oligomenorhea and abnormal eating patterns will also help prevent osteoporosis as well. Fracture prevention may be enhanced by weight-resistant exercise. If contraception is needed, oral contraception is recommended, since DMPA (depo-medroxy- progesterone acetate) can lead to bone loss.[50] The athlete with low BMD from pathophysiologic factors associated with the female athlete triad must understand that osteopenia can occur and lead to osteoporosis later in adult life, even if her weight and menstrual cycles become normal at some point later in her life. This athlete is at risk for never acquiring a normal BMD in her adolescent or adult life.

REFERENCES

1. Greydanus DE, Patel DR. The female athlete: before and beyond puberty. *Pediatric Clin No Amer.* 2002;49:553-580.
2. Griffin LY. The female athlete. In: DeLee JC, Drez D Jr, Miller MD, eds. *DeLee & Drez's Orthopaedic Sports Medicine Principles and Practice.* Philadelphia, PA: Elsevier/Saunders; 2003:505-520.
3. Nattiv A, Arendt EA, Hecht SS. The female athlete. In: Garrett WE, Kirkendall DT, Squire DL, eds. *Principles and Practice of Primary Care Sport Medicine.* Philadelphia, PA: Lippincott Williams and Wilkins; 2001:93-113.
4. Patel DR, Nelson TL. Sport injuries in adolescents. *Pediatr Clin No Amer.* 2000;84:983-1007.
5. Ireland ML. Special concerns of the female athlete. In: Fu F, Stone R, eds. *Sports Injuries: Mechanisms, Prevention and Treatment.* 2nd ed. Baltimore: Williams and Wilkins; 2000:156-187.
6. Yurko-Griffin L, Harris SS. Female athletes. In: Sullivan A, Anderson S, eds. *American Academy of Orthopedic Surgery and American Academy of Pediatrics.* 2000:137-148.
7. Nygaard I, Delancey J, Arnsdorf L, et al. Exercise and incontinence. *Obstet Gynecol.* 1990;75:848-851.
8. Bø K. Urinary incontinence, pelvic floor dysfunction, exercise and sport. *Sports Med.* 2004;34(7):451-464.
9. Nattiv A. Track and field. In: Drinkwater BA, ed. *Women in Sport.* Oxford: Blackwell Scientific; 2000:470-485.
10. Bourcier AP, Juras JC. Nonsurgical therapy for stress incontinence. *Urol Clin North Am.* 1995;22:613-627.
11. Greydanus DE, Torres AD, Wan JH. Genitourinary and renal disorders. In: Greydanus DE , Patel DR, Pratt HD, eds. *Essential Adolescent Medicine.* New York: McGraw-Hill Medical Publishers; 2006:355-359.
12. Wan J. The male genitourinary system. In: Greydanus DE, Feinberg AN, Patel DR, Homnick DN, eds. *Pediatric Diagnostic Examination.* New York: McGraw-Hill Medical Publishers; 2008:645-684.
13. Kaul P, Beach K. Breast disorders In: Greydanus DE, Patel DR, Pratt HD, eds. *Essential Adolescent Medicine.* New York: McGraw-Hill Medical Publishers; 2006:569-590.
14. Greydanus DE, Tsitsika AK, Gains MJ. The gynecology system and the adolescent. In: Greydanus DE, Feinberg AN, DR Patel DR, Homnick DN, eds. *Pediatric Diagnostic Examination.* New York: McGraw-Hill Medical Publishers; 2008: 701-749.
15. Greydanus DE, Patel DR, Baxter TL. The Breast and sports: issues for the clinician. *Adolesc Med.* 1998;9:533-550.
16. Thune I, Brenn T, Lund E, et al. Physical activity and the risk of breast cancer. *N Engl J Med.* 1997;336:1269-1275.
17. Greydanus DE, Parks DS, Farrell EG. Breast disorders in children and adolescents. *Pediatr Clin No Amer.* 1989;36: 601-638.
18. Nequin ND. More on jogger's ailments. *N Engl J Med.* 1978;298:405-406.
19. Greydanus De, Matytsina L, Gains M. Breast disorders in children and adolescents. *Prim Care Clin Office Pract.* 2006;33:455-502.
20. Haycock CE. How I manage breast problems in athletes. *Phys Sportsmed.* 1987;15:89-95.
21. Lee J. Sport support. *Women's Sports and Fitness.* 1995;17:72-73.
22. Sports bras. *Women's Sports and Fitness.* 1995;17:72.
23. Mottola MF, Wolfe LA. The pregnant athlete. In: Drinkwater BA, ed. *Women in Sport.* Oxford: Blackwell Science; 2000:194-207.
24. American College of Obstetrics and Gynecology (ACOG) Committee on Obstetric Practice. Exercise during pregnancy and the postpartum period. ACOG Committee Opinion No. 267. 2002;99(1):171-173.
25. Kelly AKW. Practical exercise advice during pregnancy: guidelines for active and inactive women. *Phys and Sports Med.* 2005;33(6):1-10.
26. Campaigne BN. Diabetes and sport. In: Drinkwater BA, ed. *Women in Sport.* Oxford, England: Blackwell Scientific; 2000:265-279.

27. Prentice A. Should lactating women exercise? *Nutr Rev.* 1994;52:358-360.

28. Greydanus DE, Tsitsika AD, Gains MJ. The gynecology system and the adolescent. In: Greydanus DE, Feinberg AN, Patel DR, Homnick DN, eds. *Pediatric Physical Diagnosis.* New York: McGraw-Hill Medical Publishers; 2008: 01-758.

29. Greenfield TP, Blythe MJ Menstrual disorders in adolescents. In: Greydanus DE, Patel DR, Pratt HD, eds. *Essential Adolescent Medicine.* New York: McGraw-Hill Medical Publishers; 2006:591-612.

30. Frankovich RJ, Lebrun CM. Menstrual cycle, contraception and performance. *Clin Sports Med.* 2000;19:1-6.

31. Constantini NW, Gubnov G, Lebrun CM. The menstrual cycle and sports performance. *Clin Sports Med.* 2005;24: 51-82.

32. Moller-Nielson J, Hammar M. Women's soccer injuries in relation to the menstrual cycle and oral contraceptive use. *Med Sci Sports Exerc.* 1989;21:152-160.

33. Greydanus DE, Patel DR, Rimsza ME. Contraception in the adolescent: an update. *Pediatrics.* 2001;107:562-573.

34. Rimsza ME. Contraception in the adolescent. In: Greydanus DE, Patel DR, Pratt HD, eds. *Essential Adolescent Medicine.* New York: McGraw-Hill; 2006:543-568.

35. Greydanus DE, Rimsza ME, Matytsina L. Contraception for college students. *Pediatr Clin No Am.* 2005;52: 135-161.

36. Lybrel A. Continuous oral contraceptive. *Med Lett Dr Ther.* 2007;49:61-62.

37. Coffee AL. Long-term assessment of symptomatology and satisfaction of an extended oral contraceptive regimen. *Contraception.* 2007;75:444-446.

38. American Academy of Pediatrics. Medical concerns in the female athlete. *Pediatrics.* 2000;106:610-613.

39. Beals KA, Meyer NL. Female athlete triad update. *Clin Sports Med.* 2007;26:69-89.

40. Brunet IIM. Female athlete triad. *Clin Sports Med.* 2005;24: 623-636.

41. Ireland ML, Ott SM. Special concerns of the female athlete. *Clin Sports Med.* 2004;23:281-298.

42. Nattive A, Louks AB, Manore MM, Sanborn CF, Sundgot-Borgen J, Warren MP. American College of Sports Medicine Position Stand. The Female Athlete Triad. *Med Sci Sports Exerc.* 2007;39(10):1867-1882.

43. Herring SA, Bergfeld JA, Boyajian-O'Neill LA, et al. Female athlete issues for the team physician: a consensus statement. *Med Sci Sports Exerc.* 2003;1785-1993. Available at http://www.acsm-msse.org. Assessed July 28, 2007.

44. Redman LM, Loucks AB. Menstrual disorders in athletes. *Sports Med.* 2005;35(9):747-755.

45. Currie A, Morse ED. Eating disorders in athletes: managing the risks. *Clin Sport Med.* 2005;24:871-883.

46. Sanborn CF, Horea M, Siemers BJ, et al. Disordered eating and the female athlete triad. *Clin Sports Med.* 2000;19:1-11.

47. *Diagnostic and Statistical Manual of Mental Disorders.* 4th ed. Text Revision. DSM-IV-TR. Washington, DC: American Psychiatric Association; 2000:583-595.

48. Eliakim A. Beyth. Exercise training, menstrual irregularities and bone development in children and adolescents. *J Pediatr Adolesc Gynecol.* 2003;16(4):201-206.

49. Kamboj MK. Metabolic bone disease in adolescents: recognition, evaluation, treatment, and prevention. *Adolesc Med.* 2007:24-46.

50. Cromer BA, Scholes D, Berenson A, et al. Depot medroxyprogesterone acetate and bone mineral density in adolescents. The black box warning: a position paper of the society for adolescent medicine. *J Adolesc Health.* 2006;39: 296-301.

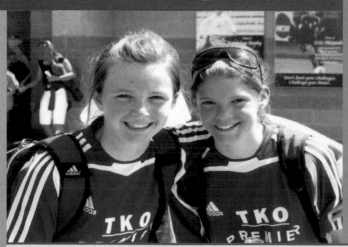

CHAPTER 10

Epilepsy

*Donald E. Greydanus and
David H. Van Dyke*

DEFINITION AND EPIDEMIOLOGY

A seizure is a discrete event with various manifestations while epilepsy (seizure disorder) is defined as a condition with recurrent seizures.[1–4] The well-known Mayo Clinic study looking at the incidence of epilepsy in their area from 1935 to 1967 reported an incidence of newly identified epilepsy as 36 to 48/100,000/y in the 10 to 19 year age cohort.[5] Various studies note that epilepsy affects approximately 1% to 2% of the general population and approximately 25% of those with epilepsy are younger than 18 years.[3,5–7] The prevalence is 3 to 5/1000 adolescents while research notes the annual incidence of a seizure disorder is 24.7/100,000 10- to 14-year-old and 18.6/100,000 15- to 19-year-old. Thus, there are many children and youth with epilepsy who may be involved in sports.

PATHOGENESIS

Epilepsy may develop *de novo* in childhood at any time; thus, in adolescence, it may be a carryover from childhood or begin anytime in the adolescent years. Table 10-1 identifies various causes for epilepsy, but most cases are idiopathic in children and also in adolescents beginning younger than 16 years. As youths get older than 16 years of age, the possibility of a space-occupying lesion increases. Evaluation can also identify seizures because of head trauma, drug abuse, cerebrovascular accidents, central nervous system infections, pseudoseizures, cancer or adverse effects of cancer treatment, syncopal complications, sleep deprivation, hyponatremia, and others (Table 10-1).[3,8] Juvenile myoclonic epilepsy and juvenile absence epilepsy are examples of epilepsy that begin in the adolescent years.[9,10]

CLINICAL PRESENTATION

A careful history and physical examination along with selected laboratory testing is necessary to identify the underlying cause of the new-onset seizure activity (Table 10-1).[3,4] It is important to pay close attention to preseizure and periseizure events, overall development, family history of epilepsy, and history of injuries (including sports-related trauma, such as concussions). Fortunately, the injury sustained by most children and adolescents is not severe enough to lead to traumatic brain injury (TBI) or seizures. A careful description of the seizure and events surrounding it is useful in classifying the type of epilepsy that has developed.

If there is a history of fainting and vision reduction, syncope may be the cause of the unconsciousness and a concomitant reduction in blood pressure leading to the appearance of a pale facies. Pay close attention to the aura, that may have developed, eye or limb movements, duration of loss of consciousness (including reactions to pain or voice), and the presence or absence of incontinence. A thorough review of associated medical and psychologic factors is important in identifying a diagnosis of pseudoseizures, either as the only diagnosis or as concomitant with idiopathic epilepsy.

The physical examination includes blood pressure assessment, both standing and lying measurements to look for orthostatic hypotension. A thorough neurologic evaluation is important including auscultation for bruits (neck, orbits, and skull) while a dermatologic assessment may reveal clues for neurocutaneous syndromes. Body or extremity asymmetry may point to a chronic neurologic abnormality.

Table 10-1.

Evaluation of Seizures in Adolescents*

Differential Diagnosis	Possible Precipitating Factors Idiopathic Seizures	Laboratory Evaluation*
Infectious: Bacterial viral meningitis, encephalitis; systemic infection with fever, sepsis	1. Puberty†	1. CBC
	2. Menses	2. Urinalysis
	3. Trauma	3. Electrolytes
Congenital defects: AV malformations, porencephaly	4. Fever	4. Glucose (fasting and tolerance)
Trauma neoplasms: CNS primary, metastatic	5. Drugs (alcohol, phenothiazines, tricyclic antidepressants, antihistamines, others)	5. BUN, creatinine
Neurocutaneous syndromes: Sturge-Weber, tuberous sclerosis, neurofibromatosis	6. Psychologic stress	6. Toxic drug screen: Urine, serum, gastric
	7. Sleep/sleep deprivation	7. Lumbar puncture‡
Metabolic: Hypoglycemia, hypoparathyroidism, hypocalcemia, hyponatremia, hypernatremia, hypomagnesemia, hypophosphatemia, inborn errors of metabolism	8. Hyperventilation (with absence types)	8. EEG
	9. Photic stimuli (flashing or flickering light, television)	9. CT scan or MRI
	10. Olfactory or tactile stimuli	10. Video EEG
Vasculitis cerebrovascular accident: Ruptured aneurysm (congenital, mycotic), AV malformation, thrombocytopenia	11. Ingestion of certain foods	11. Others: Blood culture, liver function testes, blood gases, serum anticonvulsant level, Wood's Lamp examination
	12. Reading	
	13. Music	
	14. Laughter	
Drug related: Withdrawal from anticonvulsant drugs, withdrawal from CNS depressant addiction (including alcohol, cocaine), insulin overdose, phencyclidine overdose.		
Many drugs are reported (e.g., antidepressants, antihistamines, various antibiotics, and sympathomimietics).		
Hypertensive encephalopathy: Primary, renal, coarctation		
Others: Collagen vascular diseases (SLE), porphyrias, liver disease, renal failure, Gaucher's disease, juvenile huntington's disease, mitochondrial encephalomyopathy, shuddering attacks, pseudoseizures, syncope		

*Perform those tests indicated by clinical judgment and clinical signs.
†The role of puberty in precipitating seizures remains controversial.
‡Perform lumbar puncture only with great caution, if cerebral bleed or increased pressure from other cause suspected. CT scan may be safer as first procedure. Never delay antibiotics for a lumbar puncture.
*(Used with permission from: Greydanus DE, Van Dyke D. Neurologic disorders. In: DE Greydanus, DR Patel, HD Pratt, eds. Essential Adolescent Medicine. New York: McGraw-Hill Medical Publishers; 2006:236.)

DIAGNOSIS

A number of conditions can mimic a seizure disorder, as listed in Table 10-2.

Table 10-1 lists diagnostic tests used to evaluate children and adolescents with seizure activity. Seizure types include partial seizures (simple partial, complex partial, or partial types that become secondarily gener-alized), generalized seizures (absence [including atypi-cal types], myoclonic [versus myoclonic jerks], clonic, tonic, tonic-clonic, and atonic [astatic]), and unclassi-fied types.[3,11–14]

The 16-channel electroencephalogram (EEG) is an adjunctive or confirmatory test in epilepsy diagnosis and is normal in some cases of epilepsy, as for example, in complex partial seizures or in some children with

Table 10-2.

Differential Diagnosis of Epilepsy

Chorea
Dystonia following phenothiazine ingestion
Gilles de la Tourette's syndrome
Hyperventilation
Hysteria (pseudoseizure)
Migraine headaches
Narcolepsy
Nightmares
Night terrors
Oculogyric crisis
Tardive dyskinesia
Vasomotor syncope
Vertigo

epilepsy as they enter puberty. It is the patient who is treated and not the EEG. The EEG, when performed, should be done with the child or adolescent awake and, if possible, asleep or sleep deprived, and during photic as well as hyperventilatory stimuli. Characteristic EEGs are noted in various seizure types, such as infantile spasms, absence seizures, or Lennox-Gastaut syndrome.[3,4,9,10]

Important imaging techniques include ultrasound, computed tomography (CT scan), and magnetic resonance imaging (MRI). The MRI is preferred over the CT scan to assess the spinal cord, brain stem, temporal lobe, and posterior fossa. Also, the MRI is preferred over the CT scan for assessing youth with seizures of probable focal onset. Brain mapping is an experimental and technically challenging diagnostic procedure that is of minimal proven value in epilepsy assessment. Also experimental are single-photon-emission computed tomography (SPECT)—blood flow and positron-emission tomography (PET)—glucose metabolism with EEG correlation.

TREATMENT

There has long been concern that participation in sports would be detrimental to children and adolescent athletes.[6] At one time, those with epilepsy were prevented from participation in many sports and many are less physically active than their nonepileptic peers.[13] However, research has noted the beneficial aspects of exercise and sports in all athletes, including those with a chronic illness such as epilepsy.[13,14] Reports of seizures worsening with exercise are rare and cases of sudden death during exercise are even rarer.[7,15] There is no evidence that the stress of sports participation, increased breathing or

hyperventilation associated with aerobic exercise, or injury resulting from sports (including contact or collision sports) will worsen the seizure pattern in an individual with epilepsy.[6,13,14,16] Although concern about allowing children or adolescents with epilepsy to take part in swimming often arises, there is minimal support for concern for those in good control who are well-supervised, including using a peer to always be available ("buddy system").[1,13,14]

The athlete should be in good seizure control and an adequate supervision is always important, especially in situations where a seizure could result in major injury, such as high diving, gymnastics with parallel bars, rope climbing, scuba diving, skydiving, and motor racing.[7,13,16] Those not in good control need individual assessment to see which sports may be acceptable, depending on the type of seizure the athlete has and the specific sport being played.[16] An individual with epilepsy is prohibited from becoming a pilot.[14]

Some experts have expressed concern when a seizure will injure not only the athlete, but also those who depend on him or her, such as in scuba diving, rope or mountain climbing, and others.[13,14] Careful supervision is always necessary, but especially if the athlete is swimming, water skiing, horse riding, hang-gliding, parachuting, and involved in other high-risk activities.[1,7,13] Those with mental retardation and developmental disabilities need careful supervision. Thorough discussion is important for the athlete and parents regarding theoretical risks.[6] However, these risks should not be exaggerated. For example, a seizure-related drowning by one with epilepsy is more likely when alone taking a bath than being involved in a supervised swim meet.[1,17]

Trauma and Epilepsy

An impact seizure describes seizurelike activity that occurs within seconds following head trauma. It alone does not increase any risk for development of epilepsy. Head trauma, even repetitive trauma, from contact or collision sports has not been shown to induce epilepsy in one without this diagnosis, or to worsen by itself seizure patterns in someone with diagnosed but well controlled epilepsy.[6,14] Thus, antiseizure medication is not necessary for someone with an impact seizure unless there is further evidence of idiopathic epilepsy.

Early posttraumatic epilepsy (PTE) is a disorder that may develop within 7 days of head trauma and results from acute, overt damage to the central nervous system. Later PTE develops over 7 days from head injury that causes CNS damage. PTE risk factors are noted in Table 10-3. PTE is acutely and chronically controlled with antiseizure medications. However, there is no link between head trauma in contact or

Table 10-3.

Risk Factors for Posttraumatic Epilepsy (PTE)

Cerebral edema
Subdural hematoma
Skull fracture
Focal signs
Post-traumatic amnesia lasting over 24 h
Others

Table 10-4.

Reasons for Limited Seizure Control

Mixed or complex seizure disorders
Cerebral edema
Central nervous system tumors
Severe congenital or acquired brain damage
Pubertal changes
Poor medication compliance
Use of wrong anticonvulsant medication
Subtherapeutic medication dosage
Drug interferences or interactions when two or more agents
   are combined
Malabsorption
Development of physiologic drug tolerance
Comorbid substance abuse disorder
Incorrect diagnosis

collision sports and PTE except in unusual, anecdotal situations. Adequate sports equipment, including protection of the head and neck, is always recommended for any athlete involved in sports with increased risks for head or neck injury. If head trauma does seem to provoke seizures, avoidance of contact sports is then warranted.[6] See the discussion of sports and concussions.

Education About Epilepsy

Attention to psychosocial aspects in children and youth with epilepsy is important in the development of optimal seizure control. Pediatric patients with epilepsy can be told that full sports play is usually allowed, if they stay in good seizure control. They should receive comprehensive education regarding their chronic illness to allow full compliance with management recommendations.[3,18,19] For example, children and youth with epilepsy should understand that exposure to flickering lights (as in video games or even driving through a forest with flickering sunlight) can worsen seizure patterns because of photic stimulation; specially made filtered glasses may help. Sleep deprivation, common in many youth and some children, may worsen seizure patterns. Seizure thresholds can be lowered by alcohol and drug abuse. Some adolescent females develop a seizure pattern that is worsened with menses and benefit from increased antiseizure medication to control the seizures. The influence of estrogen is usually to lower the seizure threshold while progesterone may offer some protection in this regard. An increased frequency of anovulatory menstrual cycles, decreased levels of unbound testosterone with hyposexuality in males, and low fertility rates are all described in patients with complex partial seizure disorders.

Anticonvulsant Medication and Sports

Research suggests that approximately 30% of those with epilepsy are not fully controlled with monotherapy while adding a multidrug plan leads to an additional 10% in good seizure control.[3] That leaves approximately 20% who are not well-controlled with polytherapy. Reasons for reduced seizure control despite the use of antiseizure medications are listed in Table 10-4. Caution should be exercised in recommending sports activity in which a seizure places these athletes and/or those around them at risk of injury or death.

Table 10-5 notes adverse effects of various anticonvulsant medications.[1,3,9,13,20] Some of these side effects may undermine sports performance. For example, carbamazepine and valproate can lead to weight gain, gastrointestinal symptoms, rash, and other side effects that athletes will not appreciate. Valproate can also lead to menstrual dysfunction, polycystic ovary syndrome, and hyperandrogenism. Phenobarbital and phenytoin may lead to cognitive and behavior dysfunction. Phenobarbital, for example, may increase depression and suicidal ideation, especially if there is a positive family history for depression.[21] Even side effects not directly linked to lowered sports performance may affect sports by reducing compliance with medication and resultant unstable seizure patterns. For example, the development of coarse facies or gingival hyperplasia noted with phenytoin may lead to reduced medication compliance. This unstable seizure pattern can lead to reduced self-esteem in the patient and increased family conflicts. Thus, side effects of anticonvulsant medications can have a direct and indirect effect on sports performance in athletes with epilepsy.

Clinicians caring for athletes with epilepsy must monitor side effects of these various drugs that are used to keep the patient in as seizure-free a state as possible without major compromise from drug effects. Monitoring

Table 10-5.

Anticonvulsant Medications Side Effects*

1. Phenobarbital

Drowsiness; Lethargy (tends to improve with continued administration), stupor, coma (with levels over 60 mcg/mL), fever, nystagmus, ataxia

LESS COMMON: Osteomalacia with chronic use, hepatic dysfunction, leucopenia, maculopapular or bullous rash, lymphadenopathy, Stevens-Johnson syndrome, behavioral and cognitive effects (including depression), teratogenicity

2. Phenytoin (Dilantin)

Gingival hyperplasia (can prevent with good oral hygiene), hypertrichosis, nystagmus (with levels over 25–30 µg/mL), ataxia, dysarthria, diplopia, choreoathetosis, lethargy, stupor, excitement, peripheral neuropathy, hepatic dysfunction, lymphadenopathy, hypocalcemia, osteomalacia, rickets, hyperglycemia, folic acid deficiency. Idiosyncratic reactions may occur (usually within first 1–4 wk), including exfoliative dermatitis and other rashes, a lupuslike reaction, Stevens-Johnson syndrome. Overdose results in acute cerebellar symptoms, delirium, and coma. Can interfere with cognitive functions, contributing to academic dysfunction. Also, teratogenicity.

3. Ethosuximide (Zarontin)

Nausea, vomiting, lethargy, anorexia, hiccups, irritability, GI irritation, headaches, abdominal pain, skin rash, leukopenia, eosinophilia, ataxia, nystagmus, urticaria, bone marrow depression, lupuslike syndrome, dyskinesis, emotional reaction, including psychotic reactions.

4. Carbamazepine (Tegretol)

Fatigue, malaise, dizziness, anorexia, lethargy, nausea, vomiting, diplopia, nystagmus, ataxia, hepatic dysfunction, bone marrow depression, cardiac arrhythmias, inappropriate ADH secretion, leukopenia, skin rashes, eosinophilic myocarditis, Stevens-Johnson syndrome. Emotional liability and impaired task performance is noted.

5. Primidone (Mysoline)

Lethargy, dizziness, vertigo, nausea, vomiting, ataxia, nystagmus, diplopia, megaloblastic anemia (folic acid deficiency), behavioral changes, bone marrow depression, edema, lupuslike syndrome. Tolerance develops, if previously on phenobarbital. Often used as adjunct to phenytoin and carbamazepine.

6. Acetazolamide (Diamox)

Sedation, teratogenicity, paresthesias, transient increased thirst, increased urination, hyperventilation.

7. Clonazepam (Klonopin)

Behavioral disturbances, ataxia, drooling, sedation.

8. Clorazepate dipotassium (Tranxene)

Sedation, ataxia, behavioral difficulties, drooling.

9. Valproic acid or valproate (Depakene, Depakote)

Nausea, emesis, abdominal cramps, diarrhea, lethargy, transient alopecia, abnormal clotting, reduced platelets and platelet aggregation, pancreatitis, hepatic dysfunction, hair loss, encephalopathy, teratogenicity, weight changes, increased salivation, skin rashes, insomnia, headache. Take with meals to reduce GI side effects. Minimal cognitive impairment is noted.

10. Felbamate (Felbatol)

Increasing aplastic anemia and acute hepatic failure reports have limited the use of this drug. Used alone or with other drugs for partial and secondarily generalized epilepsy and with other drugs for the complex epilepsy seen in the Lennox-Gastaut syndrome.

11. Gabapentin (Neurontin)

Usually well-tolerated. Side effects are often mild and transient: lethargy, ataxia, dizziness, and nystagmus. Does not induce or inhibit hepatic enzymes and does not interfere with other anticonvulsants. Used with other medications to control refractory partial and secondarily generalized epilepsy.

12. Lamotrigine (Lamictal)

Used with other medications for complex partial and generalized epilepsy. Side effects include lethargy, headache, dizziness, blurred vision, rash, ataxia, diplopia, nausea, and vomiting. Rash seen in 10% within 2 wk of drug initiation and disappears when the drug is stopped. Stevens-Johnson syndrome is noted in a few. Interference with valproate is seen.

13. Clonazepam (Clonopin)

Lethargy, irritability, belligerence, aggression, hyperactivity, antisocial patterns, weight gain, ataxia, dysarthria. Tolerance can develop if given with valproic acid, as may be needed in petit mal. Behavioral disorders can occur.

14. Topiramate (Topamax)

Reduce dose 50% with impaired renal function, cognitive slowing, behavioral change, word finding difficulty, may precipitate glaucoma.

15. Oxcarbazepine (Trileptal)

May produce dizziness, hyponatremia, double vision. Requires less hematologic evaluation than carbamazepine. Will occasionally give rash with carbamazepine sensitivity.

16. Levetiracetam (Keppra)

May cause or worsen behavioral abnormalities. Usually well tolerated. Effective in juvenile myoclonic epilepsy.

*(Modified with permission from: Greydanus DE, Van Dyke D. Neurologic disorders. In: Greydanus DE, Patel DR, Pratt HD, eds. Essential Adolescent Medicine. New York: McGraw-Hill Medical Publishers; 2006:243-246.)

drug effects at their therapeutic dosages includes asking about how the side effects impact the athlete's sports performance. Drug interactions are also important to monitor. For example, lamotrigine interacts only with valproate while gabapentin does not interact with others drugs.

The exact dose an individual needs for optimal seizure control is an individual matter and sometimes an increase in dose is necessary, such as during menstruation or significant infections. It should be rare if ever, that sports activity must be stopped while stabilizing an athlete with epilepsy on new medication (s). Monotherapy is the ideal, but as many as three anticonvulsant medications may be needed to control a complex seizure pattern, sometimes requiring months to years for maximal possible control.[1,3] Exercise and sports participation are generally beneficial for children and adolescents; thus, the sports activity should be continued and monitored while attempts to stabilize the seizure patterns continue.

Also, the decision to stop medication after a period of seizure-free activity should not result in preventing any sports activity that the children or youth enjoy. Gradual tapering of the antiseizure medication over 3 to 18 months is the typical pattern, and sports play should be continued during this process. If, in the process of lowering the medication, increased seizure activity occurs, exercise should not be implicated. Starting, continuing, and tapering anticonvulsant medication should always be done with an expert in neurology who appreciates the beneficial impact sports and exercise has on children and youth Box 10-1.

Anticonvulsant Medication and Driving

A rite to pubertal passage for many youth, athletic or not, is the eligibility to obtain a driver's license and operate motorized vehicles.[3,19,22] Youth must be seizure-free for a variable amount of time that varies from state to state, before being allowed to apply for and receive a valid driver's license. This seizure-free period varies from 3 months to 2 years, with an average of 1 year. A physician may be required by law to report patients with a seizure disorder to the local state motor vehicle office. Participating in sports has a beneficial effect on good seizure control. However, a youth with seizure activity may be reluctant to inform the physician in this regards out of fear of being prevented from sports play as well as driving. The restriction of a license may lead to anger, reduced self-esteem, reduced compliance with medication as well as with motor vehicle regulations, and reduced employment opportunities. Tapering or stopping antiseizure medication during the time of license procurement may not be advisable.

Anticonvulsant Medication and Contraception

Involvement in sports activity, even is she has epilepsy, does not prevent the adolescent female from being sexually active and incurring the associated risks of sexually transmitted diseases and unwanted pregnancy. Thus, the sports examination is a good time to ask if the adolescent female is sexually active, encourage abstinence if that is chosen, and provide contraception, if sexual behavior is occurring. The female athlete, who is on antiseizure medication should be educated to avoid unwanted pregnancy, since pregnancy can lower her seizure threshold, increase her antiseizure medications, and lead to limited medication compliance.[3,19] She should be educated about various contraceptive methods, such as barrier methods, oral contraception, depo-medroxy-progesterone acetate, and others, if contraception is desired.[23–25] Anticonvulsant medications induce hepatic microsomal enzymes that can interfere with oral contraceptives; Table 10-6 lists anticonvulsants that interfere with oral contraceptives and some that do not.[26]

Table 10-6.
Anticonvulsants Effect on Oral Contraceptives

Interference
Phenytoin
Phenobarbital
Primidone
Carbamazepine
Topiramate
Ethosuximide
Tiagabine
Noninterference
Valproic acid
Felbamate
Lamotrignine
Gabapentin.
Levetiracetam

Box 10-1 Referral to a Specialist

1. Seizure activity of unknown cause (Table 10-1 and 10-2)
2. Children or adolescent with established seizure patterns that are worsening (Table 10-4)
3. Children or adolescent with known epilepsy unable to tolerate side effects of medications being taken for seizure control (Table 10-5)
4. Request for an athlete with known epilepsy to participate in high-risk sports (such as scuba diving, mountain, climbing, and others)
5. Epilepsy worsened by sports trauma (Table 10-3)
6. Adolescent female with epilepsy, who requested contraception (Table 10-6)
7. Adolescent female with epilepsy who is pregnant.

Anticonvulsant Medication and Pregnancy

The female athlete, who is pregnant may continue with some physical activity. However, she must understand that risks for potential teratogenic effects of her antiseizure drugs exist. Physicians should provide adolescent females with epilepsy with folate along with antiseizure drugs to reduce the risks for neural tube defects induced by these drugs. The dosage of folate ranges from 1 mg/d to 4 mg/d and the upper limits are used, if there is a family history of neural tube defects or sickle cell disease. However, good seizure control during the pregnancy is very important and the fetus is at higher risk from the mother's seizure activity than the potential medication risks of teratogenicity. Good seizure control may require an increase in antiseizure medication during pregnancy since serum levels of these drugs may drop during pregnancy. A subsequent lowering of the dosages is usually necessary after delivery. The youth can be counseled that seizure risks are not increased in the offspring unless there is a strong family history for epilepsy.

Teratogenicity mainly develops in the first 2 months of pregnancy and a two- to threefold increase in birth defects rate is noted in offspring of the mother or father with epilepsy on antiseizure medications.[3,19] Tridione should be avoided in adolescent females at risk for pregnancy because of the associated very high rate of stillbirths and congenital anomalies. Other antiseizure medications linked to birth defects include phenytoin, valproate, and carbamazepine. The use of folate (400 mcg/d) in nonpregnant women with epilepsy lowers the incidence of neural tube defects.[27] Alpha-fetoprotein levels are monitored during pregnancy, if the patient is taking valproate because of the increased risk for spina bifida. The safety of lamotrigine and gabapentin during pregnancy is not known at this time.[28]

REFERENCES

1. Zupanc ML. Sports and epilepsy. In: DeLee JC, Drez D Jr, Miller MD, eds. DeLee & Drez's Orthopaedic Sports Medicine Principles and Practice. vol 1. Philadelphia, PA: Saunders/Elsevier; 2003:312-317.
2. Chang BS, Lowenstein DH. Epilepsy. *N Engl J Med.* 2003;349:1257-1266.
3. Greydanus DE, Van Dyke D. Neurologic disorders. In: Greydanus DE, Patel DR, Pratt HD, eds. Essential Adolescent Medicine. New York: McGraw-Hill Medical Publishers; 2006:235-279.
4. Feinberg AN. The neurology system. In: Greydanus DE, Feinberg AN, Patel DR, Homnick DN, eds. Pediatric Physical Diagnosis. New York: McGraw-Hill Medical Publishers; 2008:349-401.
5. Hauser WA, Kurland LT. The epidemiology of epilepsy in Rochester, Minnesota, 1935 through 1967. *Epilepsia.* 1975;16:1-16.
6. Sahoo SK, Fountain NB. Epilepsy in football players and other land-based contact or collision sport athletes: when can they participate, and is there an increased risk? *Curr Sports Med Reports.* 2004;3:284-288.
7. Howard GM, Radloff M, Sevier TL. Epilepsy and sports participation. *Curr Sports Med Reports.* 2004;3:15-19.
8. Dimeff RJ. Seizure disorder in a professional American football player. *Curr Sports Med Reports.* 2006;5:173-176.
9. Liebenson MH, Rosman NP. Seizures in adolescents. *Adolesc Med.* 1991;2:629-648.
10. Paolicchi JM. Epilepsy in adolescents: diagnosis and treatment. *Adolesc Med.* 2002;13:443-459.
11. Commission on Classification and Terminology of the International League Against Epilepsy. Proposal for revised classification of epilepsies and epileptic syndromes. *Epilepsia.* 1989;30:389-399.
12. Engel J Jr. A proposed diagnostic scheme for people with epileptic seizures and epilepsy: Report of the ILAE Task Force on Classification and Terminology. *Epilepsia.* 1996;37(Suppl 1):S26-S40; 2001;42:796-803.
13. DuBow JS, Kelly JP. Epilepsy in sports and recreation. *Sports Med.* 2003;33:499-516.
14. Fountain MB, May AC. Epilepsy and athletics. *Clin Sports Med.* 2003;22:605-616.
15. Harrison BK, Asplund C. Sudden unexplained death in epilepsy during physical activity. *Curr Sports Med Reports.* 2007;6:13-15.
16. Miele VJ, Bailes ME, Martin MA. Participation in contact or collision sports in athletes with epilepsy, genetic risk factors, structural brain lesions, or history of craniotomy. *Neurosurg Focus.* 2006;21:1-8.
17. Greydanus DE. Preface. Neurologic and neurodevelopmental dilemmas in the adolescent. *Adolesc Med.* 2002;13(3):13-14.
18. Parmet S, Lynm C, Glass RM. Epilepsy. JAMA Patient Page. 2004;291:654.
19. Greydanus DE, Van Dyke D. Epilepsy in the adolescent: the sacred disease and the clinician's sacred duty. *Internat Pediatr.* 2005;20(2):6-8.
20. LaRoche SM, Helmers SL. The new antiepileptic drugs. *JAMA.* 2004;291:605-614, 615-620.
21. Loring DW, Meador KJ. Cognitive and behavioral effects of epilepsy treatment. *Epilepsia.* 2001;42(Suppl 8):24-32.
22. Nordli DR Jr. Special needs of the adolescent with epilepsy. *Epilepsia.* 2001;42(Suppl 8):10-17.
23. Rimsza ME, Greydanus DE, Braverman PK. Contraception. AAP Pediatr Update. 2004;24:1-10.
24. Rimsza ME. Contraception in the adolescent. In: Greydanus DE, Patel DR, Pratt HD, eds. Essential Adolescent Medicine. New York: McGraw-Hill; 2006:543-568.

25. Greydanus DE, Rimsza ME, Matytsina L. Contraception for college students. *Pediatr Clin North Am.* 2005;52: 135-161.

26. Rageneau-Majlessi I, Levy RH. Levetiracetam does not alter the pharmacokinetics of oral contraceptives in healthy women. *Epilepsia.* 2002;43(7):697-702.

27. Yerby MP. Management of issues for women with epilepsy. Neural tube defects and folic acid. *Supplementation.* 2003;61:23-26.

28. White JR, Walczak TS, Leppik IE, et al. Discontinuation of levetiracetam because of behavioral side effects. *Neurology.* 2003;61:1218-1221.

CHAPTER 11

Concussions

Dilip R. Patel

The purpose of this chapter is to outline aspects of sport-related concussions most relevant in the management of young athletes seen in practice. At the outset, it is recognized that research-based data for the evaluation and management of sport-related concussions in children and adolescents are limited. Because no guideline or protocol has been specifically studied for its applicability in children and adolescents, a more cautious approach to management of concussions is recommended in this age group.

DEFINITION

There is no universal consensus on the definition of concussion.[1–4] In its practice parameter on concussion management in sports, the American Academy of Neurology defines concussion as a trauma-induced alteration in mental status that may or may not be associated with loss of consciousness.[5] Confusion, loss of memory, and impaired information processing speed, which may occur immediately or several minutes later, are considered to be the key features of concussion and seen in all instances.[1–8]

The Prague Conference (Second International Conference on Concussion in Sports, 2004, Prague) in its definition includes the following key elements associated with concussion as a result of trauma in sports[6]:

1. Concussion may be caused by a direct blow to the head, face, neck, or elsewhere on the body with "impulsive" force transmitted to the head.
2. Concussion typically results in the rapid onset of short-lived impairment of neurologic function that resolves spontaneously.
3. Concussion may result in neuropathologic changes, but the acute clinical symptoms largely reflect a functional disturbance rather than structural injury.
4. Concussion may result in a graded set of clinical syndromes that may or may not involve loss of consciousness. Resolution of the clinical and cognitive symptoms typically follows a sequential course.
5. Concussion is typically associated with grossly normal structural neuroimaging studies.

The term postconcussion syndrome refers to the persistence of symptoms and signs following the brain injury. Postconcussion syndrome can last for weeks, months, or years. Postconcussion syndrome indicates a more severe injury and precludes athlete's return to high-risk sports.

EPIDEMIOLOGY

In addition to direct impact to the head or other part of the body in contact/ collision sports, concussion can also occur in noncontact sports as a result of sudden acceleration, deceleration, or rotational forces imparted to the brain.[6–9] Thus, absence of a history of direct impact to the head or elsewhere on the body does not rule out the possibility of a concussion.

In high school sports in the United States, 300,000 head injuries are reported every year, and 90% of these are concussions.[1–3] Reported incidence of concussions at high school level is 0.14 to 3.66 concussions per 100 player seasons accounting from 3% to 5% of all sport-related injuries.[8] The highest number of concussion has been reported in American football (Table 11-1).[1–4]

Table 11-1.

Sports with Relatively Higher Risk for Concussion*

American football
Ice hockey
Soccer
Wrestling
Basketball
Field hockey
Baseball
Softball
Volleyball

Listed in decreasing order of risk.

Symptoms and signs of concussion are by definition transient and therefore many athletes may fail to grasp the significance of head trauma and subsequent symptoms of concussion and not seek timely medical attention. Some athletes may not report symptoms or head injury for fear of being excluded from further sport participation. Because of these reasons it is generally accepted that the reported incidence of concussion is an underestimate. Most athletes with concussion seen in a pediatric practice are adolescents, and the following discussion is most applicable to the adolescent age group.

Pathogenesis

Animal and experimental models have shown that in moderate to severe traumatic brain injuries a cascade of complex metabolic and biochemical changes in the setting of genetic overlay results in diffuse neuronal cell injury and dysfunction.[2–9] Alterations in the intracellular and extracellular potassium and calcium ions and excitatory neurotransmitter glutamate have been described. It has been proposed that concussive brain injury causes a disturbance in the autoregulation of cerebral blood flow resulting in a relative decrease in cerebral blood flow, while at the same time there is an increased metabolic demand by the neuronal cells.[2–9] The resultant mismatch between the cellular metabolic demands and cerebral blood flow is believed to be a key contributing factor leading to cellular dysfunction and increased vulnerability to further injury. There are fundamental differences between the developing brain of the child and adolescent and the mature brain of the adult making adult models of pathophysiology far less applicable to children. In broad terms, these differences include continuing neurocognitive maturation, anatomical configuration of the head and brain, structural properties of the skull, biomechanics of head trauma, vulnerability of neurons to injury, and neuronal recovery.[2–9]

CLINICAL PRESENTATION AND EVALUATION

History

Pediatricians may see an athlete with concussion on the field or more commonly in the office setting. On the sideline, the athlete may present with a history of direct blow to the head or other part of the body. The athlete may give a history of collision with another player, a fall to the ground, or being struck by an object such as a ball, a puck, or a bat. Concussion can result from indirect shearing or rotational forces imparted to the brain without direct impact. Not uncommonly, a teammate may notice that "something is not right" with the athlete and communicate that to the trainer on the sideline. The athletic trainer or the coach or less commonly a spectator may see collision and observe that the player is confused. Typically, the confused and disoriented athlete is not able to execute proper moves or follow commands as expected in the context of the play at the time.

The most common scenario for a pediatrician to see an athlete with a concussion is in the office setting when the athlete presents for a follow-up of head injury and needs a medical clearance to return to sport. The athlete may be symptomatic or asymptomatic. On the other hand, some athletes may initially present with symptoms or signs of concussion several days or weeks after the head injury; many may not realize the significance of the initial symptoms and delay seeking medical attention, or seek medical attention because of persistence or worsening or onset of new symptoms. Parents may first seek pediatrician's advice when they notice deterioration of academic performance and changes in behavior, mood, or personality in the athlete; this is critically important to recognize and a probing history of antecedent head trauma must be ascertained.

During the annual sport preparticipation evaluation (PPE), a past history of head injury should be ascertained. Detailed history should include: when did the most recent concussion occurred, what were the symptoms and signs, how long did it take for full recovery, how many concussions have occurred in the past, interval between concussions, and results of any neuropsychologic testing or neuroimaging done.[10–12] PPE visit is also the time for prevention education.

A relevant review of systems should include any known (preinjury) neurologic condition or learning disability, attention deficit hyperactivity disorder, depression, academic function before and since the injury, use of drugs or performance enhancing supplements, and use of therapeutic medications. Psychosocial history should assess athlete's interest in sports, and any evidence of parental pressure to return to sport.[13]

Table 11-2.

Symptoms and Signs of Concussion

Mental status changes
Amnesia
Confusion
Disorientation
Easily distracted
Excessive drowsiness
Feeing "dinged" or "stunned" or "foggy"
Impaired level of consciousness
Inappropriate play behaviors
Poor concentration and attention
Seeing stars or flashing lights
Slow to answer questions or follow directions

Physical or somatic
Ataxia or loss of balance
Blurry vision
Decreased performance or playing ability
Dizziness
Double vision
Fatigue
Headache
Lightheadedness
Nausea, vomiting
Poor coordination
Ringing in the ears
Seizures
Slurred, incoherent speech
Vacant star/glassy eyed
Vertigo

Behavioral or psychosomatic
Emotional liability
Irritability
Low frustration tolerance
Personality changes
Nervousness, anxiety
Sadness, depressed mood

Symptoms and Signs

The athlete with concussion may manifest any one or more of a number of symptoms or signs (Table 11-2); some immediately after the injury to the brain, whereas others may be delayed for days or weeks.[3–8,14–17] Because no one or a set of symptoms and signs is pathognomonic of concussion, and most are nonspecific in nature, a contemporaneous relationship between the time of initial injury to the brain and subsequent development of symptoms and signs should be established on the basis of history and examination.

In the evaluation of an athlete with symptoms and signs of concussion the physician should consider other conditions that can present with similar clinical features. In the acute setting, heat-related illness,

effects of dehydration, hypoglycemia, and acute exertional migraine can mimic concussion. Many of the delayed symptoms of concussion are nonspecific, making it necessary to carefully delineate the differential diagnosis or concomitant conditions such as depression, attention deficit/hyperactivity disorder, sleep disorder, cerebellar or brain stem lesions, or psychosomatic disorder. By definition a variable degree of mental status impairment is seen in all cases of concussion.

Mental Status and Cognitive Function

Assessment of cognitive functions and neurologic examination are essential components of evaluation of athletes with concussion. An athlete with concussion may continue to manifest physical and emotional symptoms even after resolution of cognitive deficits. Cognitive function can be affected by many factors other than the effects of concussion, such as baseline (preinjury) intellectual ability, learning disability, attention deficit/hyperactivity disorder, substance abuse, level of education, cultural background, lack of sleep, fatigue, anxiety, age, and developmental stage.[1,2,18,19] Cognitive assessment techniques should be appropriate for the athlete's age, level of education, and developmental stage or maturity.

A practical way to assess memory and orientation on the sidelines is Maddocks questions (Table 11-3); not able to answer or incorrect answer to any one of the Maddocks questions indicates concussion.[20,21] The following areas of cognitive functioning and assessment techniques are generally included in a brief mental status examination of athletes with sport-related concussion.[5–7,15,22,23]

1. Orientation—Orientation in person, place, and time.
2. Attention
   - Digit span: Recite a series of two digits to the athlete at a rate of about one per second. Ask the athlete to repeat the numbers back to

Table 11-3.

Maddocks Questions

Which ground are we at?
Which team are we playing today?
Who is your opponent at present?
Which quarter is it?
How far into the quarter is it?
Which side scored the last goal?
Which team did we play last week?
Did we win last week?

you. If the athlete is able to correctly repeat the two digits, recite a series of three numbers, then four, five, and so on, as long as the athlete is able to correctly repeat the digits back to you. If the athlete makes an error, try one more time with another series of the same length. Stop after the athlete fails at the second attempt. Similarly, have the athlete repeat the digits backwards starting with a series of two. Normally the athlete should be able to repeat correctly at least five digits forward and four backwards.

   ■ Serial 7s: Ask the athlete to subtract 7 from 100 and keep subtracting. Typically, the athlete should be able to complete a serial 7 in 1.5 minutes with fewer than four errors. If the athlete finds it difficult to do serial 7s, have him do serial 3s in a similar way.

   ■ Spelling backwards: Say a five-letter word, spell it, then ask the athlete to spell it backward.

3. Memory

   ■ Give the athlete five words and ask him or her to repeat them back to you. The athlete with intact registration and immediate recall should be able to correctly repeat the five words back to you. Without informing the athlete that he or she will be asked to recall these words later, move on to another task of assessment in the meantime. Five minutes later ask the athlete to recall the five words. The athlete with intact delayed recall should be able to recall the five words.

   ■ Ask the athlete to recite the months of the year in reverse order starting with a given month or the current month (other than December or January).

   ■ Ask the athlete to tell current score of the game, which quarter it is and the name of the opposing team (recent memory).

   ■ Ask the athlete to tell you the name of his or her elementary school or place of birth (remote memory).

      The onset of posttraumatic amnesia, a key feature of concussion, may be delayed for more than 20 minutes following injury to the brain.[2] Resolution of posttraumatic amnesia is best indicated by the athlete's ability to recall fully the events from before the injury to the brain to present (continuous memory).[2,8,16]

4. Higher cognitive functions—General knowledge and vocabulary are good indicators of intellectual function. Assess calculation ability by asking the athlete to perform a simple task:

how many nickels make a quarter? Or what is the square root of 64? Abstract thinking can be assessed by asking the athlete meaning of a common proverb for example: rolling stone gathers no moss; or by similarities test, for example: how are a train and an airplane similar? Constructional abilities give a good indication of visual motor abilities. To test constructional abilities ask the athlete to draw for example a clock face with numbers and hands and judge the quality of the drawing.

5. Other areas of mental status—Insight, judgment, affect, and mood are other areas of mental status that should be assessed in athletes with concussion.

Neurologic Examination

A complete neurologic examination is essential in the evaluation of athletes with concussion with specific attention to the following components: (1) Speech, (2) visual acuity, visual fields, ocular fundi, pupillary reactions, and extraocular movements, (3) muscle strength and deep tendon reflexes, and (4) tandem gait, finger-nose test, pronator drift, and Romberg test. By definition, neurologic examination should be normal in athletes with concussion, except the mental status functions. Abnormal or focal findings on neurologic examination should prompt consideration of a focal intracranial pathology and emergent evaluation and management of the athlete.

   Before the athlete is allowed to return to play, he or she must be asymptomatic both at rest as well as on exertion and the examination must be normal. The athlete should be assessed for recurrence of any symptoms or signs on physical exertion; simple exertion provocative measures (Table 11-4) can be integrated in the examination.[2,5,6,8]

Severity Grading of Concussions

Most concussion grading systems are based on the presence or absence of loss of consciousness, duration of loss of consciousness, presence or absence of confusion, and

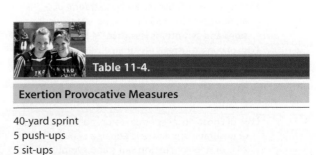

Table 11-4.

Exertion Provocative Measures

40-yard sprint
5 push-ups
5 sit-ups
5 jumping jacks

Table 11-5.

American Academy of Neurology Concussion Severity Grading System

Grade	Criteria
1	Transient confusion No loss of consciousness Symptoms and mental status abnormalities resolve in less than 15 min
2	Transient confusion No loss of consciousness Symptoms and mental status abnormalities last more than 15 min
3	Any loss of consciousness

presence or absence and duration of posttraumatic amnesia, none of which have been shown to reliably predict the severity or prognosis for recovery.[1–6,8,24] The duration of symptoms and signs following the initial brain injury has been shown to predict the severity of concussion and prognosis for recovery more reliably, hence the prevailing view is to consider the severity grading of concussion retrospectively after the clinical resolution of concussion.[2,6,8,24] Although more than 20 grading schemes for concussion have been published, the American Academy of Neurology (Table 11-5) and Cantu (Table 11-6) grading systems are the most widely known.[2,5,24]

The Prague Concussion in Sport Consensus Statement does not recommend use of conventional grading scales in the management of concussions.[6] It is recognized that the severity of concussion in an individual athlete can only be ascertained retrospectively after full clinical recovery has occurred. A simple concussion typ-

Table 11-6.

Cantu Concussion Severity Grading System

Grade	Criteria
1	No loss of consciousness and posttraumatic amnesia less than 30 min; and postconcussion signs and symptoms less than 24 h
2	Loss of consciousness less than 1 min; or posttraumatic amnesia equal to or less than 30 min and less than 24 h; or postconcussion signs and symptoms equal to or more than 24 h and less than 7 d
3	Loss of consciousness equal to or more than 1 min; or posttraumatic amnesia equal to or more than 24 h; or postconcussion signs and symptoms equal to or more than 7 d

ically resolves within 7 to 10 days and requires no further intervention, whereas a complex concussion is characterized by failure of clinical resolution and associated sequelae.

DIAGNOSTIC STUDIES

Neuroimaging

Neuroimaging is indicated in athletes with focal neurologic signs, those with progressively worsening symptoms and signs, failure of clinical resolution of symptoms (typically more than 2 weeks), severe acute headache, and loss of consciousness greater than a few seconds.[24] Static imaging with magnetic resonance imaging (MRI) or computerized tomography does not show any structural abnormalities of brain in concussion. Imaging modalities such as positron emission tomography (PET), functional MRI (fMRI), or single photon emission tomography (SPECT) provide information on brain metabolism and regional blood flow; however, their application in clinical evaluation and management of athletes with concussion is limited at best.

Neuropsychologic Testing

The important domains of cognitive function assessed by neuropsychologic (NP) testing include: memory, speed of information processing, visual spatial and visual motor abilities, and various components of executive function (including working memory, attention, planning, and organization).[25,26] Memory and speed of information processing (or reaction time) are the most important cognitive functions impaired by concussion that are measured by NP testing. Conventional (or paper and pencil) NP testing utilizes a battery of tests administered over one or more sessions (several hours) and interpreted by trained neuropsychologists. Conventional NP tests are neither specifically designed nor validated to assess athletes with sport-related concussion, cannot be easily adapted for mass application, and are relatively expensive.

During the adolescent years there is continued neurological maturation associated with increased acquisition of neurocognitive abilities as well as rapid acquisition of new skills and knowledge.[1,14] A sensitive indicator of resolution of concussion is a return to baseline neuropsychological profile following concussion; however because of continued neuomaturation during adolescence, a return to baseline NP profile may not necessarily indicate full recovery. This confounding factor should be taken into account in interpreting NP tests in adolescents.

Computerized NP testing specifically designed to assess athletes with sport-related concussion, is now

Table 11-7.

Computerized Neuropsychological Tests

Test	Contact/Web Site
Automated Neuropsychological Assessment Metrics (ANAM)	National Rehabilitation Hospital Assistive Technology and Neuroscience Center, Washington, DC http://thirlstanewest.com/CCN/ANAM.php
(1) CogSport (2) Concussion Sentinel (Specifically designed for American athletes)	CogState Ltd, 51 Leicester Street, Carlton South, Victoria 3053, Australia www.cogsport.com
(1) Concussion Resolution Index (CRI) (2) eSAC for sideline testing	HeadMinder, Inc, 15 Maiden Lane, Suite 205, New York, NY 10038, USA www.headminder.com
(1) Immediate Post Concussion Assessment and Cognitive Testing (ImPACT 2.0) (2) Sideline ImPACT for sideline testing	ImPACT Applications, Inc, P.O. Box 23288, Hilton Head Island, SC 29925, USA www.impacttest.com

Immediate Postconcussion ImPACT Applications, Inc, P.O.Box 23288, Hilton Head Island, SC
Assessment and Cognitive Testing (ImPACT 2.0) Sideline ImPACT for sideline testing www.impacttest.com

being utilized at high school, collegiate, and professional levels to obtain baseline as well as postconcussion neuropsyhological profile of athletes to monitor recovery.[1,2,25–29] Some of the advantages of computerized testing include: simple to administer, less expensive, takes only few minutes to administer, can be easily given to a group of athletes (team), and easy to interpret. Examples of currently available computerized NP tests are listed in Table 11-7. For interested physicians detailed information on each of the tests is available at their websites.

Notwithstanding the increased application of computerized NP testing, their validity and reliability has been a subject of much debate.[25] NP testing, either conventional or computerized, must not be used in isolation in the assessment or monitoring recovery of athletes with concussion, and return to play decisions should not be guided solely based on results of NP testing. With more baseline data being accumulated, properly constructed and administered computerized NP testing hold great promise as a valuable tool to objectively assess and monitor athletes with sport-related concussion. Formal NP testing is useful to delineate specific impairments in athletes who fail to recover as expected or deteriorate or those who have had multiple concussions. NP testing can be useful in guiding the management of academic difficulties in children and adolescents.

MANAGEMENT

On Field Management

Recognition, stabilization, and appropriate disposition of athletes with severe head and neck injuries should be the first priority of the physician on the field. From a practical perspective it is difficult to assess severity of injury in athletes with loss of consciousness of any duration, and therefore it is most prudent to immediately initiate stabilization and transport of the unconscious athlete to the emergency department. Fortunately severe head and neck injuries are rare in youth sports.

Once the young athlete is recognized to have a concussion he or she must be removed from the practice or game for the day.[2,4,8,14] The athlete should not be left unattended on the sideline, and must be assessed periodically for evolving symptoms and signs. Acute symptoms typically resolve within few minutes in most athletes and the athlete may be allowed to go home with appropriate instructions and a follow-up should be arranged for the next day in the office. The Prague statement recommends that the athlete should watch for the following symptoms and to seek immediate medical attention if any occurs[6]:

> headache that gets worse
> feeling drowsy or difficult to be awakened
> difficulty recognizing people or places
> repeated vomiting
> increased confusion
> increased irritability
> seizures
> weakness of arms or legs
> unsteady gait
> slurred speech

The athlete whose symptoms fail to resolve within a few minutes, whose symptoms worsen, or who is noted to have abnormal findings on neurological examination should be transferred to the emergency department for further evaluation and management Box 11-1. With the recognition of the fact that each athlete follows a variable time course to recovery from acute cerebral concussion, an individualized, stepwise plan for return to play is now considered the most preferred practice rather than following the conventional return to play guidelines. The more widely known Cantu and the AAN guidelines, base return to play decisions on the severity grading of concussions. In practice this approach is less useful because severity of a concussion can be more reliably determined retrospectively after clinical resolution of the concussion. Also, loss of consciousness used as one of the criteria to grade concussion severity has not been shown to be a reliable indicator of severity of concussion. It is now generally agreed that, although most athletes recover over a

Box 11-1 When to Refer to Specialist

*Acute**

Severe head and neck trauma
Focal neurologic signs
Acute severe posttraumatic headache
Severe persistent vomiting
Prolonged loss of consciousness
Posttraumatic seizures
Deteriorating mental status

Chronic†

Multiple concussions
Persistent postconcussion symptoms
Symptoms of depression
Changes in personality
Changes in behavior
Deteriorating academic functioning

*Appropriate specialists include neurologist, neurosurgeon, and orthopedic surgeon.
†Specialists include sports medicine physician, psychologist, or child and adolescent psychiatrist.

Table 11-8.

Concussion Symptom Inventory*

Symptom	Absent	Present
Headache	0	1
Nausea	0	1
Balance problems/dizziness	0	1
Fatigue	0	1
Drowsiness	0	1
Feeling like "in a fog"	0	1
Difficulty concentrating	0	1
Difficulty remembering	0	1
Sensitivity to light	0	1
Sensitivity to noise	0	1
Blurred vision	0	1
Feeling slowed down	0	1
Total		

Randolph C, Barr WB, McCrea M, et al: Concussion symptom inventory (CSI): an empirically derived scale for monitoring resolution of symptoms following sport-related concussion. www. smf.org/articles/hic/concussion_symptom_inventory, 2006. Accessed 2006.

period from 2 to 3 weeks to 1 to 3 months, each athlete follows a variable trajectory to recovery following a concussion, making any fixed period of time out before return to play a less valid approach.[1–3,8]

Follow-up and Subsequent Management

The athlete must be seen in the office the next day and further management should be guided by the Prague consensus statement, which recommends the following stepwise approach of management[6]:

1. No activity, complete rest, once asymptomatic, proceed to (step 2).
2. Light aerobic exercise such as walking, stationary cycling, and no resistance training.
3. Sport-specific exercise (e.g., skating in hockey, running in soccer), progressive addition of resistance training at step 3 and 4.
4. Noncontact training drills.
5. Full-contact training after medical clearance.
6. Return to sport.

With the stepwise progression, the athlete should continue to proceed to the next level if asymptomatic at the current level. If postconcussion symptoms reoccur the athlete should fall back to the previous asymptomatic step and try to progress after 24 hours.

Increasing evidence suggests that concussion-rating scales based on athlete self-report of multiple symptoms are a reliable and practical way of detecting and monitoring concussion during recovery phase.[2,6,17,29,30] The Concussion Symptom Inventory (Table 11-8) is one such scale shown to be sensitive and specific for tracking subjective symptoms following sport-related concussion, and is recommended for use during the postinjury monitoring.[17] A baseline Concussion Symptom Inventory profile (preseason) can be valuable to compare later with postinjury profile of the same athlete at various time intervals.

Children and adolescents should return to increasing level of schoolwork gradually.[4] They need cognitive rest until full cognitive recovery.[4,6,14] The school should be informed of the athlete's need for special accommodations during the recovery phase. Most student athletes recover fully from concussion within a few days or weeks, a few may need to utilize Section 504 plan, and even fewer may need implementation of the individualized education plan.

Return to play decisions should be individualized and ultimately are made based on the clinical judgment of the physician.[1,2,4,6,8,12]

Athlete with Multiple Concussions

The adverse effects of repeated concussions on the brain are cumulative and relatively greater as the interval between two successive concussions gets shorter.[30–36] Likelihood of long-term and permanent impairment in cognitive functioning is increased significantly with each repeated concussion. The effects of neurotrauma are even greater for the developing brain.[1,4,17] An athlete can sustain multiple concussions during the same day, during the same season, or over his or her career. There are no scientifically validated criteria for return to play for athletes who have sustained more than one concussion.[32,33,34]

There is no agreement as to how many concussions are too many to disqualify the athlete from further participation in high-risk sports; however some have suggested 3 concussions as the magic number.[2,3,32] For the young athlete a more conservative approach is recommended. The young athlete and his or her parents must be educated about the significance of repeated concussions on the developing brain and a serious consideration must be given not to return the athlete with multiple concussions to high-risk sports.

OUTCOME

Most young athletes recover fully from concussion. In fact 30% of high school and collegiate athletes return to play the same day, and 70% after 4 days.[2] Based on NP testing data, correlation between NP testing and clinical findings indicate that most athletes with simple (mild) concussion recover cognitive function within 7 to 10 days, and those with complex (severe) concussion show recovery over a period of 1 to 3 months.[6,26] Athletes who have recovered in terms of their neurocognitive deficits may still have persistent emotional symptoms.

Children and adolescents have a relatively more prolonged recovery course compared with adults, are significantly more likely to have another concussion, and the effects of repeated concussion are cumulative.[4,14,33–46] Children and adolescents can have lifelong implications as a result of concussion in terms of poor academic achievement, emotional symptoms, and psychosocial difficulties.

A syndrome of rapidly progressive brain edema, brain stem herniation, and high mortality within minutes of a second concussion in an athlete who still has persistent symptoms (or has not clinically fully recovered) from a previous concussion has been described in adolescent male athletes.[47] Although some recent reports have raised doubts on the occurrence or significance of second impact syndrome, the issue has neither been fully elucidated nor resolved.[1,2,4,14,47] It seems prudent at present that no athlete should return to play until fully asymptomatic and has normal examination at rest and on provocative exertion.

PREVENTION

Increased awareness among athletes, parents, coaches, and public at large, of various aspects of sport-related concussion is the most essential element of prevention strategy.[1,4,6,48,49] On an individual level the pediatrician should incorporate education about sport-related concussion in the anticipatory guidance during well visits as well as during the evaluation and management of athletes who present with concussion. Key aspects of such education include: recognition of features of concussion, importance of seeking timely medical attention, not to return to sports before recovery is complete, potential acute and known long-term consequences of concussion.

Enforcement of rules of the game play important role in prevention of head and neck injuries. Use of helmets in American football has reduced the likelihood of severe skull injury; however, helmet use has not been shown to be effective in prevention of brain concussion.[6,8,50] Appropriate use of mouth guards has been shown to reduce the incidence of orofacial injuries; their efficacy in prevention of concussion has not been established[51,52] Strong neck muscles may allow the athlete to tense these muscles and maintain the head and neck in a fixed position just prior to impact and help dissipate the forces, theoretically reducing the impact on the brain. However in real world, there is little time to anticipate the impact and fix the head and neck before the actual impact.

REFERENCES

1. Patel DR, Shivdasani V, Baker RJ. Management of sport-related concussion in young athletes. *Sports Med.* 2005; 35(8):671-684.
2. Guskiewicz KM, Bruce SL, Cantu RC, et al. National Athletic Trainers Association Position Statement: management of sport-related concusión. *J Athl Train.* 2004;39: 280-297.
3. Landry GL. Central nervous system trauma: Management of concussions in athletes. *Pediatr Clin North Am.* 2002; 49(4):723-742.
4. Kirkwood MW, Yeats KO, Wilson PE. Pediatric sport-related concussions: a review of the clinical management of an oft-neglected population. *Pediatrics.* 2006;117(4): 1359-1371.
5. Quality Standards Subcommittee of the American Academy of Neurology. The management of concussion in sports. *Neurology.* 1997;48:581-585.
6. MCrory P, Johnson K, Meeuwisse W, et al. Summary and agreement statement of the 2nd International Conference on Concussion in Sport, Prague, 2004. *Clin J Sport Med.* 2005;15(2):48-55.
7. Wojtys EM, Hovda D, Landry G, et al. Concussion in sports. *Am J Sports Med.* 1999;27(5):676-687.
8. American College of Sports Medicine. Concussion (mild traumatic brain injury) and the team physician: a consensos statement. *Med Sci Sports Exerc.* 2006;36(2)395-399.
9. Powel JW, Barber-Foss KD. Traumatic brain injury in high school athletes. *JAMA.* 1999;282:958 963.
10. Patel DR. Managing concussion in a young athlete. *Contemp Pediatr.* 2006;23(11):62-69.
11. McCrory P. Preparticipation assessment for head-injury. *Clin J Sport Med.* 2004;14:139-144.
12. American Academy of Pediatrics, American Academy of Family Medicine, American Medical Society for Sports Medicine, American College of Sports Medicine, American

Orthopedic Society for Sports Medicine. *Preparticipation Physical Evaluation Monograph.* 3rd ed. New York, NY: McGraw Hill; 2005.

13. Patel DR, Greydanus DE, Pratt HD. Youth sports: More than sprains and strains. *Contemp Pediatr.* 2001;18(3):45-76.

14. McCrory P, Collie A, Anderson V, Davis G. Can we manage sport related concussion in children the same as in adults? *Br J Sports Med.* 2004;38:516-519.

15. Kelly JP, Rosenberg JH. The diagnosis and management of concussion in sports. *Neurology.* 1997;48:575-580.

16. Maroon JC, Field M, Lovell M, et al. The evaluation of athletes with cerebral concussion. *Clin Neurosurg.* 2002; 49:319-332.

17. Randolph C, Barr WB, McCrea M, et al. Concussion symptom inventory (CSI): an empirically-derived scale for monitoring resolution of symptoms following sport-related concussion. 2006. www.smf.org/articles/hic/concussion_symptom_inventory.pdf. Accessed October 12, 2006.

18. Grindel SH, Lovell MR, Collins MW. The assessment of sport-related concussion: the evidence behind neuropsychological testing and management. *Clin J Sport Med.* 2001;11:134-143.

19. Schatz P, Zillmer EA. Computer-based assessment of sports-related concussion. *Appl Neuropsychol.* 2003;10(1): 42-47.

20. Maddocks D, Dicker G. An objective measure of recovery from concussion in Australian rules footballers. *Sport Health.* 1989;7(suppl):6-7.

21. Maddocks DL, Dicker G, Saling MM. The assessment of orientation following concussion in athletes. *Clin J Sport Med.* 1995;5(1):32-35.

22. Bickley LS. *Bates' Guides to Physical Examination and History Taking.* 9th ed. Baltimore: Lippincott Williams & Wilkins; 2006.

23. McCrea M, Kelly JP, Randolph C. Standardized assessment of concussion (SAC): on-site mental status evaluation of the athlete. *J Head Trauma Rehabil.* 1998:13(2):27-35.

24. Cantu RC. Work-up of the athlete with concussion. *Am J Sports Med.* 2002;4:152-154.

25. Randolph C, McCrea M, Barr WB. Is neuropsychological testing useful in the management of sport-related concussion? *J Athl Train.* 2005;40(3):139-154.

26. Lovell MR. The relevance of neuropsychological testing in sports-related head injuries. *Curr Sports Med Rep.* 2002;1 (1):7-11.

27. Collie A, Darby D, Maruff P. Computerised cognitive assessment of athletes with sports related head injury. *Br J Sports Med.* 2001;35:297-302.

28. Collie A, Maruff P, McStephen M, et al. Psychometric issues associated with computerized neuropsychological assessment of concussed athletes. *Br J Sports Med.* 2003; 37(6):556-559.

29. Piland SG, Motl RW, Guskiewicz KM, et al. Structural validity of a self-report concussion-related symptom scale. *Med Sci Sports Exerc.* 2006;38(1):27-32.

30. Erlanger D, Kaushik T, Cantu RC, et al. Symptom-based assessment of the severity of a concussion. *J Neurosurg.* 2003;98:477-484.

31. Collins MW, Lovell MR, Iverson GL, et al. Cumulative effects of concussion in high school athletes. *Neurosurgery.* 2002;51(5):1175-1181.

32. McCrory P. What advice should we give to athletes post-concussion? *Br J Sports Med.* 2002;36(5):316-318.

33. McCrory P. Treatment of recurrent concussion. *Curr Sports Med Rep.* 2002;1(1):28-32.

34. Cantu RC. Recurrent athletic head injury: Risks and when to retire. *Clin Sports Med.* 2003;22(3):593-603.

35. Guskiewicz KM, McCrea M, Marshall SW, et al. Cumulative effects associated with recurrent concussion in collegiate football players: the NCAA Concussion Study. *JAMA.* 2003;290:2549-2555.

36. Bruce JM, Echemendia RJ. Concussion history predicts self-reported symptoms before and following a concussive event. *Neurology.* 2004;63:1516-1518.

37. Pellman ES, Lovell MR, Viano DL, Casson IR. Concussion in professional football: recovery of NFL and high-school athletes assessed by computerized neuropsychological testing, Part 12. *Neurosurgery.* 2006; 58(2): 263-272.

38. Moser RS, Schatz P, Jordan BD. Prolonged effects of concussion in high-school athletes. *Neurosurgery.* 2005;57(2): 300-306.

39. Iverson GL. No cumulative effects of one or two previous concussions *Br J Sports Med.* 2006;40(1):72-75.

40. Bleiberg J, Cernich AN, Cameron K, et al. Duration of cognitive impairment after sports concussion. *Neurosurgery.* 2004;54(5):1073-1080.

41. McClincy MP, Lovell MR, Pardini J, et al. Recovery from sport concussion in high-school and collegiate athletes. *Brain Inj.* 2006;20(1):33-39.

42. Sterr A, Herron K, Hayward C, Montaldi D. Are mild head injuries as mild as we think? Neurobehavioral concomitants of chronic post-concussive syndrome. *BMC Neurol.* 2006;6:7-17.

43. Browne GJ, Lam LT. Concussive head injury in children and adolescents related to sports and other leisure physical activities. *Br J Sports Med.* 2006;40(2):163-168.

44. Field M, Collins MW, Lovell MR, Maroon J. Does age play a role in recovery from sports-related concussion? A comparison of high school and collegiate athletes. *J Pediatr.* 2003;142:546-553.

45. Lovell MR, Collins MW, Iverson GL, et al. Grade 1 or "ding" concussions in high school athletes. *Am J Sports Med.* 2004;32:47-54.

46. Lovell MR, Collins MW, Iverson GL, et al. Recovery from mild concussion in high school athletes. *J Neurosurg.* 2003;98:296-301.

47. McCrory PR, Berkovic SF. Second impact syndrome. *Neurology.* 1998;50(3):677-683.

48. Kelly JP, Nichols JS, Filley CM, et al. Concussion in sports: guidelines for the prevention of catastrophic outcome. *JAMA.* 1991;266(20):2867-2869.

49. McCrea M, Hammeke T, Olsen G, Leo P, Guskiewicz K. Unreported concussion in high school football players: implications for prevention. *Clin J Sport Med.* 2004;14(1):13-17.

50. McIntosh AS, McCrory P. Effectiveness of headgear in a pilot study of under 15 rugby union football. *Br J Sports Med.* 2001;35(3):167-169.

51. Wisniewski JF, Guskiewicz K, Trope M, Sigurdsson A. Incidence of cerebral concussions associated with type of mouthguard used in college football. *Dent Traumatol.* 2004;20(3):143-149.

52. Labella CR, Smith BW, Sigurdsson A. Effect of mouthguards on dental injuries and concussions in college basketball. *Med Sci Sports Exerc.* 2002;34(1):41-44.

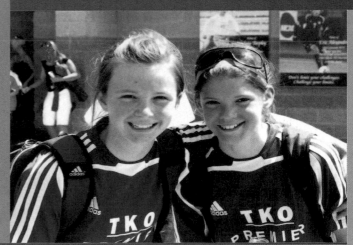

CHAPTER 12

Chest and Pulmonary Conditions

Douglas N. Homnick

INTRODUCTION

The upper and lower airways (above and below the glottis), lung, and chest wall function as an integrated unit to provide for efficient gas exchange during exercise and sports. Dysfunction in any of these components can lead to compromised exercise tolerance. This chapter will consider common conditions that affect the respiratory tract and that can lead to limitation in physical activities. Locating the site of dysfunction through physical examination and laboratory testing, particularly the evaluation of pulmonary function is the first step in solving a sports-related respiratory problem. Consideration of pulmonary function alterations together with signs and symptoms of disease and specific therapies will be the focus of this chapter. Consequently, a general discussion of respiratory exercise physiology and pulmonary function evaluation will form the basis for understanding specific conditions that affect each.

Respiratory Exercise Physiology

There is a significant and interdependent interaction of muscle, cardiovascular output, and ventilation during rest as well as during exercise. Ventilation is dependent on airway caliber, integrity of the central and peripheral nervous system, and respiratory musculature. During quiet breathing, the diaphragm and to some extent the abdominal muscles and inspiratory intercostal muscles are active. With exercise, there is considerable increase in activity of these muscle groups in addition to recruitment of other muscles including the expiratory intercostals and sternocleidomastoids. The sum total is increased ventilation to meet the metabolic demands of more vigorous exercise including increased oxygen consumption and carbon dioxide elimination.

At high levels of exercise, all respiratory muscles are participating and movement of extremities also facilitates breathing.[1] Increase in all the body's muscle activity requires increased oxygen consumption and during strenuous exercise up to 95% of oxygen demands can be accounted for by respiratory and other muscles groups.[1] The physiologic adjustments for adequate oxygen consumption to support aerobic metabolism and provide adequate elimination of carbon dioxide are dependent on the linked factors shown in Figure 12-1. These are specifically increased ventilation, increased cardiac output, and redistribution of blood flow to working muscles.[1] When oxygen requirements to support aerobic metabolism are exceeded, anaerobic metabolism begins. Increased lactate is the end product. During exercise, the point of transition from aerobic to anaerobic metabolism (the anaerobic threshold) is measured in the laboratory. This will vary with level of conditioning or with disease state (Figure 12-2).[2]

Conditioning

Physical training has many positive effects on respiratory and circulatory function (Table 12-1).[1] In the pulmonary function laboratory, measuring maximal oxygen uptake is a base measure for level of fitness. Increase in maximal cardiac output as a result of increased stroke volume relates directly to increase in maximal O_2 uptake. Muscle undergoes a number of changes including increased blood flow above pretraining levels, in increase in density of muscle capillaries, and increased oxygen extraction. Both aerobic and anaerobic work capacity increase with training as measured by increased oxygen consumption and decreased lactate production for a given work load. Maximal ventilation increases with training in some individuals but

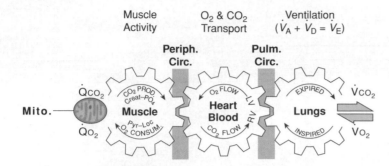

FIGURE 12-1 ■ Gas transport mechanism for the coupling of cellular to pulmonary respiration. Q_{O_2}, oxygen extraction of muscle from blood; Q_{CO_2}, carbon dioxide production from muscle activity; V_{O_2}, volume of oxygen taken up by the lung; V_{CO_2}, volume of carbon dioxide during expiration. *(Used with permission from reference 2)*

not all, however at sub maximal levels; ventilation is consistently lower after training.[1]

Pulmonary Function Testing

Pulmonary function testing (PFT) is important to quantify not only the degree (or lack) of impairment of respiratory function but also the type of dysfunction. It can also be used to monitor response to therapy whether medical, physical, or the effects of training. It is important to note that PFT supports specific diagnoses by determining the type of lung, airway, or chest wall disease but does not give specific pulmonary diagnoses. Clinical correlation is always necessary.

PFTs consist of a measure of airflow (spirometry), lung volumes (static lung volumes), diffusion capacity, and gas exchange (oximetry, blood gases); and specialized tests such as bronchial challenge with chemicals such as methacholine, exercise challenge with serial spirometry, and exercise metabolic testing. In the office setting, spirometry is the most practical measure and most problems associated with sports are supported by spirometric changes; therefore, we will focus on this test. Exercise testing (see section on exercise-induced asthma) or methacholine challenge with serial spirometry done in the hos-

pital PFT laboratory is also useful for determining sports-related respiratory dysfunction. Lung volumes are helpful in evaluating chest wall dysfunction as a cause of reduced exercise capacity and are done in the PFT laboratory.

Figure 12-3 shows a typical expiratory flow volume loop during spirometry. The patient takes as deep a breath as possible and expires as forcibly and completely as possible. For evaluation of upper airway obstruction, (see discussion of vocal cord dysfunction) it is also useful to obtain an inspiratory curve as well. An adequate forced vital capacity (FVC) maneuver is defined by less than 5% variability in three to five FVC attempts. Most children 5 years or older can perform adequate spirometry. Relative changes in FVC and the forced expiratory volume for 1 second (FEV_1) determine patterns of dysfunction including obstructive, restrictive, and mixed defects (Figure 12-4 and Table 12-2). Spirometry can suggest restrictive and mixed pulmonary disease but confirmation of this type of dysfunction is made using lung volume measurements in the PFT laboratory.

Table 12-1.

The Effects of Training on Circulatory and Respiratory Function During Exercise

Variable	Response
Maximal O_2 uptake	Increased
Work output	Increased
Mechanical efficiency	Unchanged
Cardiac output	Increased
Maximal heart rate	Unchanged
Heart rate at submaximal loads	Decreased
Stroke volume	Increased
Arteriovenous O_2 difference	Increased
Hemoglobin, hematocrit	Unchanged
Blood lactate level at maximal loads	Increased
Blood lactate level at submaximal loads	Decreased
Maximal ventilation	Unchanged
Ventilation at submaximal loads	Decreased
Pulmonary diffusing capacity	Unchanged
Capillary density in muscles	Increased
Oxidative enzymes in muscles	Increased

Adapted from Murray JF. The Normal Lung. New York: WB Saunders; 1986.

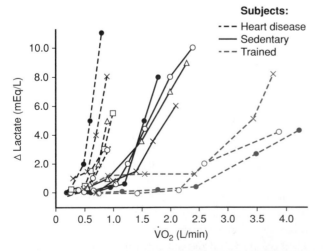

FIGURE 12-2 ■ Change in lactate level versus oxygen consumption (Vo2) in patients with heart disease, sedentary patients, and physically trained individuals. *(Used with permission from reference 2)*

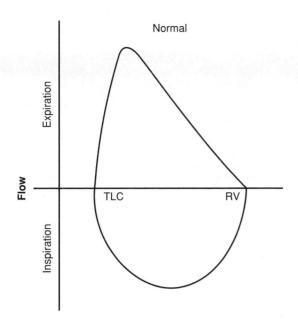

FIGURE 12-3 ■ Typical flow volume loop. TLC, total lung capacity; RV, residual volume.

A relatively simple measure of reversible airway obstruction can be done by measuring spirometry before and after 20 minutes of giving an inhaled bronchodilator such as albuterol sulfate. An increase of 12% or greater in FEV_1 is diagnostic for reversible airway obstruction. Reference to findings on spirometry with various conditions and need for further testing, if required, will be included with the various sports-related conditions discussed below.

THE UPPER AIRWAY

Vocal Cord Dysfunction

Definition and epidemiology

Vocal cord dysfunction (VCD) (paradoxical vocal cord motion, laryngeal dyskinesia, functional stridor, Munchausen's stridor, psychosomatic stridor, factitious asthma) often occurs during sports activities and is very common among adolescents, particular females.[3] The symptoms are often underrecognized and consequently VCD is under-diagnosed. Thirty to fifty percent of patients with VCD typically also have a history of asthma and may be aggressively over treated with multiple inhaled medications, systemic steroids, and even repeated hospitalizations because of the unrecognized coexisting VCD symptoms.[4,5]

Clinical presentation

A typical episode of VCD consists of the sudden onset of inspiratory stridor with accompanying throat tightness, hoarse voice, cough, and occasional wheezing.[3] VCD rarely occurs during sleep, but occurs more commonly during activity. Symptoms often remit over minutes with cessation of activity or removal or distraction from a stressful situation. On examination, stridor locates over the glottis and lung evaluation is normal unless coexisting asthma is occurring. Endoscopic examination is typical, with characteristic anterior apposition of the vocal cords with a small, posterior, diamond shape opening ("posterior glottic chink," Figure 12-5).[4,6]

Differential diagnosis

VCD is most often confused with asthma, although a careful history and examination can differentiate the two, eliminating unnecessary treatments (Table 12-3). Throat tightness and upper chest discomfort may also occur with hyperventilation associated with performance anxiety (probable panic attack) but stridor is usually absent.[3]

Diagnostic tests

Direct laryngoscopy is definitive but rarely available during an episode. Spirometry may show persistent flattening of the inspiratory portion of the flow volume loop either at rest or during bronchoprovocation with exercise, methacholine, cold air, or histamine in the hospital PFT laboratory (Figure 12-5).[4]

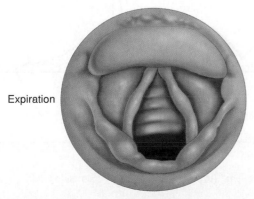
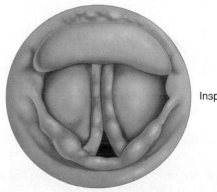

Expiration   Inspiration

FIGURE 12-4 ■ Laryngoscopic appearance of the vocal cords in VCD.

Table 12-2.

Pulmonary Function Abnormalities in Lung Disease

Type	FVC	FEV$_1$	FEV$_1$/FVC	TLC	RV
Obstructive	Normal	Decreased	Decreased	Normal or increased	Normal or increased
Restrictive	Decreased	Decreased	Normal or Increased	Decreased	Decreased or Increased
Combined	Decreased	Decreased	Decreased	Decreased	Decreased

FVC, forced vital capacity; FEV$_1$, forced expiratory volume for more than 1 second; TLC total lung capacity; RV, residual volume.

Treatment

Behavioral treatments, particularly speech therapy for hyperfunctional voice disorders, but also including hypnosis, relaxation, breathing exercises and biofeedback are shown to be helpful in this condition.[3,5,7] If there is major underlying anxiety or other psychopathology, more extensive evaluation and therapy for a specific psychological condition is warranted.

THE CHEST WALL

Chest Wall Pain

Chest wall pain in sports is common, frequently accompanying local trauma or repetitive strenuous activity and is most often of musculoskeletal origin. Localization of the pain to a specific site and observation of the chest wall for swelling can help differentiate conditions responsible for the discomfort. Most common are costochondritis, *Tietze's syndrome*, stress fracture of the rib, and slipping rib syndrome. These conditions are described individually with clinical presentation and pathophysiology where known.

Costochondritis and Tietze's Syndrome

Definitions and epidemiology

Up to 30% of patients presenting to the emergency department with chest wall pain have these conditions.[8] They occur commonly in youth of either gender, often in those undertaking stressful activity of the upper body such as weight lifting, gymnastics, etc.

Clinical presentation

The etiology is unknown although there is soft evidence of localized inflammation of the costochondral junction.[9] Localized, palpable pain over the costochondral junction without systemic symptoms is typical. If there is a localized, nonsuppurative nodule, usually located at the second or third costochondral junction, the condition is termed Tietze's syndrome.[10] The etiology of this condition is likewise unknown although inflammation

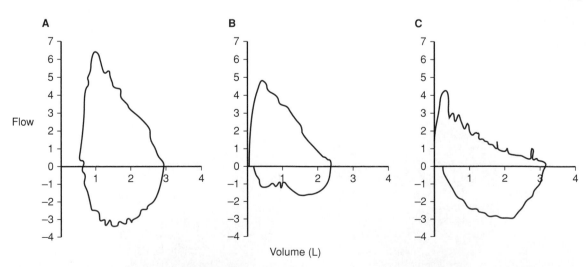

FIGURE 12-5 ■ Flow volume loop in VCD. (**a**). Normal flow volume loop. (**b**). Flattened inspiratory loop during VCD. (**c**). Scooped expiratory curve during acute asthma.

Table 12-3.

Vocal Cord Dysfunction Compared to Exercise-Induced Asthma

	VCD	EIB
Women > men	+	−
Associated psychiatric diagnosis	+	±
Exercise induced	+	+
Very short duration of symptoms	+	−
Improves with bronchodilator	−	+
Eosinophilia	−	±
Hypoxia	−	+
Syncope	−	+
Dyspnea	+	+
Stridor	+	−
Wheeze	Inspiration	Expiration > inspiration
Spirometry	Blunted inspiration portion of flow-volume loop	Normal inspiration portion of flow-volume loop
Laryngoscopy	Tonic adduction of cords during inspiration or inspiration/expiration	Abduction during inspiration
Chest x-ray	Normal	Hyperinflation

Adapted from Homnick D, Marks J. Exercise and sports in the adolescent with chronic pulmonary disease. Adolesc Med. 1998;9:467–481.

is also implicated. Diagnosis of either condition is dependent on history and clinical examination as radiographs are usually normal. Soft tissue swelling and, occasionally partial calcification of the costal cartilage may be evident.[11]

Differential diagnosis

Local palpable pain is the key to diagnosis of costochondritis, but always consider other causes of chest pain including that of cardiac, GI, and infectious origin. Spirometric evaluation should not reveal abnormalities unless pain limits the performance of a vital capacity maneuver in which case the evaluation will suggest restrictive disease based on both reduction in VC and FEV_1. Dyspnea is not usual and suggests intrinsic pulmonary disease. Chest x-ray is helpful to rule out parenchymal lung disease and rib fracture.

Treatment

These conditions are self-limited and treatment consists of reassurance, mild analgesics, such as oral nonsteroidal anti-inflammatory agents, and discontinuation of any aggravating activity. Severe pain may respond to local injection of corticosteroid, especially with Tietze's syndrome.[10]

Stress Fractures of the Ribs

Definitions and epidemiology

Stress-related rib fracture especially that of the first rib occurs in athletes engaged in strenuous activity, particularly those involving overhead activity such as baseball,

basketball, tennis, or weight lifting. Baseball pitching, golf, and surfing have all been associated with traumatic rib fracture. Collegiate rowers appear to be at particular risk with 12% of a national rowing team diagnosed with rib fracture over approximately a 1-year period.[12]

Clinical presentation

With first rib fracture, pain occurs in the shoulder, cervical triangle or clavicular region. Fracture may occur in other ribs including the so-called floating ribs (11th and 12th ribs) in cases of extreme chest wall and abdominal muscle contraction. Pain is insidious in onset progressing from ill defined to sharp pain over days to weeks. Pain may be felt in the back as the fracture site is often at the posterolateral rib angle. Examination often reveals local rib tenderness and plain chest x-ray most often is diagnostic.

Differential diagnosis

Rule out both shoulder injury and clavicular fracture with first rib fracture by careful examination and specific radiographs. Careful palpation of the spine is useful in ruling out local vertebral injury and the possibility of diskitis. The chest x-ray is most useful in diagnosing rib fracture.[13]

Treatment

Treatment for first rib fracture includes sling immobilization of the shoulder and use of a soft cervical collar. Prognosis is good with return to normal activity within 3 months.

Slipping Rib Syndrome (Painful Rib, Clicking Rib Syndrome)

This occurs in up to 3% of patients presenting with rib pain.[14] Sharp pain is often described in the lower chest or upper abdomen along with a tender spot on palpation of the lower costal margin. The etiology is thought to be caused by hyper mobility of the anterior ends of ribs 11 and 12 with a tendency of one rib to slip under the other. The development of this condition may follow chest trauma as might be found in sports activities.[10] Pain is likely caused by impingement on the intercostal nerve or strain of the lower costal cartilage.[15] The excess rib movement may be accompanied by a snap, click, or pop associated with sharp intermittent pain. The "hooking maneuver" (the examiner hooks his or her fingers under the lower costal margin and pulls anteriorly) will reproduce the pain accompanied by a typical click. There is neither specific radiological diagnostic test nor changes in lung function in this condition. Conservative management consists of rib strapping, avoidance of precipitating activities, and use of mild analgesics. Occasionally local nerve block and injection of corticosteroid may be necessary to relieve severe pain. Excision of the anterior end of the rib and costal cartilages may provide definitive relief in extreme cases.[16,17]

CHEST DEFORMITY

Pectus Excavatum

Pectus deformities (pectus excavatum and carinatum, Figure 12-6) occur in approximately 1% of the population with boys affected in a 4:1 ratio to girls.[18] Pectus excavatum (funnel chest) is the most common with inward indentation of the sternum readily apparent on chest inspection. With adolescent growth acceleration, the defect becomes more severe but stops progressing once one attains adult growth. Dystrophic growth of the costal cartilages appears to be the cause of the sternal depression.[18] There is often a familial tendency toward this defect. Although specific symptoms are not routinely associated with pectus excavatum, adolescents may complain of fatigue, decreased exercise tolerance, and chest and back discomfort. Mitral valve prolapse may occur in up to 20% of children with pectus excavatum and resolves about half the time with repair.[19–25] Pectus deformities are also seen in connective tissue disorders including Marfan and Ehlers-Danlos syndromes.[18] Embarrassment as a result of the cosmetic nature of the deformity most often leads to the patient seeking medical or surgical evaluation of the deformity. Surgery is indicated for primarily cosmetic purposes. Although mild restrictive defects in pulmonary function may accompany severe pectus excavatum deformities, functional improvement in lung function and exercise tolerance is quite variable after surgery.[26] The reduced exercise capacity seen in some patients with severe pectus excavatum appears to be primarily caused by impaired cardiovascular performance rather than from ventilation limitation.[27] In one large study, FVC, FEV_1, and the FEF^{25-75} (forced expiratory flow rate between 25% and 75% of vital capacity) improved postoperatively in the majority of patients.[28] Subjective improvement in exercise tolerance may be noted by patient and family.

Pectus Carinatum (Pigeon Chest)

This defect characterized by anterior protrusion of the sternum, with or without torsion, is less common than

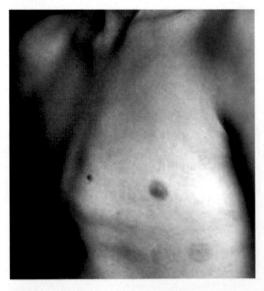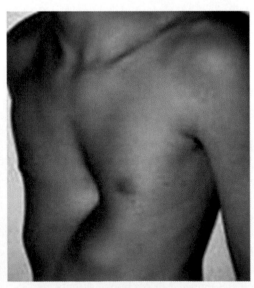

FIGURE 12-6 ■ Pectus carinatum (left) and pectus excavatum.

pectus excavatum. It also occurs more commonly in males than in females and progresses during adolescent growth.[18] It has not been associated with consistent cardiorespiratory symptoms and similar to pectus excavatum, surgery is primarily for cosmetic reasons. Several different surgical techniques are available for treatment of the pectus deformities.[23]

Scoliosis

Definitions and epidemiology

Scoliosis is a lateral curvature of the spine with associated rib cage deformity that can result in progressive pulmonary disability. Although scoliosis can be congenital or caused by an underlying process (e.g., neuromuscular disease, spinal cord tumor, or trauma), 80% to 85% of cases are idiopathic.[24] Idiopathic scoliosis (IS) can begin in infancy, childhood, or more frequently in adolescence. In contrast with pectus excavatum, adolescent IS occurs more frequently in girls than in boys. The prevalence of scoliosis in the general population is thought to be 2% to 3%; however, school screening programs have reported prevalence as high as 15%.[25] The severity of scoliosis is assessed by radiographic measurement of the spinal curve (Cobb angle). IS results in restrictive lung disease because of decreased chest wall compliance, impaired lung growth, and reduced respiratory muscle strength.[24] These factors lead to an increased dead space to tidal volume ratio (V_D/V_T) and an abnormal ventilation/perfusion ratio ($\dot{V}/\dot{Q}$). Although, there is a negative linear correlation between the degree of curvature and forced vital capacity, the relationship between severity of scoliosis and lung function is complex. Pulmonary impairment is related to angle of scoliosis, number of vertebrae involved, cephalad location of the curve, and loss of normal thoracic kyphosis. Reduction in vital capacity is associated with increasing angle of scoliosis, longer curves, curves higher in the thoracic spine, and decreased kyphosis.[26] FVC and exercise capacity are usually normal or only mildly reduced in patients with mild deformity (Cobb angle <35 degrees).[27] Tidal volume response to exercise may be reduced with an increased frequency of respirations used to maintain normal exercise capacity.[28] Exercise testing may therefore be a useful way to demonstrate early pulmonary impairment in asymptomatic patients with normal resting pulmonary function. As curves progress to moderate (50–60 degrees), resting pulmonary function abnormalities and ventilatory limitation in response to exercise become evident. Severe curves (>90 degrees) are associated with alveolar hypoventilation and risk of cardiorespiratory failure.

Interestingly, one study noted a greater participation in gymnastics in children and adolescents with IS.[29] Increased joint laxity preceding the patient's decision to undertake this sport appears to be a common factor between scoliosis and participation in gymnastics even excluding those patients with connective tissue disorders (Marfan's and Ehler-Danlos). The authors proposed that young patients with scoliosis and joint laxity could adapt to the rigors of the sport more easily than those without joint laxity and therefore participated at higher rates.

Clinical presentation

Patients with severe scoliosis and thoracic muscle weakness and contracture will show typical thoracic deformities leading to restrictive pulmonary dysfunction and possible ventilatory compromise. This often occurs in children with severe developmental disabilities or neuromuscular disease. In IS, a careful back examination including review of shoulder height combined with confirming x-rays will delineate the type and degree of curve. Back pain is not a consistent feature of IS and in one study[29] 80% of patients reported no back pain associated with IS and 86% did not change sports practice habits because of the deformity.

Differential diagnosis

Chest wall deformity as a result of abnormal rib placement (pectus), rib anomalies (e.g., bifid rib, missing rib, etc.), and anomalous chest wall musculature (e.g., Poland anomaly) may mimic the chest wall deformity seen in severe scoliosis. Again, careful examination combined with confirmatory x-ray will reveal the diagnosis.

Treatment

Scoliosis with mild curves of less than 25 degrees is usually followed closely. If the curve becomes greater than 25 degrees, bracing is instituted.[24] A prescribed exercise program had no effect on change in curve after several months and wearing a brace does not improve exercise performance.[30,31] In general, sports participation does not need to be restricted in patients with mild curves. Rapidly progressing curves or curves greater than 50 degrees usually require surgical treatment. Pulmonary function may improve partially after surgery, but the improvement may not be evident for up to 2 years. Sports participation of surgically treated patients will depend on the degree of pulmonary impairment and limitation of motion due to the surgery. Referral to an orthopedic physician with interest in back deformity is advisable particularly during early teenage growth years when IS may worsen.

THE LUNG

Primary Spontaneous Pneumothorax

The incidence of primary spontaneous pneumothorax is estimated at approximately 18/100,000 population in men and 6/100,000 in women.[32] The typical patient is an

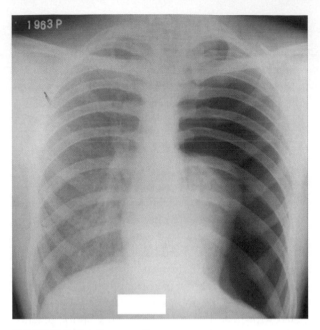

FIGURE 12-7 ■ Left pneumothorax.

otherwise normal tall, thin male between 10 and 30 years. Smoking increases the risk of spontaneous pneumothorax by up to a factor of 20.[33] Subpleural emphysematous bullae or blebs are commonly found when patients proceed to thoracoscopic surgery. This contrasts to the infected, fibrotic, and cystic lung apices found in patients with cystic fibrosis.

Most episodes of spontaneous pneumothorax occur at rest with the sudden onset of pleuritic (sharp) chest pain and dyspnea. The examination may be normal with small pneumothoraces. Those with air occupying more than 15% of the pleural cavity are accompanied by decreased movement of the chest wall, decreased breath sounds, distant cardiac tones, and hyper resonance on percussion. Tachycardia is common and if accompanied by cyanosis and hypotension indicates tension pneumothorax, a medical emergency (Figure 12-7).

The diagnosis is made with a combination of physical examination and upright chest x-ray. Treatment depends on the size of the pneumothorax, the clinical presentation, and whether it is recurrent. With a pneumothorax that is less than 15% of the hemi thoracic volume and the patient has minimal symptoms, simple observation may be sufficient. The addition of supplemental oxygen hastens the reabsorption of the pleural gas by a factor of four by replacing less well-absorbed nitrogen with more diffusible oxygen.[32] A larger primary pneumothorax, especially when accompanied by symptoms, requires evacuation of the intrapleural air. Simple aspiration of air with a small-bore catheter, with or without water seal, may be sufficient with a one-time leak. With reacummulation of intrapleural air or with development of a tension pneu-

mothorax, placement of a thoracostomy tube will be necessary either under radiographic guidance by an interventional radiologist or at the bedside by skilled pulmonary or critical care staff. Attach the tube to a water seal device or Heimlich valve for a day or two until the persistent leak is resolved. Persistent leaks of more than about 4 to 5 days require surgical intervention.

Recurrence of pneumothorax is quite common occurring in 30% to 50% of patients.[32] Thoracoscopy with resection of bullae and local pleurodesis by pleural abrasion or instillation of a sclerosing agent, such as talc, has generally replaced the administration of sclerosing agents through a chest tube.[34] The recurrence rate for primary pneumothorax with this method is 5% to 9%.[35] In secondary pneumothorax such as occurs in cystic fibrosi (CF), the recurrence rate appears to be somewhat higher probably because of forceful cough and extreme lung and airway inflammation. A consensus document on the management of spontaneous pneumothorax was published by the American College of Chest Physicians in 2001.[36]

Exercise-Induced Asthma

Definitions and epidemiology

Asthma is a chronic, inflammatory disease that includes bronchospasm (increased airway hyper reactivity), increased mucus production, cellular infiltration into airway and airway sub mucosa, airway edema and narrowing, and, in some cases, deposition of submucosal collagen. It involves increased airway responsiveness to a variety of both immunologic (e.g., animal dander, pollen, dust mite, etc.) and nonimmunologic stimuli (e.g., viruses, cold air, exercise, etc.). In the United states, asthma is the most common chronic disease of children and adolescents numbering approximately five million below the age of 18 years. Children and adolescents miss approximately 10 million school days per year and parents often miss work caring for these youngsters. This has significant social and economic costs (approximately 11 billion dollars per year in direct and indirect costs). Many children and adolescents with chronic asthma will experience exacerbations during exercise-limiting activities and interfering with their participation in sports.

Pathophysiologically there may or may not be evidence of airway inflammation or increased airway hyper responsiveness and therefore either term, exercise-induced bronchospasm (EIB) or exercise-induce asthma (EIA), may be used. Although the exact mechanism of induction of EIA is unknown, several plausible hypotheses have been put forth. Increased minute ventilation during exercise (increased volume of air inspired and expired over 1 minute) leads to evaporative and conductive cooling of the lower airway.[37] This especially occurs during the transition from nose breathing to mouth breathing with reduced contribution of air

Table 12-4.

Hypotheses of the Mechanisms in Exercise-Induced Asthma

Hypothesis	Mechanism
Heat loss from airway	Direct bronchoconstrictive effect
Water loss from airway	Hypersomolarity of periciliary fluid leads to:
	Increased mucosal blood flow leading to vascular engorgement and airway edema
	Direct release of preformed mediators of inflammation (e.g., histamine) from inflammatory and airway structural cells
Airway rewarming	Heat loss during exercise leads to temporarily deceased bronchial blood flow. At cessation of exercise, rewarming leads to reactive hyperthermia with vascular engorgement and airway edema

Adapted from: Homnick D, Marks J. Exercise and sports in the adolescent with chronic pulmonary disease. Adolesc Med. 1998;9:467–481.

humidification and warming from the upper airway. The hypotheses for development of EIA include direct effects of airway cooling, effects of evaporative water loss, and effects of rewarming of airway after exercise and are summarized in Table 12-4.[38]

As EIA can be induced by warm, humidified air and occur during the exercise period itself, and increases in mucosal osmolarity in vivo may not be sufficient to cause inflammatory mediator release demonstrated in vitro, it is likely that all three proposed mechanisms of induction of EIA occur together to a greater or lesser degree in any individual.

Clinical presentation

Symptoms of EIA include shortness of breath or complaints of breathlessness, chest pain, chest tightness, cough, or wheeze usually associated with short periods of intense physical activity. A typical pattern for EIA includes a short (5–10 minutes) period of bronchodilation at the start of exercise, possibly because of release of endogenous catecholamines, followed by symptoms of progressive bronchconstriction peaking at 5 to 10 minutes after cessation of exercise. Spontaneous remission of symptoms and gradual return to baseline typically occur 30 to 60 minutes after the end of the exercise period. Some individuals with EIA reach a clinical refractory period ("second wind") sometime during exercise and are able to "run through" initial symptoms to reach this point. The existence of this refractory period may be used in some individuals as a therapeutic strategy and induced by warm up exercises prior to more vigorous activity (see section "Treatment").[39]

Differential diagnosis

Diagnosis of EIA is best done with a combination of respiratory tract directed history and physical examination and a quantitative exercise challenge test under controlled, supervised conditions with a standard proto-col.[40,41] Alternative diagnoses such as anxiety associated hyperventilation and VCD may mimic asthma and a careful evaluation will differentiate these conditions. Quantization of EIA is important to evaluate response to therapy in a safe and systematic manner. It may also be important where adequate history cannot be obtained from the young patient because of perceived pressure to withhold or underplay symptoms. Patients, parents, and coaches may perceive EIA as lack of conditioning and quantitative demonstration of pulmonary function changes as well as response to therapy is important.

Prior to undertaking exercise challenge testing, one should eliminate the presence of bone, joint, or cardiac conditions by examination and specific testing, if required. Withhold asthma medications prior to the test. After performing baseline spirometry, the patient exercises on a treadmill with predetermined speed and inclination for more than 6 to 8 minutes to attain 80% of maximum heart rate. Cardiac and oximetric monitoring is maintained throughout the test. Symptoms are noted and FEV_1 is determined at 5-minute intervals up to 30 minutes after the cessation of the exercise period. A drop in FEV_1 of 15% is diagnostic. Nonquantitative exercise testing such as running around the block outside the office is neither safe nor helpful for later evaluation of response to therapy. Direct observation of the patient under controlled conditions can also reveal alternative diagnoses such as VCD or the combination of VCD and EIA where symptom presentation may be confusing.

Treatment

Asthma management protocols and guidelines have been available in the United States since the 1991 publication of the Expert Panel Report 1, Guidelines for the Diagnosis and Management of Asthma, National Institutes of Health, National heart, Lung, and Blood Institute. Additional evidence-based guidelines including updates were published in 1997 as the Expert Panel Report 2 (with a further update in 2002),[42,43] and the joint American Academy of Pediatrics and American Academy of Allergy, Asthma, and Immunology, Pediatric Asthma, Guide for Managing Asthma in Children in 1999.[44]

One will not control EIA without controlling underlying chronic asthma and most patients presenting with symptoms of EIA will reveal upon careful questioning that they have symptoms at other times such as with upper respiratory tract infection or cold air exposure. Therefore daily anti-inflammatory therapy (inhaled corticosteroid) with or without a long acting beta-adrenergic agent or leukotriene modifier combined with intermittent use of short acting beta-adrenergic agent will be necessary for many patients. In addition, it is imperative that environmental controls be instituted including avoidance of asthma triggers such as dust mite and second-hand smoke. Bear in mind that many adolescents and even middle school age children are occult smokers and questioning them away from parents can reveal this aggravating factor.[45]

Avoidance of dry and cool air through nose breathing, use of masks and scarves, and avoiding outdoor exercise can be simple means of controlling symptoms. However, when sports activities require the adolescent to participate in less than ideal environmental circumstances, a more active approach is required. This includes the attempted induction of the refractory period by undertaking carefully graded warm-up exercises for 45 to 60 minutes before actual sports participation and judicious use of medications. The use of medications considers that the adolescent has been properly instructed on their use including technique of administering metered dose and dry powder inhalers and timing of their administration. First line medications include beta-adrenergic agents with short to medium duration of action (2–4 hours) such as albuterol, terbutaline, and pirbuterol which are administered as two puffs 15 to 20 minutes before exercise. The alternatives for longer duration of action (8–12 hours) are the long-acting beta-adrenergic agent, salmeterol, and fomoterol. Salmeterol must be given 1 hour before anticipated exercise (two puffs) because of slow onset of peak activity but fomoterol (1 inhalation) may be given 20 minutes before activities, similar to short-acting agents. If EIA is incompletely controlled, addition of a second pre-exercise medication may be necessary. The anti-inflammatory medications nedocromil sodium and cromolyn sodium have been shown to be effective as first line therapy in mild EIA and as adjunctive therapy to beta-adrenergic agents in more refractory EIA.[46] These are given as two puffs 15 to 20 minutes prior to sports participation. Additional adjunctive therapy includes the use of sustained release preparations of theophylline, the leukotriene inhibitors and receptor antagonists (zileuton, montelukast, zafirlukast) and

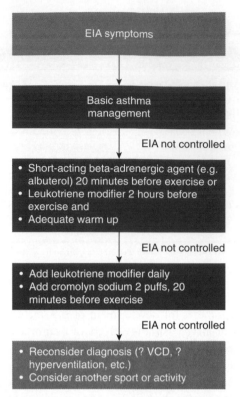

FIGURE 12-8 ■ Flow diagram for the treatment of exercise-induced asthma.

inhaled corticosteroids to assure baseline asthma control and decrease adverse response to exercise. The use of these medications before the onset of exercise has not been shown to be specifically beneficial in the prevention of EIA with the exception of the leukotriene receptor antagonists. Montelukast given 2 hours before an exercise challenge has been shown to be more effective than placebo in preventing EIA symptoms.[47] In cases where satisfactory control of EIA symptoms cannot be achieved with standard pharmacologic and nonpharmacologic methods, exercise testing with various combinations of medications may be useful. In the final analysis, some forms of exercise may not be physiologically suited for a particular individual and persistence in trying to achieve unrealistic goals may lead to problems in self-esteem, especially where peer relationships are based on sports performance. Finding an alternative sport that is less asthmogenic, i.e., those with lower minute ventilation, such as baseball, or those done in more humid and warm environments, such as swimming, may be the ultimate solution for EIA in individual cases. Figure 12-8 shows an algorithm for treatment of EIA.

Cystic Fibrosis

Definitions and epidemiology

Cystic fibrosis (CF) remains the most common lethal genetic disease among Caucasians with over 30,000 patients in the United States. Although lethal, the predicted survival of CF individuals has improved significantly over the last decade with median age at death about 35 years.[48] Ninety percent of CF deaths are caused by respiratory disease from chronic infection and inflammation secondary to airway obstruction from tenacious secretions. However, many children with CF enter teen and young adult years with normal lung function and the desire to participate in sports activities similar to their normal peers. As exercise capacity correlates with resting lung function in CF, those patients with normal lung function would be expected to be able to fully participate in sports.[49,50] Greater aerobic fitness leads to improved survival in CF and a greater sense of well-being.[51,52] Additional factors that affect lung function and exercise capacity in CF include nutritional status, CF-related diabetes, lung microbiology, and thermal stress. Because of the sweat defect in CF, large amounts of electrolytes and water may be lost with high sweat rates under warm ambient conditions leading to reduced capacity to sustain activities and increasing the risk of heat exhaustion.

Clinical presentation

Diagnosis of CF is usually made in infancy as a result of increasing numbers of state newborn screening programs and/or clinical presentation of recurrent respiratory infection and failure to thrive because of pancreatic insufficiency. Therefore, most children and adolescents desiring to undertake sports will already have a confirmed diagnosis. Patients with mild to moderate pulmonary disease will usually have normal or near normal exercise tolerance. With severe pulmonary disease, physical working capacity and maximal oxygen consumption are significantly reduced with patients at risk of hemoglobin-oxygen desaturation. However, even patients with severe disease may tolerate sub maximal exercise which can be done with or without supplemental oxygen.[53,54]

Normal individuals are limited by cardiovascular fitness rather than ventilation but CF patients with decreased lung function may attain exercise limitation owing to ventilatory demands before cardiovascular limits are reached.[55] This means that for a given workload, ventilation is greater than normal owing to increased pulmonary dead space and wasted ventilation. Female athletes with CF demonstrate a greater resting energy expenditure than their normal peers despite similar peak aerobic capacity and nutritional status.[56] Decreased peripheral muscle strength in young males with CF correlates with airflow limitation.[57] In addition, many athletes with CF have coexisting asthma, that, if untreated may limit their exercise capacity.[58]

Differential diagnosis

Most CF patients are known by the time they begin participation in sports and are rarely diagnosed in later childhood and adulthood. Exceptions to this may be adults with mild CF gene mutations with little or no intestinal malabsorption and who also have normal lung function and exercise tolerance. Diseases similar to CF with airway inflammation and progressive decline in lung function include primary ciliary dyskinesia (Kartagener's if with situs inversus) and recurrent pulmonary infection because of congenital or acquired immunodeficiency.

Treatment

The basic treatment of CF involves nutritional support, aggressive antimicrobial therapy of chronic endobronchial infection, and enhancement of airway clearance. The goals of treatment are to sustain adequate nutrition, prevent decline in pulmonary function, and maintain as normal a lifestyle as possible for CF patients.

Exercise has been advocated in CF to improve pulmonary function, increase ventilatory muscle strength and endurance, and supplement or replace standard chest physiotherapy.[59,60] Patients with greater aerobic fitness are also found to have better survival.[61] Exercise tolerance also correlates with patients' sense of well-being.[52] Specific ventilatory muscle training can improve ventilatory muscle endurance, pulmonary function and exercise tolerance.[62] Supervised vigorous exercise programs have resulted in improved exercise capacity and aerobic fitness with or without improvement in pulmonary function .[63] A home exercise program improved physical performance and ability to perform activities of daily living and the benefits persist even without exercise supervision.[64] Replacing standard chest physiotherapy with exercise sessions in hospitalized CF patients resulted in improvement in pulmonary function, suggesting that some patients may use daily exercise as a form of airway clearance.[65]

Patients with CF should be encouraged to exercise regularly to maintain or improve fitness and pulmonary function. Prior to starting an exercise program, pulmonary function and exercise testing should be done to develop the best exercise prescription for the patient. Patients with hyper reactive airways should use inhaled bronchodilators before exercise. Patients with more advanced lung disease may need supplemental oxygen during exercise. Increased salt and water intake should be encouraged during exercise in high ambient temperatures to prevent hyponatremic dehydration.

SUMMARY

Children and adolescents with thoracic and respiratory disease can very effectively participate in sports and attain greater levels of fitness leading to increased exercise tolerance. In fact, up to 15% of elite athletes with chronic respiratory disease in high schools, colleges, and in the United States Olympic team very effectively compete with their normal peers.[55] Prompt diagnosis and appropriately directed treatment can aid in rehabilitation of respiratory system injury and prevent the development of debilitating limitation in exercise tolerance allowing youngsters to fully participate in sports (Box 12-1).

REFERENCES

1. Murray JF. *The Normal Lung.* New York: WB Saunders; 1986.
2. Wasserman K, Whipp BJ. Exercise physiology in health and disease. *Am Rev Respir Dis.* 1975;112:219-249.
3. Homnick D, Pratt H. Respiratory disease with a psychosomatic component. *Adolesc Med.* 2000;11(3):547-566.
4. Newman KB, Mason UG III, Schmaling KB. Clinical features of vocal cord dysfunction. *Am J Respir Crit Care Med.* 1995;152:1382-1386.
5. Wood PW, Milgrom H. Vocal cord dysfunction. *J Allergy Clin Immunol.* 1996;98:481-485.
6. Landwehr LP, Wood RP II. Vocal cord dysfunction mimicking exercise-induced bronchospasm in adolescents. *Pediatrics.* 1996;98:971-974.
7. Wilson JJ, Wilson EM. Practical management of vocal cord dysfunction in athletes. *Clin J Sport Med.* 2006; 16(4):357-360.
8. Disla E, Rhim HR, Reddy A, et al. Costochondritis: a prospective analysis in an emergency department setting. *Arch Intern Med.* 1994;154(21):2466-2469.
9. Miller JH. Accumulation of gallium-67 in costochondritis. *Clin Nucl Med.* 1980;5(8):362-363.
10. Gregory PL, Biswas AC, Batt ME. Musculoskeletal problems of the chest wall in athletes. *Sports Med.* 2002; 32(4):235-250.
11. Honda N, Machida K, Mamiya T, et al. Scintigraphic and CT findings of Tietze's syndrome: report of a case and review of the literature. *Clin Nucl Med.* 1989;14(8): 606-609.
12. Christiansen E, Kanstrup IL. Increased risk of stress fractures of the ribs in elite rowers. *Scand J Med Sci Sports.* 1997;7(1):49-52.
13. Lord MJ, Ha KI, Song KS. Stress fractures of the ribs in golfers. *Am J Sports Med.* 1996;24(1);118-122.
14. Scott EM, Scott BB. Painful rib syndrome—a review of 76 cases. *Gut.* 1993;34(7):1006-1008.
15. Arroyo JF, Vine R, Reynaud C, et al. Slipping rib syndrome: don't be fooled. *Geriatrics.* 1995;50(3):46-49.
16. Spence EK, Rosato EF. The slipping rib syndrome. *Arch Surg.* 1983;118(11):1330-1332.
17. Porter GE. Slipping rib syndrome: an infrequently recognized entity in children: a report of three cases and review of the literature. *Pediatrics.* 1985;76(5):810-813.
18. Williams AM, Crabbe DCG. Pectus deformities of the anterior chest wall. *Paediatr Respir Rev.* 2003;4:237-242.
19. Shamberger RC, Welch KJ, Sanders SP. Mitral valve prolapse associated with pectus excavatum. *J Pediatr.* 1987;111: 404-407.
20. Rowland T, Mariarty K, Banever G. Effect of pectus excavatum deformity on cardiorespiratory fitness in adolescent boys. *Arch Pediatr Adolesc Med.* 2005;159:1069-1073.
21. Malek MH, Fonkalstrud EW, Cooper CB. Ventilatory and cardiovascular responses to exercise in patients with pectus excavatum. *Chest.* 2003;124:870-872.
22. Lawson ML, Mellins RB, Tabangin M, et al. Impact of pectus excavatum on pulmonary function before and after repair with the Nuss procedure. *J Pediatr Surg.* 2005;4: 174-180.
23. Robicsek F. Surgical treatment of pectus carinatum [review]. *Chest Surg Clin N Am.* 2000;10(2):357-376,viii.
24. Canet E, Praud JP, Bureau MA. Chest wall diseases and dysfunction in children. In: Chernick V, Boat T, eds. *Kendig's Disorders of the Respiratory Tract in Children.* Philadelphia, PA: WB Saunders; 1997:794-799.
25. Lonstein JE. Screening for spinal deformities in Minnesota schools. *Clin Orthop.* 1977;126:33.
26. Kearon C, Viviani GR, Kirkley A, Killian KJ. Factors determining pulmonary function in adolescent idiopathic thoracic scoliosis. *Am Rev Respir Dis.* 1993;148:288-294.
27. Leech JA, Ernst P, Rogola EJ, Gurr J, Gordon I, Becklake MR. Cardiorespiratory status in relation to mild deformity in adolescent idiopathic scoliosis. *J Pediatr.* 1985;106: 143-149.
28. Smyth RJ, Chapman KR, Wright TA, Crawford JS, Rebuck AS. Ventilatory patterns during hypoxia, hypercapnia, and exercise in adolescents with mild scoliosis. *Pediatrics.* 1986;77:692-697.
29. Meyer C, Cammarata E, Haumont T, et al. Why do idiopathic scoliosis patients participate more in gymnastics? *Scand J Med Sci Sports.* 2006;16:231-236.
30. Stone B, Beekman C, Hall V, Guess V, Brooks HL. The effect of an exercise program on change in curve in adolescents with minimal idiopathic scoliosis. A preliminary study. *Phys Ther.* 1979;59:759-763.
31. DiRocco PJ, Breed AL, Carlin JI, Reddan WG. Physical work capacity in adolescent patients with mild idiopathic scoliosis. *Arch Phys Med Rehabil.* 1983;64:476-478.
32. Montgomery M. Air and liquid in the pleural space. In: Chernick V, Boat T, eds. *Disorders of the Respiratory Tract*

in Children. 6th ed. Philadelphia, PA:.WB Saunders Company; 1998:389-414.

33. Gobbel WG, Rhea W, Nelson IA, Daniel RA. Spontaneous pneumothorax. *J Thoracic Cardiovasc Surg* 1963;46:331-345.

34. Yim APC, Ng CSH. Thorascopy in the management of pneumothorax. *Pulm Med.* 2001;7:210-214.

35. Tschopp M, Brutsche M, Frey JG. Treatment of complicated spontaneous pneumothorax by simple talc pleurodesis under thorascopy and local anesthesia. *Thorax.* 1997;52:329-332.

36. Bauman MH, Strange C, Heffner JF, et al. Management of spontaneous pneumothorax-consensus conference. *Chest.* 2001;119:590-602.

37. Mcfadden ER, Gilbert FA. Exercise induced asthma. *N Engl J Med.* 1994;330:1362-1367.

38. Deal EC, Mcfadden ER, Ingrom RH, et al. Role of respiratory heat exchange in production of exercise-induced asthma. *J Appl Physiol.* 1979;46:467-475.

39. Kyle JM, Walker RB, Hanshaw SL, Leaman JR, Frobase JK. Exercise-induced bronchospasm in the young athlete: guidelines for routine screening and initial management. *Med Sci Sports Exerc.* 1992;24(8):856-859.

40. Eggleston, PA. Laboratory evaluation of exercise-induced asthma: methodologic considerations. *J Allergy Clin Immunol.* 1979;64(6, pt 2):604-608.

41. Cropp GJA. The exercise bronchoprovocation test: standardization of procedures and evaluation of response. *J Allergy Clin Immunol.* 1979;64(6, pt 2):627-633.

42. *Guidelines for the Diagnosis and Management of Asthma.* Expert panel report #2. National Institutes of Health, National Heart, Lung and Blood Institute. April 1997. NIH publication 97-4051.

43. *Guideline for the diagnosis and Management of Asthma—Update on Selected Topics 2002.* NIH/NHLBI #5074, 2002.

44. *Pediatric Asthma—Promoting Best Practice. Guide for Managing Asthma in children.* Milwaukee, WI: AAAAI/ AAP; 1999.

45. Patel DR, Homnick DN. Pulmonary effects of smoking. *Adolesc Med.* 2000;11(3):567-576.

46. Morton AR, Ogle SC, Fitch KD. Effects of nedocromil sodium, cromolyn sodium, and placebo in exercise-induced asthma. *Ann Allergy.* 1992;68:143-148.

47. Pearlman DS, van Adelsberg J, Phillip G, et al. Onset and duration of protection against exercise induced bronchoconstriction by a single dose of montelukast. *Ann Allergy Asthma Immunol.* 2006;97(1):98-104.

48. *2005 Patient Registry Data.* Cystic Fibrosis Foundation, Bethesda, MD.

49. Cropp GJ, Pulliano TP, Cerny FJ, Nathason IT. Exercise tolerance and cardiorespiratory adjustment of peak work capacity in cystic fibrosis. *Am Rev Respir Dis.* 1982;126: 211-216.

50. Stranghelle JK, Skyberg D. Cystic fibrosis patients running a marathon race. *Int J Sports Med.* 1988;1(37):37-40.

51. Nixon PA, Orenstein DM, Kelsey S, Doershuk C. The prognostic value of exercise testing in patients with cystic fibrosis. *N Eng J Med.* 1992; 327:1785-1788.

52. Orenstein DM, Nixon PA, Ross EA, Kaplan RM. The quality of well-being in cystic fibrosis. *Chest.* 1989;95:344-347.

53. Nixon PA, Orenstein DM, Curtis SE, Ross EA. Oxygen supplementation during exercise in cystic fibrosis. *Am Rev Respir Dis.* 1990;142:807-811.

54. Freeman W, Stableforth DE, Cayton RM, Morgan MDL. Endurance exercise capacity in adults with cystic fibrosis. *Respir Med.* 1993;87:541-549.

55. Orenstein DM. Pulmonary problems and management concerns in youth sports. *Pediatr Clin North Am.* 2002;49: 709-721.

56. Selvaduri H, Allen J, Sachinwalla T, Macauley J, Blimkie CJ, Van Asperen PP. Muscle function and resting energy expenditure in female athletes with cystic fibrosis. *Am J Respir Crit Care Med.* 2003;168:1476-1480.

57. Hussey J, Gormley J, Leen G, Greally P. Peripheral muscle strength in young males with cystic fibrosis. *J Cyst Fibros.* 2002;1(3):116-121.

58. Balfour-Lynn IM, Elborn JS. "CF asthma": what is it and what do we do about it? *Thorax.* 2002;57:742-748.

59. Freeman W, Stableforth DE, Cayton RM, Morgan MDL. Endurance exercise capacity in adults with cystic fibrosis. *Respir Med.* 1993;87:541-549.

60. Strauss GD, Osher A, Wang CI, et al. Variable weight training in cystic fibrosis. *Chest.* 1987:92:273-276.

61. Nixon PA, Orenstein DM, Kelsey S, Doershuk C. The prognostic value of exercise testing in patients with cystic fibrosis. *N Eng J Med.* 1992;327:1785-1788.

62. Sawyer EH, Clanton TL. Improved pulmonary function and exercise tolerance with inspiratory muscle conditioning in children with cystic fibrosis. *Chest.* 1993;104:490-497.

63. Orenstein DM, Franklin BA, Doershuk CF, et al. Exercise conditioning and cardiopulmonary fitness in cystic fibrosis. *Chest.* 1981;80:392-398.

64. deJong W, Grevink RG, Roorda RJ, Kaptein AA, van der Schans CP. Effect of a home exercise training program in patients with cystic fibrosis. *Chest.* 1994;105:463-468.

65. Cerny FJ. Relative effects of bronchial drainage and exercise for in-hospital care of patients with cystic fibrosis. *Phys Ther.* 1989;69:633-639.

CHAPTER 13

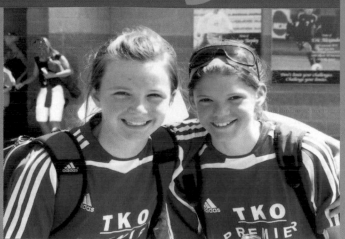

Disorders of the Kidneys

Donald E. Greydanus and Alfonso Torres

This chapter reviews relevant aspects of renal disease that have implications for sport participation by adolescents, including solitary kidney, hypertension, hyponatremia, proteinuria, hematuria, exercise-related acute renal failure, and chronic/end-stage renal disease (ESRD).[1] The effects of creatine and protein supplementation, including renal effects, are reviewed in Chapter 6.[2,3]

SOLITARY KIDNEY

Definition and Epidemiology

Solitary kidney refers to the occurrence of one kidney instead of the normal situation with two kidneys. Approximately 1 in 1500 children and adolescents have a solitary kidney.[4] The concern is whether sports activity should be avoided or limited for fear of injuring the one kidney the child or teen has and then having no kidney at all.

Pathogenesis

Solitary kidney may result from congenital or acquired causes (Table 13-1). Congenital causes include renal fusion anomalies. Acquired causes include the removal of a kidney because of malignancy or trauma.

Renal trauma from sports is fortunately an unusual condition and most of these are seen as a result of blunt trauma in contact/collision sports.[4] Recreational bicycle riding is the most common cause of sports-related kidney injury in children, sometimes leading to major renal injury; team contact sport activity is an unusual cause of major renal injury.[5] Also, the incidence of renal trauma from motor vehicle accidents is significantly higher in adolescents than renal trauma from sports activities.[6]

Clinical Presentation

Solitary kidney is typically asymptomatic and often is not known. Renal anomalies may be suspected in infants, if there is only one umbilical artery or other anomalies are present, such as congenital heart disease or multiple anomalies (such as imperforate anus, scoliosis, external ear defects, and others). Clinically, there are no specific manifestations of a solitary functioning kidney including renal agenesis. However, because of the generalized use of prenatal ultrasound, the diagnosis is commonly made prenatally and confirmed after delivery by repeated

Table 13-1.

Causes of Solitary Functioning Kidney

Congenital
Unilateral renal agenesis
Multicystic dysplastic kidney
Hypoplastic kidney

Nephrectomy
Renal trauma
Hydronephrosis
Vesicoureteral reflux
Renal artery thrombosis
Renal vein thrombosis
Kidney donation
Malignancy
Wilms tumor
Neuroblastoma

ultrasonography or nuclear renal scan. Unilateral renal agenesis in otherwise healthy individuals is compatible with normal longevity. Hypertension, proteinuria, hyperuricemia, focal segmental sclerosis, and decreased glomerular filtration rate (GFR) developing in individuals with a solitary functioning kidney are well documented in the literature. Renal hyperfiltration has been implicated as the cause of these abnormalities.

Diagnostic Studies

A renal sonogram may be done in cases of suspected renal anomalies or if an enlarged kidney is palpated.

More advance studies are undertaken in consultation with nephrologists as indicated based on initial clinical evaluation Box 13-1.

Management

There is no consensus among nephrology consultants regarding whether or not children or adolescents with one normal kidney should be involved in contact/collision sports.[4,7–10] In a survey of pediatric urologists published in 2002, 68% recommended the avoidance of contact sports in this situation, though 88% (182 out of 231) of those who answered the survey noted that the risk of loss the single kidney from sports trauma was less than 1%.[4] Another survey of sports medicine clinicians noted that 54% agreed with contact sports activity in these patients after reviewing potential risks of kidney damage with the athlete and family, though only 41.6% would allow such participation if this patient was their child.[11]

Other than the motor-vehicle-related injuries, the most frequent causes of severe renal injuries were associated with bicycle riding, being struck by the handlebars seems to be the mechanism of injury and may occur even when the speed of the riding is low. Renal injuries occur in team sports at much lower rate and severity than with other external causes of injury, and seldom are associated with loss of a kidney. Because of these observations, some pediatric urologists allow these children to participate in contact sports.

Besides the solitary functioning kidney, other renal disorders may predispose to renal trauma. We have seen a 12-year-old girl who after a mild trauma, when playing at school presented with gross hematuria. Family history and renal ultrasound revealed autosomal dominant polycystic kidney disease. Renal abnormalities such as hydronephrosis and horseshoe kidney as well as cross ectopia with fusion may predispose to blunt trauma resulting in renal injury.

The AAP Committee on Sports Medicine and Fitness recommendation for contact/collision sports is a "qualified yes" and based on "clinical judgment." Most pediatric urologists differ from these recommendations.

The reasons are not clear. Contact sports are often not related to high-grade renal injury, at least in individuals with two normally functioning kidneys. A few cases of solitary functioning kidney being injured during physical activities have been reported. The solitary functioning kidney is usually hypertrophic and it is not known, if this characteristic makes it more susceptible to blunt trauma.

In general, children or adolescents with one healthy kidney can be allowed participation in contact/collision sports if they wish such after careful explanation is provided to the athletes and their family of the low, but potential risks.[12–14] The importance of proper protection with recommended sports equipment and an appropriate supervision should be emphasized in these discussions. Some might say that one has only one brain and it needs proper protection as well in any sports activity. However, contact/collision sports activity should not be allowed, if there is a multicystic kidney, if hydronephrosis is present, if a pelvic or iliac location is present, or if there are uteropelvic junction abnormalities.[12]

HYPERTENSION

Definition and Epidemiology

Hypertension is defined as an average systolic blood pressure (SBP) and/or diastolic blood pressure (DBP) ≥95th percentile for gender, age, and height on ≥3 occasions.[15] Prehypertenion in children is defined as average levels of SBP or DBP that are ≥90th percentile but <95th percentile. Teenagers with blood pressure readings ≥120/80 are considered to be prehypertensive. The prevalence of hypertension is adolescents is approximately 5%.

Pathogenesis

Blood pressure results from the interaction between cardiac output and peripheral resistance, and it is increased if either of these factors increase. If no overt cause for the hypertension is found, the term primary or essential hypertension is used. If another disease is found to cause the rise in blood pressure, it is called secondary hypertension. White-coat hypertension refers to elevated blood pressure in the office setting (or other anxiety-provoking situations) but normal blood pressure readings otherwise. Table 13-2 lists causes for hypertension in adolescents.

Clinical Presentation

Most adolescents with hypertension are asymptomatic and the finding of an increased blood pressure is typically noted during a sports preparticipation or other

Table 13-2.

Causes of Hypertension in Adolescents*

Primary (essential) hypertension
White coat hypertension
Secondary causes of hypertension
- Renal
    Renal parenchymal diseases: Acute and chronic glomerular diseases, chronic interstitial disease, polycystic kidney disease, reflux nephropathy, obstructive uropathy
    Renovascular disease: Renovascular hypertension caused by renal artery muscular dysplasia.
    Extramural compression of renal artery: Neurofibromatosis
- Endocrine
    Congenital adrenal hyperplasia, adrenal adenoma, bilateral adrenal
    Hyperplasia
    Cushing syndrome
    Pheochromocytoma of the medulla of the adrenal glands, extra-adrenal chromaffin cell tumor
    Hyperthyroidism, hypothyroidism
- Medications and illicit drugs
    Glucocorticoids, mineralocorticoids, cyclosporin, erythropoietin, sympathomimetics, contraceptives, NSAIDs, monoaminooxydase inhibitors, licorice, herbal remedies, heavy metals, cocaine, alcohol, etc.
- Exogenous obesity
    Insulin resistance, sleep apnea
- Spinal cord injury
    Paraplegia, quadriplegia
    Peripheral neuropathy; Guillain-Barre syndrome
- Mendelian forms of hypertension
    Apparent mineralocorticoid excess (AME)
    Glucocorticoid-remediable hyperaldosteronism (GRH)
    Liddle's syndrome
    Gordon Syndrome

*Used with permission from Greydanus DE, Torres AD, Wan JH. Genitourinary and renal disorders. In: Greydanus DE, Patel DR, Pratt HD, eds. Essential Adolescent Medicine. New York: McGraw-Hill Medical Publishers; 2006;347.

Table 13-3.

Tests for Evaluation of Secondary Hypertension in Adolescents*

- Renal parenchymal
    Proteinuria, hematuria, RBC casts, complement C3, C4, ASO titers, ANA, antidouble strand DNA, ANCA titers, renal biopsy
- Reflux nephropathy
    Proteinuria, urine culture, VCUG, DMSA renal scan
- Renal artery stenosis
    Plasma rennin activity, captopril renogram, spiral computed tomographic angiography, magnetic resonance angiography
- Endocrine causes
    Pheochromocytoma: Plasma metanephrines, clonidine suppression test, localization of tumor by CT scan, MRI, metaiodobenzyl guanidine (MIBG)
    Primary aldosteronism: Serum potassium, serum aldosteron/plasma renin ratio, CT scan, MRI of adrenal glands
    Cushing syndrome. Morning serum cortisol after dexamethasone suppression
    Hyperthyroidism/hpothyroidism. Total and free thyroxin TSH
- Medications/drug abuse
    History of prescribe and not prescribed medications, herbal remedies. Drug screening.

*Used with permission from Greydanus DE, Torres AD, Wan JH. Genitourinary and renal disorders. In: Greydanus DE, Patel DR, Pratt HD, eds. Essential Adolescent Medicine. New York: McGraw-Hill Medical Publishers; 2006:347.

sion. Those with presumed primary hypertension can have a work-up including a complete blood count, electrolytes, blood urea nitrogen, creatinine, and urinalysis. Other tests include serum uric acid (often increased in primary hypertension), fasting lipid profile, electrocardiogram, and echocardiographic examination. Table 13-3 lists tests used for evaluation of adolescents with secondary hypertension.

Treatment

Children or adolescents who have severe, symptomatic hypertension should be immediately and rapidly treated to bring their blood pressure down to safer levels even before diagnostic tests are ordered. Those with mild to moderate hypertension should receive nonpharmacologic intervention that consists of lifestyle modifications to improve exercise patterns, diet, and overweight or obesity, if present. The patient should be counseled to avoid cigarette smoking if using this substance. Adolescents who are in a prehypertensive state, should receive instruction in lifestyle modifications as well.

Regular exercise is a key part of systemic hypertension management in adolescents. The benefits of exercise

preventive examination. The physical examination is typically normal except for the elevated blood pressure. Those with severe, sustained hypertension eventually develop retinopathy, left ventricular hypertrophy, and other hypertensive complications.

In general, patients younger than 10 years with hypertension have secondary hypertension and adolescents typically have essential or primary hypertension. An adolescent with mild to moderate hypertension and a positive family history for primary hypertension usually has primary or essential hypertension.

Diagnostic Studies

The patient should have at least three elevated blood pressure measurements before using the term hyperten-

on hypertension are supported by research and these youth should be instructed in being physically active and given full guidance in exercise and sports participation.[16–19] The 36th Bethesda Conference[20] and the American Academy of Pediatrics[16] have published their recommendations for sports participation by athletes with systemic hypertension. Full athletic participation is allowed for those with hypertension in the 95th to 98th percentile for age and gender (significant hypertension) who have no evidence of target organ damage or other cardiovascular disease. Adolescent athletes with hypertension in the 99th percentile for age and gender (severe hypertension) are recommended to avoid competitive sports and activities with high-static loads until the blood pressure is controlled and there is no evidence for target organ damage. Table 13-4 reviews medications used to treat hypertension in adolescents.[15]

HYPONATREMIA

Definition and Epidemiology

The normal serum sodium concentrations or $[Na^+]$ is between 138 and 142 mmol/L and is maintained within these narrow limits despite large variations in water intake. Hyponatremia is defined by a serum sodium level that is below 135 mEq/L. Hyponatremia develops when there is an increased ratio of water to sodium that involves the total body water and total body sodium.

Pathogenesis

Causes of hyponatremia in athletes are listed in Table 13-5.[21,22] Mildly symptomatic or asymptomatic hyponatremia is a common phenomenon in athletes and an incidence as high as 30% has been reported in long-distance runners.[21] However, rare deaths caused by hyponatremia have been reported in long-distance runners.[21,22]

Hypotonic or dilutional hyponatremia is the main situation seen in athletes and is owing to excessive water intake before and during the sporting event or physical activity, particularly when occurring in hot and humid conditions.[9] Most cases of exercise-associated hyponatremia (EAH) are owing to a combination of increased fluid intake with modest increases of plasma arginine vasopressin (AVP) levels from various stimuli during prolonged exercise.[23] Those at increased risk for hyponatremia are athletes with smaller total body surface area and who sweat excessively. The potentially fatal outcome of hyponatremia should be understood by athletes who seek to keep themselves properly hydrated during sports events and other physical activities.

Numerous factors acting in the concentrating and diluting mechanisms in the kidney contribute to the regulation of the normal serum $[Na^+]$. Most of the changes in serum sodium concentration that occur acutely are the result of changes in the total body water content, rather than rapid changes in total body sodium content. Significant amount of water loss relative to sodium loss will result in an increase in serum sodium concentration, whereas a decrease in water excretion, because of disorders of renal diluting capacity without a significant change in solute $(Na^{2+} K^+)$ will result in dilutional hyponatremia.

There are a few conditions in which the serum sodium does not reflect serum osmolality, when osmotically active substances (i.e., glucose, mannitol, glycine) are present in the extracellular fluid. Increased serum osmolality without changes in sodium concentration is seen when osmolytes (i.e., urea, ethanol, methanol, ethylene glycol) are distributed in the total body water. Pseudohyponatremia is present when the solid content of plasma is increased (hyperlipidemia, dysproteinemias), and the sodium is measured by flame photometer rather than specific sodium electrode.

Clinical Presentation

Most athletes remain asymptomatic with sodium levels between 125 mEq/L and 135 mEq/L. Mild cases of hyponatremia may result in nausea, emesis, headaches, lethargy, confusion, irritability, edema of hands, as well as feet. However, rapid decreases in sodium levels, especially if rapid drop off are noted, can result in significant osmotic fluid shifts with resultant cerebral edema, seizure activity, coma, and rarely, death.

Hypotonic hyponatremia causes increase in water content in all body cells. However, the central nervous system swelling causes most relevant clinical manifestations. The severity of the neurologic manifestations correlates with the rapidity with which the hyponatremia develops. The more rapid the hyponatremia develops, the more severe the clinical manifestations occur. Rapidly developing cerebral edema causes increased intracranial pressure and the risk of brain herniation, death, or severe neurologic sequelae. Although the brain has the ability to adapt to hyponatremia by extruding electrolytes and organic osmolytes out of the brain cells, this adaptive response requires time, an average of 48 hours.

The development of moderate, asymptomatic hypernatremia correlates with body weight loss, whereas hyponatremia correlates with weight gain. Acute symptomatic hyponatremia results from both excessive fluid intake and decreased urine formation contributing to its rapid onset. Life-threatening complications secondary to pulmonary edema and cerebral edema may result. Susceptibility for the development of exercise associated hyponatremia includes female gender, medications that interfere

Table 13-6.

Characteristic Findings in SIADH

Hypotonic hyponatremia.
Normal or slightly expanded extracellular volume.
Inappropriate urine concentration more than 100 mOsm/L of H_2O in the presence of hypo-osmolality in serum.
Elevated urinary sodium concentration in the presence of normal salt and water intake, negative electrolyte free water excretion, absence of thyroid, adrenal disease, use of diuretic, or renal insufficiency.

Treatment

Treatment of symptomatic hyponatremia depends on its severity and associated complications; these patients should be transferred to appropriate medical centers for careful monitoring and management to correct the electrolyte imbalance. However, prevention of sports-related hyponatremia is an important part of sports guidance for children and adolescents.

One guideline for fluid replacement recommend that adolescents ingest 400 to 600 mL (14–22 oz) of fluid approximately 2 hours before, and 200 to 350 mL (6–12 oz) every 20 minutes during exercise sessions.[24,25] Fluid intake will be variable from athlete to athlete and depend on factors such as body surface area, rate of sweating, and fitness level. Athletes should be educated to avoid drinking "as much water or other fluids as possible." They should check their body weight before and after the exercise session to aid in identifying how much fluid replacement is needed.

Fluid replacement with cold water is recommended for short duration sessions (as less than 1 hour). Carbohydrate and electrolyte balanced drinks are recommended for sessions that are longer; an added benefit for these balanced drinks is that they are usually more palatable to the youth and thus, they are more likely to consume them.

Symptomatic patients present a therapeutic dilemma, because the treatment is different in acute hyponatremia and chronic hyponatremia. A careful history and physical examination continue to be the corner stone in clinical assessment and therapeutic decision. Young individuals in normal health until hours before becoming symptomatic most likely, but not always represent cases of acute hyponatremia.

The treatment of exercise-associated hyponatremia depends on the severity of the symptoms. For mild symptomatic hyponatremia, restriction of hypotonic fluids until the runner is urinating normally, and consumption of oral hypertonic solutions are sufficient. For severely symptomatic individuals, 3% sodium chloride intravenous administration will speed recovery and improve outcome. Prerun education includes addressing early symptoms, expected weight changes, and avoidance of over hydration. Gone are the days of the advice "drink as much as you can" before the race.

HYPOKALEMIA

Definition

Hypokalemia is defined as $[K^+]$ of less than 3.5 mEq/L. The total body K content in a healthy individual is estimated to be 50 mEq/kg of body weight. It is estimated that 98% of K is located in the intracellular space and 2% in the extracellular space. The normal plasma potassium concentration is between 3.5 mEq/L and 5.5 mEq/L. The minimal dietary K requirement is 40 to 50 mEq/d.

Pathogenesis

The causes of hypokalemia are listed in Table 13-7.

Clinical Presentation

Most patients with mild hypokalemia are asymptomatic and the hypokalemia may be discovered as an incidental finding and suspected based on electrocardiogram or laboratory evaluation. It may be anticipated in individuals

Table 13-7.

Symptomatic Hypokalemia

Associated with cardiac arrhythmias, electrocardiogram findings with inversion of T wave, prominent U waves, and abnormal S-T segment.
Neuromuscular manifestations include muscular weakness, muscular cramps, depressed deep tendon reflexes, paresthesia, and paralysis.
Gastrointestinal manifestations of hypokalemia include constipation and even paralytic ileus that may develop during an acute episode of gastroenteritis.
The renal manifestations of chronic hypokalemia include hyposthenuria, polyuria, polydipsia, renal cysts formation, interstitial nephritis, and hypochloremic, hypokalemic, metabolic alkalosis.
Neurologic manifestations including encephalopathy associated with hyperammonemia particularly in the presence of hepatic disease.
Pulmonary manifestations are progressive respiratory failure resulting from respiratory muscle weakness and paralysis.

with predisposing factors such as a history of diuretic intake, family history of periodic hypokalemic paralysis, Bartter syndrome, and Gitelman syndrome. Symptomatic hypokalemia is infrequently seen in practice of sport, when it occurs, it may manifest as acute life-threatening event, and usually is associated with predisposing factors.

One of the most dramatic presentations of hypokalemia is that of *primary hypokalemic periodic paralysis*. It may occur as a sporadic event usually in young adults or adolescent males during intense exercise, or after ingesting a high carbohydrate containing meal after exercise. The individual complains of an acute, progressive, generalized weakness developing within a few hours after ingestion of the carbohydrates meal progressing to paralysis and deteriorating mental status. The weakness and paralysis affect the proximal muscles more than distal ones. Cardiac arrhythmias and abnormalities in the ECG (inverted T waves, prominent U waves, and S-T segment depression) are seen. Respiratory insufficiency develops because of weakness or paralysis of the respiratory muscles. The disease follows an autosomal dominant pattern of inheritance in 60% of cases with the rest following a sporadic occurrence. The condition has an estimated prevalence of 1 in 100,000.

Treatment

Urgent management of these patients in the intensive care setting is needed. The goal in treating hypokalemia is to prevent life-endangering complications resulting from injudicious therapies. The route and speed of therapy is determined by the severity and manifestations of the hypokalemia. Serum [K] <2.5 mEq/L, may require immediate therapy because of the increased risk of cardiac arrhythmias. Before initiating K replacement therapy, it is prudent to evaluate and judge the adequacy of renal function to prevent dangerous hyperkalemia. Oral potassium replacement is safe and effective in most cases. Intravenous potassium is used when the oral route cannot be used. IV potassium chloride is generally the preparation used. Other potassium chloride preparations are available for special needs as when there is hypokalemia and hypophosphatemia; potassium acetate is used in cases in which parenteral nutrition is necessary.

Symptomatic hypokalemia associated with electrocardiographic changes, myocardial infarction, respiratory insufficiency because of respiratory muscle paralysis, digitalis intoxication, and hepatic coma because of hyperammonemia require intravenous administration of KCl to restore K levels to a safe concentration. Replacement of the total potassium deficit will require a longer period of time.

PROTEINURIA

Definition and Epidemiology

The upper normal limit of protein excretion in the urine of children and adolescents is 100 mg/m^2 per 24 hours.[15] Approximately 1 in 10 patients, aging between 8- to 15-year-old will have a positive urine dipstick for protein.[26] Orthostatic (postural) proteinuria is the most common cause of persistent proteinuria in adolescents, noted in 60% of cases.[26]

The protein excretion is 10-fold higher in the upright versus supine position.[26] The precise incidence of exercise-related proteinuria in athletes is unclear, but it is commonly seen in children and adolescent athletes involved in swimming, running football, rowing, cross-country skiing, and other sports.

Pathogenesis

Table 13-8 lists causes of proteinuria. The pathogenesis for postexercise proteinuria is not known, though it is common and correlates to the intensity of the physical activity.[27] Some research implicates prostaglandins and the renin-angiotensin system in the development of postexercise proteinuria.[27]

Clinical Presentation

Proteinuria is asymptomatic and noted by urinalysis. Table 13-9 notes causes of false-positive urine protein by dipstick.

Treatment

In general, exercise-induced proteinuria is a benign finding and not associated with chronic problems. In

Table 13-8.

Causes of Proteinuria

- Orthostatic (postural) proteinuria
- Glomerular diseases (acute or chronic)
    Acute or chronic glomerulonephritis
    Cystic kidney diseases
    Focal sclerosis
    IgA nephropathy
    Hereditary nephritis
- Tubulointerstitial diseases
- Overflow proteinuria caused by abnormal production of low molecular weight proteins
- Reflux nephropathy (VUR, renal scarring, hypertension, increased creatinine)
- Pregnancy
- Congestive heart failure

Table 13-9.

Causes of False-Positive Urine Protein by Dipstick*

Highly buffered urine from alkaline medications or storage
Leaving dipstick in urine too long thereby washing out buffer
Contamination of urine by quaternary ammonium cleaning
   compounds
Treatment with phenazopyridine (in some dipstick brands)
Urine pH >7.0

*Used with permission from Greydanus DE, Torres AD, Wan JH. Genitourinary and renal disorders. In: Greydanus DE, Patel DR, Pratt HD, eds. Essential Adolescent Medicine. New York: McGraw-Hill Medical Publishers; 2006:335.

Table 13-10.

Causes/Mechanisms of Hematuria in Athletes

- Relative renal ischemia : Strenuous exercise results in increase blood flow to skeletal muscles at the expense of decreased renal blood flow.
- Exercise-induced increase in catecholamines: Result in renal arteriolar vasoconstriction.
- Hypoxia and increased lactic acid associated damage to nephrons.
- Skeletal muscle damage from exercise combined with dehydration predisposes to rhabdomyolysis.
- NSAIDs use associated with hematuria in half of the athletes.
- Foot-strike hemolysis: Repetitive trauma to the heel from running and jumping cause rupture of RBCs and release of hemoglobin. Hemoglobin is excreted in urine once excess haptoglobin binding sites are saturated by excess Hb.
- Indirect trauma to bladder from repetitive jarring motions.
- Direct blunt trauma to kidneys in contact/collision sports: Rare.
- Dehydration: Increased blood viscosity leads to increased RBC and plasma osmolality resulting in increased hemolysis of older RBCs.
- Decreased RBC membrane resistance: Because of increased body temperature and circulation associated with strenuous exercise.
- Free radical damage: Increased free radical production associated with exercise may contribute to renal tissue damage.
- Lysolecithin: Strenuous exercise is associated with increased catecholamines that cause spleen contraction and release of lysolecithin. Lysolecithin causes destruction of RBCs.

*Used with permission from Patel DR, Torres AD, Greydanus DE. Kidneys and sports. Adolesc Med Clin. 2005;16(1):111-119.

most situations, another urinalysis examined 1 to 2 days after the exercise activity will be normal.[15,26] It is recommended that a consultation with a nephrologist occur for the athlete with persistent asymptomatic proteinuria and those with symptomatology suggestive of renal or other chronic illness Box 13-1.

HEMATURIA

Definition and Epidemiology

Hematuria is defined as over three red blood cells (RBCs) per high-power field.[28,29] Significant hematuria is defined as the presence of over 50 RBCs/μL of urine. The precise prevalence of hematuria in adolescent athletes is not known, though it is felt to be considerably higher than in nonathletes; some research have reported hematuria in 20% of marathon runners, 55% of football players, and 80% of swimmers.[28]

Pathogenesis

Table 13-10 lists various mechanisms and etiologies for exercise-associated hematuria.[27,28]

Hematuria, gross or microscopic, is a common finding in athletes participating in many types of sport activities. Gross hematuria may be the result of direct trauma to organs of the urinary tract including the kidneys and is seen in individuals falling from bikes, horses, motorcycles, and skating. Direct trauma to the kidney can occur in football or boxing; direct trauma to the bladder may occur during long-distance running, particularly when the bladder is empty.

The athlete may not be aware of the existence of abnormalities of the urinary tract predisposing to bleeding with relatively minor trauma such as seen in polycystic kidneys or hydronephrosis. Coagulation defects may be manifested with minor trauma during a sporting event or when children are playing. Glomerular hematuria can occur with the participation in sports not directly associated with trauma. The presence of dysmorphic RBC and RBC casts in the urine, as seen during the participation in sports, particularly long-distance running is well documented.

Alterations in renal hemodynamics occur during intensive physical activities, resulting in the shunting of blood from the kidneys to skeletal muscles. With vigorous exercise, there is an increase in sympathetic nerve activity resulting in renal vasoconstriction and increase in renin-angiotensin II activity. There is an increase in the glomerular vascular resistance particularly at the level of the efferent arteriole that increases transglomerular filtration pressure, facilitating extrusion of RBC through the glomerular basement membrane.

We have seen the case of a 16-year-old cross-country runner, who predictably developed bouts of gross asymptomatic hematuria during his cross-country

Table 13-11.

Conditions Associated with Transient Hematuria*

Infections (generalized, urinary, prostatic, vulvovaginal)
Genitourinary foreign bodies
Coagulation defects
Sickle cell trait or anemia
Post-trauma (both recognized and unrecognized, as may occur in contact sports)

Used with permission from Greydanus DE, Torres AD, Wan JH. Genitourinary and renal disorders. In: Greydanus DE, Patel DR, Pratt HD, eds. Essential Adolescent Medicine. New York: McGraw-Hill Medical Publishers; 2006:341.

running practices. Extensive urologic and nephrologic evaluation was unrewarding. A renal biopsy disclosed thin basal membrane nephropathy. The patient was treated with a long-acting angiotensin converting enzyme inhibitor (ACE) with disappearance of the gross hematuria associated with running.

Clinical Presentation

The patient with microscopic hematuria is often asymptomatic and the individual with discolored urine is also typically asymptomatic. A microscopic analysis of 10 to 15 mL of fresh centrifuged urine is essential to confirm the diagnosis of hematuria.[29] Table 13-11 lists conditions associated with transient hematuria and Table 13-12 shows extraparenchymal causes of urinary bleeding. Red urine may occur in the presence of myoglobin or hemoglobin. In rhabdomyolysis, myoglobinuria is noted without hematuria, while

Table 13-12.

Causes of Extraparenchymal Urinary Bleeding*

Urinary infection
Hypercalciuria ± urolithiasis
Abdominal or flank trauma
Urinary tract structural malformations
Medical/nonmedical instrumentation of the lower urinary tract
Hemoglobinopathies
Medications
Tumors
Hemorrhagic diatheses

Used with permission from Greydanus DE, Torres AD, Wan JH. Genitourinary and renal disorders. In: Greydanus DE, Patel DR, Pratt HD, eds. Essential Adolescent Medicine. New York: McGraw-Hill Medical Publishers; 2006:343.

Table 13-13.

Common Components of the Clinical Evaluation of Hematuria*

History of:	Suggests:
dysuria, fever	upper or lower UTI
headache, rash, arthralgias, others	systemic infection, vasculitis, collagen vascular diseases, Henoch-Schönlein nephritis
sinusitis, cough, headache, epistaxis	Wegener's granulomatosis
flank pain	renal calculus, acute urinary obstruction, subacute pyelonephritis, cystic diseases
intermittent gross hematuria	IgA and IgG nephritis; urethritis, foreign body, hypercalciuria, neoplasm (rare)
antecendent viral illness	postinfectious nephritis, IgA nephropathy, other nephritis
cola-colored urine, edema, hypertension	glomerulonephritis
bloody diarrhea	hemolytic uremic syndrome (serotoxin-producing E coli and others)
Family history of:	
microhematuria	Thin basal membrane disease, hereditary nephritis, hypercalciuria
hearing loss	hereditary nephritis
renal failure	hereditary nephritis, cystic kidney disease
anemia	sickle cell disease or trait
Physical findings of:	
hypertension	acute or chronic glomerulonephritis
edema, ascites	glomerulonephritis, membranous nephropathy, focal sclerosis
bruising	coagulopathy, collagen vascular disease,
heart murmur, fever	subacute bacterial endocarditis
purpura	systemic infection, Henoch-Schönlein nephritis
flank mass	polycystic kidney disease, obstructive uropathy, renal tumor, multicystic dysplastic kidney

Used with permission from Greydanus DE, Torres AD, Wan JH. Genitourinary and renal disorders. In: Greydanus DE, Patel DR, Pratt HD, eds. Essential Adolescent Medicine. New York: McGraw-Hill Medical Publishers; 2006:342.

hemoglobinuria is found in hemolytic anemia without hematuria.[15,27,29]

Diagnostic Studies

The typical situation is that hematuria is first noted during a screening urinalysis in an athlete who has no symptoms. Table 13-13 provides principles of evaluation for hematuria.

Treatment

The athlete is usually asymptomatic with benign hematuria and the hematuria resolves in 1 to 2 days after the exercise activity with rest.[28,29] The presence of anemia in athletes with only exercise-associated hematuria is unusual. Proper hydration is recommended to help prevent bladder contusions that are caused by indirect trauma-related jarring motions.[27] Urethral injury in cyclists can be prevented by using proper cushioning along with a lowered seat height. It is recommended that the asymptomatic athlete consult with a nephrologist if the hematuria persists for 14 days or more; a nephrology consult should also occur if there are associated symptomatology, such as proteinuria, high blood pressure, edema, and anemia Box 13-1.

EXERCISE-ASSOCIATED ACUTE RENAL FAILURE

There are case reports of acute renal failure that develop after strenuous physical activity; however, these cases are quite unusual.[27]

Causes of acute renal failure in children and adolescents are noted in Table 13-14. Blood is preferentially shunted to skeletal muscles that are exercising; glomerular filtration rate and urine output decrease by 30% to 60% as the intensity of exercise approaches 50% VO_2 max.[30] The

Table 13-14.

Causes of Acute Renal Failure in Children and Adolescents*

Ages 2–12 y
Hemolytic-uremic syndrome
Multiple organ dysfunction due to sepsis
Drug toxicity
Surgery for congenital heart diseases
Primary renal diseases
Malignancies
Tumor lysis syndrome
Postbone marrow transplantation (including kidney transplantation)

Ages 13–21 y
Multiple organ dysfunction due to sepsis
Trauma
Ingestion of nephrotoxic agents
Drugs
Malignancies
Solid organ transplantation
Postbone marrow transplantation

*Used with permission from Torres AD, Greyanus DE. The renal system. In: Greydanus DE, Feinberg AD, Patel DR, Homnick DN, eds. The Pediatric Diagnostic Examination. New York: McGraw-Hill Medical Publishers; 2008:478.

risk of acute renal failure is increased when other factors contribute to further decreased renal blood flow. Such factors include the presence of dehydration, sickle cell disease, renal hypouricemia, and rhabdomyolysis; there can also be nonsteroidal anti-inflammatory drugs (NSAIDs) effects.[27, 31–34]

NSAIDs are commonly used by both athletes and nonathletes.[34] NSAIDs inhibit cyclooxegenase leading to prevention of prostaglandin (PGE_2 and PGI_2) production. Reduced levels of these prostaglandins lead to renal vasoconstriction and decreased renal blood flow that are further exaggerated during exercise, heat stress, and dehydration.[30] Prevention of exercise-associated acute renal failure involves maintaining appropriate hydration by using balanced carbohydrate electrolyte solutions and avoiding heat stress; it is also critical to identify precipitating factors such as sickle cell disease and avoid using amphetamines, alcohol, and NSAIDs.[31–34]

RHABDOMYOLYSIS

Definition

Rhabdomyolysis is injury to skeletal muscle cells of sufficient severity that results in cell disruption leading to leakage of intracellular contents into the blood stream and their appearance in the urine.

Pathogenesis

Exertional rhabdomyolysis develops in situations with strenuous exercise (such as marathon running) induces release of massive amounts of myoglobin (a muscle protein) into the blood which precipitates in the kidneys leading to acute renal failure.[31] The risk of rhabdomyolysis in increased with ingestion of alcohol and amphetamines. The unusual case of exertional rhabdomyolysis may be because of a combination of factors, including strenuous exercise, use of drugs or analgesics (as NSAIDs, amphetamines, others), dehydration, heat stress, infection (viral or bacterial), and others.[31]

Multiple mechanisms injurious to the skeletal muscle alter the sarcolemma permeability resulting in edema. Generalized ATP depletion affects all the ion transporters, specifically in the muscle cells. The decreased activity of the Na^+ K^+ ATP-ase, inhibits the function of the $2Na^+/Ca^{2+}$ exchanger responsible for the extrusion of Ca^{2+} from the cell. It also induces opening of the K^+ channels, blocking the Ca^{2+} uptake by the sarcolemma reticulum, these changes result in increased intracellular Ca^{2+} concentration that directly damage the mitochondria resulting in the production of oxygen radicals and oxidative stress. Intracellular calcium activates cytolytic enzymes causing cell death by necrosis or apoptosis. The

Table 13-15.

Examples of Rhabdomyolysis Associated with Sporting Activities

Violent calisthenics (such as "wind sprinting," weight lifting, pushups)

Long-distance running in hot humid conditions

Long walks especially when using eccentric muscle contractions (such as walking downhill)

most common cause of rhabdomyolysis is vigorous exercise, such as squat jumping, prolonged marches, and running (Table 13-15).

Clinical Presentation

Clinical manifestations include myalgias, muscle tenderness and swelling, stiffness, weakness, and even paralysis. The physical findings include muscle tenderness exacerbated by attempt to move the muscle involved and firm edema. In nontraumatic rhabdomyolysis, the physical findings are not prominent. Acute renal failure has been described with heat stroke associated with rhabdomyolysis, under circumstances likely to interfere with glycolysis (including fever and hypokalemia). The onset is abrupt with cardiovascular collapse, hypotension, agitation, disorientation, and convulsion. The most common cause of pigment-induced acute renal failure is myoglobinuria resulting from rhabdomyolysis (Table 13-16).

Diagnostic Studies

In acute rhabdomyolysis, total creatinine kinase (CK) in plasma is elevated. More than 90% of the CK in skeletal muscle is CK-MM fraction and only 6% represents

Table 13-16.

Causes of Myoglobin-Induced Acute Renal Failure

Muscle trauma—postexertional, crush syndrome, ischemic, grand mal seizures

Myopathy—McArdle disease, Tarui disease, and alcohol-induced

Drug overdose—alcohol, narcoticsm sedatives, heroin

Prolonged hyperosmolar coma

Heat stroke

Carbon monoxide poisoning

Severe hypokalemia

Severe hypophosphatemia

Idiopathic paroxysmal myoglobinuria

CK-MB; therefore, in the presence of markedly elevated total CKs, the existence of elevated CK-MB does not signify myocardial damage. There is no troponin I in skeletal muscle. The level of CK-MM peaks between 24 and 48 hours. Persistent elevation or increasing levels of CK-MM implicate ongoing muscle injury. Other enzymes that may be markedly elevated during rhabdomyolysis include lactic dehydrogenase (LDH), aspartate transaminase (AST), alanine transaminase (ALT), and aldolase; these enzymes are less specific.

Early during myoglobinuria, a transient glycosuria may be observed in the absence of hyperglycemia, because of decreased glucose reabsorption in the proximal tubule. This transient glycosuria reflects proximal tubular dysfunction and in most cases disappears in 12 hours. In most cases of rhabdomyolysis, there is an elevation of plasma creatinine out of proportion to the elevation of BUN. During rhabdomyolysis, creatine normally present in the skeletal muscle cells, leaks out into the blood where it converted into creatinine. Elevation of creatinine between 2 mg/dL and 4 mg/dL in the presence of normal levels of BUN usually normalizes in 2 to 3 days.

Because of its low molecular weight (around 17,000 Da), myoglobin is rapidly filtered by the normal glomeruli and is cleared from the serum more rapidly than hemoglobin; except in the most severe cases of rhabdomyolysis, the serum remains clear. When the urine concentration of myoglobin is >100 mg/dL, it becomes visible. Because myoglobin contains a heme group, lower concentrations may be detected by dipstick technology, giving a positive reaction for blood in the absence of RBC or hemoglobin. The diagnosis of rhabdomyolysis in general, does not require specific immunoassay methods.

Treatment

Management of rhabdomyolysis includes appropriate management of fluids and electrolytes and rapid restoration of the extracellular volume in the inpatient setting. Alkalinization of the urine to prevent precipitation of myoglobin in the renal tubules as consequence of an acid pH is important in the initial management. Careful monitoring of potassium, phosphorus, uric acid, and acid base balance are necessary. Early hemodialysis should be initiated when indicated.

HEMOGLOBINURIA

Definition

Hemoglobinuria is characterized by the presence of hemoglobin in the urine that has been filtered through the glomerular basal membrane and has escaped uptake and metabolism by the tubular epithelial cells.

Pathophysiology

Hemoglobinuria associated with repetitive trauma to RBCs is seen with the use of cardiovascular prosthesis, in the microangiopathic diseases particularly those affecting the kidneys (hemolytic uremic syndrome, thrombotic thrombocytopenic purpura), and in individuals with membrane abnormalities of RBCs. Enzyme abnormalities in the RBC membrane predispose to mechanical rupture of the RBC. The lack or deficiency of haptoglobin that is normally bound to hemoglobin in the circulation may facilitate the filtration of hemoglobin in the glomeruli. Many other causes of hemoglobinuria are described. Hemoglobinuria associated with an acute renal failure is rare. Other causes of intravascular hemolysis include infections and venoms, drugs and chemicals, genetic diseases, immunologic processes, and mismatched blood transfusions.

The presence of hemoglobin in the renal circulation induces renal vasoconstriction. Tubular obstruction and tubular cell injury are well demonstrated findings in experimentally induced hemoglobinuria and myoglobinuria. Heme is cytotoxic and free iron can induce mitochondrial damage. In sport activities, hypovolemia and acidosis predispose to pigment-induced renal tubular injury. Another contributing factor is mechanical tubular obstruction by the formation of pigment casts in the presence of decreased urine flow and an acid urine pH.

Diagnostic Studies

Laboratory findings in hemoglobinuria reveal an evidence of hemolysis: decreased haptoglobin, elevated lactate dehydrogenase, elevated unconjugated bilirubin, reticulocytosis, and pink supernatant in the serum because of binding of hemoglobin to haptoglobin. In myoglobinuria, the supernatant is clear because of the rapid filtration of the myoglobin by the glomeruli. The peripheral smear demonstrates fragmented erythrocytes.

Treatment

Management of hemoglobinuria requires appropriate fluid and electrolyte administration, management of acid base disturbances, and prevention of the triggering mechanisms for hemolysis. Fortunately sport associated hemoglobinuria and ARF is a rare event.

CHRONIC/END-STAGE RENAL DISEASE

Causes of chronic renal diseases in those aged 10 years though adolescence are noted in Table 13-17, the most

Table 13-17.

Causes of Chronic Renal Diseases in Those Aged 10 Years Through Adolescence*

Glomerular disorders
Focal segmental glomerulosclerosis
Membraneous nephropathy
Membranoproliferative glomerulonephritis
IgA nephropathy
Small blood vessel vasculitis
Lupus nephritis
Hereditary nephritis (Alport syndrome)
Renal tubular diseases
Bartter syndrome
Gitelman syndrome
Diabetic nephropathy

*Used with permission from Torres AD, Greyanus DE. The Renal System. In: Greydanus DE, Feinberg AD, Patel DR, Homnick DN, eds. The Pediatric Diagnostic Examination. New York: McGraw-Hill Medical Publishers; 2008:480.

important of which are the glomerular diseases.[35] In patients with chronic renal failure, the exercise capacity is impaired for various reasons. These include general deconditioning, limited state of nutrition, side effects of medications, hypertension, chronic anemia, acid-base dysfunction, metabolic disorders, and postkidney transplant obesity.[36]

Athletes with chronic renal disease should consult with their nephrologist and renal care team with regards to participation in a specific sport and it is made on a case by case basis after looking at the specific sport and what risks are inherent in that activity Box 13-1. Potential risks of sport participation by athletes who have chronic renal disease include dehydration, electrolyte dysfunction, syncope, seizures, and increased risk for traumatic fractures, if metabolic bone disease is present.[36] Other risk factors include trauma-induced injury to the renal allograft, arteriovenous fistula, vascular access catheter, or the peritoneal catheter. Kidney transplant patients participate in sports activities much less than their peers who have not had these transplants.[37]

Box 13-1 When to Refer

When to Refer to Nephrology
Hypertension
Persistent proteinuria
Persistent hematuria
Renal failure
Rhabdomyolysis
Evaluation of hemoglobinuria
Chronic renal disease
Renal neoplasms
Complex fluid and electrolyte problems
Congenital renal anomalies

A survey of British and Irish pediatric kidney transplantation facilities (17 out of 26 surveyed programs responded) noted that they recommended their patients not take part in sports such as rubgy football, judo, karate, boxing, and kick boxing; six percent also felt that their patients should not play volleyball, basketball, or soccer (association football).[38] All the centers that responded agreed that their kidney transplant athletes could be involved in rowing, golf, sailing, cricket, netball, cycling, canoeing, skiing, swimming, track sports, field hockey, tennis, and badminton.[38] Certainly more research in this area is needed and recommended in the area of sports participation by children and youth with chronic renal disease.[39]

REFERENCES

1. Patel DR, Torres AD, Greydanus DE. Kidneys and sports. *Adolesc Med Clin.* 2005;16(1):111-119.
2. Greydanus DE, Patel DR. Sports doping in the adolescent athlete: the hope, hype, and hyperbole. *Pediatr Clin N Am.* 2002;49:829-855.
3. Greydanus DE, Patel DR. Sports doping in the adolescent athlete. *Asian J Paediatr Pract.* 2000;4:9-14.
4. Sharp DS, Ross JH, Kay R. Attitudes of pediatric urologists regarding sports participation by children with solitary kidney. *J Urol.* 2002;168:1811-1815.
5. Gerstenbluth RE, Spirnak JP, Elder JS. Sports participation and high grade renal injuries in children. *J Urol.* 2002;168:2575-2578.
6. Johnson B, Christensen C, DiRusso S, et al. A need for reevaluation of sports participation recommendations for children with a solitary kidney. *J Urol.* 2005;174:686-689.
7. Heffernan A, Gill D. Sporting activity following kidney transplantation. *Pediatr Nephrol.* 1998;12:447-448.
8. Wan J, Corvino TF, Greenfield SP, DiScala C. Kidney and testicle injuries in team and individual sports: data from the national pediatric trauma registry. *J Urol.* 2003;170:1528-1532.
9. McAleer IM, Kaplan GW, LoSasso BE. Renal and testis injuries in team sports. *J Urol.* 2002;168:1805-1807.
10. Gerstenbluth RE, Spirnak JP, Elder JS. Sports participation and high grade renal injuries in children. *J Urol.* 2002;168:2575-2578.
11. Anderson CR. Solitary kidney and sports participation. *Arch Fam Med.* 1994;4:886.
12. American Academy of Pediatrics, American Academy of Family Physicians, American Medical Society for Sports Medicine, American Orthopedic Society for Sports Medicine, American Osteopathic Academy of Sports Medicine. *Preparticipation Physical Evaluation.* Minneapolis: McGraw Hill; 2005.
13. Grimsell MM, Schwalter S, Gordon KA, Norwood VF. Single kidney and sports participation: perception versus reality. *Pediatrics.* 2006;118:1019-1027.
14. Psooy K. Sports and the solitary kidney: how to counsel parents. *Can J Urol.* 2006;13(3):3120-3126.
15. Greydanus DE, Torres AD. Genitourinary and renal disorders. In: Greydanus DE, Patel DR, Pratt HD, eds. *Essentials of Adolescent Medicine.* New York: McGraw-Hill Medical Publishers; 2005:250-285.
16. American Academy of Pediatrics (Committee on Sports Medicine and Fitness Position Statement). Athletic participation by children and adolescents who have systemic hypertension. *Pediatrics;* 1997;99:637-638.
17. Sachtleben T, Fields KB. Hypertension in the athlete. *Curr Sports Med Rep.* 2003;2(2):79-83.
18. Feld LG, Springate JE, Waz WR. Special topics in pediatric hypertension. *Semin Nephrol.* 1998;18(3):295-303.
19. Flynn JT. Hypertension in adolescents. *Adol Med Clin.* 2005;16(2):46-57.
20. Maron BJ, Zipes DP. 36th Bethesda Conference. Recommendations for determining eligibility for competition in athletes with cardiovascular abnormalities. Task Force 4: Systemic hypertension. *J Am Coll Cardiol.* 2005;45:1318-1321.
21. Murray B, Stofan J, Eichner ER. Hyponatremia in athletes. *Sports Sci Exchange.* 2003;16(1):1-6.
22. Noakes TD. Hyponatremia in distance runners: fluid and sodium balance during exercise. *Curr Sports Med Rep.* 2002;4:197-207.
23. Verbalis JG. Renal function and vasopressin during marathon running. *Sports Med.* 2007;37:455-458.
24. American Academy of Pediatrics. Climatic heat stress and the exercising child. *Pediatrics.* 2000;106:158-159.
25. American College of Sports Medicine. Position Stand on exercise and fluid replacement. *Med Sci Sports Exerc.* 2007;39:377-390.
26. Vogt BA, Avner ED. Conditions particularly associated with proteinuria. In: Kliegman RM, Behrman RE, Jenson HK, Stanton BF, eds. *Nelson Textbook of Pediatrics.* Philadelphia, PA: WB Saunders; 2004:1751-1752.
27. Trojian TH, McKeag DB. Renal problems in the athlete. In: Garrett WE, Kirkendall DT, Squire DL, eds. *Principles and Practice of Primary Care Sports Medicine.* Philadelphia, PA: Lippincott Williams & Wilkins; 2001:299-310.
28. Jones GR, Newhouse I. Sport-related hematuria: a review. *Clin J Sport Med.* 1997;7(2):119-125.
29. Davis ID, Avner ED. Clinical evaluation of the child with hematuria. In: Kliegman RM, Behrman RE, Jenson HK, Stanton BF, eds. *Nelson Textbook of Pediatrics.* Philadelphia, PA: W B Saunders; 2004:1735-1736.
30. Farquhar B, Kenney WL. Anti-inflammatory drugs, kidney function, and exercise. *Sports Sci Exch.* 1997;11(4):1-6.
31. Clarkson PM. Exertional rhabdomyolysis and acute renal failure in marathon runners. *Sports Med.* 2007;37:361-363.
32. Schaller S, Kaplan BS. Acute nonoliguric renal failure in children associated with nonsteroidal anti-inflammatory agents. *Pediatr Emerg Care.* 1998;14(6):416-418.
33. Enriquez R, Sirvent AE, Antolin A, et al. Acute renal failure and flank pain after binge drinking and non-steroidal anti-inflammatory drugs. *Nephrol Dial Transplant.* 1997;12:2034-2035.
34. Nakahura T, Griswold W, Lemire J, et al. Nonsteroidal anti-inflammatory drug use in adolescence. *J Adolesc Health.* 1998;23(5):307-310.
35. Torres AD, Greyanus DE. The renal system. In: Greydanus DE, Feinberg AD, Patel DR, Homnick DN, eds. *Pediatric Physical Diagnosis.* New York: McGraw-Hill Medical Publishers; 2008:443-488.

36. Kennedy TL III, Siegel NJ. Chronic renal disease. In: Goldberg B, ed. *Sports and Exercise for Children with Chronic Health Conditions.* Champaign, IL: Human Kinetics; 1995: 265-278.

37. Van der Mei SF, Van Sonderen ELP, Van Son WJ, et al. Social participation after successful kidney transplantation. *Disabil Rehabil.* 2007;29(6):473-483.

38. Heffernan A, Gill D. Sporting activity following kidney transplantation. *Pediatr Nephrol.* 1998;12:447-448.

39. Johansen KL. Exercise and chronic kidney disease: current recommendations. *Sports Med.* 2005;35(6):485-499.

Additional Readings

Chorley JN. Hyponatremia: identification and evaluation in the marathon medical area. *Sports Med.* 2007;37(4-5): 451-454.

Michel Conchol, Tomas Berl. Hyponatremia. In: Thomas D, DuBose L Jr, Lee Hamm, eds. *Acid-Base and Electrolyte Disorders: A companion to Brenner & Rector's the Kidney.* Philadelphia, PA: Saunders; 2002:229-239.

Alan Dubrow. Walter Flamenbaum acute renal failure associated with myoglobinuria and hemoglobinuria. In: Barry M, Brenner J, Michael Lazarus, eds. *Acute Renal Failure.* 2nd ed. New York:Churchill Livingstone; 1988:279-293.

Johnson B, Christensen C, DiRusso S, Choudhury M, Franco I. A need for reevaluation of sports participation recommendations for children with a solitary kidney. *J Urol.* 2005;174(2):686-689.

James P. Knochel Nontraumatic rhadomyolysis. In: Bruce A, Molitoris, William F. Finn, eds. *Acute Renal Failure: A companion to Brenner and Rector's The Kidney.* 1st ed. Philadelphia, PA: Saunders. 2001:220-235.

Gertstenbluth RE, Spirnak JP, Elder JS. Sports participation and high grade renal injuries in children. *J Urol.* 2002; 168(6):257-258.

GÖkhan M. Mutlu and Phillip Factor Acute-onset quadriplegia, respiratory failure, and ventricular tachycardia is a 21-year-old man following a soccer match. *Chest.* 2002;121:2036-2039.

Linda N Peterson, Moshe Levi. Disorders of potassium metabolism. In: *Renal and Electrolyte Disorders.* 5th ed. Lippincott-Raven.1997:192-240.

Psooy K . Sports and the Solitary Kidney: how to counsel parents. *Can J Urol.* 2006;13(3):3120-3126.

Siegel AJ, Verbalis JG, Clement S, et al. Hyponatremia in marathon runners due to inappropriate arginine vasopressin secretion. *Am J Med.* 2007;120(461):e11-e17.

Siegel AJ. Hypertonic (3%) sodium chloride for emergent treatment of exercise-associated hypotonic encephalopathy. *Sports Med.* 2007;37(4-5):459-462.

Stuart B, Bauer MD. Anomalies of the upper urinary tract. In: Retik AB, Vaughan ED Jr, Weing AJ, eds. *Campbell's Urology.* 8th ed. Philadelphia, PA: Saunders; 2002:1885-1924.

Tracz MJ, Alam JA, Nath K. Physiology and pathophsyology of heme: implications for kidney disease. *J Am Soc Nephrol.* 2007;18:414-420.

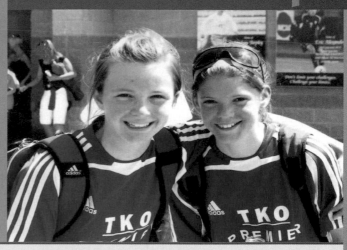

CHAPTER 14

Cardiovascular Considerations

Dilip R. Patel

CARDIOVASCULAR SCREENING

Annual preparticipation cardiovascular screening of athletes is a generally accepted practice.[1,2,3] The main objective of the screening is to identify risk factors that predispose a previously asymptomatic and apparently healthy athlete to sudden cardiac arrest and death.

History

History is the most important aspect of cardiovascular screening of young athletes. The history has been shown to have the most yield for identifying potential risk factors for adverse cardiac outcome. The key elements of cardiovascular screening history are summarized in Table 14-1.[14]

Physical Examination

A general physical examination may reveal some important clues to cardiovascular disease, exemplified by the wide ranging clinical features seen in Marfan syndrome (Table 14-2).[5] Key elements of cardiovascular examination are summarized in Table 14-3. Heart murmurs are a common finding in children and adolescents and it is important to appropriately distinguish the benign from pathologic murmurs that will indicate need for further evaluation. A simple classification of heart murmurs is presented in Table 14-4, the effects of certain physiologic maneuvers on cardiac auscultatory events are summarized in Table 14-5, and clinical clues that help identify benign heart murmurs are summarized in Table 14-6.[4,6]

Laboratory Studies

No screening laboratory studies are recommended as part of cardiovascular screening of athletes. Screening of all

Table 14-1.

Cardiovascular Screening History

Symptoms
Fatigue
Exercise-related chest pain
Presyncope or syncope during exercise
Dizziness
Heart racing or skipping beats during exercise
Exercise-related shortness of breath
Recent febrile illness

Past history
Heart surgery
Congenital heart disease
Kawasaki disease
Rheumatic fever

Personal history
Known heart murmur
Known high cholesterol or lipid disorder
Systemic hypertension
Diabetes mellitus
Marfan syndrome
Any diagnosed heart disease
Any previous or currently recommended physical activity restrictions
Current use of therapeutic medications, dietary supplements, over-the-counter medications
Current or past history of substance abuse, smoking, or other forms of tobacco use

Family history
Death of close family relatives before age 50 y from a cardiac or unknown cause
Congenital heart disease including Marfan syndrome, cardiomyopathy, long-QT syndrome
Systemic hypertension
Diabetes mellitus
Lipid disorders

Table 14-2.

Criteria for Marfan Syndrome

System	Major Criteria	Minor Criteria	Requirements for System Involvement
Skeletal	Medial displacement of the medial malleolus causing pes planus Pectus carinatum Pectus excavatum requiring surgery Protrusio acetabulae of any degree (ascertained on radiographs) Reduced extension of the elbow Reduced upper-to-lower segment ratio or arm-span-to-height ratio >1.05 Wrist and thumb sign	Facial appearance (dolichocephaly, down-slanting palpebral fissures, enophthalmos, malar hypoplasia, retrognathia) High-arched palate with crowding teeth Joint hypermobility Pectus excavatum of moderate severity	2 major or 1 major plus 1 minor criteria
Note: 4 of 8 major criteria for the skeletal system are required to confirm the diagnosis of Marfan syndrome.			
Ocular	Ectopia lentis	Abnormally flat cornea (as measured by keratometry) Hypoplastic iris or hypoplastic ciliary muscle causing decreased miosis Increased axial length of globe (as measured by ultrasound)	At least 2 minor criteria
Cardiovascular	Dilation of the ascending aorta with or without aortic regurgitation and involving at least the sinuses of Valsalva Dissection of the ascending aorta	Mitral valve prolapse with or without mitral valve regurgitation Dilatation of the main pulmonary artery in the absence of valvular or peripheral pulmonic stenosis or any obvious cause if patient is younger than 40 y Calcification of the mitral annulus (if patient is younger than 40 y) Dilation or dissection of the descending thoracic or abdominal aorta, if patient is younger than 50 y	1 major or 1 minor criterion
Pulmonary	None	Spontaneous pneumothorax Apical blebs (ascertained by chest radiograph)	1 minor criterion
Skin and integument	None	Recurrent incisional hernia Stria atrophicae (stretch marks) not associated with marked weight changes, pregnancy, or repetitive stress	1 minor criterion
Dura mater	Lumbosacral dural ectasia visible on CT scan or MRI	None	1 major criterion
Family/genetic history	Parent, child, or sibling who meets diagnostic criteria independently Presence of mutation in fibrillin-1 gene, known to cause the Marfan syndrome Presence of a haplotype around fibrillin-1 gene inherited by descendant known to be associated with unequivocally diagnosed Marfan syndrome	None	1 major criterion

Table 14-3.

Key Elements of Cardiovascular Screening Examination

- Heart rate, rhythm, character
- Blood pressure
- Femoral pulses palpated simultaneously with radial or brachial pulses (delay or diminished in coarctation of aorta)
- Heart sounds
- Systolic ejection murmur that intensifies with standing or Valsalva maneuver and decrease with squatting suggest hypertrophic cardiomyopathy
- Decrescendo diastolic (aortic insufficiency) or holostystolic (mitral insufficiency) murmurs may be noted in Marfan syndrome
- Midsystolic click may be noted in mitral valve prolapse

asymptomatic apparently healthy young athletes with electrocardiogram, echocardiogram, or more advanced testing including exercise stress testing are not recommended. Laboratory cardiovascular evaluation is based on any significant findings on the history and physical examination.

Screening Recommendations

The American Heart Association recommendations for preparticipation cardiovascular screening of competitive athletes are listed in Table 14-7.[1,2] Significant findings on screening evaluation generally indicate need for cardiology consultation for further evaluation and recommendations (Box 14-1).

Determination of Eligibility to Participate

In order to match the athlete with a cardiovascular condition to appropriate physical activity, the cardiovascular demands of a given sport is the main consideration. A classification of sports based on cardiovascular demands, exercise type, and intensity is presented in Table 14-8.[1,7]

Exercise types

The two types of exercises based on the mechanical action of the muscles involved are dynamic (isotonic) and static (isometric).[1,7] Dynamic exercise is characterized by

Table 14-4.

Classification of Heart Murmurs*

Timing	Class	Description	Characteristic Lesions
Systolic	Ejection	Begins in early systole; may extend to mid or late systole; crescendo-decrescendo pattern; often harsh in quality	Valvular, supravalvular, and subvalvular aortic stenosis; HCM; pulmonic stenosis; aortic or pulmonary artery dilation; malformed but nonobstructive aortic valve; transvalvular flow (e.g., aortic regurgitation, hyperkinetic states, ASD, physiologic flow murmur)
	Holosystolic	Extends throughout systole; relatively uniform in intensity	MR; tricuspid regurgitation; ventricular septal defect
	Late	Variable onset and duration, often preceded by a nonejection click	MVP
Diastolic	Early	Begins with A2 or P2; decrescendo pattern with variable duration; often high-pitched, blowing	Aortic regurgitation
	Mid	Begins after S_2, often after an opening snap; low-pitched "rumble" heard best with bell of stethoscope Presystolic accentuation of mid-diastolic murmur	Mitral stenosis; tricuspid stenosis; ↑ flow across-AV valves (e.g., MR, tricuspid regurgitation, ASD)
	Late		Mitral stenosis; tricuspid stenosis
Continuous		Systolic and diastolic components; "machinery" murmurs	Patent ductus aerteriosus; coronary AV fistula; ruptured sinus of Valsalva aneurysm into right atrium or ventricle; mammary soufflé; venous hum

HCM = hypertrophic cardiomyopathy; ASD = atrial septal defect; MR = mitral regurgitation; MVP = mitral valve prolapse; AV = atrioventricular
*Used with permission from Carpenter CJ, Griggs RC, Loscalzo eds. Cecil Essentials of Medicine. 6th ed. Philadelphia, PA: Saunders Elsevier; 2003;45.

Table 14-5.

Effects of Physiologic Maneuvers on Auscultatory Events*

Maneuver	Major Physiologic Effects	Useful Auscultatory Changes
Respiration	↑ Venous return with inspiration	↑ Right heart murmurs and gallops with inspiration; splitting of S2
Valsalva (initial ↑ BP, phase I; followed by ↓ BP; phase 2)	↓ BP, venous return, LV size (phase 2)	↑ HCM ↓ AS, MR MVP click earlier in systole, murmur prolongs
Standing	↓ Venous return	↑ HCM; ↓ AS, MR; MVP click earlier in systole, murmur prolongs
Squatting	↑ Venous return, systemic vascular resistance, LV size	↑ AS, MR, AI: ↓ HCM; MVP click delayed, murmur shortens
Isometric exercise (e.g., handgrip)	↑ Arterial pressure, cardiac output	↑ MR, AI, MS ↓ AS, HCM
Post PVC or prolonged R-R interval	↑ Ventricular filling, contractility	↑ AS; little change in MR
Amyl nitrate	↓ Arterial pressure, LV size ↑ Cardiac output	↑ HCM, AS, MS ↓ AI, MR, Austin Flint murmur; MVP click earlier in systole, murmur prolongs
Phenylephrine	↑ Arterial pressure, LV size ↓ Cardiac output	↑ MR, AI; ↓ AS, HCM; MVP click delayed, murmur shortens

↑ = increased intensity; ↓ = decreased intensity; AI = aortic insufficiency; AS = aortic stenosis; BP = blood pressure; HCM = hypertrophic cardiomyopathy; LV = left ventricular; MR - mitral regurgitation; MS = mitral stenosis; MVP = mitral valve prolapse; PVC = premature ventricular contraction; R-R = interval between the R waves on an ECG

*Used with permission from Carpenter CJ, Griggs RC, Loscalzo eds. Cecil Essentials of Medicine. 6th ed. Philadelphia, PA: Saunders Elsevier; 2003;43.

rhythmic contractions of muscles accompanied by change in muscle length (shortening or lengthening) with movement of the joint over which the muscles act and minimal intramuscular force. Static exercise, on the other hand is characterized by contractions of muscles not accompanied by change in muscle length or joint movement and generation of large intramuscular force.

Table 14-6.

Clues to Benign Character of the Murmur

Usually early to midsystolic murmur
Best heard over the left sternal border
Crescendo-decrescendo murmur
Intensity of less than three-sixths
Intensity changes with position of the patient
Musical or vibratory quality
Venous hum
Arterial bruit or murmur in carotid vessels at or above the clavicle in adolescents
Normal heart sounds
Patient is asymptomatic
Negative family history for cardiac disease
Normal heart rate
Normal peripheral arterial pulses

Based on the muscle metabolism or the energy system utilized, exercise can also be categorized as either predominantly aerobic or predominantly anaerobic types. Aerobic exercise is oxygen-dependent, long-term energy system with unlimited time to fatigue. Anaerobic exercise that utilizes the phosphocreatine-ATP pathway provides immediate energy for muscle action with a time to fatigue from 5 to 10 seconds, whereas anaerobic exercise that utilizes the glycogen-lactic acid (glycolytic) pathway provides energy for short-term action with time to fatigue from 60 to 90 seconds.

Although most dynamic, long-term exercises predominantly utilize the aerobic energy system and most static, short-term exercises utilize the anaerobic energy system, these are not synonymous terms and the energy system utilized depends on the nature of the particular activity.

Exercise intensity

Although there are many methods utilized to measure exercise intensity, two parameters are used in the classification of sports presented in Table 14-8, namely maximal oxygen uptake ($VO_{2\,max}$) and maximum voluntary contraction (MVC). $VO_{2\,max}$ or maximal oxygen uptake is defined as the greatest amount of oxygen consumed during exercise and is expressed as milliliters of oxygen consumed per kilogram of body weight per minute.[7]

Table 14-7.

The 12-Element AHA Recommendations for Preparticipation Cardiovascular Screening of Competitive Athletes

Medical history
(Parental verification is recommended for high school and middle school athletes)

Personal history
1. Exertional chest pain/discomfort
2. Unexplained syncope/near syncope (judged not to be neurocardiogenic or vasovagal; of particular concern when related to exertion)
3. Exessive exertional and unexplained dyspnea/fatigue associated with exercise
4. Prior recognition of a heart murmur
5. Elevated systemic blood pressure

Family history
6. Premature death (sudden and unexplained, or otherwise) before age 50 y because of heart disease in one or more relative

7. Disability from heart disease in a close relative younger than 50 y
8. Specific knowledge of certain cardiac conditions in family members: hypertrophic or dilated cardiomyopathy, long-QT syndrome, or other ion channelopathies, Marfan syndrome, or clinically important arrhythmias

Physical examination
9. Heart murmur (auscultation should be performed in both supine and standing positions [or with Valsalva maneuver], specifically to identify murmurs of dynamic left ventricular outflow tract obstruction)
10. Femoral pulses to exclude aortic coarctation
11. Physical stigmata of Marfan syndrome
12. Brachial artery blood pressure (sitting position) preferably taken both arms

Table 14-8.

American Heart Association and American College of Cardiology Classification of Sports

Increasing Static Component		A. Low (<40% Max O₂)	B. Moderate (40-70% Max O₂)	C. High (>70% Max O₂)
III. High (>50% MVC)		Bobsledding/Luge*†, Field events (throwing), Gymnastics*†, Martial arts*, Sailing, Sport climbing, Water skiing*†, Weight lifting*†, Windsurfing*†	Body building*†, Downhill skiing*†, Skateboarding*†, Snowboarding*†, Wrestling*	Boxing*, Canoeing/Kayaking, Cycling*†, Decathlon, Rowing, Speed-skating*†, Triathlon*†
II. Moderate (20-50% MVC)		Archery, Auto racing*†, Diving*†, Equestrian*†, Motorcycling*†	American football*, Field events (jumping), Figure skating*, Rodeoing*†, Rugby*, Running (sprint), Surfing*†, Synchronized swimming†	Basketball*, Ice hockey*, Cross-country skiing (skating technique), Lacrosse*, Running (middle distance), Swimming, Team handball
I. Low (<20% MVC)		Billiards, Bowling, Cricket, Curling, Golf, Riflery	Baseball/Softball*, Fencing, Table tennis, Volleyball	Badminton, Cross-country skiing (classic technique), Field hockey*, Orienteering, Race walking, Racquetball/Squash, Running (long distance), Soccer*, Tennis

Increasing Dynamic Component ⟶

Classification is based on peak static and dynamic components achieved during completion. It should be noted, however, that higher values may be reached during training. The increasing dynamic component is defined in terms of the estimated percent of maximal oxygen uptake (Max O₂) achieved and results in an increasing cardiac output. The increasing static component is related to the estimated percent of maximal voluntary contraction (MVC) reached and results in an increasing blood pressure load. The lowest cardiovascular demands (cardiac output and blood pressure) are shown in green and the highest in red. Blue, yellow, and orange depict low moderate, moderate, and high moderate total cardiovascular demands.
Danger of bodily collision.
†Increased risk, if syncope occurs.

Table 14-9.

Conditions that Predispose Young Athletes to Sudden Cardiac Death

Anomalous origin of coronary arteries (Second most common cause in US)

Aortic stenosis

Aortic dissection

Arrythmogenic right ventricular dysplasia (most common cause in Italy)

Brugada syndrome (most prevalent in those of Asian descent)

Cardiomyopthay, hypertrophic (most common cause in the US)

Cardiomyopathy, dilated

Coarctation of aorta

Congenital heart block (Mobitz type 2, complete or third-degree heart block)

Congenital and acquired long-QT syndrome

Congenital short–QT syndrome

Commotio cordis (unique to young children with pliable chest wall as a result of blunt impact)

Coronary artery disease (most common cause after age 35 y)

Endocarditis

Ehlers-Danlos syndrome

Ion channelopathies

Marfan syndrome

Mitral valve prolapse

Muscular dystrophies

Myocarditis

Pericarditis

Postoperative tetralogy of Fallot

Postoperative atrial switch transposition of great vessels

Postoperative atrial septal defect

Wolff-Parkinson-White syndrome

$VO_{2\ max}$ can be either measured directly or estimated indirectly by various methods and is a good indicator of functional aerobic capacity or overall cardiorespiratory fitness.

Muscle strength, expressed in *Newtons* (sometimes in kg) is the maximal intramuscular force generated by a muscle or group of muscles.[1,7] Static (isometric) muscle strength is specific for a given muscle or group of muscles and can be measured by various devices. Maximum voluntary contraction (MVC) refers to the peak intramuscular force generated by a muscle or group of muscles.

For specific eligibility recommendations for competitive athletes with cardiovascular abnormalities, the reader should refer to the 36th Bethesda Conference report available at www.acc.org.

SUDDEN CARDIAC DEATH

Sudden cardiac death is defined as "nontraumatic and unexpected sudden death that may occur from a cardiac arrest within 6 hours of a previously normal state of health."[1] The incidence of sudden cardiac death in high school athletes is estimated to be 1 in 200,000 high school age athletes per year.[8] In the United States, the male to female ratio for sudden cardiac death is 9:1, and most deaths have been reported in basketball and football players.[9,10] In Europe, most sudden deaths in young athletes have been reported in soccer player.

Conditions that increase the risk of sudden cardiac death are listed in Table 14-9.[1–4,11–18] The most common underlying identified disease in young athletes (those younger then 35 years of age) in the United States is hypertrophic cardiomyopathy followed by anomalous origin of the coronary artery. The cardiac arrest is triggered by lethal arrhythmias in the presence of underlying heat disease. Commotio cordis is unique condition in children in which a direct blow to the chest during a vulnerable period of cardiac cycle triggers ventricular fibrillation leading to sudden death.

MANAGEMENT OF CARDIAC ARREST

The algorithm presented in Figure 14-1 provides an approach recommended by the Inter-Association Task Force for the management of sudden cardiac arrest in case of witnessed collapse.[19]

The detail description of pathophysiology and management of cardiac arrest are out of scope of the present discussion and for those with further interest, the Inter-Association Task Force consensus recommendations on emergency preparedness and management of sudden cardiac death in college and school athletes report can be accessed at www.nata.org.

The critical element influencing the survival rate is the time to defibrillation and ready access to automated external defibrillator (AED) units at venues hosting athletic events is now recommended.[20–25] The use of AED is illustrated in Figure 14-2 (Box 14-1).

Box 14-1 When to Refer

When to Refer to Cardiology

- Exercise-related chest pain, presyncope, syncope
- Excessive dyspnea with exercise
- Palpitations
- Kawasaki disease
- Rheumatic disease
- Congenital heart disease
- Ongoing management after heart surgery
- Pathologic heart murmur
- Delayed or diminished femoral arterial pulses
- Marfanoid features
- Marfan syndrome
- Family history of sudden cardiac death before age 50

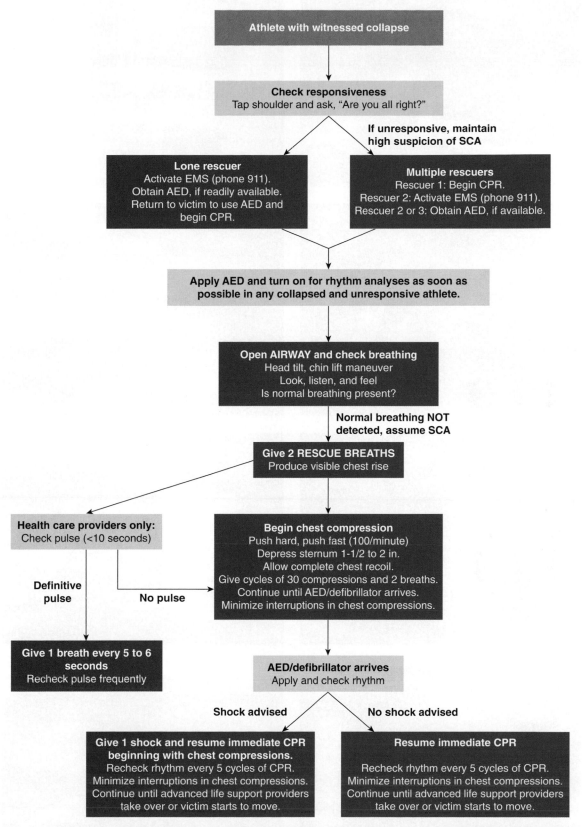

FIGURE 14-1 ■ Management of sudden cardiac arrest. SCA indicates sudden cardiac arrest; EMS, emergency medical services; AED, automated external defibrillator; CPR, cardiolpulmonary resuscitation. *Source: Inter-Association Task Force Recommendations on Emergency Preparedness and Management of Sudden Cardiac Arrest, 2007.*

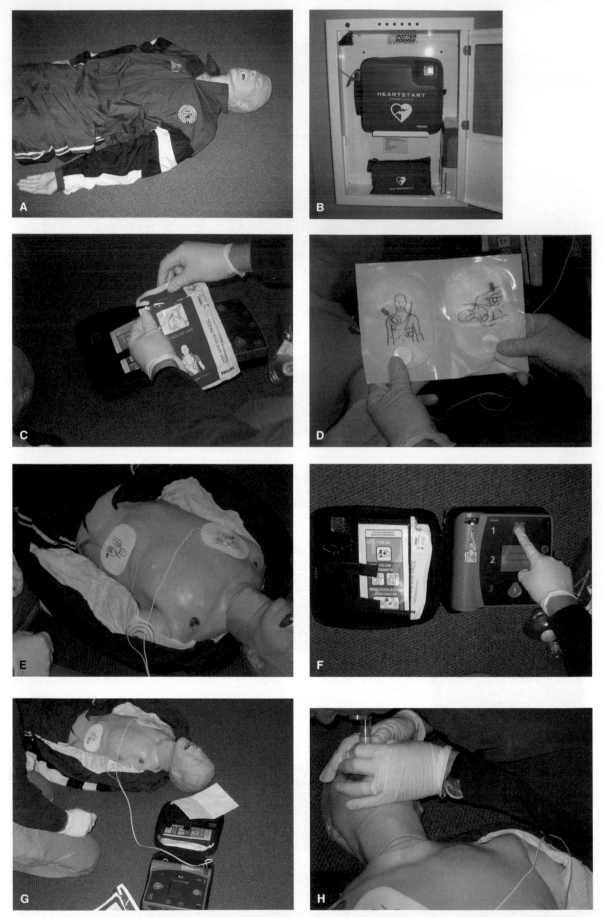

FIGURE 14-2 ■ Use of AED. In an athlete with witnessed collapse (**A**), check responsiveness. The lone rescuer should first activate EMS, and obtain AED (**B**). Open the AED and apply chest pads as shown (**C–E**). Turn AED on (**F** and **G**) for rhythm analysis. Open airway, check breathing and give two rescue breaths (**H**). *(continued)*

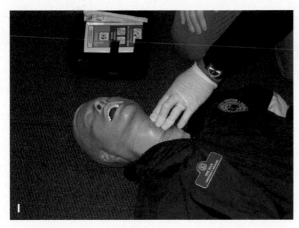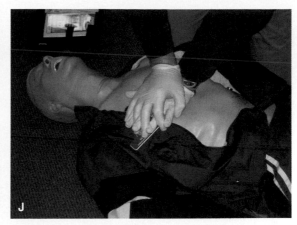

FIGURE 14-2 ■ *(Continued)* The health care provider should check the pulse (**I**). If no pulse is detected, then begin chest compressions (**J**). Based on AED rhythm analysis, if a shock is advised give one shock and resume CPR beginning with chest compressions. If no shock is advised, then resume immediate CPR. (*Courtesy of Stu Myer, Human Resuscitation Learning Laboratory, Department of Emergency Medicine, Michigan State University Kalamazoo Center for Medical Studies*).

ACKNOWLEDGEMENT

Author acknowledges Saad Siddiqui, MD, for providing research assistance for this chapter.

REFERENCES

1. Bethesda Conference Report. 36th Bethesda Conference: eligibility recommendations for competitive athletes with cardiovascular abnormalities. *J Am Coll Cardiol.* 2005;45(8): 1313-1375.
2. Maron BJ, Thompson PD, Ackerman MJ, et al. Recommendations and considerations related to preparticipation screening for cardiovascular abnormalities in competitive athletes: 2007 update: a scientific statement from the American Heart Association Council on Nutrition. Physical Activity, and Metabolism: endorsed by the American College of Cardiology Foundation. *Circulation.* 2007;115:1643-1655.
3. Basilico FC. Cardiovascular disease in athletes. *Am J Sports Med.* 1999;27:108-121.
4. Luckstead EF Jr. Cardiac risk factors and participation guidelines for youth sports. *Pediatr Clin North Am.* 2002;49(4):681-708.
5. De Paepe A, Devereux RB, Dietz HC, et al. Revised diagnostic criteria for the Marfan syndrome. *Am J Med Genet.* 1996;62(4):417-426.
6. Luckstead EF. The cardiovascular system. In: Greydanus DE, Feinberg AN, Patel DR, Homnick DN, eds. *The Pediatric Diagnostic Examination.* New York: McGraw Hill; 2008:227-265.
7. Whaley MH, Brubaker PH, Otto RM, eds. *ACSM's Guidelines for Exercise Testing and Prescription.* Philadelphia: Lippincott Williams & Wilkins, 2006.
8. Maron BJ, Gohman TE, Aeppli D. Prevalence of sudden cardiac death during competitive sports activities in Minnesota high school athletes. *J Am Coll Cardiol.* 1998;32: 1881-1884.
9. Maron BJ. Sudden death in young athletes. *N Engl J Med.* 2003;349:1064-1075.
10. Maron BJ, Shirani J, Poliac LC, et al. Sudden death in young competitive athletes: clinical, demographic and pathological profiles. *JAMA.* 1996;276:199-204.
11. Maron BJ, Gohman TF, Kyle SB, Estes NA III, Link MS. Clinical profile and spectrum of Commotio Cordis. *JAMA.* 2002;287:1142-1146.
12. Maron BJ, Wentzel DC, Zenovich AG, Estes NA III, Link MS. Death in a young athlete due to commotio cordis despite prompt external defibrillation. *Heart Rhythm.* 2005;2:991-993.
13. Maron BJ, Carney KP, Lever HM. Relationship of race to sudden cardiac death in competitive athletes with hypertrophic cardiomyopathy. *J Am Coll Cardiol.* 2003;41: 974-980.
14. Corrado D, Basso C, Rizzoli G, Thiene G. Does sport activity enhance the risk of sudden death in adolescents and young adults? *J Am Coll Cardiol.* 2003;41: 974-980.
15. Corrado D, Thiene G, Nava A, et al. Sudden death in young competitive athletes. *J Am Coll Card.* 1986;7:204-214.
16. Van Camp SP, Bloor CM, Mueller FO, et al. Nontraumatic sports death in high school and college athletes. *Med Sci Sports Exerc.* 1995;27:641-647.
17. Maron BJ. Triggers for sudden cardiac death in athlete. *Cardiol Clin.* 1996;:195-210.
18. Cantu RC. Congenital cardiovascular disease: the major cause of athletic death in high school and college. *Med Sci Sports Exerc.* 1992;24:279-280.
19. Drezner JA, Courson RW, Roberts WO, Mosesso VN, Link MS, Maron BJ. Inter-association task force recommendations on emergency preparedness and management of sudden cardiac arrest in high school and college athletic programs: a consensus statement. *J Athlet Train.* 2007; 42(1):143-158.
20. Rea TD, Eisenberg MS, Sinibaldi G, White RD. Incidence of EMS-treated out-of-hospital cardiac arrest in the United States. *Resuscitation.* 2004;63:17-24.

21. White RD, Russell JK. Refibrillation, resuscitation and survival in out of-hospital sudden cardiac arrest victims treated with biphasic automated external defibrillators. *Resuscitation.* 2002;55:17-23.

22. Berg MD, Clark LL, Valenzuela TD, Kern KB, Berg RA. Postshock chest compression delays with automated external defibrillator use. *Resuscitation.* 2005;64:287-291.

23. Drezner JA, Rogers KJ. Sudden Cardiac arrest in inter-collegiate athletes: detailed analysis and outcomes of resuscitation in nine cases. *Heart Rhythm.* 2006;3: 755-759.

24. Drezner JA. Practical guidelines for automated external defibrillators in the athletic setting. *Clin J Sport Med.* 2005;15(5):367-369.

25. Rothmier JD, Drezner JA, Harmon KG. Automated external defibrillators in Washington State high school. *Br J Sport Med.* 2007;42:301-305.

CHAPTER 15

Diabetes Mellitus

Manmohan K. Kamboj and
Martin B. Draznin

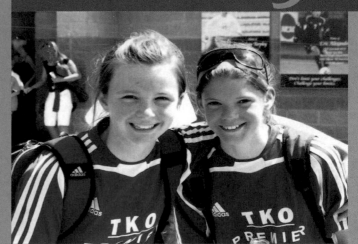

Athough the incidence of type 2 diabetes mellitus (type 2 DM) in chidren and adolescents has increased in recent years, type 1 diabetes mellitus (type 1 DM) is the most prevalent type seen in this age group and is reviewed in more detail here. Within the context of sport participation, most patients seen by pediatricians are adolescents and although the following discussion mostly refers to adolescents, it is equally applicable to children unless otherwise specified.

TYPE 1 DIABETES MELLITUS

Definitions

The diagnostic criteria for diabetes mellitus are shown in Table 15-1.

Epidemiology

There are 20.8 million individuals in the United States with diabetes mellitus, comprising 7% of the total population; 176,500 of them are children and adolescents younger than 20 years of age. One in 400 to 600 children and adolescents have insulin-dependent diabetes, also called type 1 DM.[1]

Pathogenesis

A brief summary of the pathophysiology of diabetes mellitus as it relates to sports participation is essential to better understand the principles of management of diabetes in children and adolescents.

The availability of carbohydrates is important for use by the exercising muscles. Nondiabetic children and adolescents have full muscle and liver glycogen stores at

Table 15-1.

American Diabetic Association Diagnostic Criteria for Diabetes Mellitus		
Normoglycemia	**IFG or IGT**	**Diabetes***
FPG ≤100 mg/dL	FPG≥ 100 and ≤126 mg/dL (IFG)	FPG ≥126 mg/dL
2-h PG†≤140 mg/dL	2-h PG†≥140 and ≤200 mg/dL (IGT)	2-h PG†≥200 mg/dL
		Symptoms of diabetes and casual plasma glucose concentration ≥200 mg/dL

*In the absence of unequivocal hyperglycemia, a diagnosis of diabetes must be confirmed, on a subsequent day, by measurement of FPG, 2-h PG, or random plasma glucose (if symptoms are present). The FPG test is greatly preferred because of ease of administration, convenience, acceptability to patients, and lower cost. Fasting is defined as no caloric intake for at least 8 h.
†This test requires the use of a glucose load containing the equivalent of 75 g anhydrous glucose dissolved in water. 2-h PG, 2-h postload glucose.
Source: American Diabetes Association Position Statement. Diagnosis and Classification of Diabetes Mellitus. Diabetes Care. 2004;27:S5-S10.

rest. During exercise, muscle glycogen is used first to release lactic acid for the Cori cycle, followed quickly by liver glycogenolysis. As insulin levels decrease, liver glycogenolysis is continued; at the same time, with increased blood flow, binding of insulin to receptors in skeletal muscles is increased causing increased glucose uptake and metabolism during exercise. The glycogen stores in muscles and liver are then replenished from blood glucose following completion of physical activity.[2–4]

It is believed that hepatic glucose production is the same in children and adolescents with diabetes and those without diabetes. However, there are some basic metabolic differences in carbohydrate metabolism between children and adolescents with and without diabetes.[2] Compared with children and adolescents without diabetes, in children and adolescents with diabetes:

- Gluconeogenesis may be increased up to three times the normal
- There is reduced mitochondrial pyruvate dehydrogenase activity, which may lead to compromised glucose oxidation in muscles, and
- Relatively higher fatty acid oxidation occurs in the exercising muscles.

The effects of exercise will vary in the adolescent with diabetes depending on the level of the metabolic control and the amount of insulin available in the body. It has also been shown that the adolescent with diabetes will have a consistent response to similar level of exercise activity, metabolic control and insulin dosing.

Insulin may be more rapidly absorbed if administered in the exercising limb. If there is excessive insulin available, muscle and liver glycogenolysis is suppressed, compromising the availability of glucose, whereas the glucose requirement in the exercising muscle is increased. This leads to hypoglycemia, which can occur during the activity, soon after the activity, or hours later.[3]

There is no significant change in the "counter-regulatory" hormone response to physical activity in adolescents with well-controlled diabetes compared with adolescents without diabetes. In hypoinsulinemic states, the response of the counter-regulatory hormones is exaggerated with an abnormal increase in glucagon, cortisol, growth hormone and catecholamines, which may lead to worsening of hyperglycemia, lipolysis, and ketosis. In scenarios of under-insulinization, hepatic glycogenolysis is promoted while glucose utilization in the muscle may be decreased, again causing hyperglycemia.[3] Ketogenesis is also promoted by stimulation of lipolysis as result of escape from insulin inhibition by hormone sensitive lipase.[2,5]

Clinical Presentation

Within the context of sports participation, the previously undiagnosed adolescent may first present with

Table 15-2.

Symptoms and Signs of Hypoglycemia and Hyperglycemia

Hypoglycemia

Mild	Moderate	Severe
Headaches	Pallor	Unresponsive
Shakiness	Blank stare	Unconscious
Excessive sweating	Refusal to eat	seizures
Dizziness	Slurring of speech	
Pallor	Uncontrollable crying	
Tachycardia	Staggering gait	
Poor concentration		
Inappropriate emotions (laughing, crying)		
Anger, restlessness, confusion		
Quite, withdrawn		

Hyperglycemia
Increased urination
Increased thirst
Headaches
Tiredness
Sleepiness
Fruity odor to breath
Rapid shallow breathing

Source: http://wwwchildrenwithdiabetes.com/d_0q_590.htm. Accessed May 14, 2007.

symptoms of diabetes mellitus. On the other hand, and least commonly, the adolescent with type 1 DM may present with symptoms and signs of macro- and microvascular complications. Most commonly though, the adolescent with type 1 DM who is participating in sports is likely to be seen for symptoms and signs of either hypoglycemia or hyperglycemia with or without ketoacidosis. Additionally, adolescents who are deficient in insulin may develop postexercise hyperglycemia that may persist for several hours. A state of ketosis may develop quite rapidly in this scenario, leading to diabetic ketoacidosis and that may necessitate hospitalization. The symptoms and signs of hypoglycemia and hyperglycemia are listed in Table 15-2.

Diagnosis

Adolescents with diabetes should have the same comprehensive sports preparticipation evaluation as do adolescents without diabetes. The history should ascertain associated chronic illness, factors that may limit the ability to exercise, general well-being and overall health. Physical examination should ascertain any physical limitations or disabilities (congenital or acquired), cardiovascular or respiratory limitations, limitations of range of limb mobility and control, and deficits in central or peripheral neurological function that would cause difficulties during participation in sports. Adolescents with diabetes mellitus should have additional screening for any evidence of micro- or macrovascular complications that may predispose them to injury and compromise safety, or exacerbate the underlying disease.

Physical examination should include vital signs, careful blood pressure measurements to look for hypertension as well as orthostatic changes. A detailed neurological examination should be done to detect peripheral or autonomic neurological deficits. An yearly detailed retinal examination should be done by an ophthalmologist to identify early diabetic retinopathy. Microvascular complications are not commonly seen in adolescents prior to 10 or more years' duration of diabetes. The incidence of micro- as well as macrovascular complications in adolescents is not very high, but adolescents who were diagnosed in early childhood may have already had 10 years' duration of the disease and may have evidence of these complications.[6]

Laboratory Tests

For all adolescents with type 1 DM after 5 years' duration and type 2 DM at the time of diagnosis, laboratory tests should include HgbA1c; urine analysis for protein, glucose and ketones; and urine for microalbuminuria (spot) in adolescents with proteinuria on urine dipstick. Annual thyroid function tests, lipid profile and antiendomysial antibodies should be performed for screening and early detection of hypo-/hyperthyroidism, hyper-/dyslipidemias and celiac disease, all of which are seen with increased incidence in Type 1 DM.[7]

Management

The management of type 1 DM for the adolescent must be individualized, with appropriate consultations (Box 15-1), to allow for safe participation and optimal

Table 15-3.
Factors Determining Recommendations for Diabetes Management during Sports Participation

Individual factors
Motivation to achieve tight metabolic control
Adherence to treatment recommendations

Metabolic control
Metabolic response to exercise
Metabolic control with current treatment regimen
Average blood glucose
Average glycated hemoglobin levels

Physical activity
Metabolic demands of sport
Duration and intensity of physical activity
Frequency of physical activity
Timing of physical activity in relation to meals

Insulin regimen
Continuous subcutaneous insulin infusion
Intensive–flexible insulin regimen
Three injections per day regimen

Plan of action for hypogycemia
Identification of individuals responsible for emergency administration of glucagon
Identification of personnel responsible for accessing EMS
On site availability of glucagons
On site availability of intravenous 50% dextrose and supplies for administration

performance in sports. Factors that determine recommendations for diabetes management during sports participation are presented in Table 15-3.[8]

Preparticipation Management

Preparticipation assessment of the diabetes treatment regimen is outlined in Table 15-4.[9] Every athlete requires an individualized plan of care. Safe participation in sport at any level is possible with adequate self-monitoring of blood glucose (SMBG) in order to make suitable adjustments to the therapeutic regimen, including insulin dosing and modification of carbohydrate intake. Adolescents (and primary care takers of young children) need education about appropriate modifications in the insulin and diet regimens based on SMBG to avoid immediate, as well as, delayed hypoglycemia and hyperglycemia.

Baseline Metabolic Control

Sports participation may need to be delayed until satisfactory glycemic control has been achieved based on SMBG and HgbA1c levels. Factors determining the metabolic response to exercise are listed in Table 15-5.

Box 15-1 When to Refer to Specialist	
Condition	**Ideally Managed in Consultation wtih**
Poor metabolic control	Pediatric endocrinologist
Acute diabetic ketoacidosis	Pediatric endocrinologist and intensivist
Diabetic retinopathy	Ophthalmologist
Diabetic nephropathy	Pediatric nephrologist
Diabetic neuropathy	Pediatric neurologist
Nutrition	Registered dietician
All diabetes patients	Diabetes educator

Table 15-4.

Preparticipation Assessment of Diabetes Treatment Regimen

Type of insulin regimen used

Continuous subcutaneous insulin infusion
Intensive–flexible insulin regimen
Three injections per day regimen

Assessment of adolescent's undertanding of self-management

Dose, onset, peak, duration of action of insulin used
Technical ability to use blood glucose monitoring device
Blood glucose testing schedule
Knowledge to recognize and manage hypoglycemia and hyperglycemia
Sick day management
Knowledge for nutritional management including routine carbohydrate intake, carbohydrate counting, and amount of carbohydrate necessary for a given level of exercise

Assessment of the demands of the sport

Frequency of games and practices per wk
Length of each session
Schedule of the activity in relation to time of the meal

Other aspects

Support of the peers and staff
Preferable to have team members trained in diabetes management
Adequate facility to test blood glucose, treat hypoglycemia and administer insulin if needed
Availability of sources of carbohydrate at all times

Failure to do so may result in frequent episodes of hypoglycemia and/or hyperglycemia with or without ketosis. However, a balanced approach is needed because requiring "perfect" control before allowing participation may frustrate the athlete and result in a missed opportunity to engage in a healthy and fun activity.

Table 15-5.

Factors Determining Metabolic Response to Exercise

Baseline glycemic control
Level of exercise intensity
Time spent in exercise
Levels of circulating insulin in blood
Glycogen available
Blood glucose before exercise
Carbohydrate intake

Hypoglycemia

Exercise-induced hypoglycemia may occur during, soon after, or over the subsequent 6 to 24 hours following the cessation of exercise.[8,10] Appropriate modifications should be made in insulin dosing and carbohydrate intake, along with more frequent monitoring of blood glucose levels, to avoid hypoglycemia. The Diabetes Research in Children Network (DirecNet) Study Group demonstrated the need for modification of insulin regimen to prevent hypoglycemia following afternoon exercise.[11] In addition to the hypoglycemia caused by exercise, other causes of hypoglycemia in adolescents with type 1 DM include accelerated absorption of rapid-acting insulin from an exercising limb within 1 to 2 hours of injection, blunting of glucagon response to hypoglycemia as may be seen in type 1 diabetes of more than 5 years duration, and blunting of epinephrine response to exercise seen in some adolescents with tightly controlled type 1 DM.

Hyperglycemia

Hyperglycemia may result from the effects of increased counter-regulatory hormone response especially in conjunction with a state of relative hypoinsulinemia. The question in sports and exercise settings is whether this hyperglycemia should be treated with supplemental insulin. If insulin is used, postexercise hypoglycemia may be precipitated; therefore, a smaller or lower correction factor should be used if at all, and blood glucose measurements should be followed over subsequent few hours.

Attempting to keep preexercise blood glucose levels at elevated levels to compensate for exercise-related hypoglycemia may be counter productive by precipitating ketosis. Symptoms suggestive of hypoglycemia should always be validated by blood glucose testing as symptoms of precontest anxiety may mimic symptoms of hypoglycemia, and if carbohydrates are present hyperglycemia and ketosis may occur.

Blood Glucose Assessment

Blood glucose should be assessed prior to the start of exercise or sports session. Many blood glucose testing devices with varied technological features are available (Figure 15-1). A pre-exercise snack may need to be taken based on this blood glucose value (Table 15-6).[5] Blood glucose testing should be done at intervals during the sports session, especially if the session is prolonged or if symptoms of hypoglycemia occur. This should be followed by blood glucose checks after activity, as well as, for several hours after completion of the session. Overnight (2 AM) blood glucose checks may be needed to detect nocturnal hypoglycemia. The American

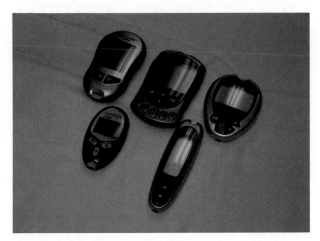

FIGURE 15-1 ■ Blood glucose testing devices with varied technological features.

Diabetes Association (ADA) general safety guidelines for regulating glycemic response to physical activity are summarized in Table 15-7.[12]

Management of the Insulin Regimen

Modifications in the insulin regimen depend on the specific type of insulin or insulin regimen being used (Tables 15-8 to 15-10).[7,13] Changes can be planned if the level of activity is known; but adolescents are frequently involved in unplanned physical activity as well. The modification in the insulin dose depends on the intensity and duration of exercise, as well as type and peak time of the particular insulin (Table 15-11).[4,14,15]

Table 15-6.

General Guidelines for Exercise Based on Preexercise Blood Glucose

Preexercise Blood Glucose	Recommended Action
Less than 100 mg/dL	Ingest 15 g of carbohydrates snack with protein
Between 250 mg/dL and 300 mg/dL	Test urine for ketones
	Exercise if urine negative for ketones
	If urine positive for ketones, delay exercise until negative
More than 300 mg/dL	May exercise with caution if urine negative for ketones
	If urine positive for ketone, delay exercise until negative

Modified with permission from American Diabetes Association. Position statement. Physical activity/exercise in diabetes. Diabetes Care. 2004;27(suppl 1):S58–S62.

Table 15-7.

Exercise Safety Guidelines

Medic Alert—to alert others in case of emergency about the person's diabetes status

Preferably exercise with a partner—"buddy up"

Maintain adequate hydration during exercise

Avoid extremes of temperature; proper attire, footwear

Blood glucose testing before, during, and more frequently after exercise

Watch for hypoglycemia during and after exercise

Avoid exercising during peak insulin action

Insulin to be administered away from site of exercising limb

Lower dose of rapid-acting insulin just before exercise

Simple carbohydrate/sugar should be available for immediate use if needed

Check blood glucose before, during, and after prolonged/intense physical activity

Identify need for changes in insulin dosing and/or food intake based on blood glucose levels

Try to gauge the glycemic response to different physical activities based on blood glucose levels

Consume additional carbohydrate snacks to avoid hypoglycemia

Sources of carbohydrate should be available for using during and after physical activity

Modified with permission from American Diabetes Association. Position statement. Physical activity/exercise in diabetes. Diabetes Care. 2004;27(suppl 1):S58–S62.

Table 15-8.

Continuous Subcutaneous Insulin Infusion Regimen (CSII)

Insulin pump used for continuous subcutaneous administration of rapid-acting insulin

Varying basal rates over 24 h period to mimic basal secretion. This may be helpful in preventing nocturnal hypoglycemia and down phenomena

Variable bolus option for meal coverage dependent on meal content e.g., immediate, square wave or dual wave

Pump may be suspended during prolonged physical activity to avoid hypoglycemia

Extreme motivation, commitment, and technical expertise necessary for maximum benefit

Mechanical failures are possible and appropriate trouble shooting techniques need to be in place

Adequate carbohydrate counting skills essential

Intensive self-monitoring of blood glucose remains a prerequisite

With permission from Kamboj MK, Draznin MB. Office management of the adolescent with diabetes mellitus. Prim Care Clin Office Pract. 2006;33:581–602.

Table 15-9.

Three Injections a Day Insulin Regimen

Insulin regimen	Intermediate acting (NPH) prebreakfast and before bedtime PLUS rapid/short acting (Lispro, Aspart, Glulisine) prebreakfast and predinner time
Dosing	• Calculate total daily insulin dose (based on body weight) • 2/3 dose prebreakfast (2 parts intermediate + 1 part rapid acting) • 1/3 dose in the evening (1 part rapid acting predinner and 2 parts NPH at bedtime) • Usually no lunchtime insulin required
Meals/carbs	• Consistency in meal timings required • Consistency in carbohydrate content of meals required • Meal content needs to be more or less similar from day-to-day

Modified with permission from: Kamboj MK. Diabetes on college campus. Pediatr Clin North Am. 2005;52: 279–305.

Insulin pump/continuous subcutaneous insulin infusion (CSII)

There are no absolute guidelines available for proper adjustments of the insulin pump during exercise and an individualized approach must be followed. One study

Table 15-10.

Flexible Dose Insulin Regimen

Insulin regimen	Long-acting insulin (e.g., Glargine. Detemir) once a day subcutaneous (usually at bedtime) for basal insulin coverage PLUS rapid/short acting (Lispro, Aspart, Glulisine) as bolus for meal coverage
Dosing	• Calculate total daily insulin dose (based on body weight) • 40%–60% of dose as long-acting insulin
Meals/carbs	• Insulin—carbohydrate ratio calculated initially using 1800 rule (1800 ÷ total daily insulin = correction factor – CF) • CF ÷ 3—insulin: carbohydrate ratio • Correction factor is used to correct for hyperglycemia • Insulin required with any carbohydrate ingestion (meal/snack) • More flexible with regards to meal timings as well as content

Modified with permission from: Kamboj MK. Diabetes on college campus. Pediatr Clin North Am. 2005;52:279–305.

Table 15-11.

Onset, Peak, and Duration of Action of Insulin Preparations

Insulin	Onset of Action (hours)	Peak of Action (hours)	Duration of Action (hours)
Rapid acting			
• Lispro	0.25–0.5	0.5–2.5	≤5
• Aspart	≤0.20	1–3	3–5
• Glulisine	Rapid	0.9	Not listed
Short acting			
• Regular	0.5–1	2–3	3–6
Intermediate acting			
• NPH (Isophane)	2–4	4–10	10–16
Long acting			
• Glargine	2–4	Peakless	20–24
• Detemir	?	?	?

Sources: American Diabetes Association. Tools of therapy: Exercise. In: BW Bode, ed. Medical Management of Type I Diabetes Mellitus. 4th ed. Alexandria, VA: American Diabetes Association. LEVEMIR Insulin detemir [rDNA origin] injection; Product insert; Robinson, DM, Wellington, K: Insulin glulisine. Drugs. 2006;66(6): 861–869.

concluded that turning the insulin pump off during unplanned physical activity was convenient, obviated the need to change basal insulin rates, and possibly lowered the risk of hypoglycemia.[6] It was also reported that the late onset hypoglycemia was more common than hypoglycemia during exercise and the overall chance of hypoglycemia was higher if the insulin pump continued to deliver insulin during exercise.[6]

Others have recommended decreasing the pump basal rate to 50% of the athlete's baseline dosage during exercise, while monitoring blood glucose before, during, and after the exercise. Pre-exercise bolus coverage (if planned) may be lowered by 30% to 50% from baseline dosage, and postexercise adjustments in bolus dosing may be made based on the adolescent's blood glucose pattern. Also, the use of a long acting form of insulin, given the night before planned athletic activities that may last many hours, has been suggested to replace a fraction of the pump basal rate.[16] This will allow the athlete to disconnect the pump for extended periods during water and contact sports while still having enough insulin to suppress ketogenesis. Insulin pump devices are continually being modified to offer advanced features, comfort and ease of use (Figure 15-2).

Intensive flexible insulin regimen with Glargine/Detemir and Aspart/Lispro/Glulisine

Doses of rapid-acting insulin used for meal coverage prior to scheduled exercise may need to be lowered by 30% to 50% from the athlete's baseline dosage, or occasionally

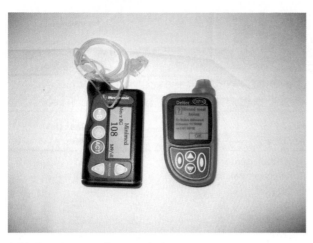

FIGURE 15-2 ■ Insulin pump devices.

may be omitted altogether if the activity is going to be intense and prolonged. For unplanned activities, insulin adjustment may not be possible; in those instances taking an extra carbohydrate snack may be an appropriate option. For planned periods of prolonged exercise such as an all day athletic event or a marathon, it may be helpful to lower the basal insulin (Glargine/Detemir) dose by 50% the night prior to the event. Further rapid-acting insulin administration and carbohydrate snacking will be based on close blood glucose monitoring throughout the day.[4,17] Insulin pen devices offer increased convenience for insulin administration versus the traditional syringe and vial methods (Figure 15-3).

Three insulin injections/day regimen with NPH and Aspart/Lispro/Glulisine

In this regimen modification of doses of insulin will depend on the time of scheduled activity in relation to peak action time of the insulin. For example, if the exercise activity is scheduled for mid-morning, the morning

dose of rapid-acting insulin may be lowered by 30% to 50%; if activity is in mid-afternoon or predinner, the dose of NPH would be lowered; activity in the postdinner period requires lowering the dose of the rapid-acting insulin used for dinner coverage. For early morning or prebreakfast activity, the bedtime NPH may need to be decreased.[4,17]

Other considerations

Other insulin combinations may be in use and will need to be modified with attention to time of action of insulin in comparison to time of activity. Insulin dose should be taken at least 1 hour prior to time of exercise. Insulin may need to be administered in a nonexercising limb, preferably anterior abdominal wall if taken within a few hours prior to exercise. This may avoid increased insulin absorption from the site of actively exercising limb, and thus minimize risk for hypoglycemia.

Modification of Meals or Snacks with Exercise

The athlete requires carbohydrates to meet the energy needs of exercise and may require additional carbohydrate in order to maintain normal blood glucose levels during exercise (Table 15-6).[12] Specific recommendations will vary depending on the timing of exercise in relation to prior meal, intensity and duration of exercise, levels of circulating insulin and timing of prior insulin dose. Alternatively, when exercise is planned ahead of time, prior insulin dosing may be lowered. A planned session of exercise ideally should be timed 1 to 2 hours after a meal or a snack. If a longer time period has elapsed between the meal or snack and exercise activity, blood glucose should be checked and guidelines for the snack coverage recommended should be followed (as noted earlier). A carbohydrate snack may be consumed prior to and for each half hour of activity. It is recommended that the carbohydrate snack should be consumed in conjunction with blood glucose level monitoring.

To prevent early and delayed onset of postexercise hypoglycemia, blood glucose should be checked with increased frequency over the subsequent 12 to 24 hours. If the activity was intense and prolonged, increased carbohydrate intake may be encouraged during this time as well. A bedtime snack comprised of complex carbohydrate and protein may be consumed to prevent overnight/early morning hypoglycemia on days of intense exercise in the afternoon/evening.[4,8,12]

Energy expenditures depend on the specific sports activity as well as body mass of the adolescent (Table 15-12).[18] The amount of energy expended by an adolescent therefore can be estimated based on his or her body mass, particular sport played, and the duration of play. Exercise "exchanges" have been developed based

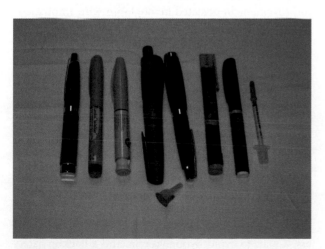

FIGURE 15-3 ■ Insulin pen devices.

Table 15-12.

Energy Expenditures (kcal/min) of Various Activities in Children Based on Body Mass

Activity	Body Mass (kg)		
	20	40	60
Basketball (game)	5.0	10.0	15.0
Cross-country skiing (leisure)	2.3	4.7	7.0
Cycling			
10 km/h	1.5	2.5	4.0
15 km/h	2.2	4.0	6.0
Figure skating	4.0	8.0	12.0
Ice hockey (ice time)	5.0	10.0	15.0
Running			
8 km/h	3.7	6.7	9.0
12 km/h	—	9.0	12.3
Snow shoeing	3.3	6.7	10.0
Soccer	3.7	7.2	10.7
Swimming			
30 m/min breast stroke	3.0	6.0	11.5
Tennis	2.5	4.3	6.3
Walking			
4 km/h	1.9	2.6	3.4
6 km/h	2.6	3.4	4.3

(With permission from. Riddell MC, Barr-Or O. Children and adolescents., In: Riderman N, ed. Handbook of Exercise in Diabetes. American Diabetes Association; 2001:547–566.)

Table 15-13.

Exercise Exchanges of 100 kcal (420 kJ) in Children Based on Body Mass

Activity	Body Mass (kg)		
	20	40	60
Basketball (game)	30	15	10
Cross-country skiing	40	20	15
Cycling			
10 km/h	65	40	25
15 km/h	45	25	15
Figure skating	25	15	10
Ice hockey (ice time)	20	10	5
Running			
8 km/h	25	15	10
12 km/h	—	10	10
Snow shoeing	30	15	10
Soccer	30	15	10
Swimming			
30 m/min breast stroke	55	25	15
Tennis	45	25	15
Walking			
4 km/h	60	40	30
6 km/h	40	30	25

Values shown are the estimated number of minutes that a certain activity should be sustained to be equivalent to one exercise exchange. Assuming that, on average, 60% of total energy is provided by carbohydrate, one exchange is equivalent to 60 kcal or 15 g carbohydrate.
With permission from Riddell MC, Barr-Or O. Children and adolescents, In: Riderman N, ed. Handbook of Exercise in Diabetes. American Diabetes Association; 2001:547–566.

on these estimates (Table 15-13).[18] Therefore the amount of carbohydrate can be individualized based on these exercise exchanges in order to reduce the incidence of hypoglycemia. Others have shown the success of similar algorithms where extra carbohydrate replacement during physical activity and sports is based on the duration and intensity of the activity.[19]

Additional Considerations for Sport Participation

Adolescents with diabetes should be able to perform at par with adolescents without diabetes as long as they maintain adequate metabolic control and use precautions to avoid hyper- or hypoglycemia. Optimal everyday metabolic control, in addition to careful blood glucose monitoring, appropriate modifications of insulin regimen and adequate carbohydrate ingestion should enable adolescents with type 1 DM to be able to participate in virtually any exercise regimen or sports activity.

The long-term benefits of exercise in the metabolic control of type 1 DM are not well-defined. Nevertheless, all the other benefits of exercise and sports participation remain the same as in nondiabetic athletes. Improvements in cardiovascular risk factors and appro-

priate weight management may serve to lower the risk of onset of chronic macro- and microvascular complications of diabetes mellitus. Studies have shown that regular exercise results in lower average blood glucose and glycohemoglobin concentrations with unchanged or decreased plasma insulin levels.[12,20,21] Other studies have failed to document a well-defined, consistent improvement in glycated hemoglobin with implementation of exercise regimens. Careful planning is essential to avoid the potential risks that may be associated with participation in sports by adolescents with diabetes.[22]

Hypoglycemia

Adolescents experiencing hypoglycemia may cause undue injury to themselves and/or others because of diminished ability to concentrate, compromised judgment, and loss of consciousness or even frank seizures. Motor vehicle racing, collision sports, swimming, diving, scuba diving, rock climbing and other inherently hazardous activities may pose significant risks in this regard.[9] A frank assessment of the risk to self and others, a plan to avoid hypoglycemia, and a backup safety plan in case hypoglycemia occurs, should be mandatory

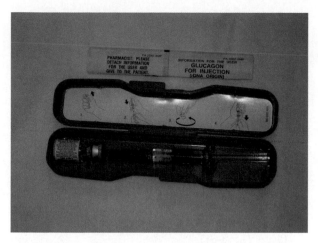

FIGURE 15-4 ■ Glucagon administration setup.

for adolescents taking on these challenges. It is recommended that selected other personnel, including other team members or coach, be trained to administer glucagons if needed for severe hypoglycemic reaction (Figure 15-4).

Hyperglycemia

Adolescents with hyperglycemia may risk worsening of hyperglycemia and development of diabetic ketoacidosis. Therefore it is very important to check blood glucose prior to physical exercise, not only to rule out hypoglycemia but to check for hyperglycemia as well. The ADA recommends that physical activity be avoided if blood glucose is more than 250 mg/dL with ketones, or blood glucose more than 300 mg/dL with or without ketones.

Retinopathy

Annual screening for retinopathy and nephropathy is recommended for all adolescent with diabetes mellitus. Adolescents with evidence of proliferative retinopathy should avoid those strenuous static exercises that require Valsalva-like maneuvers. The intense elevation of blood pressure from the Valsalva maneuver may precipitate vitreous or preretinal hemorrhage.[20]

Nephropathy

Adolescents with nephropathy and hypertension may already have reduced capacity for physical activity and may need to avoid intensive physical activity.[4] Although no specific guidelines exist, low to moderate dynamic exercise with careful monitoring may be well tolerated.

Neuropathy

Neuropathy is not usually seen in adolescence. Peripheral neuropathy, if present, may lead to loss of touch, temperature and vibration sensations, predisposing the

adolescent athlete to ulcerations, fractures and other injuries, especially of feet and legs.[4] Autonomic neuropathy may also limit exercise tolerance in the presence of cardiac autonomic neuropathy. There may be interference with food absorption in gastrointestinal neuropathy causing erratic glycemic control, especially hypoglycemia.

TYPE 2 DIABETES MELLITUS

The incidence of type 2 DM in children and adolescents is probably increasing but has not to date been accurately assessed.[1] In type 2 DM, the epinephrine and glucagon responses are preserved, which is probably why athletes with type 2 DM do not have as high an incidence of hypoglycemia.

In the current "obesity epidemic," there are concerns that onset of prediabetes and type 2 DM will be seen at an increasingly early age. Hence, "life style" modifications, including increased physical activity and healthy dietary patterns to avoid obesity, especially in adolescents with a family history of type 2 DM, may be crucial in preventing the early onset of type 2 DM in adolescence.[23] The emphasis should be on promoting healthy living from early childhood.

Exercise is the cornerstone in the management of type 2 DM, where it not only causes improvement of glycemic control by virtue of increased insulin effectiveness from increased insulin receptor sensitivity, but also is important for weight control, lowering of cardiovascular risk factors, and improvement in self-image and confidence.[8,12,24] Physical activity increases the insulin sensitivity in type 2 DM but exercise may not fully replace the insulin requirement. It is prudent, therefore, that good metabolic control be maintained in all adolescents with diabetes as a prerequisite for sports participation.

The significant impact of exercise on the improvement of glycemic control in type 2 DM occurs in part from weight loss, but also at exercise levels that merely yield weight maintenance. The long-term beneficial effects on metabolic abnormalities have been documented in multiple studies. The regulation of glycemic control during exercise and sports participation in type 2 DM is much easier as long as there is the presence of endogenous insulin secretion.[24]

Adolescents with type 2 DM may be taking one of the (or sometimes two) oral hypoglycemic agents and, less commonly, insulin. Increased exercise improves insulin sensitivity and glycemic control, more so when accompanied by weight stabilization and weight loss. In adolescents whose diabetes is diet controlled, there should be very little risk of hypoglycemia thus they may not need additional snacking except in very vigorous and prolonged exercise regimens. Adolescents taking sulfonylureas, thiazolidinediones and/or insulin are more likely to experience exercise-induced hypoglycemia.

Obese adolescents on low calorie diets need to ensure that at least 35% of their calorie intake is from carbohydrates.[8] Physical exercise is generally well tolerated by these adolescents. Obese adolescents with type 2 DM may need detailed evaluation to rule out evidence of micro- and macrovascular complications and assess suitability for particular sports program.[25] The exercise regimens should be gradually started and slowly built up to ensure adaptation and safety. Dyslipidemia screening is needed in Type 2 DM generally at the time of diagnosis and then at least annually.[7]

ACKNOWLEDGMENT

Authors thank Ms Amy Esman for her expert administrative assistance.

REFERENCES

1. Centers for Disease Control. National Diabetes Fact Sheet. http://www.cdc.gov/diabetes/pubs/factsheet05.htm. Accessed January 24, 2007.

2. Dorchy H, Poortmans JR. Juvenile diabetes and sports. The child and adolescent athlete (Encyclopaedia of Sports Medicine). In: Bar-Or O, IOC Medical Commission Staff, International Federation of Sports Medicine Staff, eds. *Disease and the Young Athlete*. Malden, MA: Blackwell Publishing; 2005:455.

3. DeLee JC, Drez D, Miller MD. *DeLee and Drez's Orthopaedic Sports Medicine: Principles and Practice*. 2nd ed. Philadelphia, PA: Saunder 2003.

4. Bode BW, ed. *Tools of Therapy—Exercise, in Medical Management of Type I Diabetes Mellitus*. 4th ed. Alexandria, VA: American Diabetes Association; 2004:108-119.

5. Berg K. The athlete with type I diabetes. In: Garrett WE, Jr, Kirkendall DT, Squire DL, eds. *Principles and Practice of Primary Care Sports Medicine*. Philadelphia, PA: Lippincott Williams & Wilkins; 2001:287-291.

6. Admon G, Weinstein Y, Falk B, et al. Exercise with and without an insulin pump among children and adolescents with type I diabetes mellitus. *Pediatrics*. 2005;116(3):348-355.

7. Kamboj MK. Diabetes on the college campus. *Pediatr Clin North Am*. 2005;52:279-305.

8. Steppel J, Horton ES. Exercise. In: American Diabetes Association, ed. *Therapy for Diabetes Mellitus and Related Disorders*. 4th ed. Alexandria, VA: American Diabetes Association; 2004:149-156.

9. Draznin MB. Type I diabetes and sports participation, strategies for training and competing safely. *Phys Sportsmed*. 2000;28(12):49-56.

10. Steppel J, Horton E. Exercise for the patient with type I diabetes. In: LeRoith D, Olefsky J, Taylor S, eds. *Diabetes Mellitus: A Fundamental and Clinical Text*. Philadelphia, PA: Lippincott-Raven; 2003:671-681.

11. The Diabetes Research in Children Network (DirecNet) Study Group. Impact of exercise on overnight glycemic control in children with type I diabetes mellitus. *J Pediatr*. 2005;147:528-534.

12. American Diabetes Association. Position Statement. Physical activity/exercise in diabetes. *Diabetes Care*. 2004;27 (Suppl 1):S58-S62.

13. Kamboj MK, Draznin MB. Office management of the adolescent with diabetes mellitus. *Prim Care Clin Office Pract*. 2006;33:581-602

14. LEVEMIR (Insulin detemir [rDNA origin]) injection – Product insert 2005.

15. Robinson DM, Wellington K. Insulin glulisine. *Drugs*. 2006;66(6):861-869.

16. Edelman S. The Un-Tethered Regimen. http://www.childrenwithdiabetes.com/clinic/untethered.htm. Accessed January 23, 2007.

17. Toni S, Reali MF, Barni F, et al. Managing insulin therapy during exercise in type I diabetes mellitus. *Acta Biomed Ateneo Parmense*. 2006;77(Suppl 1):34-40.

18. Riddell MC, Barr-Or O. Children and adolescents. In: Riderman.N, ed. *Handbook of Exercise in Diabetes*. Alexandria, VA: American Diabetes Association; 2001: 547-566.

19. Grimm JJ, Ybarra J, Berné C, et al. A New table for prevention of hypoglycaemia during physical activity in type I diabetic patients. *Diabetes Metab*. 2004;30(5):465-470.

20. American Diabetes Association. Position Statement. Physical activity. *Diabetes Care*. 2006;29(Suppl 1):S14-S16.

21. Schneider SH, Guleria PS. Diabetes and exercise. In: Warren MP, Constantine NW, eds. *Contemporary Endocrinology: Sports Endocrinology*. Totwa, NJ: Humana Press Inc; 2000:227-238.

22. Chipkin SR, Klugh SA, Chasan-Taber L. Exercise and diabetes. *Cardiol Clin*. 2001;19(3):489-505.

23. Steppel J, Horton E. Exercise in patients with type 2 diabetes. In: LeRoith D, Olefsky J, Taylor S, eds. *Diabetes Mellitus: A Fundamental and Clinical Text*. Philadelphia, PA: Lippincott-Raven; 2003:1099-1105.

24. Kelley DE, Goodpaster BH. Effects of exercise on glucose homeostasis in type 2 diabetes mellitus. *Med Sci Sports Exerc*. 2001;33(Suppl 6):S495-S501; Discussion S528-S529.

25. Zierath JR, Wallberg-Henriksson H. Exercise training in obese diabetic patients. Special considerations. *Sports Med*. 1992;14(3):171-189.

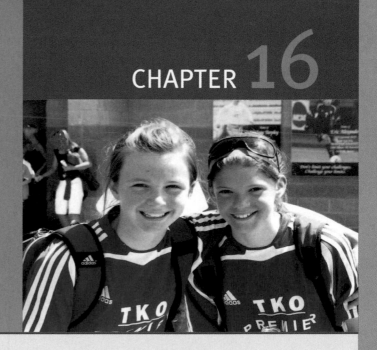

CHAPTER 16

Hematologic Conditions

Dilip R. Patel

HEMOPHILIA

Definition and Epidemiology

Hemophilia A and B are X-linked recessive inherited bleeding disorders affecting 1:5000 males with no racial predilection.[1-3] Hemophilia A is caused by deficiency of factor VIII and hemophilia B is caused by deficiency of factor IX. The normal plasma levels of factor VIII or factor IX range between 50% and 150%. The severity of hemophilia is predictive of risk for bleeding and is based on plasma levels of the factor VIII or IX (Table 16-1).[1]

Pathogenesis

Hemophilias are X-linked inherited bleeding disorders resulting from deficiency of clotting factors VIII or IX. Two examples of how hemophilia can be inherited are illustrated in Figures 16-1 and 16-2.[2] Female carriers have adequate levels of clotting factors because of the one normal X chromosome and do not manifest the clinical disease. In a very rare circumstance, a girl may be born with hemophilia when her father has hemophilia and the mother is a carrier. Hemophilia can also

occur in males who are not born to mothers who are not carriers of the abnormal gene because of mutation in the gene.

Clinical Presentation

Clinically hemophilia A and B are indistinguishable and the differentiation is based on factor assays. The clinical presentation depends upon the severity of the hemophilia. Patients with hemophilia may present with a history of easy bruising, spontaneous bleeding in the joints or muscles, and prolonged bleeding after trauma[1-3] They are also at risk for intracranial bleeding and internal bleeding at various other sites such as gastrointestinal tract and kidneys. Hemophilia should be differentiated from the most common inherited bleeding disorder, von Willebrand disease resulting from von Willebrand factor abnormality. The characteristics and differences between hemophilias and von Willebrand disease are summarized in Table 16-2.[1]

Diagnosis

Diagnosis is suspected based on positive family history and clinical presentation and confirmed by factor assays. An approach to laboratory diagnosis to a bleeding patient is presented in Figure 16-3.

Treatment

Patients should be managed in consultation with a hematologist at hemophilia treatment centers (Box 16-1). Treatment is directed at raising and maintaining the factor levels above which the risk of bleeding is minimized.[1,2,4-6] For minor bleeding such as joint or muscles the factor level should be raised up to 30% and for

Table 16-1.

Severity of Hemophilia

Severity	Plasma Level of Factor VIII or IX
Mild	More than 5%
Moderate	Between 1% and 5%
Severe	Less than 1%

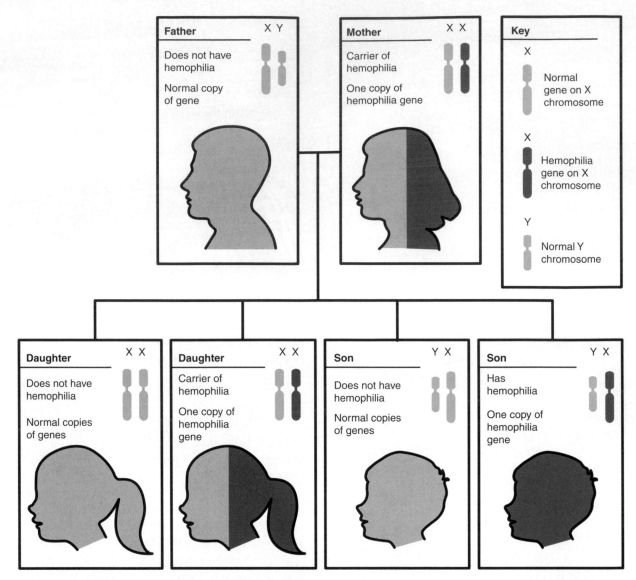

FIGURE 16-1 ■ Mode of inheritance of hemophilia. The mother is a carrier of hemophilia. Each daughter has a 50% chance of inheriting the abnormal gene from her mother and being a carrier. Each son has a 50% chance of inheriting the abnormal gene from his mother and having hemophilia. (*From: www.nhlbi.nih.gov.*)

major bleeding such as internal organ bleeding it should be raised up to 100%. The factor level is raised by intravenous administration (either bolus or continuous infusion) of specific factor (factor VIII or IX or von Willebrand) concentrate. One unit per kilogram of body weight will raise plasma factor VIII by 2%, factor IX by 1.5%, and von Willebrand facor (Ristocetin cofactor activity) by 1.5%.[1,4] The typical dose for prophylactic regimen for factor VIII is 25 to 40 U/kg body weight every other day and for factor IX is 25 to 40 U/kg body weight two times per week.

Desmopressin has been shown to effectively raise the plasma levels of factor VIII and von Willebrand factor by two- to sixfold and is used to treat mild hemophilia A and von Willebrand disease.[1,4] Epsilon amino caproic acid or tranexamic acid are used as adjunct hemostatic therapy for mucosal bleeds.

Sports participation and regular exercise are encouraged for patients with hemophilias and von Willebrand disease.[1,2,5,6] Sport participation and regular physical activity have been shown to have significant positive effect on joint health, overall health, and psychosocial

---

Box 16-1 When to Refer

When to Consult Hematologist

Bleeding disorders
Sickle cell disease and other hemoglobinopathies
Thrombotic disorders and thrombophilia
Thrombocytopenias
Severe iron deficiency anemia with complications
Chronic anemia not responding to treatment
Hemolytic anemias
Aplastic anemias

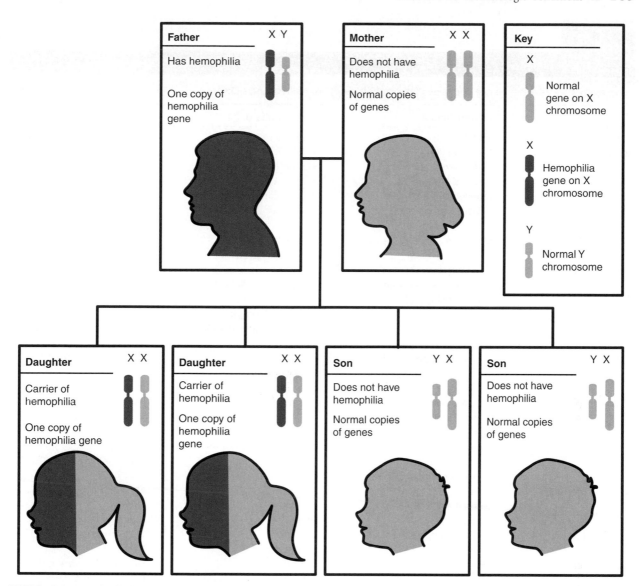

FIGURE 16-2 ■ Mode of inheritance of hemophilia. The father has hemophilia. The mother is not a carrier of hemophilia. Each daughter will inherit the abnormal gene from her father and be a carrier. None of the sons will inherit the abnormal gene from their father, and, therefore, none will have hemophilia. (*From: www.nhlbi.nih.gov.*)

well being. Category 1 sports such as swimming, golf, and running are considered safe to allow full participation; category 2 sports such as bowling, weight lifting, and biking in which the benefits outweigh the risks are also generally appropriate to allow participation; and category 3 sports such as football and skateboarding in which the risks outweigh the potential benefits are generally not considered safe to allow participation. Athletes should maintain their factor levels in the normal range and administration of factor concentrate before the anticipated physical activity is also recommended. Factors to be considered in planning athletic participation include preparticipation evaluation and clearance by hematologist, ready availability of appropriate factor concentrate, knowledge by the athlete and the staff involved of the location and contact information of

nearest hemophilia center while traveling for away games, and specific emergency action plan in case of bleeding.[5] Specific sport related issues are summarized in Table 16-3.

SPORTS ANEMIA

Definition and Epidemiology

Sports anemia is a benign, self-limited, pseudoanemia resulting from training induced plasma volume expansion and hemodilution, with mild decrease in measured hemoglobin levels, not associated with any other abnormal laboratory parameters.[7–10] Although the exact incidence is not known, it is the most common

Table 16-2.

Characteristics and Differences Between Hemophilias and von Willebrand's Disease

	Hemophilia A	Hemophilia B	von Willebrand's Disease
Incidence	1:5,000	1:30,000	1%–3% of US population
Abnormality	Factor (F) VIII deficiency. Normal levels: 50%–150%	F IX deficiency Normal levels: 50%–150%	VWF abnormality
Inheritance	X-linked, affects males Gene at the tip of X-chromosome	X-linked, affects males	Autosomal dominant (gene on chromosome 12). Affects males and females
Site of production	Unknown	Liver, vitamin K depended protein	Megakaryocytes and endothelial cells
Function of protein	Cofactor; forms "tenase" complex with FIX and activate FX	Clotting protein (zym ogen). Activated by F XI or VIIa and forms a "tenase" complex with FVIII and activates FX	Platelet adhesion, protection of F VIII
Classification (Normal plasma levels of FIII and IX = 50–150%)	Mild (>5%) Moderate (1%–5%) Severe (<1%)	Mild (>5%) Moderate (1%–5%) Severe (<1%)	Types 1 Type 2 (2A, 2B, 2M, 2N) Type 3
Clinical manifestations	Positive family history (30% new mutation). Hemarthroses, hematomas, intracranial hemorrhages, hematuria, gastrointestinal hemorrhage, and so forth	Positive family history (30% new mutation). Milder disease, though identical hemorrhage sites as hemophilia A	Positive family history Mucocutaneous (epistaxis, menorrhagia, postdental bleeding). Type 3 may present as hemophilia A
PFA/Bleeding time	Normal	Normal	May be prolonged
PT	Normal	Normal	Normal
APTT	Prolonged	Prolonged	Prolonged or normal
F VIII assay	Decreased or absent	Normal	↓ or Normal
F IX assay	Normal	Decreased or absent	Normal
VWF: antigen	Normal	Normal	Decreased or absent (type 3)
VWF R: Co	Normal	Normal	Decreased or abnormal
VWF multimers	Normal	Normal	Normal or abnormal
Specific treatment	Recombinant (r) F VIII (preferred), virally safe plasma derived concentrates	Recombinant F IX, virally safe plasma derived concentrates	DDAVP (intranasal or intravenous) VWF concentrates (plasma derived)
Inhibitor patients	rFVIIa, FEIBA	rFVIIa	Rare
Adjunct treatment	Antifibrinolytics	Antifibrinolytics	Oral contraceptives, antifibrinolytics

Kulkarni R, Gera R, Scott-Emuakpor AB. Adolescent hematology. In: Greydanus DE, Patel DR, Pratt HD, eds. Essential Adolescent Medicine. New York, NY: McGraw Hill; 2006:371–390.

type of "anemia" (pseudoanemia) seen in athletes, especially endurance athletes.

Pathogenesis

During moderate to vigorous exercise there is a decrease in plasma volume between 6% and 20%.[8–10] Three mechanisms have been postulated to explain this decrease: (1) increase in systemic arterial blood pressure and muscle contractions increase the capillary hydrostatic pressure, moving fluid into extravascular space, (2) movement of fluid from intravascular space into the muscle tissue because of generation of lactic acid and other metabolites that occurs as a result of muscular activity, and (3) insensible loss of fluid in the sweat.[6–10]

On cessation of the physical activity the plasma volume typically returns to normal within a few hours and then it begins to expand. The degree of plasma volume expansion depends up on the intensity and

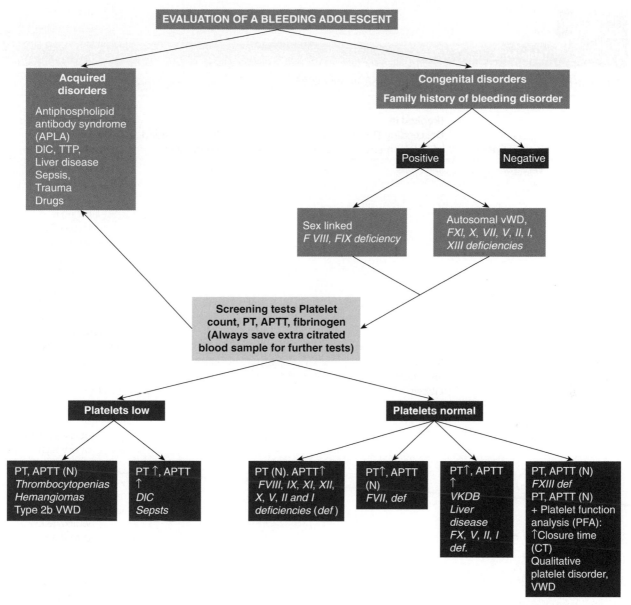

FIGURE 16-3 ■ Evaluation of bleeding patient. Screening tests assess the degree of hemorrhage and the adequacy of hemostasis in a bleeding patient. (*Used with permission from Kulkarni R, Gera R, Scott-Emuakpor AB. Adolescent hematology. In: Greydanus DE, Patel DR, Pratt HD, eds. Essential Adolescent Medicine. New York: McGraw Hill; 2006:371-390.*)

duration of the endurance activity. The plasma volume and hemoglobin concentration generally return to normal levels within 1 week. It is believed that this adaptive plasma volume expansion may in fact be beneficial to the athlete as it will increase the cardiac output, stroke volume, delivery of oxygen to the tissues, decrease blood viscosity, and improve thermoregulation.[7–10]

Clinical Presentation

Athletes with dilutional pseudoanemia generally remain asymptomatic and have normal findings on physical examination. Athletes with findings suggestive of anemia such as fatigue, pallor, shortness of breath, hepatosplenomegaly, should be thoroughly investigated for other causes of anemia such as iron deficiency and hemolysis.

Diagnosis

Laboratory studies show a mild decrease in hemoglobin concentration. Hemoglobin level is generally reported to be 1 to 1.5 g/dL lower in endurance athletes compared to population norm. All other hematologic laboratory parameters are normal.

Table 16-3.

Canadian Hemophilia Society Guidelines for Sport Participation

Sport	Risk of Sport	Joints Involved (Ranked in Descending Order of Involvement)	Degree of Stress to Joints	Recommended Equipment	Additional Comments
Swimming	Very low	Shoulders	+	None	Swimming is a low-risk sport assuming no diving is involved. Stress to joints is directly related to intensity and duration of swimming. Whipkick may irritate knees.
Waterskiing	High	Knees Shoulders Elbows	+++ ++ ++	Life jacket	Very stressful on muscles. The overall risk is high because of outside forces over which skier has no control (examples: speed at which he hits the water, being hit by a ski).
Windsurfing	Medium	Spine Shoulders Elbows	++ ++ +	Life jacket	Lessons useful initially to learn proper technique. High winds increase risk especially if inexperienced.
Golf	Low	Shoulders Elbows Knees	+ + +	Appropriate footwear	
Tennis	Low	Knees Ankles Elbows	++ ++ +	Tennis shoes	
Squash/Racquetball	Medium	Knees Ankles Elbows Shoulders	+++ +++ ++ ++	Appropriate footwear	Protective eyeglasses. Contact with ball, racquet could be harmful.
Volleyball	Low/medium	Knees Hands (fingers/wrists) Ankles	++ ++ +	Knee pads High-top running shoes	Increased risk with higher level of competition.

(continued)

Table 16-3. (Continued)

Canadian Hemophilia Society Guidelines for Sport Participation

Basketball	Low/medium	Knees	+++	High-top running shoes	High-top running shoes may prevent ankle sprains. Knee pads provide some form of cushioning when falling on knees.
		Ankles	+++	Knee pads	
		Fingers	++		
Baseball	Medium	Shoulders	++	Knee pads	Higher risk of soft tissue injuries
		Knees	++	Appropriate footwear	
		Elbows	++	Helmet (batting)	
		Ankles	++		
Soccer	Medium	Ankles	+++	Appropriate footwear	Higher risk of soft tissue injuries
		Knees	++	Shin pads	
		Hips	++		
Football (tackle)	High	Knees	+++	Helmet	High risk of head injuries and traumatic bleeds because of repeated heavy physical contact in tackle football.
		Ankles	+++	Protective pads	
		Shoulders	+++		
Rugby	High	Knees	+++	Generally not used in this sport	Harmful because of high risk of physical contact. Increased risk of head injury and jarring injury to the spine.
		Ankles	+++		
		Shoulders	+++		
Weight lifting	Medium	Elbows	+++		Proper lifting techniques can lessen risk of injury. Recommended lifting through mid-range only. Increase number of repetitions rather than weight. Train regularly. Not recommended for young children.
		Shoulders	+++		
		Back	+++		
Skating	Low	Knees	++	Proper fitting skates with good ankle support.	Helmet is advisable during initial learning period. Knee pads or snow pants.
		Ankles	++		
Skateboarding	High	Knees	+++	Helmet	Risk of fracture and head injury owing to falling.
		Ankles	+++	Knee and elbow pads	

(continued)

Table 16-3.

Canadian Hemophilia Society Guidelines for Sport Participation

Sport	Risk of Sport	Joints Involved (Ranked in Descending Order of Involvement)	Degree of Stress to Joints	Recommended Equipment	Additional Comments
Roller skating/ roller blading	High	Spine	Stress on joints related to falling.	Helmet Knee, elbow and shin pads	Risk of injury is high owing to risk of falling on hard surfaces. Rough surfaces, hills, and ramps increase risk.
Road hockey	Medium	Knees Ankles	++ ++	Helmet and knee pads may be beneficial.	Contact with stick and other players could be harmful.
Ice hockey	High	Knees Shoulders Ankles	+++ +++ ++	Proper fitting skates with good ankle support. Protective padding (shoulder, elbows, knees). Helmet	Contact with puck, stick, boards, other players could be harmful.
Nordic skiing (cross-country)	Low/medium	Knees Ankles Shoulders	++ ++ +	Skis and poles of appropriate length. Boots with good support.	The difficulty of the course will directly affect the degree of stress on joints and overall risk such as risk of falling.
Alpine skiing (downhill)	High	Knees	+++	Helmet Ski boots	Appropriate length of skis and poles. The risk of head injury is high owing to the inherent risk of falling at high speeds.
Horseback riding	High	Spine	++	Helmet	The risk of head injury and serious muscle or joint injury is high owing to the possibility of falling off or being thrown from the horse. Jumping should be avoided.
Bicycling	Low	Knees	+	Properly adjusted bike with seat at proper height. Bicycle helmet. Toe straps.	To minimize stress on knees: 1. Keep seat high. 2. Avoid hills. 3. Stay in lower gears. 4. Pedal at high revolution (80–100/min).

(continued)

Table 16-3. (Continued)

Canadian Hemophilia Society Guidelines for Sport Participation

| Running | Low/medium | Ankles Knees | + + | | Appropriate footwear (need good shock absorption, firm heel-counter, arch support). | Running surface (e.g., concrete or uneven ground) will affect risk. Intensity of running (such as distance, speed, frequency) will also affect risk. |
| Karate/Judo | Medium/high | Knees Elbow Ankles | + + + + + | | | None. If there is contact, the risk of injury is high. Without contact, the training can be good for improving muscle flexibility, coordination and balance. |

Scale: + Low degree of stress
+ + Moderate degree of stress
+ + + High degree of stress
Source: Canadian Hemophilia Society. http://www.hemophila.ca.

Treatment

No treatment is required for dilutional psuedoanemia as this is considered to be an adaptive response to exercise and is self limited typically resolving within 1 week.

IRON DEFICIENCY ANEMIA

Definition and Epidemiology

Iron deficiency anemia is characterized by a decrease in total body iron resulting in a lower than normal hemoglobin for age and gender (Table 16-4).[1,11] The reported prevalence of iron deficiency anemia in the United States is 2% in females ages 12 to 19 years. Anemia is less common in males than in females. The exact prevalence of iron deficiency anemia in athletes is not known. The reported prevalence of iron deficiency anemia in athletes ranges between 4% in male endurance athletes to 20% in female athletes.[6–8]

Pathogenesis

Iron deficiency anemia is the result of depletion of body iron stores that leads to iron-deficient erythropoiesis.

Table 16-4.

Normal Values for Hemogoblin, Hematocrit, and MCV for Adolescents

Age (yr)	Hemoglobin (g/dL)		Hematocrit (%)		MCV (μ³)	
	Mean	Lower Limit	Mean	Lower Limit	Mean	Lower Limit
12–14						
Female	13.5	12	41	36	85	78
Male	14	12.5	43	37	84	77
15–17						
Female	14	12	41	36	87	79
Male	15	13	46	38	86	78

Iron-deficiency erythropoiesis eventually results in the production of microcytic hypochromic red blood cells that are iron-deficient, characteristic of iron deficiency anemia. Iron deficiency can result from chronic blood loss, inadequate dietary iron intake or inadequate dietary iron absorption.[11–14] Gastrointestinal and genitourinary bleeding, poor dietary habits, high expenditure of energy, increased demands for iron, exertional hemolysis, and some losses in the sweat have been implicated that result in iron deficiency in athletes.[6,7,11] In female athletes who participate in sports that require a thin body habitus, lack of sufficient dietary calories and nutrients is further exacerbated contributing to a higher prevalence of iron deficiency in these athletes. Consumption of antacids and other antiulcer drugs that reduce the gastric pH also result in reduced iron release from food. Iron from meat has a higher bioavailability and vitamin C enhances iron absorption.

In individual with iron deficiency anemia, less iron is available for the synthesis of hemoglobin and myoglobin. There is reduced oxygen carrying capacity of the blood, reduced work capacity, reduced aerobic capacity, and decreased endurance performance.[6,11,13] In athletes this will have negative effect for continued ability to participate effectively in sports because of their inability to meet the increased metabolic and oxygen demands.

Clinical Presentation

The clinical manifestations of iron deficiency anemia in athletes are the same as in nonathletes. Fatigue, exercise intolerance, decreased performance are of particular importance in athletes.[6,7,15–24] Other clinical manifestations of iron deficiency anemia include headaches, dizziness, palpitations, heart murmurs, craving for nonfood items, pallor, aphthous ulcers, angular cheilitis, glossitis, stomatitis, fatigue, shortness of breath, koilonychia, restless legs syndrome, irritability, poor appetite, and poor concentration.[11,13,15–24] Rarely severe anemia may lead to cardiomyopathy and splenomegaly.

Diagnostic Studies

A complete blood count with indices and hemoglobin levels are the most useful initial tests. A low mean corpuscular volume (less than 82 fL in adolescents and adults) indicates microcytic anemia.[11,14] In iron deficiency anemia the hemoglobin level is below that is normal for age and gender (Table 16-4). In nonpregnant adolescents and adult women a hemoglobin level of equal to or less than 12 g/dL and in males equal to or less than 12.5 to 13.5 g/dL is consistent with anemia.[11–14] Serum ferritin levels less than 15 ng/mL is a good indicator of depleted iron stores, although it may be higher in inflammatory conditions and some malignant conditions. With progression of iron deficiency total serum iron level is decreased and total iron-binding capacity is increased.

The sTfR/Log Ferritin Index (ratio of sTfR to the log of ferritin) is considered a more sensitive measure of iron deficiency before the stage of iron-deficient erythropoiesis.[1] In iron deficiency anemia the value is typically more than 1.5. Peripheral smear will show characteristic microcytic hypocrhmoc red cells. The spectrum of body iron content is presented in Table 16-5.[11]

Treatment

A mild to moderate anemia (hemoglobin 8–11 g/dL) can be presumptively treated with iron supplementation of 3 to 6 mg of elemental iron per kg of body weight per day (adult maximum is 240 mg/d).[1,14,20] An increase in hemoglobin of 1 g/dL after 4 week of therapy is consistent with iron deficiency obviating the need for further work up. Hemoglobin should be measured at 1 month and 3 month once the treatment is initiated. Treatment should be continued for 3 months following normalization of hemoglobin level.

The preferred iron preparations are ferrous iron salts (ferrous fumarate, ferrous sulfate, and ferrous gluconate). Because the amount of iron absorbed decreases with increasing doses, it is recommended that the total

Table 16-5.

Spectrum of Body Iron Content

Iron Status	Stored Iron	Transport Iron	Functional Iron
Iron-deficiency anemia	Low	Low	Low
Iron-deficient erythropoiesis	Low	Low	Normal
Iron depletion	Low	Normal	Normal
Normal	Normal	Normal	Normal
Iron overload	High	High	Normal

daily dose be taken in two or three divided doses. Side effects associated with therapeutic doses of iron include nausea, vomiting, constipation, diarrhea, dark colored stools, and abdominal distress.[11,14] The side effects can be minimized by gradually increasing the dose to reach the recommended therapeutic dose and by taking the iron supplement with food in two to three divided doses during the day. Enteric coated or delayed release preparations are less well absorbed and are generally not preferred even though they may have fewer gastrointestinal side effects.

Patients with severe anemia (hemoglobin less than 8 mg/dL) and those with clinical symptoms should be worked up fully to identify the type and cause of the anemia to guide the treatment decisions. Causative factors should be identified and corrected, especially improved dietary intake of iron and avoiding unhealthy weight control practices. A diet high in iron is recommended (Tables 16-6 and 16-7).

The Recommended Daily Allowance for iron in adolescents and adults and nonpregnant females is approximately 12 to 15 mg/d.[11,12,14] Some studies suggest that those who engage in regular vigorous physical activity may need up to 30% more than RDA for iron.[11]

Most athletes with adequate dietary iron intake, those who are asymptomatic, and those with mild to moderate anemia being treated tend to continue to participate in sports as tolerated although their capacity to sustain physical activity may be significantly affected.

Iron deficiency without anemia

Iron deficiency without anemia is more prevalent than anemia affecting between 9% and 11% of adolescent females and 5% of adolescent males in the United States.[14] Screening of all asymptomatic athletes to identify iron deficiency without anemia is controversial and there is no consensus to routinely supplement otherwise well athletes with iron.[19–24]

SICKLE CELL TRAIT

Definition and Epidemiology

Sickle cell trait (SCT) results from the inheritance of one normal and one abnormal gene for hemoglobin. It is usually considered to be a benign disorder that does

Table 16-6.

Selected Food Sources of Nonheme Iron

Food	Milligrams per Serving	% DV*
Ready-to-eat cereal, 100% iron fortified, ¾ cup	18.0	100
Oatmeal, instant, fortified, prepared with water, 1 cup	10.0	60
Soybeans, mature, boiled, 1 cup	8.8	50
Lentils, boiled, 1 cup	6.6	35
Beans, kidney, mature, boiled, 1 cup	5.2	25
Beans, lima, large, mature, boiled, 1 cup	4.5	25
Beans, navy, mature, boiled, 1 cup	4.5	25
Ready-to-eat cereal, 25% iron fortified, ¾ cup	4.5	25
Beans, black, mature, boiled, 1 cup	3.6	20
Beans, pinto, mature, boiled, 1 cup	3.6	20
Molasses, blackstrap, 1 tablespoon	3.5	20
Tofu, raw, firm, ½ cup	3.4	20
Spinach, boiled, drained, ½ cup	3.2	20
Spinach, canned, drained solids ½ cup	2.5	10
Black-eyed peas (cowpeas), boiled, 1 cup	1.8	10
Spinach, frozen, chopped, boiled, ½ cup	1.9	10
Grits, white, enriched, quick, prepared with water, 1 cup	1.5	8
Raisins, seedless, packed, ½ cup	1.5	8
Whole wheat bread, 1 slice	0.9	6
White bread, enriched, 1 slice	0.9	6

*DV = Daily value. DVs are reference numbers developed by the Food and Drug Administration (FDA) to help consumers determine if a food contains a lot or a little of a specific nutrient. The FDA requires all food labels to include the percent DV (% DV) for iron. The percent DV tells you what percent of the DV is provided in one serving. The DV for iron is 18 mg. A food providing 5% of the DV or less is a low source, while a food that provides 10%–19% of the DV is a good source. A food that provides 20% or more of the DV is high in that nutrient. It is important to remember that foods that provide lower percentages of the DV also contribute to a healthful diet. For foods not listed in this table, refer to the US Department of Agriculture's Nutrient Database Web site: http://www.nal.usda.gov/fnic/cgi-bin/nut search.pl.

Table 16-7.

Selected Food Sources of Heme Iron

Food	Milligrams per Serving	% DV*
Chicken liver, cooked, 3½ ounces	12.8	70
Oysters, breaded and fried, 6 pieces	4.5	25
Beef, chuck, lean only, braised, 3 ounces	3.2	20
Clams, breaded, fried, ¾ cup	3.0	15
Beef, tenderloin, roasted, 3 ounces	3.0	15
Turkey, dark meat, roasted, 3½ ounces	2.3	10
Beef, eye of round, roasted, 3 ounces	2.2	10
Turkey, light meat, roasted, 3½ ounces	1.6	8
Chicken, leg, meat only, roasted, 3½ ounces	1.3	6
Tuna, fresh bluefin, cooked, dry heat, 3 ounces	1.1	6
Chicken, breast, roasted, 3 ounces	1.1	6
Halibut, cooked, dry heat, 3 ounces	0.9	6
Crab, blue crab, cooked, moist heat, 3 ounces	0.8	4
Pork, loin, broiled, 3 ounces	0.8	4
Tuna, white, canned in water, 3 ounces	0.8	4
Shrimp, mixed species, cooked, moist heat, 4 large	0.7	4

*DV = Daily Value. DVs are reference numbers developed by the Food and Drug Administration (FDA) to help consumers determine if a food contains a lot or a little of a specific nutrient. The FDA requires all food labels to include the percent DV (%DV) for iron. The percent DV tells you what percent of the DV is provided in one serving. The DV for iron is 18 mg. A food providing 5% of the DV or less is a low source while a food that provides 10%–19% of the DV is a good source. A food that provides 20% or more of the DV is high in that nutrient. It is important to remember that foods that provide lower percentages of the DV also contribute to a healthful diet. For foods not listed in this table, refer to the US Department of Agriculture's Nutrient Database Web site: http://www.nal.usda.gov/fnic/cgi-bin/nut search.pl.

not result in sickling under normal homeostatic condition. SCT is found in 8% of African Americans in the United States and has a higher prevalence rate in persons of Mediterranean, Middle Eastern, Indian, Caribbean, and Central and South American descent.[25] The prevalence of SCT in athletes is not known but is estimated to be approximately the same for the general population.

Pathogenesis

The substitution of the amino acid valine for glutamic acid at position 6 of the beta chain of hemoglobin or heme molecule results in the sickle hemoglobin. Under deoxygenated conditions such as hypoxia, dehydration, infection, fever, and acidosis, hemoglobin molecule assumes the deoxygenated or reduced form, which is less soluble.[25–35] This sickling state is usually reversible in the initial 10 to 15 seconds if these changes in homeostasis can be reversed. Failure to do so results in the formation of tactoids that lead to the alteration of the red blood cell (RBC) resulting in the formation of sickled RBC. The sickled RBC is unable to perform its normal functions and is increasingly adhesive to the endothelium. There is blocking of small vessels of vital organs leading to ischemia. The extent of sickling depends on the amount of Hb S present. In SCT, the excess amount of

sickled Hb required to cause symptoms that will be fatal under severe exertion has not been fully elucidated, since there is significant sickling in the postmortem period.[27,28]

In SCT it is estimated that approximately 60 % of the hemoglobin is Hb A and 40% is Hb S. This, under normal physiological conditions does not lead to any symptoms because of the amount of Hb A present. When there is dehydration, high intensity exercise, a state of low oxygen tension, such as high altitudes, underlying illness, high humidity and temperatures, sickling may occur.[25] This, coupled with the hyperviscosity may lead to obstruction of blood flow to vital organs. This may persist or worsen up to 24 hours after cessation of exercise.[29]

Lactate is a by-product of anaerobic metabolism employed my muscle. Its accumulation likely plays a key role in muscle fatigue and poor performance. The role of lactate levels in the process of sickling is not clearly established; while some studies have reported increased levels, others have shown no changes or even decreased levels after strenuous physical exercise.[30]

Clinical Presentation

Under normal homeostatic conditions athletes with SCT are asymptomatic. Risk factors for exercise-related death of young athletes include environmental heat stress during the preceding 24 hours, inadequate acclimation, excessive clothing that interfere with heat loss, dehydration, obesity, poor conditioning for the given physical activity, sustained extreme ("heroic") physical exertion, lack of adequate rest and sleep, and failure to recognize and treat exertional heat illness in a timely manner.[25,27,31,32,34,35] The most consistent factor that increases the risk of exercise-related death in athletes with SCT is the intensity and/or the duration of the physical activity for which the athlete is not adequately conditioned or trained for.[25] The reported causes of sudden death in athletes with SCT include acute extertional rhabdomyolyis, heat stroke, and cardiac arrhythmia.

Diagnostic Studies

Definitive diagnosis of SCT and disease is confirmed by quantitative hemoglobin electrophoresis.

Treatment

Athlete's SCT can be ascertained based on history or laboratory investigation. Routine screening of asymptomatic athletes to identify those with SCT is neither universally recommended nor practiced.[25]

Asymptomatic athletes with SCT do not require any active medical intervention and are allowed full sports participation. Athletes should be appropriately educated about the nature of their condition, to recognize early symptoms, to seek immediate medical attention, and potential for complications under certain physiologic and environmental conditions. All athletes must be appropriately conditioned for the sport, stay well hydrated, and avoid strenuous physical exertion in extremes of environmental conditions. Sickling collapse is a medical emergency and on-field response must be prompt and aggressive provided by appropriately trained staff on site and the athlete must be transported to emergency department.

Sickle cell disease

Patients with sickle cell disease should be managed in consultation with a hematologist. Their participation in sports will depend on the severity of the disease, state of their general health, and the presence of complications (Table 16-8). The level of physical activity should be individualized based on the overall assessment of athlete working with the treating hematologist.

ACKNOWLEDGMENT

We thank Samuel Anim, MD, for assistance with preparation of this chapter.

Table 16-8.

Major Clinical Features of Sickle Cell Disease at Various Stages

	Infancy	Childhood	Adolescent
A. Impairment of circulation	Pain, hand and foot syndrome	Pain, stroke, arthralgia, hematuria, hyposthenuria	Chronic pain, stroke, autosplenectomy, renal insufficiency, avascular necrosis
B. Red blood cell destruction (Hemolysis)	Pallor, jaundice, lethargy	Pallor, jaundice, lethargy, splenomegaly, cardiomegaly, shortness of breath	Exercise intolerance pallor, jaundice, gall stones, chronic lung disease, chronic transfusion, and iron overload
C. Stagnation of blood in organs	Sequestration	Sequestration	Priapism, hepatomegaly, chronic leg ulcers
Combination of A, B, and C	Fever, pneumonia, osteomyelitis, susceptibility to infections (*Pneumococcus* and *Haemophilus influenzae*)	Fever, pneumonia, osteomyelitis, susceptibility to infections (*Pneumococcus* and *H. influenzae*)	Fever, osteomyelitis (*Salmonella* sp.), acute chest syndrome, pulmonary hypertension, retinopathy delayed sexual maturation, pregnancy complications, depression , pain intolerance, narcotic dependence, increase school absenteeism

Kulkarni R, Gera R, Scott-Emuakpor AB. Adolescent hematology. In: Greydanus DE, Patel DR, Pratt HD, eds. Essential Adolescent Medicine. New York: McGraw Hill; 2006:371–390.

REFERENCES

1. Kulkarni R, Gera R, Scott-Emuakpor AB. Adolescent hematology. In: Greydanus DE, Patel DR, Pratt HD, eds. *Essential Adolescent Medicine*. New York, NY: McGraw Hill; 2006:371-390.

2. United States Department of Health and Human Services. National Heart, Lung, and Blood Institute. Hemophilia. www.nhlbi,nih.gov. Accessed July 9, 2008.

3. Bolton M, Pasi KJ. Hemophilias A and B. *Lancet.* 2003;36:1801.

4. National Hemophilia Foundation Medical and Scientific Advisory Council. *Treatment Recommendations*. New York, NY: National Hemophilia Foundation; 2006. www.hemophilia.org. Accessed July 9, 2008.

5. Fiala KA, Hoffmann SJ, Ritenour DM. Traumatic hemarthrosis of the knee secondary to hemophilia A in a collegiate soccer player: a case report. *J Athl Train.* 2002; 37(3):315-319.

6. Mercer KW, Densmore JJ. Hematologic disorders in the athlete. *Clin Sports Med.* 2005;24:599-621.

7. Shaskey DJ, Green GA. Sports haematology. *Sports Med.* 2000;29(1):27-38.

8. Davidson RJ, Robertson JD, Galea F, et al. Hematological changes associated with marathon running. *Int J Sports Med.* 1987;8(1):19-25.

9. Eichner ER. Sports anemia, iron supplements, and blood doping. *Med Sci Sports Exerc.* 1992;24(9S):S315-S318.

10. Balaban EP. Sports anemia. *Clin Sports Med.* 1992;11(2): 313-325.

11. National Institutes of Health, Office of Dietary Supplements Fact Sheet. Iron. 2007. http://ods/od.nih.gov/factsheets/iron.asp. Accessed July 9, 2008.

12. Institute of Medicine. Food and Nutrition Board. *Dietary Reference Intakes for Vitamin A, Vitamin K, Arsenic, Boron, Chromium, Copper, Iodine, Iron, Manganese, Molybdenum, Nickel, Silicon, Vanadium and Zinc*. Washington, DC: National Academy Press; 2001.

13. US Department of Health and Human Services, National Heart Lung and Blood Institute. Iron deficiency anemia. 2007. http://www.nhlbi.nih.gov. Accessed July 9, 2008.

14. Centers for Disease Control and Prevention. Recommendations to prevent and control iron deficiency in the United States. *MMWR.* 1998;47(RR-3):1-36.

15. Stoltzfus RJ. Iron deficiency: global prevalence and consequences. *Food Nutr Bull.* 2003;24(suppl 4):S99-S103.

16. Wright RO, Tsaih S-W, Schwartz J, Wright RJ, Hu H. Association between iron deficiency and blood lead level in a longitudinal analysis of children followed in an urban primary care clinic. *J Pediatr.* 2003;142:9-14.

17. Shafir T, Angulo-Barroso R, Calatroni A, Jimenez E, Lozoff B. Effects of iron deficiency in infancy on patterns of motor development over time. *Hum Mov Sci.* 2006; 25(6):821-838.

18. Hegde N, Rich MW, Gayomali C. The cardiomyopathy of iron deficiency. *Tex Heart Inst J.* 2006;33(3):340-344.

19. Suedekum NA, Dimeff RJ. Iron and the athlete. *Curr Sports Med Rep.* 2005;4(4):199-202.

20. Chatard JC, Mujika I, Guy C, Lacour JR. Anaemia and iron deficiency in athletes. Practical recommendations for treatment. *Sports Med.* 1999;27(4):229-240.

21. Raunikar RA, Sabio H. Anemia in the adolescent athlete. *Am J Dis Child.* 1992;146(10):1201-1205.

22. Nielsen P, Nachtigall D. Iron supplementation in athletes. Current recommendations. *Sports Med.* 1998;26(4): 207-216.

23. Cowell BS, Rosenbloom CA, Skinner R, Summers SH. Policies on screening female athletes for iron deficiency in NCAA division I-A institutions. *Int J Sport Nutr Exerc Metab.* 2003;13(3):277-285.

24. Fallon KE. Utility of hematological and iron-related screening in athletes. *Clin J Sport Med.* 2004;14(3):145-152.

25. United States Department of Health and Human Services National Heart, Lung, and Blood Institute. *Management of Sickle Cell Disease*. 2002. NIH Publication 02-2117.

26. Bitanga E, Rouillon JD. Influence of the sickle cell trait heterozygote on energy abilities. *Pathol Biol (Paris).* 1998;46(1):46-52.

27. Bock H, Seidl S, Hausmann R, Betz P. Sudden death due to a haemoglobin variant. *Int J Legal Med.* 2004;118(2):95-97.

28. Wirthwein DP, Spotswood SD, Barnard JJ, Prahlow JA. Death due to microvascular occlusion in sickle-cell trait following physical exertion. *J Forensic Sci.* 2001;46(2): 399-401.

29. Monchanin G, Connes P, Wouassi D, et al. Hemorheology, sickle cell trait, and alpha-thalassemia in athletes: effects of exercise. *Med Sci Sports Exerc.* 2005;37(7):1086-1092.

30. Sara F, Hardy-Dessources MD, Voltaire B, Etienne-Julan M, Hue O. Lactic response in sickle cell trait carriers in comparison with subjects with normal hemoglobin. *Clin J Sport Med.* 2003;13(2):96-101.

31. Le Gallais D, Bile A, Mercier J, Paschel M, Tonellot JL, Dauverchain J. Exercise-induced death in sickle cell trait: role of aging, training, and deconditioning. *Med Sci Sports Exerc.* 1996;28(5):541-544.

32. Hedayati B, Anson KM, Patel U. Focal renal infarction: an unusual cause of haematuria in a patient with sickle cell trait. *Br J Radiol.* 2007;80(953):e105-e106.

33. Eichner ER. Sickle cell trait. *J Sport Rehabil.* 2007;16(3): 197-203.

34. Dowling MM. Sickle cell trait is not a risk factor for stroke. *Arch Neurol.* 2005;62(11):1780-1781.

35. Golomb MR. Sickle cell trait is a risk factor for early stroke. *Arch Neurol.* 2005;62(11):1778-1779.

CHAPTER 17

Gastrointestinal Conditions

Robert J. Baker

Gastrointestinal (GI) symptoms affect as many as 65% of long-distance runners.[1] Exercise-related complaints for young athletes can include abdominal pain "stitch in the side," diarrhea "runner's trots." Exercise-related ischemic colitis can lead to GI blood loss in young endurance athletes under extreme conditions. Constipation, gastroesophageal reflux, and gastroenteritis can affect young athletes. Traveler's diarrhea can affect young athletes that travel for competition. Exercise in can uncover underlying conditions such as irritable bowel syndrome or inflammatory bowel disease.

GASTROINTESTINAL PHYSIOLOGY

Exercise is associated with reduced gastric emptying, malabsorption of water and nutrients, delayed transit time, and a decrease in splanchnic blood flow. Although small bowel transit time may be decreased, there is no clear effect on overall gastrointestinal (GI) transit time. Esophageal peristalsis is altered by exercise, but there is no consensus of effect on motility (Table 17-1).

Gastric emptying has been shown to decrease with increasing intensity of activity. Gastric emptying is impeded by exercise intensity of greater than 70% VO_{2max}.[2] Consumption of a high-carbohydrate load (>7%) can slow gastric emptying as well.[2] Dehydration and hyperthermia will both further impair gastric emptying. Slowed gastric emptying may lead to symptoms such as nausea vomiting, reflux, heartburn, side ache, and chest pain.

A direct mechanical effect of exercise has been suggested. Muscle hypertrophy, for example, of the psoas muscle may alter GI motility directly.[3] The role of physical activity on motility is not clear. Only heavy activity may have an impact on motility. No significant change in motility has been found because of transmitted movements with running.[3] However, increased intra-abdominal pressures related to exertion of lifting and increased activity of the abdominal muscles can lead to reflux of gastric contents.

Overall, there is no change in small colon transit time or absorption related to exercise. Small bowel transit time and propulsion decline with increasing exercise intensity.[3] Exercise may have no effect on large bowel transit time. Therefore, it is likely that exercise has no overall effect on GI motility. One study showed small bowel and colonic transit times were similar in trained and sedentary subjects at the rest and with exercise. The diarrhea seen in this study did not result from accelerated colonic transit.[4] Small colon transit time has been shown to increase in some studies, decrease in other studies. No total reduction in absorption in spite of

Table 17-1.

Regional Physiologic GI Tract Effects of Exercise

Region	Physiologic Effect
Esophagus	Increased peristalsis
	Decreased lower esophageal sphincter tone
Stomach	Decreased gastric emptying
	Decreased blood flow
Small colon	Possible decreased transit
	Minimal decrease in absorption
	Decreased blood flow
Large colon	No change in transit time
	Decreased blood flow

decreased blood flow, is probably because of length of colon. Small colon distension may feedback to stomach to decrease emptying.

Sympathetic tone relaxes colon and decreases blood flow to the GI tract. Hormones such as catecholamines, secretin, glucagon, motilin, gastrin, beta-endorphin, and vasoactive intestinal peptide (VIP) are altered by exercise and play a role in GI motility.[3] Decreased splanchnic blood flow is the result of increased sympathetic tone. Visceral blood flow is therefore significantly impacted by exercise. Heavy exercise can decrease blood flow to the point of bowel ischemia. Hyperthermia can further increase the likelihood of GI ischemia. Dehydration can lead to even further stress and ischemia to the gut. Sympathetic tone is increased by hyperthermia, hypovolemia, hypoglycemia, and exhaustion. The GI tract is resilient to a decrease in blood flow of 75% up to 12 hours.[2] However, exercise can lead to ischemia, hypoxia, and hyperthermia leading to loss of functional integrity, necrosis, and increased permeability. There have been reported cases of ischemic colitis for triathletes under extreme conditions.

There is an evidence that training can improve gut functioning (Table 17-2).[2] The stomach has great ability to increase volume to accommodate larger intake. Gastric emptying can improve with training. There may be a "learning effect" of the stomach where athletes become accustomed to training with fluid in stomach. Endurance athletes have shown enhanced gastric emptying and GI transit time. Splanchnic blood flow improves with training. Further, loose stools often improve with adaptation to training. Rehydration with beverages of higher carbohydrate and electrolyte content will lead to GI symptoms because of delayed gastric emptying.

Table 17-2.

Training Recommendations for Improved GI Functioning

Acclimatize to improve visceral blood flow
Maintain hydration to avoid hypovolemia
Drink training to tolerance greater fluid intake without symptoms
Limit overeating prior to activity
Limit concentrated energy consumption immediately prior to activity
Days prior to participation ingest high-energy high-carbohydrate diet
Avoid high-fiber diet
Limit NSAIDs, alcohol, caffeine, antibiotics, and nutritional supplements
Urinate and defecate prior to exercise
Consult a physician, if GI symptoms persist

Endotoxins may play a role in exercise-related GI symptoms. With increased trauma, the mucosal barrier of the colon can be compromised in response to activity. Breakdown of the mucosa may allow entry of the lipopolysaccharide (LPS) from the cell wall of the normal bowel flora. The resulting endotoxemia may either directly or indirectly lead to GI complaints.[5]

Although scientific evidence for an ergogenic effect of probiotics is lacking, probiotics may provide athletes with secondary health benefits. Enhanced recovery from fatigue, improved immune function, and maintenance of healthy gastrointestinal tract function have been attributed to probiotics. They may also play a role in preventing GI conditions such as traveler's diarrhea. Improved GI function could positively affect athletic performance.[6]

ABDOMINAL PAIN OR "STITCH IN THE SIDE"

Definitions and Epidemiology

Localized pain in the abdomen associated with exercise may be referred to as the "stitch in the side" or exercise-related transient abdominal pain (ETAP). Abdominal pain is common in endurance athletes, especially runners. Surveys have reported that one-third of runners experience the stitch in the side.[7] This pain is most common among younger, possibly inexperienced, athletes. Incidence decreases with age. There appears to be no differences in incidence based on gender, but a majority of athletes experience the pain on the right side compared to the left.[7]

Pathogenesis

There is no direct evidence of the cause of exercise-related transient abdominal pain. Several hypotheses have been proposed. One of the most accepted theories is that hypoperfusion and ischemia of the viscera or diaphragm leads to pain. Direct, frequent jolting of the abdominal contents along with ischemia may lead to diaphragmatic spasm. Motion of the visceral organs during activity could lead to strain of peritoneal ligaments at the site of attachment to the diaphragm, leading to abdominal pain.[8] An exertional peritonitis from irritation and friction between the relatively mobile abdominal organs has been hypothesized as a cause for ETAP. Psychologic factors may also play a role.

Clinical Presentation

Affected athletes complain of abdominal pain often localized to the lateral aspect of the midabdomen. This pain may be described as sharp, stabbing, cramping, aching, or pulling. The intensity can vary from intense and severe to a mild annoyance. Symptoms are often worse when a meal is consumed just prior to activity.

Differential Diagnosis

Other conditions to consider include: splanchnic pain, renal colic, rib stress fracture, abdominal wall strain, and intestinal ischemia. Pain that localizes to the left upper quadrant would implicate the spleen as a source of pain. This could include enlargement of the spleen caused by infectious mononucleosis or splanchnic infarct. Acute pain in the flank could indicate renal colic possibly because of nephrolithiasis. Pain localized to the lower ribs at the attachment of muscle could indicate stress fracture of the rib. Stress fracture should be considered especially in rowers. Strain of congenital supernumery ligament of the abdominal wall has been reported in the literature.[8]

Diagnosis

The diagnosis is based on a detailed history and physical examination. Symptoms of ETAP classically occur only with activity. The physical examination is without findings in the office setting. New complaints that occur during exertion in an experienced, previously asymptomatic young athlete should raise concern. Absence of triggering factors such as trauma or dietary changes could suggest an underlying disorder.

Based on significant findings on physical examination, laboratory studies such as complete blood count, liver function tests, and pancreatic enzymes may assist in diagnosis of an underlying GI disorder. Abdominal ultrasound or CT scan can identify structural abnormalities of the internal organs or masses. Endoscopy may be necessary to identify upper or lower GI tract abnormalities. Rarely, exploratory laparoscopy may be necessary in the case of severe persistent abdominal pain.[9] All studies will be negative in athletes with ETAP.

Treatment

Lay literature is replete with anecdotal treatments for ETAP. There are no systematically studied treatments. Young athletes should avoid large meals just prior to activity, especially competitions. Fluid should be consumed regularly, but in small amounts. Techniques such as bending forward while tightening the abdominal muscle, breathing through pursed-lips or stopping activity, and raising the arms over the head have been suggested to relieve the stitch.[7] Some authors have recommended switching breathing patterns with running so that inhalation and exhalation occurs while striking alternating feet. A program to strengthen abdominal muscles may also relieve the symptoms on a long-term basis. Symptoms will resolve with discontinuation of activity, but most young athletes prefer to participate.

DISMOTILITY OR "RUNNER'S TROTS"

Diarrhea

Definitions and epidemiology

Diarrhea is defined as an increase in frequency and/or looser consistency of stools. This disorder of motility is often related to disorders of the lower GI tract. Runner's diarrhea, or "runner's trots" is a disorder related to increased motility of the lower GI tract. The prevalence of diarrhea reported among runners is 8% to 60% compared to 40% in control subjects.[10] Diarrhea is more common in runners than cyclists, swimmers, skaters, or skiers. The mechanisms of this disorder are not clearly understood.

Pathogenesis

Diarrhea is most often associated with gastroenteritis, which is usually caused by a viral infection. Strenuous exercise may not have a net effect on bowel motility. Meals high in fat, protein, and fiber taken prior to exercise can worsen symptoms. Regional decrease in blood flow may cause ischemia leading to GI bleeding and diarrhea. This may only be of significance for ultraendurance athletes under extreme environmental conditions. Mechanical stimulation of the intestinal mucosa during running may result in a release of vasoactive intestinal peptide (VIP) and prostaglandins, which promote colonic contraction and could cause abdominal cramps and secretory diarrhea.[3] Underlying bowel pathology may be uncovered in young athletes.

Clinical presentation

The increased frequency or loose consistency of stool may be associated with other symptoms such as cramping and urgency. These symptoms most often accompany infectious causes of diarrhea, but rarely are associated with runner's diarrhea. Symptoms often increase with increasing exercise intensity. Symptoms may also occur only with competition and not training and bowel function is normal at other times.

Differential diagnosis

Acute onset diarrhea is often infectious in nature. Chronic diarrhea may be caused by irritable bowel syndrome or inflammatory bowel syndrome as well. Runner's diarrhea is a diagnosis of exclusion.

Diagnosis

The diagnosis is commonly made based on history. Stool studies for ova, parasites, *Clostridium difficile* antigen, stool culture, Gram's stain, as well as cell counts can identify an infectious cause. These studies are often negative in runner's diarrhea. Because dehydration is a common complication for athletes with diarrhea, the clinician should evaluate the athlete's risk. Diarrhea is a contraindication for participation in physical activity. Occasionally, colonoscopy may be indicated to rule out serious causes of diarrhea.

Treatment

The athlete with diarrhea should be fully evaluated to rule out treatable causes of diarrhea. Often, young athletes may experience infectious diarrhea. Infectious causes may require specific treatment with antibiotics or, as in many cases, may simply run its course and resolve on its own. Generally, supportive care is all that is required. Fluid replacement to prevent dehydration is the initial treatment. The athlete should avoid caffeine as well as high fat, high-protein meals prior to activity.[1] A low-fiber liquid diet may decrease symptoms on days of competition. An antidiarrheal such as lopermide or bismuth subsalicylate may help slow bowel motility. During acute episodes, physical activity should be strictly limited if not curtailed totally.

Constipation

Definitions and epidemiology

Constipation is marked by the infrequent passage of dry hard stools or straining on defecation. Frequency of bowel movements in the adult population ranges from three bowel movements per day to three bowel movements per week. Between 1 and 5 years, one to two bowel movements per day is normal.[11]

Pathogenesis

Overall, exercise may have no effect on GI transit times. While some young athletes may experience frequent loose stools, others may experience infrequent or hard stools. Exercise can slow transit time of the small bowel. Participation in extreme conditions of heat can result in dehydration and hypokalemia leading to constipation. Hemorrhoids experienced by weight lifters could result in avoidance of defecation.

Clinical presentation

The young athlete may present with an acute onset of change in frequency of stool. This may be associated with poorly localized abdominal pain, spasm, distention, or tenesmus. Occasionally, there may also be vomiting and decreased flatus. Children may experience encopresis. On physical examination, digital rectal examination should show normal rectal tone usually with hard stool present. However, the rectum may be empty. Bowel sounds should be normal though frequency may be decreased. Abdominal distention or peritoneal signs are not necessarily seen with constipation and may be an evidence of a more serious abdominal condition is present.

Differential diagnosis

Colonic disorders such as intussusception, inflammatory bowel disease, diverticulum, bowel obstruction, and irritable bowel may present with constipation. Other systemic conditions such as hypothyroidism, Addison's disease, Cushing's syndrome, diabetes, and hypercalcemia may need to be ruled out. Hirschsprung's disease may present as constipation, though often in younger children. The athlete should be questioned regarding use of antiacids, opiates, iron supplements, anticholinergics, and antispasmotics.

Diagnosis

Specific laboratory testing for constipation is not necessary. However, further evaluation may be necessary to rule out other causes of constipation. Complete blood counts may indicate inflammatory process. Electrolyte studies will identify hypokalemia or hypercalcemia. Thyroid function studies would be appropriate for athletes with symptoms consistent with hypothyroidism. Abdominal films may show large amounts of stool in the colon. These films may help rule out tumor or obstruction.

Treatment

Rarely will symptom be severe enough to require hospital admission. The initial treatment is to clear the bowel then maintain motility while attempting behavior modification. Enemas or suppositories can be used to clear the bowel. Once the bowel is clear, the athlete should be encouraged to increase fluids and fiber in diet. Stool softeners can help maintain colon clearance; any constipating medications should be stopped. The athlete should be warned to avoid persistent use of laxatives. The young athlete can gradually return to activity. Medical supervision may be necessary to monitor for return of symptoms.

Irritable Bowel Syndrome

There is minimal data regarding participation and young athletes with irritable bowel syndrome (IBS). A study showed participation in physical activity is associated with less fatigue for female with IBS. Females with irritable bowel were less likely to be active.[5] In general, athletes with IBS can participate to their tolerance. Dehydration because of vomiting or diarrhea would be the one exception.

Inflammatory Bowel Disease

As with IBS, there is a minimal evidence regarding inflammatory bowel disease (IBD) and exercise in young athletes. Patients with Crohn's disease have been shown to tolerate low-intensity training without a flare. Strenuous activity should be avoided during time of exacerbation. Young athletes with IBD may be at higher risk of dehydration, electrolyte deficiency, vitamin deficiency, and blood loss, especially at time of flare. A low-intensity walking program may have a beneficial effect in patients with Crohn's disease and improve their quality of life with no exacerbations in disease symptoms.[12]

Gastroesophageal Reflux Disease (GERD)

Definitions and epidemiology

Gastroesophageal reflux (GERD) occurs when stomach contents is regurgitated across the lower esophageal sphinter. Prevalence in general increases with increasing age. GERD is fairly common even in young athletes, though not often performance limiting. This is often referred to as "exertional heartburn." Even in conditioned athletes, strenuous exercise induces significant reflux and related symptoms of GERD.[13]

Pathogenesis

Physically active individuals tend to have greater relaxation of the lower esophageal sphincter compared to their sedentary counterparts. High-intensity exercise can lead to a decrease in upper GI motility. This is thought to result in increased gastric contents. Relative ischemia of the bowel may contribute to decreased sphincter tone and possibly interfere with protective luminal function of the gastric wall. In addition, contraction of the abdominal wall associated with intense exercise will increase intra-abdominal pressure.[3] These two factors then would result in greater pressure across the lower esophageal sphincter and likely resulting in reflux of stomach contents and acid. It has been hypothesized that increased breathing related to intense exercise could result in increased air trapping in the stomach. This would further increase pressure across the lower esophageal sphincter.

Clinical presentation

As the stomach contents along with acids are refluxed into the esophagus, many symptoms may be associated with GERD. Because the acid is irritating to the esophageal mucosa, a burning type pain or "heartburn" is often associated with this disease. The acid can lead to foul taste, foul-smelling breath, sore throat, and difficulties swallowing. Aspiration of even small amounts can result in reactive airway disease resulting in wheezing and cough. In fact, GERD can be a major contributor to worsening symptoms in young athletes with asthma.

Differential diagnosis

The symptoms of GERD, heartburn difficulty swallowing, and breathing could be related to more serious conditions of the cardiac or pulmonary systems. Poorly controlled asthma can result in increased abdominal muscle work as well as increased abdominal pressures, which in turn can worsen GERD. A gastric ulcer, peptic ulcer, or gastritis from infection or chemical cause can result in the same symptoms of GERD. Even many young athletes will take NSAIDs for musculoskeletal injuries. While these medications are considered to be safe as over the counter medications, even low doses can result in gastritis and even ulcers. Chronic reflux can lead to damage of the lower esophagus including esophagitis, stricture, or pathologic mucosal changes known as Barrett's esophagitis.

Diagnosis

The diagnosis is commonly made based on symptoms. Placement of a pH probe in the lower esophagus is rarely needed to make the diagnosis if conservative treatment fails. Significant signs such as weight loss, persistent regurgitation, hematemesis, and hematochezia are indications for upper endoscopic study. If the primary feature is difficulty swallowing, upper GI barium contrast study may identify other causes of dysmotility.

Treatment

Treatment initially is supportive with antacids, acid blockers, and specific food avoidance. Avoiding caffeine, peppermint, high fat, and high-calorie foods, which tend to decrease lower esophageal sphincter tone will help. Smoking also decreases sphincter tone and should be discouraged. Many medications for heartburn are available over the counter and young athletes may have already tried these previously. However, the over the counter acids blockers are generally half strength, so the athlete can try doubling the dose. Decreasing the intensity of exercise remains an option though most athletes are not compliant with this recommendation.

Gastrointestinal Bleeding

Definitions and epidemiology

Gastrointestinal bleeding has been known to occur in athletes. This bleeding is generally not significant enough to cause major problems. Athletes in higher intensity activities such as marathon triathalon, ironman, and ultramarathon are at greatest risk. Occult blood has been detected in up to 87% of participants of endurance events.[14] Hematochezia has been noted in

Treatment

Priority of treatment is fluid replacement. Oral rehydration with a mixture of water, sodium chloride, potassium chloride, glucose, and bicarbonate is preferred. Although the diarrhea is self-limited, antibiotic may be necessary if the athlete experiences severe diarrhea, fever, or bloody stools, and they can shorten the duration of disease by 1 day.[16] Azithromycin is the best antibiotic choice for children. Antimotility agents such as loperamide can lend symptom relief. Prophylactic antibiotic use is not recommended because of increased risk of resistance. Probiotics may reduce the risk of traveler's diarrhea.[16] Participation should be limited, if there are any signs of dehydration.

REFERENCES

1. Simmons SM, Kennedy RG. Gastrointestinal problems in runners. *Curr Sports Med Rep.* 2004;3:112-116.
2. Murray R. Training the gut for competition. *Curr Sports Med Rep.* 2006;5:161-164.
3. Paluska SA. Gastrointestinal system. In: McKeag DB, Moeller J, eds. *ACSM's Primary Care Sports Medicine.* 2nd ed. Philadephia, PA: Lippincott Williams & Wilkins; 2007:173-184.
4. Rao KA, Yazaki E, Evans DF, Carbon R. Objective evaluation of small bowel and colonic transit time using pH telemetry in athletes with gastrointestinal symptoms. *Br J Sports Med.* 2004;38:482-487.
5. Casey E, Mistry DJ, MacKnight JM. Training room management of medical conditions: sports gastroenterology. *Clin Sports Med.* 2005;24:525-540.
6. Nichols AW. Probiotics and athletic performance: a systematic review. *Curr Sports Med Rep.* 2007;6:269-273.
7. Eichner ER. Stitch in the side: causes, workup, and solutions. *Curr Sports Med Rep.* 2006;5:289-292.
8. Dimeo FC, Peters J, Guderian H. Abdominal pain in long distance runners: case report and analysis of the literature. *Br J Sports Med.* 2004;38:e24.
9. Dimeff RJ. Abdominal pain in a cross country runner. *Curr Sports Med Rep.* 2004;3:189-191.
10. Harmon K. Exercise-induced diarrhea. In: Bracker MD, ed. *The 5-Minute Sports Medicine Consult.* Philadelphia, PA: Lippincott Williams & Wilkins; 2001:416-417.
11. Best A. Constipation. In: Bracker MD, ed. *The 5-Minute Sports Medicine Consult.* Philadephia, PA: Lippincott Williams & Wilkins; 2001:398-399.
12. Ng V, Millard W, Lebrun C, Howard J. Low-intensity exercise improves quality of life in patients with crohn's disease. *Clin J Sport Med.* 2007;17:384-388.
13. Collings KL, Pratt FP, Rodriguez-Stanley S, Bemben M, Miner P. Esophageal reflux in conditioned runners, cyclists, and weightlifters. *Med Sci Sports Exerc.* 2003; 35(5):730-735.
14. Moses FM. Exercise-associated intestinal ischemia. *Curr Sports Med Rep.* 2005;4:91-95.
15. Nasr I. Gastroenteritis. In: Bracker MD, ed. *The 5-Minute Sports Medicine Consul.* Philadephia, PA: Lippincott Williams & Wilkins; 2001:428-429.
16. Boggess BR. Gastrointestinal infections in the traveling athlete. *Curr Sports Med Rep.* 2007;6:125-129.

CHAPTER 18

Infectious and Dermatologic Conditions

Dilip R. Patel, Ashir Kumar, and Cynthia Feucht

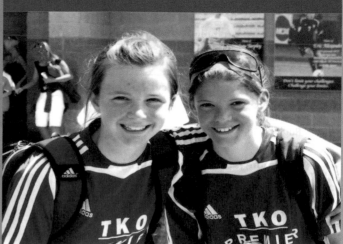

DEFINITIONS AND EPIDEMIOLOGY

A number of common contagious diseases (Table 18-1) have special significance in the athletic setting. For the athletes, this may mean not being able to continue participation, subpar performance, or risk of potentially serious complications as a result of continued physical stress.

Sports in which outbreaks or clusters of contagious diseases have been reported are listed in Table 18-2.[1] Infections in the athletic settings can be transmitted via either person-to-person spread or common-source spread (Table 18-3).[1-6] The most common infection transmitted by direct contact is *Herpes simplex virus* infection among wrestlers and rugby players. Outbreaks associated with person-to-person spread have also been caused by *Staphylococcus aureus*, Group A *Streptococci*, and fungi and involve participation in wrestling, basketball, football, rugby, and orienteering.[2] The most frequently reported common-source infections are owing to enteroviruses. Outbreaks of aseptic meningitis and pleurodynia have been documented in football and soccer players associated with oral contamination of shared water sources and drinking containers.[2] Most cases of aseptic meningitis are caused by echoviruses (types 5, 9, 16, 24) and Coxsackie viruses (types B1, B2, B4, B5) from sharing of common contaminated source of drinking water.[1,5] Epidemics of measles among athletes and spectators have been reported, spread by air-borne droplets in crowded confined environments in basketball, wrestling, and other sports necessitating mass immunizations and relocation or cancellation of events.[3]

Table 18 -1.

Common Contagious Diseases in Athletic Setting

Upper respiratory tract infections
Systemic viral illnesses
Acute viral syndrome
Infectious mononucleosis
Human immunodeficiency virus infection
Hepatitis B virus infection
Influenza A infection
Measles
Hepatitis A infection

Skin and soft tissue infections
Bacterial
Impetigo
Folliculitis, furuncles, carbuncles
Methicillin resistant staphylococcal aureus infections
Hidradenitis suppurativa
Viral
Herpes simplex virus
Herpes zoster
Warts
Molluscum contagiosum
Fungal
Tinea corporis, pedis, capitis
Zoonosis
Pediculosis
Scabies

Other infectious illnesses
Enteric pathogens
Otitis externa
Conjunctivitis
Streptococcal pharyngitis
Sexually transmitted infections
Tuberculosis

Table 18-9.

General Guidelines for Sport Participation by Athletes with Skin Infections*

Before participation in contact sports all athletes must be examined for any skin lesions, including the pubic area, and scalp.

The presence of a communicable skin disease is sufficient reason for disqualification in wrestling.

Open wounds and skin conditions that cannot be adequately covered are considered a cause for disqualification from practice or competition in contact sports.

All equipment, mats, and shared common areas, such as locker rooms should be routinely cleaned.

The athlete who has infectious skin disease (boils, herpes, impetigo, scabies, molluscum), while contagious, not participate in gymnastics with mats, martial arts, or other collision/contact or limited contact sports.

*Based on NCAA, NFSHA, AAP.

Splenomegaly occurs in 50% to 75% of cases of infectious mononucleosis.[27,29] The enlarged speen is more prone to rupture; however, this is a rare complication with an estimated prevalence of less than 0.2%.[4,37–39] Splenic rupture is most likely between day 4 and 21 of the illness.[39,40] Most ruptures have been reported to occur during nonathletic activity such as defecating and lifting, or spontaneously without any trauma. The athletes should refrain from all types of strenuous physical activity and contact sports, until complete clinical resolution of the illness and return of the spleen to normal size.[40] It is generally recommended that the athletes not return to sports for at least 4 weeks from the onset of the illness. The spleen can be assessed by either palpation or ultrasonography or MRI scans. There is no clear consensus as to when one should obtain imaging studies to assess splenomegaly. In most cases, the baseline or preillness size of the spleen is not known and this may be a confounding factor in determining the resolution of splenomegaly based on imaging of the spleen.[39,40] The athlete should return to activity with gradually increasing intensity and duration over a period of several weeks to months. There is generally a prolonged period of 3 months or more before the athlete may reach his or her optimal preillness performance level.

Human Immunodeficiency Virus Infection

HIV infection is transmitted via blood and blood products, semen, vaginal and cervical secretions, breast milk,

Table 18-10.

Guidelines for Minimizing the Risk of Transmission of Blood-Borne Infections in Athletic Settings

1. Athletes should be examined prior to competition or practice to assess any wounds or weeping or open lesions. These wounds and lesions must be cleaned, and securely covered with an occlusive dressing.
2. Team physicians, athletic trainers, and others involved in taking care of the athletes should have any similar wounds appropriately covered.
3. Appropriate equipment and supplies should be readily available to implement universal precautions: These include gloves, disinfectants and antiseptics, containers for soiled equipments and uniforms, bandages and dressings, and a container for proper disposal of sharps.
4. An injured athlete with a bleeding wound should be immediately identified during a competition or practice session.
5. Athletes should be educated about the significance and responsibility of reporting any bleeding injury to the officials immediately. Recognition of the bleeding athlete is also the responsibility of the officials, and medical personnel.
6. Bleeding athlete should be removed from the game or practice for evaluation and treatment. The wound should be assessed for severity and first aid care initiated to control bleeding. Prior to the athlete returning to participation, the bleeding must have stopped and the wound been securely covered with an occlusive dressing.
7. The uniform must be changed, if contaminated with blood. It should be appropriately disposed of and laundered. Some experts suggest that minor blood stains may not require a change of uniform and interruption of the game.
8. Life-threatening injuries should receive appropriate emergency care and treatment not delayed for fear of contaminated blood. Gloves and pocket masks should be used. Universal precautions should be followed when handling blood or body fluids.
9. Blood on the skin of the injured athlete and other participants must be washed with soap and water.
10. Athletic equipment surfaces or environments contaminated with blood must be cleaned thoroughly with household bleach (1 part bleach to 10 parts of water prepared fresh daily). Any spill must first be contained in as small an area as possible using absorptive material.
11. Needles, scalpels, and other sharps must be appropriately disposed of in designated containers.
12. Athletes should shower thoroughly after each practice or game. All surfaces and equipment must be cleaned with disinfectant and uniforms should be bagged and laundered.
13. If blood or body fluids are transmitted from injured athlete to another athlete, the game or practice must be stopped, the skin of the athlete must cleaned with antimicrobial wipes, and washed with soap and water.
14. Any contaminated linens must be washed at the end of the competition with hot water at 160°F (71°C) for 25-min cycles.

Table 18-11.

Treatment Guidelines That Suggest Minimum Treatment Before Return to Wrestling*

Infection	Minimum Treatment Before Return to Wrestling
Bacterial skin diseases (non CA-MRSA)	All lesions scabbed over. No oozing or discharge. No new lesions for preceding 48 h. 3 d of appropriate oral antibiotics.
CA-MRSA skin lesions	All lesions scabbed over. No oozing or discharge. No new lesions for preceding 48 h. 14 d of appropriate oral antibiotics.
Primary herpes	All lesions scabbed over. No oozing or discharge. No new lesions for preceding 48 h. 10 d of appropriate oral antiviral medications.
Recurrent herpes	All lesions scabbed over. No oozing or discharge. No new lesions for preceding 48 h. Full 5 d or 120 h of appropriate oral antiviral medications.
Primary herpes with constitutional or systemic signs and symptoms	All lesions scabbed over. No oozing or discharge. No new lesions for preceding 48 h. 14 d of appropriate oral antiviral medications
Molluscum contagiosum	24 h after curettage of all lesions
Tinea corporis	3 d of appropriate oral or topical antifungal medication
Tinea capitis	14 d of appropriate oral antifungal medication
Bacterial conjunctivitis	24 h of topical or oral antibiotic and no eye discharge
Scabies	24 h after appropriate topical treatment
Pediculosis	

*Based on National Federation of State High School Associations Guidelines, 2007.

and amniotic fluid but is not known to be transmitted via tears, saliva, sweat, urine, sputum, and respiratory droplets.[7,27–29] It is not acquired by hand shaking, swimming pool or communal bath water, toilet seats, food, or drinking water. In the athletic environment, it is not known to be spread via contact with potentially contaminated surfaces such as wrestling mats, taping, tables, sinks, or other surfaces.[28,29] Mast, et al. have noted that for successful transmission of HIV in athletes, there must be an infected athlete with an open bleeding wound, and a susceptible individual with exposed skin lesions or a mucous membrane that could serve as a portal of entry; and sustained contact between the infective material and the portal of entry.[29] The athlete is more likely to acquire HIV infection in nonathletic activity such as unprotected sex and via IV or IM injections of illicit drugs or anabolic steroids using shared needles.[29,30]

The risk for the athlete of contracting HIV infection during sports is extremely low. A theoretical risk of acquiring HIV during contact/collision sports exists in which there is more likelihood of sustaining bleeding injuries, for example, ice hockey, karate, and football. The overall risk of HIV transmission in professional football was estimated to be 1/85 million game contacts in one study.[30] The HIV+ athletes will benefit from continued participation in sports and exercise and studies suggest enhanced immune function and a sense of mental well being from exercising by HIV+ persons.[22] Immune function may also be adversely affected by strenuous physical exertion in the HIV+ athletes as it would in other athletes. Thus, an HIV+ athlete who is asymptomatic can participate in all activities. The risk of infection to the team physician and other medical personnel working with HIV+ athletes is minimal and considered similar to that of a health provider in the health care setting in general.

Major sports medicine organizations and sports governing bodies have promulgated recommendations addressing sport participation by HIV+ athletes.[27,28,41–43] It is generally agreed that an HIV+ athletes be allowed to participate in all sports, and that routine testing of asymptomatic athletes is not recommended. It is recommended that physicians let the HIV+ athletes who want to participate in contact sports know of the theoretical risk of transmission to others and strongly encourage consideration of noncontact sport.[42] The team physician should advise all athletes of the possibility that there may be an HIV+ athlete among participants but must maintain confidentiality and not disclose the athlete's HIV+ status to others. There have been instances where courts have allowed exclusion of an HIV+ athlete from contact sports to avoid exposure to other participants if reasonable accommodations will not eliminate such a risk but legally an HIV+ athlete cannot be excluded from participation solely on the basis of his or her HIV status.[44]

Major professional medical societies and sports governing bodies have published general guidelines to minimize the risk of transmission of infection by contact with blood or other body fluids. These are based on a common sense approach emphasizing good hygienic practices and standard precautions. Major elements taken from guidelines published by the National Collegiate Athletic Association (NCAA), AAP, Canadian Academy of Sports Medicine, American College of Physicians, and American Medical Society for Sport Medicine are summarized in Table 18-10.[27,28,41–43]

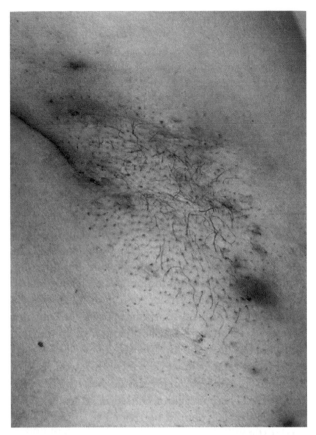

FIGURE 18-5 ■ Hidradenitis suppurativa. (With permission from Fitzpatrick's Color Atlas and Synopsis of Clinical Dermatology. 5th ed. New York: McGraw Hill Medical; 2005.)

cause the common wart (verruca vulgaris), plantar wart, flat wart, and genital wart (condyloma acuminata). Transmission occurs via direct skin-to-skin contact, autoinoculation, and by contact with contaminated fomites. Because the virions are most abundant early in the course of infection, the lesions are most contagious at this stage and infection is most commonly seen adolescents.

Plantar warts tend to be the most painful and disabling for the athlete. Infection can be acquired from contaminated mats, equipment, and clothing. Because, calluses are more susceptible to infection than normal skin, gymnasts, football players, and wrestlers are commonly affected. Swimming in public pools also seems to be a contributing factor for plantar warts. Spontaneous resolution is common in healthy athletes, in 6 months to 2 years, and only a few persist over 5 years. Since, the presence of warts may result in disqualification of the athletes from contact sports such as wrestling, treatment is warranted in many athletes. Its aim is to destroy the lesions by various methods (Table 18-4). Salicylic acid paint or plaster, or cryotherapies are the most preferred modes of treatment for common and plantar warts. The lesions must be completely and securely covered before participation in contact sports

is allowed. If lesions are extensive and cannot be covered adequately, the athletes may not be allowed to participate in contact sports.

Molluscum Contagiosum

Molluscum contagiosum is caused by a poxvirus. The lesions are highly contagious and spread by direct contact, contaminated fomites, or autoinoculation. The infection is transmitted by person-to-person contact, in gyms and swimming pools, and is common in swimmers and wrestlers. Lesions are benign and in most cases resolve spontaneously over 6 to 9 months. Curettage is curative. Topical application of cantharidin 0.7%, salicylic or lactic acid application, or tretinoin 0.025%, may be also be effective. Cryotherapy with liquid nitrogen applied directly to lesions has also been used. A lesion free period of approximately 4 months is generally considered an evidence of cure.

Herpes Simplex Virus

Herpes simplex virus (HSV) type 1 is the cause of herpes gladiatorum reported in wrestlers and scrum pox in rugby. The infection is highly contagious and spreads via direct contact with infected lesions. Transmission via fomites is questionable but HSV can be transmitted by the saliva of asymptomatic athletes. Systemic antiviral treatment initiated early (within 6 days of onset) in the course of the infection may diminish the acuity and duration of the infection. For adolescents and adults, acyclovir, famciclovir, and valacyclovir can be used. If there is inadequate response to this treatment or there is involvement of the eyes, infectious disease, and ophthalmology, consultations should be considered. Those with a history of severe recurrent herpes labialis or gladiatorum should be considered for daily suppressive therapy.

Fungal Infections

Infection of the skin, nails, and hair is caused by various dermatophytes. Fungal infections of the skin are common because of the presence of increased moisture from sweat, occlusive footwear, shared towels, contaminated locker room floors, and breakdown of skin. Superficial fungal infections are spread by direct contact, fomites, and autoinoculation.

Tinea pedis (athlete's foot), affecting the feet, is the most common fungal infection of skin among athletes. A dermatophid or id reaction often occurs with athlete's foot, appearing as dyshidrotic eczema with pruritic vesicles or annular plaques on the hands. Therefore, if dermatitis on the hands is recognized, the feet should be examined carefully. Tinea unguium (onychomycosis) can be associated with tinea pedis. Affected nails, left untreated, may become yellow, opaque, thick, and brittle.

Tinea cruris (jock itch) occurs more frequently in men and during warm weather when the groin area is kept warm and moist for prolonged periods of time. Lesions tend to be bilateral and on the medial and upper part of the thighs as well as the pubic area. The penis and scrotum are usually spared of lesions. Tinea corporis (ringworm of the body) can occur on any part of the body and outbreaks have been reported in wrestling.

Tinea capitis (ringworm of the scalp) and barbae are transmitted via direct contact and by sharing of hats, caps, combs, brushed, or shaving razors. Infection of the skin generally responds well to topical antifungal treatment, whereas infection of the hair shaft and nails typically require systemic antifungal (Table 18-6).

Before allowing a wrestler to participate, the athlete must be on topical treatment for at least 3 days for skin lesions and 2 weeks of systemic treatment for scalp lesions. Lesions should be covered. Wrestlers with extensive and active lesions may not be allowed to participate.

Pediculosis

Pediculosis is caused by *Pediculus humanus* and the infestation primarily affects the head (pediculosis capitis) or the body (pediculosis corporis). In the genital area, (pediculosis pubis) it is caused by *Phthirus pubis* and is known as crabs. Crowded conditions are most conducive to transmission of the infestations via person-to-person contact, including sharing of hairbrushes, caps, or clothes. In general, a good hygienic routine should be followed, clothing and bedding changed, laundered, and dried in hot temperatures. Contacts should be examined. Pediculosis is treated by topical application of permethrin 1% cream rinse (Nix[R]) for 10 minutes and may repeat in 7 days; or pyrethrin shampoo (RID[R]) or 1% lindane (Kwell[R]) shampoo which are used similarly. The athlete must have received complete treatment and be examined for evidence of cure before allowing participation in contact sports.[24]

Scabies

Scabies is caused by the human mite, *Sarcoptes scabiei.* Transmission requires direct human contact; occasionally, female mites survive 2 to 3 days in fomites and may transmit the infestation. Scabies is highly contagious, and can be spread by casual contact. Humans are the only reservoirs of *Sarcoptes scabies.* Close contacts should be treated and clothes and bedding changed and laundered thoroughly. Topical application of 5% permethrin (Elimite[R]) for 8 to 14 hours, lindane lotion 1% (Kwell[R], Scabene[R]) for 8 to 12 hours, or crotamiton 10% (Eurax[R]) for 48 hours are effective.

OTHER INFECTIOUS ILLNESSES

Enteric Pathogens

Enteroviral infections are spread via oral–oral and fecal–oral routes. Epidemics are commonly seen during the summer and fall with a high-attack rate and may present with a variety of syndromes that can affect almost any system of the body. The health care practitioner taking care of young athletes must be especially aware of the hand, foot, and mouth syndrome of vesicular lesions caused by enteroviruses. The Norwalk virus, rotaviruses, and bacterial infections by *Salmonella, Shigella, Campylobacter, Yersinia,* and *E. coli* (traveler's diarrhea) also are common causes of diarrhea. Person-to-person and common source spread is known to occur in the athletic setting. Symptomatic individuals with bacterial gastroenteritis are highly contagious. Athletes should avoid potentially contaminated food, water, and ice, and wash hands thoroughly. Their continued participation in sports is generally guided by clinical resolution and well-being.

Otitis Externa

Also commonly known as swimmer's ear, because of its association with water sports and common occurrence in swimmers, otitis externa is primarily a result of sustained retention of moisture in the ear canal.[50] Cerumen normally acts as a water repellent, but frequent use of ear drops and cleaning results in its loss, and infection most commonly with *Pseudomonas aeruginosa.* Poorly chlorinated water has been implicated in an outbreak of otitis externa. The degree of head submersion is also an important factor, the condition being seen more often in divers than swimmers. The athlete should avoid frequent cleaning and use of ear drops and keep the ear canals dry by keeping water out. Otitis externa is effectively treated with topical use of Vosol[R] 2% solution or ciprofloxacin or corticosporin otic drops for 5 days. Ideally, the athlete should abstain from water sports until acute infection is resolved; but in practice, return to competition is allowed within 3 days of starting the treatment.

Conjunctivitis

Infectious conjunctivitis can be caused by viruses or bacteria. Infection is spread via direct contact or contaminated hands leading to autoinoculation. Respiratory spread can also occur from droplets. A bacterial etiology is uncommon after 5 years of age and viruses are the predominant cause of conjunctivitis. Nonetheless, any athlete with conjunctivitis is considered contagious until symptoms have resolved. On occasion, it is difficult to differentiate self-limited viral infection from bacterial conjunctivitis, which should be treated with appropriate topical antibiotics. Sports participation may be allowed after 24 hours of treatment. The spread of pathogens can be minimized by regular hand washing and proper disposal of fomites. Bacterial conjunctivitis is treated effectively with erythromycin, gentamicin, or other ophthalmologic antibiotic preparations used daily for approximately 5 days.

Streptococcal Pharyngitis

Streptococcal pharyngitis caused by group A Beta-hemolytic streptococci (*Streptococcus pyogenes)* and is spread by contact with a person who has pharyngeal streptococcal infection. Transmission of GABHS infection, including major outbreaks, can occur in schools, colleges, and athletic teams, via respiratory secretions. Patients are not contagious after 24 hours of specific antimicrobial treatment. Droplet precautions are recommended during the first 24 hours of therapy. Thus participation in activities with a potential for droplet spread should be restricted till 1 day of appropriate treatment has been given. Streptococcal pharyngitis is effectively treated with oral penicillin V or amoxicillin daily for 10 days.

Sexually Transmitted Infections

Sexually transmitted infections including HIV and HBV infections can occur in athletes as well as nonathletes. All athletes should be educated and provided information about transmission during unprotected sex and abstinence must be discussed. Recommendations should also be made regarding condom use. These diseases are acquired during travel and leisure time activities by athletes but whether this group as a whole engages in more high-risk health behavior compared to nonathletes in general remains controversial.

Tuberculosis

There has been an increase in the incidence of tuberculosis in recent years in some groups and we must maintain vigilance to contain its spread. Pulmonary tuberculosis caused by *Mycobacterium tuberculosis* is an airborne infection. The adolescent or the adult with the infection can spread it via air droplets. Children younger than 12 years of age are not usually contagious because their pulmonary lesions are small, and cough and expulsion of bacilli is minimal. Adolescent athletes should be tested for tuberculosis, if they are in a high-risk group, and appropriate evaluation and treatment initiated. The majority of adult and adolescent patients are noncontagious after a few weeks of treatment and their continued participation in sports depends on their overall well being since no specific recommendations are available.

Table 18-14.

Noninfectious Dermatologic Conditions

Inflammatory
Contact dermatitis

Traumatic
Calluses, corns, blisters
Abrasions (turf burn, mat burn, raspberry etc)
Acne mechanica (occlusive folliculitis) (Figure 18–6)
Benign nodules (e.g., skate bites, surfer nodules, Nike nodules)
Piezogenic pedal papules (Figure 18–7)
Subungual hematoma (jogger's nails/toe, skier's toe, tennis toe etc)
Jogger's nipples
Talon noire (black heel) (Figure 18–8)
Mogul's palms

Related to environmental exposure
Cold-related conditions e.g., frost bite
Heat-related conditions e.g., sunburns
Green hair

NONINFECTIOUS DERMATOLOGIC CONDITIONS

A number of noninfectious skin conditions seen in athletes should be distinguished from infectious lesions to plan appropriate treatment. These conditions can be inflammatory, traumatic, or related to environmental exposure (Table 18-14).[45,46]

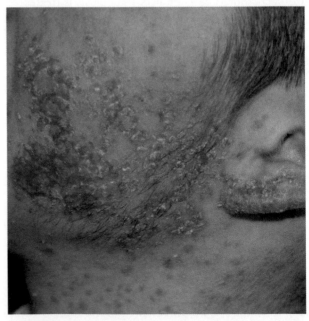

FIGURE 18-6 ■ Acne mechanica is characterized by inflammatory skin lesions in areas of friction, pressure, and sweating because of sports uniforms, padding, and equipment.

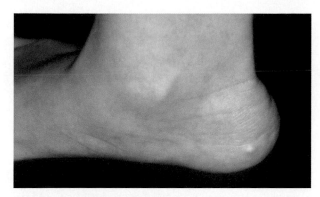

FIGURE 18-7 ■ Piezogenic pedal papules are benign lesions that represent extruded subcutaneous fat resulting from localized repetitive trauma. Similar lesions can be seen in children with certain genetic conditions such as Ehlers-Danlos syndrome.

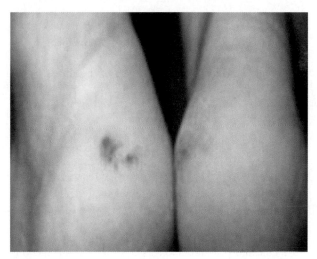

FIGURE 18-8 ■ Talon noir or black heel represents areas of subcutaneous bleeding from capillaries because of significant repetitive friction, pressure, and shearing forces applied locally in various sport activities.

ACKNOWLEDGEMENT

This chapter is partly adapted from author's previous work, Patel DR, Gordon RC. Contagious diseases in athletes. Contemporary Pediatrics 1999;16(9):139-164.

REFERENCES

1. Tuberville SD, Cowan LD, Greenfield RA. Infectious disease outbreaks in competitive sports: a review of literature. *Am J Sports Med.* 2006;34(11):1860-1865.
2. Goodman RA, Thacker SB, Solomon SL, Osterholm MT, Hughes JM. Infectious diseases in competitive sports. *JAMA.* 1994;271:862.
3. Mast ER, Goodman RA. Prevention of infectious disease transmission in sports. *Sports Med.* 1997;24:1.
4. Sevier TL. Infectious diseases in athletes. *Med Clin N Am.* 1994;78:389.
5. Hughes WT. The Athlete: an immunocompromised host. In: Aronoff SC, Hughes WT, Kohl S, Wald ER, eds. *Advances in Pediatric Infectious Diseases.* vol 13. St. Louis: Mosby-Yearbook; 1996:79-99.
6. Sharp JCM. Infections in sport. *BMJ.* 1994;308:1702.
7. American Academy of Pediatrics Committee on Infectious Diseases Report. *Red Book.* 27th ed. Elk Grove Village, IL: American Academy of Pediatrics; 2006,
8. Nieman DC. Exercise immunology: practical applications. *Int J Sports Med.* 1997;18(suppl. 1):S91.
9. Peters EM. Exercise, immunology and upper respiratory tract infections. *Int J Sports Med.* 1997;18(suppl. 1):S69.
10. Weidner TG. Literature review: upper respiratory illness and sport and exercise. *Int J Sports Med.* 1994;15:1.
11. Brenner IKM, Shek NP, Shephard RJ. Infections in athletes. *Sports Med.* 1994;17:86.
12. Metz JP. Upper respiratory tract infections: who plays, who sits? *Curr Sports Med Rep.* 2003;2:84-90.
13. Council on Sports Medicine and Fitness. American academy of pediatrics. Medical conditions affecting sports participation. *Pediatrics.* 2008;121:841-848.
14. Drug Facts & Comparisons [database on the Internet]. Indianapolis, IN: Facts & Comparisons 4.0; 2007—[cited 2007 September 22]. Drug Monographs [about 11 pages]. http://0-factsandcomparisons.com.libcat.ferris.edu/Search.aspx?search=antifungalagents.
15. Popovich N, Newton G. Warts. In: Berardi R, Kroon L, McDermott J, et al. eds. *Handbook of Nonprescription Drugs, An Interactive Approach to Self Care.* 15th ed. Washington, DC: American Pharmacist Association; 2006:907-916.
16. American Academy of Dermatology [homepage on the Internet]. Washington, DC: American Academy of Dermatology; c 2006 [cited 2007 September 24]. Flash! Duct tape can help clear up warts; [about 1 screen]. http://www.aad.org/NR/rdonlyres/EA8AE6CF-DA83-4714-991A-9C5AD450B07E/o/Ducttapeforwarts.pdf.
17. Drug Facts & Comparisons [database on the Internet]. Indianapolis, IN: Facts & Comparisons 4.0; 2007—[cited 2007 September 22]. Drug Monographs [about 11 pages]. http://0-factsandcomparisons.com.libcat.ferris.edu/Search.aspx?search+dermatologic agents.
18. Lexi-comp, Inc. Lexi-Drugs [Comp+Specialties"]. Lexi-Comp.; September 22, 2007.
19. Newton G, Popovich N. Fungal skin infections. In: Berardi R, Kroon L, McDermott J, et al. eds. *Handbook of Nonprescription Drugs, An Interactive Approach to Self Care.* 15th ed. Washington, DC: American Pharmacist Association; 2006:889-905.
20. Drug Facts & Comparisons [database on the Internet]. Indianapolis, IN: Facts & Comparisons 4.0; 2007—[cited 2007 September 22]. Drug Monographs [about 4 pages]. http://0-factsandcomparisons.com.libcat.ferris.edu/Search.aspx?search=antifungalagents.
21. Lexi-comp, Inc. Pediatric Lexi-Drugs®. Lexi-Comp.; September 22, 2007.
22. Drug Facts & Comparisons [database on the Internet]. Indianapolis, IN: Facts & Comparisons 4.0; 2007—[cited 2007 September 22]. Drug Monographs [about 12 pages]. http://0-factsandcomparisons.com.libcat.ferris.edu/Search.aspx?search=antibiotics.

23. Schlager SI. Skin and soft tissues. *Clinical Management of Infectious Diseases.* Baltimore, MD: Williams & Wilkins; 1998:1-66.

24. National Federation of State High School Associations. www.NFSHAorg website. Accessed 2007

25. Foster DT, Rowendder LJ, Reese SK. Management of sports-induced skin wounds. *J Athletic Train.* 1995;30:135.

26. Honsik KA, Romeo MW, Hawley CJ, et al. Sideline skin and wound care for acute injuries. *Curr Sports Med Rep.* 2007;6:147-154.

27. Kordi R, Wallace WA. Blood borne infections in sport: risks of transmission, methods of prevention, and recommendations for hepatitis B vaccination. *Br J Sports Med.* 2004;38:678-684.

28. Canadian Academy of Sport Medicine. HIV as it relates to sport. *Clin J Sport Med.* 1993;63:63.

29. Mast EE, Goodman RA, Bond WW, Favero MS, Drotman DP. Transmission of blood-borne pathogens during sports: risk and prevention. *Ann Intern Med.* 1995;122:283.

30. Feller A, Flanigan TP. HIV-Infected Competitive Athletes. What are the risks? What precautions should be taken? *J Gen Intern Med.* 1997;12:243.

31. Eichner ER, Calabrese LH. Immunology and exercise. physiology, pathophysiology, and implications for HIV infection. *Med Clin North Am.* 1994;78:377.

32. Immunization of Adolescents Recommendations of the Advisory Committee on Immunization Practices, the American Academy of Pediatrics, the American Academy of Family Physicians, and the American Medical Association. MMWR Recommendations and Reports. 2007

33. Friman G, Wesslen L, Fohlman J, Karjalainen J, Rolf C. The epidemiology of infectious myocarditis, lymphocytic myocarditis and dilated cardiomyopathy. *Eur Heart J.* 1995;16(suppl. 0):36.

34. Fitzgerald L. Overtraining increases the susceptibility to infection. *Int J Sports Med.* 1991;12:S5.

35. Budgett R. Fatigue and underperformance in athletes: the overtraining syndrome. *Br J Sports Med.* 1998;32:107.

36. Shepard RJ, Shek PN. Acute and chronic overexertion: do depressed immune responses provide useful markers. *Int J Sports Med.* 1998;19:159.

37. Eichner ER. Infectious mononucleosis. Recognizing the condition, reactivating the patient. *Physician Sports med.* 1996;24:49.

38. Terrell TR, Lundquist B. Management of splenic rupture and return-to-play decisions in a college football player. *Clin J Sports Med.* 2002;12:400-402.

39. Kinderknecht JJ. Infectious mononucleosis and the spleen. *Curr Sports Med Rep.* 2002;1:116-120.

40. Waninger KN, Harcke HT. Determination of safe return to play for athletes recovering from infectious mononucleosis. *Clin J Sport Med.* 2005;15(6):410-416.

41. American Medical Society for Sports Medicine (AMSSM) and the American Academy of Sports Medicine (AASM). Human immunodeficiency virus and other blood-borne pathogens in sports. *Clin J Sport Med.* 1995;5:199.

42. Committee on Sports Medicine and Fitness. American academy of pediatrics. human immunodeficiency virus [Acquired Immunodeficiency Syndrome (AIDS) Virus]. *Pediatrics.* 1991;88:640.

43. National Collegiate Athletic Association. *1998-1999 NCAA Sports Medicine Handbook.* Overland Park, KS: National Collegiate Athletic Association; 2005-2006.

44. Mitten JM. HIV-Positive Athletes. When medicine meets the law. *Physician Sports med.* 1994;22:63.

45. Adams BB. Dermatologic disorders of the athlete. *Sports Med.* 2002;32(5):309-321.

46. Cordoro KM, Ganz JE. Training room management of medical conditions: sports dermatology. *Clin Sports Med.* 2005;24:565-598.

47. Holtom P, Lu Doanh D. Community-acquired methicillin-resistant staphylococcus aureus: a new player in sports medicine. *Curr Sports Med Rep.* 2005;4:265-270.

48. Elston DM. Community-acquired methicillin-resistant staphylococcus aureus. *J Am Acad Derm.* 2007;56(1): 1-16.

49. Rihn JA, Michaels MG, Harner CD. Community-acquired methicillin-resistant Staphylococcus aureus: an emerging problem in the athletic population. *Am J Sports Med.* 2005;33(2):1924-1929.

50. Schelkun PH. Swimmers Ear. Getting patients back in the water. *Physician Sports Med.* 1991;19:85.

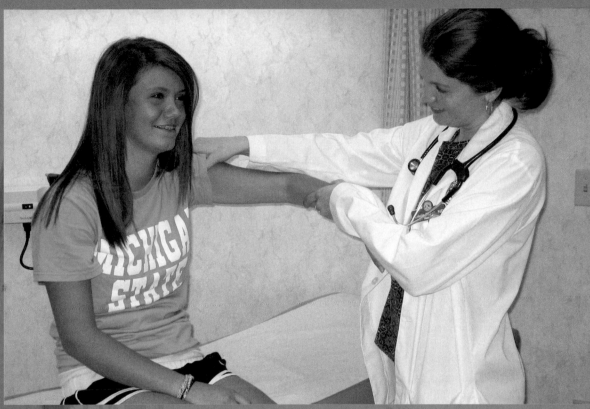

Musculoskeletal Injuries

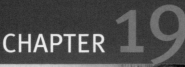
Musculoskeletal Injuries: Basic Concepts

Dilip R. Patel

MUSCULOSKELETAL INJURIES IN YOUTH SPORTS

Definitions and Epidemiology

Very little data are available on the epidemiology of sport-related musculoskeletal injuries in children and adolescents.[1–6] It is estimated that approximately 30 million children and adolescents participate in organized sports each year in the United States.[3] The Centers for Disease Control and Prevention High School Sports-Related Injury Surveillance Study was conducted in 2005–2006. There were 7.2 million students who participated in high school sports in 2005–2006. It is estimated that high school sports account for two million injuries,

500,000 physician visits, and 30,000 hospitalizations every year. In the CDC study, sports injuries were defined as those (1) resulting from participation in an organized high school athletic practice or competition, (2) requiring medical attention from a certified athletic trainer or a physician, and (3) restricting the athlete's participation for 1 or more days beyond the day of injury. An athlete exposure was defined as one athlete participating in one practice or competition during which the athlete was exposed to the possibility of athletic injury.

Sports-specific injury rates are shown in Table 19-1, proportion of injuries in practice and competition by diagnosis is shown in Figure 19-1, and proportion of injuries by sport and number of days lost are shown in Figure 19-2.

Table 19-1.

Sport-Specific Injury Rates* in Practice, Competition, and Overall—High School Sports-Related Injury Surveillance Study, United States, 2005–2006 School Year

| | Rate | | |
Sport	Practice	Competition	Overall
Boys' football	2.54	12.09	4.36
Boys' wrestling	2.04	3.93	2.50
Boys' soccer	1.58	4.22	2.43
Girls' soccer	1.10	5.21	2.36
Girls' basketball	1.37	3.60	2.01
Boys' basketball	1.46	2.98	1.89
Girls' volleyball	1.48	1.92	1.64
Boys' baseball	0.87	1.77	1.19
Girls' softball	0.79	1.78	1.13
Total	**1.69**	**4.63**	**2.44**

*Per 1,000 athlete exposures (i.e., practices or competitions).

Practice
(n = 683,199)

Competition
(n = 759,334)

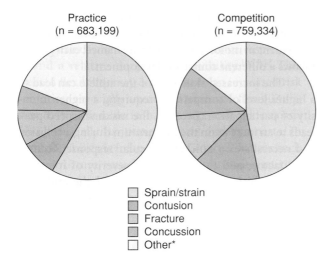

☐ Sprain/strain
◩ Contusion
◪ Fracture
◩ Concussion
☐ Other*

* Includes other injuries (e.g., lacerations or dislocations) and reportable health-related events (e.g., heat illness, skin infections, or asthma attacks).

FIGURE 19-1 ■ Proportion of injuries in practice and competition by diagnosis. *(From Centers for Disease Control and Prevention. Sport-related injuries among high school athletes – United States, 2005-06 school year. MMWR. 2006;55(38):1037-1040.)*

Based on the CDC study, the overall injury rate in all high school sports combined was 2.44 injuries per 1000 athlete exposures. Football has the highest injury rate at 4.36 injuries per 1000 athlete exposures. In each of the nine sports for which data were collected, approximately 80% of the injuries reported were new injuries. Overall, the injury rates were higher for competition compared to practice. Approximately 50% of the injuries resulted in less than 7 days of time lost from participation. No deaths were reported in the study.

Much less is known about the epidemiological characteristics of specific injuries and these are reviewed where information is available in specific chapters in this section of the book.

Mechanisms

In order to understand the mechanism and pathoanatomy of injuries in children and adolescents it is useful to briefly consider some unique aspects related to growth and development (Table 19-2). Implications of childhood growth and development for sport participation are reviewed in Chapters 1 and 2. Certain aspects unique to the adolescent age group that have implications for sport injuries include somatic growth, presence of growth cartilage, and properties and growth characteristics of bones are considered here.[7-27]

PHYSICAL GROWTH

Height and Weight

The adolescent growth spurt in weight and height contributes to increased momentum and force in collision between athletes, for example, in football. Also, the axial skeleton must support the increased weight, and increased load.[11] This increased weight and load increases the risk and severity of injuries. It has been observed that the number of football injuries increases with age throughout adolescence as the athletes get bigger. The matching of athletes based on their chronologic age and grade levels may contribute to an increased risk of injury for the late maturing athlete competing against the larger early maturing athlete.[13]

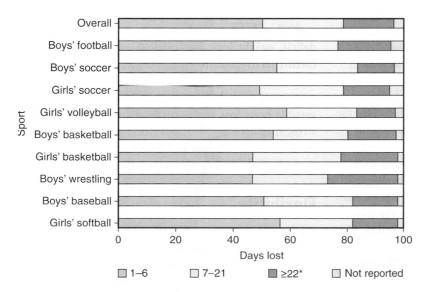

FIGURE 19-2 ■ Proportion of injuries by sport and number of days lost. *(From Centers for Disease Control and Prevention. Sport-related injuries among high school athletes–United States, 2005-06 school year. MMWR. 2006;55(38):1037-1040.)*

* Includes athletes who returned to their teams after ≥22 days and athletes who were out for the remainder of the season as a result of their injuries.

Table 19-3.

Key Elements of Musculoskeletal Injury History

When did the injury occurred or symptoms started

Sport, playing conditions, position played

Level of competition

Recent change in the type, volume, intensity of the activity

How did the injury occurred or the symptoms started

Immediate pain, swelling, deformity, loss of movement

Ability to move, walk, bear weight, continue to play

Immediate intervention if any, such as ice application

Subsequent intervention, such as physical therapy

Need for taking pain medications

Characteristics of pain—onset, duration, severity, quality, localization, radiation, modifying factors

Previous injury to the same area

injury or symptom are summarized in Table 19-3. The examination should focus on the area injured as well as other areas or systemic examination based on the history. Specific aspects of examination are reviewed in the discussion of various injuries in subsequent chapters.

Clinical presentations of musculoskeletal injuries will vary based on the type of injury and the predominant area involved. Clinically sport-related musculoskeletal injuries can be categorized as follows: overuse injuries, acute soft tissue injuries, acute and chronic growth plate injuries, acute bone fractures, stress fractures, and joint dislocations, the general concepts of which are reviewed below.

When an athlete presents with a history of musculoskeletal injury or symptom or sign, the differential diagnosis should include a wide range of conditions in addition to different injuries as summarized in Table 19-4.

Diagnostic Studies

Plain radiographs are the most common imaging study indicated in the evaluation of most musculoskeletal injuries and are sufficient in most cases. In general computed tomography (CT) scans are especially useful in delineating bone lesions, whereas magnetic resonance imaging (MRI) scans are most useful in the evaluation of soft tissue injuries. Nuclear scans are used for initial localization of the area of pathology and often suggest likely nature of the pathology when correlated clinically. There is also increasing trend to use office-based ultrasound in the evaluation of soft tissue injuries. Laboratory studies are indicated when the differential diagnosis includes considerations of conditions other than trauma (see Table 19-4).

Treatment

General approach to treatment of the broad categories of musculoskeletal injuries is described in sections below and individual injuries covered in various other chapters in this section of the book. Therapeutic exercises are integral component of treatment and rehabilitation following sport injuries and some of the exercises are illustrated in Appendix C. Various thermal and electric modalities are also used widely in the treatment and rehabilitation of sports injuries to treat pain, inflammation, muscle spasm, and swelling (Table 19-5, Figures 19-4 to 19-7). Application of superficial cold therapy (ice application or other cold medium) and superficial heat are common therapeutic modalities.[28,29]

Osteopathic manipulative treatment has also been used effectively by those with osteopathic training in the management of many sport-related injuries.

The nature of the specific injury as well as the personal experience and expertise of the pediatrician are major determinants of when to and from whom to seek specialist consultation in the management of sports injuries (Box 19-1). Most sport-related musculoskeletal injuries can be treated conservatively and do not require surgical intervention. These can be managed in consultation with a sports medicine physician. A small percentage of injuries will need further evaluation and likely surgical intervention and should be referred to orthopedic surgeon with expertise in orthopedic sports medicine. Depending on the expertise available in the local community certain injuries of the head, neck, and spine will be managed by spine surgeon or neurosurgeon as appropriate. Consultation and referral to a physiatrist should also be considered, especially when electrodiagnostic studies are indicated and questions related to aspects of physical rehabilitation arise.

Box 19-1 When to Refer

General Guidelines for Orthopedic Referral of Sports Injuries

Acute trauma with neurovascular compromise

Open fractures

Most displaced fractures

Most growth plate fractures

Most joint dislocations

Complete acute muscle or tendon ruptures

Most complete tears of joint ligaments with joint instability

Acute or chronic compartment syndromes

Acute fracture dislocations of the spine

Acute posttraumatic hemarthrosis

High-risk stress fractures

Chronic posttraumatic joint pain

Advanced osteochondritis dissecans

Table 19-4.

Broad Categories Conditions with Musculoskeletal Symptoms and Signs

Category	Selected Conditions	Laboratory and Imaging and Consultation
Developmental variations Seen in early childhood, these are physiologic conditions that correct with normal growth	External femoral or tibial torsion (out-toeing); internal femoral torsion or internal tibial version(in-toeing); physiologic genu varum or valgum	A careful observation is needed. If the condition is unilateral or associated with other signs or symptoms or developmental delay, further evaluation is needed.
Congenital and developmental conditions Characteristic abnormalities noted on examination at birth or soon thereafter during infancy.	Developmental dysplasia of the hip; congenital club foot; Klippel-Feil syndrome	Pediatric orthopedic consultation
Rheumatic diseases Typically present as inflammatory arthritis affecting one or more joints or other articular structures and systemic symptoms such as fever, fatigue, or weight loss. Disease may evolve over months to years. Family history may be positive (e.g., spondyloarthropathy, psoriasis and gout). Predominant age at onset may vary depending upon particular type of the disease	Chronic juvenile arthritis; systemic arthritis; juvenile ankylosing spondylitis; psoriatic arthritis; juvenile dermatomyositis; scleroderma	CBC, ESR, CRP are nonspecific indicators of inflammation. Specific rheumatologic tests should be considered in consultation with a pediatric rheumatologist. Plain films may show characteristic findings late in the disease and may not be useful in the initial diagnosis in most cases.
Chronic pain syndromes Characterized by a chronic, intermittent course of variable intensity of widespread or regional noncharacteristic pain. Most likely to be seen in older children and adolescent age group. Family history may be positive in hypermobility syndrome.	Fibromyalgia; hypermobility syndrome; complex regional pain syndrome	No specific laboratory or imaging studies are characteristic of a specific disease. Depending upon personal experience of the pediatrician further consultations may be needed to comanage these patients.
Vasculitis Characteristic symptoms and signs of particular syndrome. Fever, abdominal pain, petechiae and palpable purpura; mucus membrane inflammation are some of the features.	Henoch-Schonlein purpura; Kawasaki disease	CBC, ESR specific tests such as echocardiogram indicated in Kawasaki disease and pediatric cardiology consultation indicated.
Infections Characterized by a history of exposure followed by joint pain, systemic symptoms, typically of acute onset. Can affect any age group except sexually transmitted diseases that affect adolescents. A history of unprotected sex in adolescents or IVDU should be ascertained.	Disseminated gonococcal infection and arthritis; Lyme arthritis; postinfectious reactive arthritis; viral synovitis/arthritis; bacterial osteomyelitis	CBC, ESR, CRP are nonspecific. Culture of appropriate body fluid or tissue for specific etiologic diagnosis. Serology for specific diagnosis in conjunction with typical syndrome.
Overuse sydnromes Most common in the adolescent age group involved in sports and other physical activities. Can affect any soft tissue, bone, joint, or cartilage, growth plate. Characterized by activity-related pain of gradual onset, deteriorating sport performance, and localizing signs such as swelling and tenderness.	Stress injury of the distal physis of radius; stress injury of proximal physis of the humerus; juvenile osteochondritis dissecans; Osgood-Schlatter disease; stress fractures; tendonitis affecting various tendons; bursitis affecting various bursae; lateral epicondylitis; idiopathic anterior knee pain	Plain radiographs are indicated in: growth plate injury, juvenile OCD, stress fractures, joint pain and swelling. A bone scan may be indicated to make early diagnosis of stress fracture. An MRI or CT scan may be indicated in some cases of juvenile OCD in consultation with orthopedic surgeon.

(continued)

Table 19-4. (Continued)

Broad Categories Conditions with Musculoskeletal Symptoms and Signs

Category	Selected Conditions	Laboratory and Imaging and Consultation
Orthopedic conditions Each of the various orthopedic conditions present with characteristic localizing symptoms and signs.	Legg-Calve-Perthes disease; Slipped capital femoral epiphysis; Scheueremann's disease	Plain radiography is indicated. Orthopedic consultation for further evaluation and definitive treatment.
Systemic disease Systemic diseases affecting bone and joint (arthropathy) present with other typical characteristics of the systemic syndrome.	Sickle cell disease; hemophilia; diabetes mellitus; sphingolipidoses	Specific laboratory tests are indicated and management may need specialist consultation.
Metabolic bone disease A metabolic bone disease should be suspected with poor growth, poor nutritional status, recurrent fractures, and progressive joint deformities.	Rickets; idiopathic juvenile osteoporosis; osteogenesis imperfecta; hypophosphatasia; hypothyroidism	Metabolic and endocrinology work up in consultation with pediatric endocrinologist
Benign neoplasms of the bone Most are asymptomatic and incidental findings on plain radiographs, e.g., aneurismal bone cysts, fibrous dysplasias, nonossifying fibromas. There may be localized pain. In osteoid osteoma the pain is characteristically relieved by aspirin.	Osteoid osteoma; osteoblastoma; nonossifying fibromas; aneurysmal bone cysts; fibrous dysplasia	Plain radiographs or CT scan may be indicated. Orthopedic consultation. Most do not need further evaluation or intervention.
Malignant neoplams of the bone Nighttime pain, dull aching bone pain; adolescents most affected.	Osteogenic sarcoma; Ewing' sarcoma	Plain radiographs are characteristic. Orthopedic and oncology consultation
Psychosomatic Important considerations in all adolescents.	Various somatic complaints	Further evaluation may require mental health consultation
Peripheral neuropathy Characterized by neuropathic pain, paresthesia, sensory–motor dysfunction in the distribution of the affected nerve. Uncommon in pediatric age group	Median nerve (carpal tunnel syndrome); ulnar neuropathy; meralgia paresthetica; tarsal tunnel syndrome	Electromyography, physiatrist consultation
Muscle disease Characterized by true insidious and progressive muscle weakness; stretch reflexes affected; sensation remains intact except in sensory–motor diseases; can be seen at any age, however, the particular type may be more prevalent or first recognized in different age groups	Muscular dystrophies; myopathies	Creatine kinase; genetics and neurology consult and testing; metabolic workup
Acute trauma Characteristic history and mechanism of injury with specific localized findings on examination	Soft tissue injuries; bone fractures; ligament sprains; intra-articular cartilage injuries	Plain radiography is indicated in severe injuries or when fracture is suspected. MRI is indicated in severe musculotendinous and ligament and cartilage injuries in consultation with orthopedic surgeon

CBC, complete blood count; ESR, erythrocyte sedimentation rate; CRP, C-reactive protein; OCD, osteochondritis dissecans.
Used with permission from Patel DR. Musculoskeletal system. In: Greydanus DE, Feinberg AN, Patel DR, Homnick DN eds. Pediatric Diagnostic Examination. New York, NY: McGraw Hill Medical; 2008:344-348.

Table 19-5.

Therapeutic Modalities

Superficial heat using heat pads or whirlpool
Superficial cold such as application of ice or immersion in cold water
Use of ultrasound
Phonophoresis
Iontophoresis
Various modes of electrical stimulation

OVERUSE INJURIES

Definitions and Epidemiology

Musculoskeletal overuse injuries are the most common injuries in the pediatric athlete (Table 19-6).[30–35] Overuse injury is a result of excessive stress to normal tissue leading to a localized chronic inflammatory reaction. Tendons and tendon-apophyseal junctions are common sites for such injuries in the young. Overuse injuries of bone manifest as stress fractures.

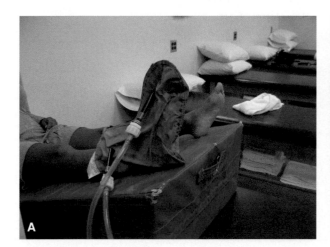
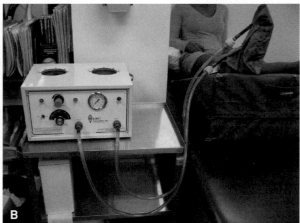

FIGURE 19-4 ■ JOBST unit. Used for intermittent compression to reduce swelling. Typically foot and ankle are place in the bag, the foot is elevated and cold water is intermittently run through the system by the machine as shown.

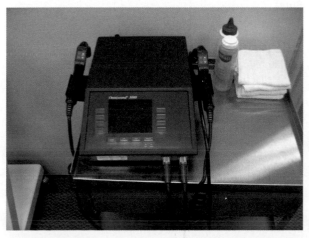

FIGURE 19-5 ■ Ultrasound. Used to apply superficial heat and to deliver topical medications to the tissue by the process of phonophoresis.

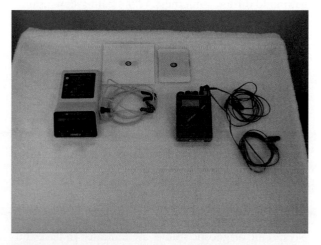

FIGURE 19-6 ■ Iontophoresis unit. Used to deliver topical drugs to the tissue by using electrical current.

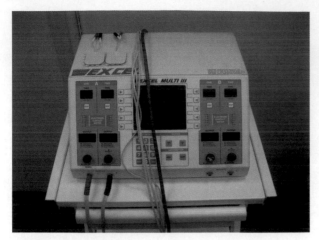

FIGURE 19-7 ■ Electrical stimulation unit. Stationary and portable units can be used for pain relief, decrease edema, muscle stimulation, or decrease inflammation.

Mechanisms

Overuse injuries are commonly seen in the athlete who is engaged in regular training and exercise and who has recently increased the intensity of training. Also a poorly conditioned recreational athlete and an athlete early in the season are prone to such injuries. A number of factors have been postulated to contribute to overuse syndromes (Table 19-7),[30–35] however, the most consistent factor contributing to an overuse injury is a rapid increase in overall intensity and volume of training.

Clinical Presentation

Clinically it is useful to consider the process of overuse as a spectrum of injuries on a continuum of clinical severity (Table 19-8).[32] In grade 1 injuries the pain or soreness is diffuse and occurs hours after the activity, with mild diffuse tenderness. When pain follows immediately after the activity it is considered a grade 2 injury. Pain is usually present for approximately 2 to 3 weeks and tenderness may localize to the affected area. This is the most common presentation of an overuse syndrome. In grade 3 injury pain is felt during the activity, is well localized, severe, and persistent. In grade 4 injury the pain is present at rest or before the activity, interfering with function. Tenderness is severe and well localized. In grade 3 and 4 injuries, a stress fracture should be strongly considered.

Diagnostic Studies

No specific diagnostic studies are indicated in the evaluation of most overuse injuries. Failure of appropriate course of treatment to resolve the symptoms may indicate

Table 19-6.

Major Overuse Injuries

Growth plate
Distal radial physis (gymnast's wrist)
Proximal humeral physis (little leaguer's shoulder)

Articular cartilage and subchondral bone
Juvenile osteochondritis dissecans (medial condyle of femur, patella, talus, capitellum)

Apophysis
Osgood-Schlatter's disease (tibial tubercle)
Sever's disease (posterior calcaneal)
Iselin disease (5th metatarsal)
Iliac crest apophysitis

Bone (stress fractures)
Low-risk stress fractures
    Medial tibia
    Fibula
    Ribs
    Radius
    2nd and 3rd metatarsals
High-risk stress fractures
    Femoral neck
    Mid-anterior tibia
    Patella
    Medial malleolus
    Talus
    Tarsal navicular
    5th metatarsal
    Pars interarticularis (spondylolysis)

Tendons
Rotator cuff tendonitis
deQuervain's (extensor pollicis longus and abductor pollicis brevis)
Popliteus tendinitis
Iliotibial band friction syndrome
Patellar tendonitis
Achilles tendonitis

Bursa
Subacromial bursitis
Olecranon bursitis
Iliopectineal bursitis
Trochanteric bursitis
Prepatellar bursitis
Pes anserine bursitis

Other
Little leaguer's elbow
Lateral epicondylitis (tennis elbow)
Osteitis pubis (affecting symphysis pubis)
Scheueremann's disease (vertebral endplates)
Idiopathic anterior knee pain
Sinding-Larsen-Johansson syndrome (distal pole of patella)
Hoffa's fat pad syndrome (infrapatellar fat)
Medial tibial stress syndrome (shin splints)
Chronic exertional compartment syndromes of the leg
Plantar faciitis

Table 19-7.

Contributing Factors for Overuse Injuries

Most consistent factors

Rapid increase in the intensity, duration and frequency of training

Inadequate sport-specific training and conditioning

Faulty sport-specific techniques (e.g., tennis serve, pitching in baseball, fast bowling in cricket, improper use of sport equipment)

Equipment that is not right for the athlete (e.g., incorrect racket grips, gymnastic dowel rings)

Qualitatively inadequate equipment (e.g., worn out shoes with poor shock absorption)

Relatively less consistent factors

Playing on hard surface

Anatomic variations (e.g., pes cavus, tarsal coalition, metatarsus adductus, hyperpronation

Genu valgus, varum, recurvatum, femoral anteversion, leg-length inequality)

Presence of growth cartilage

Myo-osseous disproportional growth and decreased flexibility

Presence of neuromuscular disorder, arthritis or other musculoskeletal conditions

Table 19-8.

Spectrum of Overuse Injuries

Grade 1

Pain follows hours after activity

Diffuse pain and "soreness"

Mild, poorly localized tenderness

Usually less than 2 wk duration

Resolves rapidly with rest from inciting activity

Grade 2

Pain immediately following activity

Pain may localize to affected area

Usually more than 2–3 wk duration

Poorly localized tenderness

Most athletes present at this stage

Takes longer to resolve

Grade 3

Pain during activity and recurs with activity

Pain localizes to affected area

Increase in severity of pain

Localized tenderness

May limit activity

Sport performance deteriorates

Grade 4

Pain at rest, continuous, also with daily activity

Localized severe tenderness

Functional disability

Usually more than 4 wk duration

Consider stress fracture or other etiology

Need longer period of rest to resolve

---

further studies that include imaging studies as well laboratory studies depending upon the nature of the injury and differential diagnostic considerations.

Treatment

Treatment of an overuse injury begins with a decrease in or cessation of the offending activity and control of pain. Local application of ice in the form of ice massage directly over the area of pain and tenderness two to three times a day is recommended. Short-term use of anti-inflammatory medication may be considered. The application of ultrasound and other physical therapy modalities are effective in controlling pain and inflammation in some patients.[29] The athlete should decrease the intensity, amount, duration, or frequency of the training to a level that does not produce the pain. This may mean a period of complete cessation of the particular activity. The athlete should be allowed to continue aerobic training and strength training of the uninjured extremity. Alternative activities such as cycling and swimming should be encouraged. The physician should work closely with sports physical therapist or athletic trainer and institute an individualized progressive rehabilitation program for the athlete, which will allow the athlete to return to a gradually increasing level of activity. Preventive measures include education of the athlete regarding the proper training regimen, and identifying and correcting vari-

ous contributing factors, especially faulty techniques, to the best extent possible.

ACUTE SOFT TISSUE INJURIES

Definitions and Epidemiology

Most acute injuries are soft tissue injuries and include sprains, strains, contusions, and lacerations. *Sprains and strains* are the most common acute injuries of the soft tissue. A sprain refers to an injury to a ligament usually resulting from excessive stretching. A strain refers to an injury to a muscle or muscle tendon unit as a result of forceful contraction against resistance. These injuries can be graded according to the degree of severity. A grade 1 injury is the mild injury and indicates stretch or pull of the ligament or muscle fibers, a grade 2 injury is a moderate injury and indicates partial tear of the tissue involved, and a grade 3 injury is a severe injury and indicates a complete tear of the tissue involved. Contusions are injuries resulting from direct impact on the tissue involved that lead to localized internal bruise and bleeding in the tissue. Superficial abrasions involve disruption of the epidermis, whereas deep abrasions involve disruption of epidermis and subdermal layer. A laceration is also an open injury or wound that involve the disruption of the muscle.

Mechanisms

Acute soft tissue injuries can result either from a direct impact to the area or an indirect injury resulting from a shear force applied to the tissue. A direct impact to the anterior thigh will result in a contusion of the quadriceps, whereas a lateral impact to the knee may indirectly result in a sprain of the medical collateral ligament.

Clinical Presentation

Sprains and strains

In grade 1 injury the tissue damage is minimal, resulting in minimal initial swelling. Usually less than 25% of the fibers are injured. There is mild pain and discomfort, full range of motion is maintained, and there is no instability. Grade 1 injuries resolve over a period of 1 to 2 weeks. In grade 2 injuries, between 25% and 50% of the tissue is damaged. There is a partial tear of ligament or muscle resulting in moderate swelling, localized tenderness, pain on movement, and some functional loss. Joint instability may be present. Recovery usually takes 4 to 6 weeks. In grade 3 injuries the tissue damage is usually more than 50% causing severe acute pain, rapid onset of swelling, localized tenderness, joint instability and some loss of function. There is a high incidence of injuries to adjacent structures. A complete tear of the ligament or muscle-tendon unit may require referral to an orthopedic surgeon for definitive treatment. Depending upon the injury, recovery may take few weeks to months.

Contusions

Contusion results from a direct blow to the tissue. Clinically significant contusions involve large muscles, a common injury being that to the anterior thigh involving the quadriceps (Charley horse). Because of its vascularity, a contusion to muscle results in significant bleeding and hematoma formation. There is localized pain and tenderness and ecchymosis develops. There is a functional loss affecting the injured muscle.

Severe muscle contusion may result in the development of *myositis ossificans traumatica*, which refers to the development of calcification and new bone formation in the area of a contusion hematoma. Possible factors that can predispose to the development of myositis ossificans include a severe injury and hematoma,

continued activity following the injury, application of heat and massage to the area, forceful stretching of the injured muscle, return to sports too soon after the injury, and reinjury to the same area.

Diagnostic Studies

Generally no specific studies are indicated. In compete rupture or grade 3 sprains or strains MRI scan may be indicated in planning surgical intervention.

Treatment

Any skin abrasion should be appropriately cleaned and dressed if warranted. Lacerations should be evaluated carefully for associated deep injuries and the treatment will be guided by the degree, site and nature of the laceration. The area should be cleaned, compression dressing applied to control bleeding, and the laceration should be closed with appropriate method such steristips or sutures and dressed.

The goals of initial approach to the treatment of soft tissue injuries are to prevent further injury, control the pain and acute inflammatory reaction, control bleeding and edema, and reduce muscle spasm. The injured area should be rested. This may require nonweight bearing and use of crutches for leg injuries. Immobilization of the extremity using temporary splint may be necessary for short periods, however prolonged immobilization should be avoided. After a period of rest of 2 to 3 days a significant improvement in symptoms may be noted.

Immediate application of ice to the tissues causes vasoconstriction and helps decrease the amount of bleeding, edema, and swelling of the tissue. Cooling of the tissue results in decreased muscle spasms and decreased pain sensation. The preferred mode of application of ice is in the form of crushed ice placed in a plastic bag placed directly over the skin. Usually each application should last 15 to 20 minutes and may be repeated three to four times or more per day for the first 2 to 3 days. Elastic compression bandage application to the area may further help reduce edema. Compression bandage may be applied over the ice bag. The injured area should be kept elevated to facilitate venous and lymphatic drainage. Short-term use of NSAID may help decrease acute pain.

After symptomatic improvement the athlete should begin rehabilitation program. The goals of the rehabilitation are to regain full range of motion with no pain, to restore muscle strength and endurance and to restore agility. Because of a period of decreased activity aerobic capacity may be decreased and need to be restored. The athlete should be allowed gradual return to previous level of activity when full range of motion with no pain is restored, there is no swelling or tenderness, and no residual loss of function.

ACUTE GROWTH PLATE INJURIES

Definitions and Epidemiology

An estimated 15% to 20% of injuries to long bones involve the growth plate and a significant number of these injuries are sports injuries.[36–38] Growth plate injuries are more common in soccer, alpine skiing, gymnastics, weight lifting, and baseball. Growth plate injuries are twice as common in the upper extremities then in the lower extremities, injury to the distal radial physis being the most common injury.[37] The peak incidence of growth plate injuries is during early adolescence. Some authors cite increased sports participation, and weakening of the growth plate as possible factors for an increased number of such injuries during the period of rapid growth.

Mechanisms

Acute injuries can result from direct impact or indirect shear forces and are commonly classified according to the Salter-Harris classification based on radiographic appearance (Figure 19-8).[38]

Clinical Presentation

Possibility of an injury to the growth plate should be strongly considered when there is a moderate or severe injury to the adjacent ligaments. A localized swelling and tenderness over the site of the growth plate is elicited on palpation. In severe injuries one may note a deformity.

Diagnostic Imaging

Plain films in two views with comparison films of the uninjured extremity should be obtained.

Treatment

The specific treatment depends upon the type of the injury and any associated injuries to the adjacent structures. Usually uncomplicated type I and II injuries can be treated with closed reduction and immobilization. It is important to restore the normal anatomic configuration in type III and IV injuries. A careful long-term follow up is essential to detect and treat delayed complications.

A partial or complete growth arrest is a known complication of injuries to the growth plate. Fortunately the majority of injuries heal without clinically significant growth disturbance. Growth arrest and deformity may result following type III or IV injuries, if anatomic configuration cannot be restored. Growth arrest commonly occurs after type V injuries. A complete growth arrest in lower extremity may result in a clinically significant leg length inequality requiring subsequent corrective surgery.

CHRONIC STRESS OR OVERUSE INJURIES OF THE GROWTH PLATE

Definitions and Epidemiology

Commonly described stress injuries of the growth plate are injury to the distal radius in gymnasts, the proximal humerus in pitchers, and injuries to the distal femur and proximal tibia in runners.[39–42]

Mechanisms

Chronic repetitive microtrauma from intense training and sports participation can result in an overuse type of injury of the growth plate.

Clinical Presentation

The athlete presents with localized pain of gradual onset which may worsen with continued activity. Localized tenderness can be elicited over the area. Other important causes of chronic bone and joint pain such as infection, tumor or arthritis should be included in the differential diagnosis.

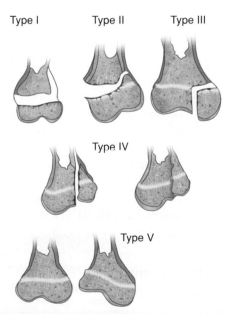

Type I   Type II   Type III

Type IV

Type V

FIGURE 19-8 ■ Salter-Harris classification system of growth plate fractures. Type I, separation of the physis; type II, fracture through the physis and adjacent metaphysis; type III, fracture through the physis and adjacent epiphysis; type IV, fracture through the physis, adjacent metaphysic and epiphysis; type V, crush injury of the physis.

Diagnostic Imaging

A radiographic examination with comparison views of the opposite side is indicated which typically shows widening of the physis.

Treatment

Prompt recognition of the injury followed by cessation of the offending activity, up to 3 months in many cases, usually results in a rapid resolution of symptoms and the majority of such injuries heal without complications. Upon resolution of the pain the athlete can return to gradually increasing level of activity and avoid excessively intensive training to prevent recurrence. Recurrence of pain should be evaluated promptly.

ACUTE FRACTURES

Definitions and Epidemiology

The anatomical structure of the immature bone is shown in Figure 19-9.

Fractures of the immature bone in children are common in general and it is estimated that 40% of boys and 25% of girls sustain an acute fracture by age 16 years.[43] The exact incidence of specific fractures in various sports is not known. In a recent study by CDC fractures were the third commonest injury in high school sports with incidence ranging between 8% and 12% of all injuries.[1]

Mechanisms

Direct impact, collision, or falls are the main mechanisms that cause acute fractures. The immature bone has a relatively greater capacity to absorb the energy from an impact and therefore is more likely to undergo a plastic deformation before it breaks. The unique physical and biomechanical characteristics of the immature bone result in unique fracture patterns. The plastic deformation can result in a buckle or torus fracture (Figure 19-10a) that most commonly affects the metaphyseal-diaphyseal junction of the growing bone. Buckle fracture may be partial or complete. The relatively thicker periosteum and flexibility of the immature bone allows it to bend to a certain degree before it breaks. This results in a greenstick fracture (Figure 19-10b), in which one side of the cortex breaks (tension side), whereas the opposite side of the cortex remains intact (compression side). In addition to the buckle and greenstick fractures, children and adolescents also sustain complete fractures that may be simple, communited, displaced or nondisplaced, open or closed.

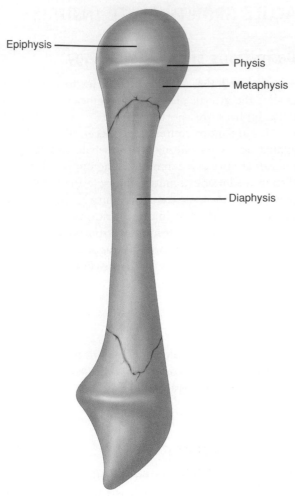

FIGURE 19-9 ■ Schematic diagram showing structure of the growing bone.

Clinical Presentation

The athlete will present with a history of direct trauma or a fall, a collision, localized pain and often deformity depending upon the type and severity of the fracture. There will be localized bony tenderness. A thorough neurovascular assessment should be done in all cases of acute injury. It is not uncommon for a buckle fracture to go undiagnosed initially because of lack of significant deformity and often mild symptoms.[43] The athlete with buckle fracture may present several weeks following the injury because of persistent pain or localized swelling.

Diagnostic Imaging

In all cases of suspected fractures x-rays are indicated. A minimal of two views at right angle to each other should be obtained. Additional specific views should be obtained depending upon the site being evaluated. Comparison views of the uninjured side should also be obtained.

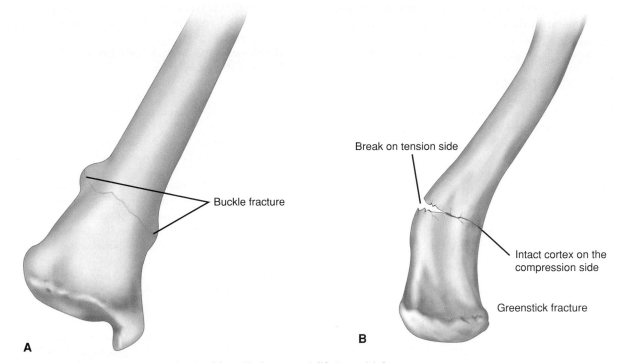

Break on tension side

Buckle fracture

Intact cortex on the
compression side

Greenstick fracture

A

B

FIGURE 19-10 ■ Schematic diagram showing **(a)** Buckle fracture and **(b)** Greenstick fracture.

Treatment

Most nondisplaced simple fractures can be treated by a period of splint or cast immobilization. The type of immobilization, the type of casting, and the duration of immobilization will depend upon specific fracture. The growing bones have a greater remodeling potential. Most pediatric fractures should be managed in consultation with orthopedic surgeon with expertise in pediatric orthopedics. Athletes with significant trauma and open fractures will typically present to the emergency department where appropriate orthopedic consultation is obtained. The pediatrician in the office setting is most likely to encounter less severe, closed injuries and should keep a high index of suspicion because many athletes may first present few to several days following the injury.

STRESS FRACTURES

See Chapter 31.

JOINT DISLOCATIONS

Major joint dislocations are reviewed in subsequent chapters on specific injuries.

PSYCHOLOGY OF SPORT INJURY

Sports play a central role in the lives of many adolescents. They participate in sports for many reasons—fun, prove themselves their own capabilities, socialize, parental and social pressures, or financial reasons (scholarships).[7] Factors such as external pressure to participate and excel in sports, and not being able to play because of an injury can be potentially stressful situations for adolescent athletes.[7,23–25] The emotional reaction to injury and coping abilities of the young athlete to injury and not being able to play should be kept in mind while treating these athletes.[7,23–25] Most adolescent athletes are motivated enough to get well soon and return to sports. They go through the rehabilitation and recovery phase with no negative feelings or consequences.[26] However, a few will despair and need extra support. Athletics is a family affair in many families, and often the physician has to manage parents more diligently than the athlete, allaying parental disappointment and anxiety. The athlete may go through a series of reactions following an injury, not unlike those described in the context of death or other loss, namely, disbelief, denial, and isolation; anger; bargaining; depression; and acceptance and resignation with hope, in that order of progression.[22,23] This pattern is believed to be seen far less commonly in adolescents than in adults, and young adolescents seem to proceed rather rapidly from anger and frustration to acceptance.[26] During this process of recovery from injury, the physician plays an important role in motivating the athlete, helping him realize realistic outcomes, and recognizing these reactions and help mange them.[23,25] Some athletes may find injury as a convenient excuse to quit without embarrassment and this may be an indication for further psychosocial investigation.

ACKNOWLEDGMENT

Partly adapted with permission from Patel DR, Baker RJ. Musculoskeletal injuries. *Prim Care.* 2006;33(2):545-580, Saunders Elsevier.

REFERENCES

1. Centers for Disease Control and Prevention. Sport-related injuries among high school athletes–United States, 2005-06 school year. *MMWR.* 2006;55(38):1037-1040.

2. National Federation of State High School Associations (NFHS). *2005-2006 High School Athletics Participation Survey.* Indianapolis, IN: NHFS; 2006. http://www.nfhs.org/sports/aspx. Accessed July 14, 2008.

3. Gotsch K, Annest JL, Holmgreen P, Gilchrist J. Nonfatal sports- and recreation-related injuries treated in emergency departments–United States, July 2000-June 2001. *MMWR.* 2002;51:736-740.

4. National Collegiate Athletic Association (NCAA). *Injury Surveillance System.* Indianapolis, In: NCAA; 2006. http://www1.ncaa.org/membership/ed_outreach/health-safety/iss/index.html. Accessed July 14, 2008.

5. Caine D, Caine C, Maffulli N. Incidence and distribution of pediatric sport-related injuries. *Clin J Sport Med.* 2006;16(6):500-513.

6. Powell JW, Barber-Foss KD. Injury patterns in selected high school sports: a review of the 1995-1997 seasons. *J Athl Train.* 1999;34(3):277-284.

7. Pratt HD, Patel DR, Greydanus DE. Sports and the neurodevelopment of the child and adolescent. In: DeLee JC, Drez D Jr, Miller MD, eds. *Orthopaedic Sports Medicine.* Philadelphia, PA: Saunders; 2003:624-642.

8. Sigel EJ. Adolescent growth and development. In: Greydanus DE, Patel DR, Pratt HD, eds. *Essential Adolescent Medicine.* New York, NY: McGraw Hill; 2006:3-16.

9. Kreipe RE. Normal somatic adolescent growth and development. In: McAnarney et al, eds. *Textbook of Adolescent Medicine.* Philadelphia, PA: WB Saunders; 1992:44.

10. Beunen G, Malina RM. Growth and physical performance relative to the timing of the adolescent spurt. *Exerc Sport Sci Rev.* 1988;16:503.

11. Burgess-Milliron MJ, Murphy SB. Biomechanical considerations of youth sports injuries. In: Bar-Or O, ed. *The Child and Adolescent Athlete.* Oxford, England: Blackwell Science; 1996:173.

12. Linder MM, Townsend DJ, Jones JC, et al. Incidence of adolescent injuries in junior high school football and its relationship to sexual maturity. *Clin J Sport Med.* 1995; 5:167.

13. Luckstead EF, Greydanus DE. *Medical Care of the Adolescent athlete.* Los Angeles, CA: Practice Management Corporation; 1993.

14. Malina RM. Physical growth and biological maturation of young athletes. *Exerc Sport Sci Rev.* 1994;22:389.

15. Malina RM. Effects of physical activities on growth in strature and adolescent growth spurt. *Med Sci Sports Exerc.* 1994;26:759.

16. Hergenroeder AC. Body composition in adolescent athletes. *Pediatr Clin North Am.* 1990;37:1057.

17. Micheli LJ. Overuse injuries in children's sports: the growth factor. *Orthop Clin North Am.* 1983;14:337.

18. Pappas AM. Osteochondroses: diseases of growth centers. *Phys Sportsmed.* 1989;17:51.

19. Micheli LJ, Fehlandt AF. Overuse injuries to tendons and apophyses in children and adolescents. *Clin Sports Med.* 1992;11(4):713.

20. Hergenroeder AC. Bone mineralization, hypothalamic amenorrhea, and sex steroid therapy in female adolescents and young adults. *J Pediatr.* 1995;126:683.

21. Bailey DA, Faulkner RA, McKay HA. Growth, physical activity, and bone mineral acquisition. *Exerc Sport Sci Rev.* 1996;24:233.

22. Kubler-Ross E. *On Death and Dying.* New York, NY: McMillan; 1969.

23. Heil J. *Psychology of Sport Injury.* Champaign, IL: Human Kinetics; 1993.

24. Tofler IR, Stryer BK, Micheli LJ, et al. Physical and emotional problems of elite female gymnasts. *N Engl J Med.* 1996;335:281.

25. Rostella RJ. Psychological care of the injured athlete. In: Kulund DN, ed. *The Injured Athlete.* Philadelphia, PA: Lippincott-Raven; 1988.

26. Smith AD. Rehabilitation of children following sport and activity related injuries. In: Bar Or O, ed. *The Child and Adolescent Athlete.* London, England: Blakwell Science; 1996:224.

27. Speer DP, Braun JK. The biomechanical basis of growth plate injuries. *Phys Sportsmed.* 1985;13:72.

28. Prentice WE, ed. *Rehabilitation Techniques for Sports Medicine and Athletic Training.* 4th ed. New York: McGraw Hill; 2004.

29. Prentice WE, ed. *Therapeutic Modalities for Sports Medicine and Athletic Training.* 5th ed. New York: McGraw Hill; 2003.

30. Stanitski CL. Overuse injuries in the skeletally immature athlete. In: DeLee JC, Drez D Jr, Miller MD, eds. *Orthopaedic Sports Medicine.* Philadelphia, PA: Saunders; 2003:703-711.

31. Outerbridge AR, Micheli LJ. Overuse injuries in the young athlete. *Clin Sports Med.* 1995;14(3):503.

32. McKeag DB. The concept of overuse : the primary care aspects of overuse syndromes in sports. *Prim Care.* 1984; 11:43.

33. Krivickas LS. Anatomical factors associated with overuse sports injuries. *Sports Med.* 1997;24:132.

34. Micheli LJ. Overuse injuries in the young athlete: stress fractures. In: Bar-Or O, ed. *The Child and Adolescent Athlete.* Oxford, England: Blackwell Science; 1996:189.

35. Hutchinson MR, Ireland ML. Overuse and throwing injuries in the skeletally immature athlete. *Instr Course Lect.* 2003;52:25-36.

36. Caine D, DiFiori J, Maffulli. Physeal inuries in children's and youth sports: reasons for concern? *Br J Sports Med.* 2006;40:749-760.

37. Wascher DC, Stazzone EJ, Finerman GAM. Physeal injuries in young athletes. In: DeLee JC, Drez D Jr, Miller MD, eds.

Orthopaedic Sports Medicine. Philadelphia, PA: Saunders; 2003:712-729.

38. Salter RB, Harris WR. Injuries involving the epiphyseal plate. *J Bone Joint Surg*. 1963;45A:587.

39. Boyd KT, Batt ME. Stress fracture of the proximal epiphysis in an elite junior badminton player. *Br J Sports Med*. 1997;31:252.

40. Carson WG, Gasser SI. Little leaguer's shoulder: a report of 23 cases. *Am J Sports Med*. 1998;26:575.

41. Rettig AC. Athletic injuries of the wrist and hand: Part II: overuse injuries of the wrist and traumatic injuries to the hand. *Am J Sports Med*. 2004;32(1):262-273.

42. Shih C, Chang CY, Penn I, et al. Chronically stressed wrists in adolescent gymnasts: MR imaging appearance. *Radiology*. 1995;195:855.

43. Herring JA. General principles of managing orthopaedic injuries. In: Herring JA, ed. *Tachdjian's Pediatric Orthopaedics*. 3rd ed. Philadelphia, PA: Saunders Elsevier; 2002:2057-2086.

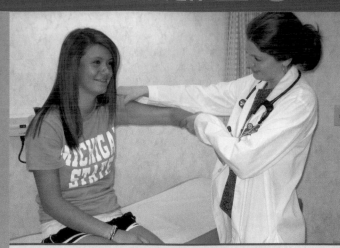

CHAPTER 20

Acute Injuries of the Shoulder Complex and Arm

Steven Cline

ANATOMY

The anatomy of the shoulder (Figures 20-1 and 20-2) is complex because of the unconstrained nature of the joint, which allows an arc of motion greater than any other joint in the body. The shoulder is stabilized by both bony and soft tissue restraints (Table 20-1). The glenoid forms a small cup, which minimally constrains and stabilizes the humeral head (Figure 20-3). The glenoid labrum, a fibrocartilage lip, adds to the depth and width of the glenoid and is commonly injured in shoulder dislocations and in biceps tendon attachment injuries. The superior, middle, and inferior glenohumeral ligaments stabilize the shoulder through different arcs of motion, and are commonly injured along with the labrum in both adult and younger athletes.[1]

The rotator cuff (Figures 20-4 and 20-5) provides secondary and dynamic stability to the shoulder, as do the periscapular muscles, which aid in stabilizing

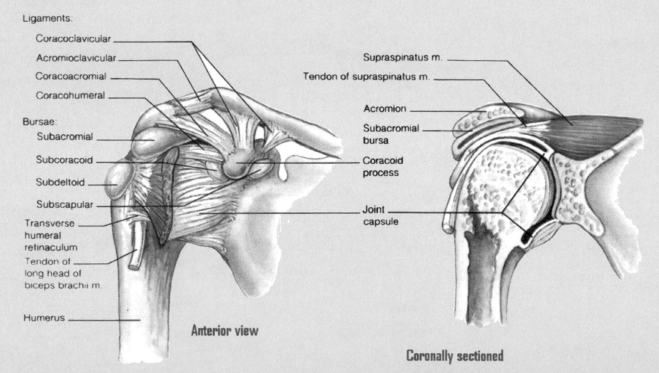

Ligaments:
Coracoclavicular
Acromioclavicular
Coracoacromial
Coracohumeral

Bursae:
Subacromial
Subcoracoid
Subdeltoid
Subscapular
Transverse humeral retinaculum
Tendon of long head of biceps brachii m.
Humerus

Anterior view

Supraspinatus m.
Tendon of supraspinatus m.
Acromion
Subacromial bursa
Coracoid process
Joint capsule

Coronally sectioned

FIGURE 20-1 ■ Anatomy of shoulder. (*Used with permission from Van De Graaff KM. Human Anatomy. 6th ed. New York:McGraw Hill;2002: Figure 8-25, p 216.*)

the shoulder and position it in space. There is some debate as to whether the biceps and its long head provide significant dynamic shoulder stability or not, but the biceps tendon and associated muscles are commonly injured in association with other patterns of shoulder injury. Although significant portion of shoulder motion is caused by the motion of the shoulder girdle itself, the scapula, the acromioclavicular (AC) joint, clavicle and the sternoclavicular (SC) joint, all contribute to the scapulothoracic and shoulder motion, and this needs to be addressed in detail when considering shoulder injuries. Basic movements of the shoulder are depicted and described in Figure 20-6.

Definitions and Epidemiology

Injuries resulting from acute macrotrauma to the shoulder, scapulothoarcic region and proximal arm in the young athlete are listed in Table 20-2. Although sport-related acute injuries to the shoulder and arm are most

common in contact—collision sports, such injuries also occur in noncontact throwing sports and weight lifting and similar activities.

Mechanisms

The mechanisms of shoulder injuries are reviewed with specific injuries below.

Clinical Presentation

The history should ascertain the mechanism of injury. The athlete with acute shoulder area injury will present with localized pain that is exacerbated by movements. There will be localized tenderness and characteristic deformity depending upon the nature of the injury. Because of the pain, the movements are restricted. The shoulder area is examined based on the methods described under the "Physical Examination" section below. Abnormal findings are further described under specific injuries.

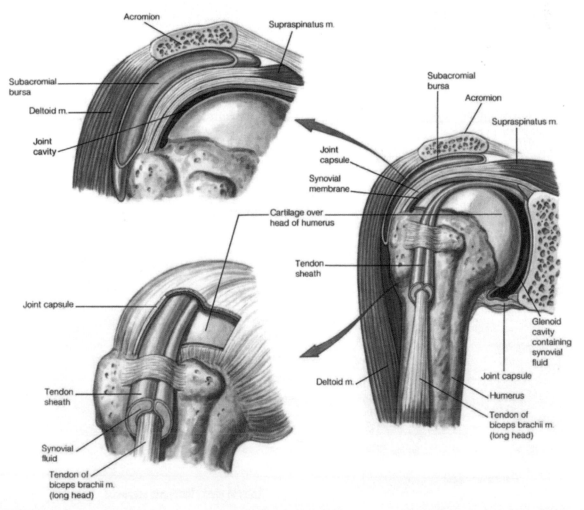

FIGURE 20-2 ■ Anatomy of shoulder. (*Used with permission from Van De Graaff KM. Human Anatomy. 6th ed. New York:McGraw Hill;2002: Figure 8-25, p 216.*)

Table 20-1.

Glenohumeral Stabilizers

Static
Humeral head (ball) plus glenoid (socket)
Glenohumeral ligaments
Glenoid labrum

Dynamic
Rotator cuff musculotendinous complex
Long head of the biceps brachii

Physical Examination

Always examine the neck and cervical spine in a patient with shoulder and arm symptoms. Neurovascular examination of the entire upper limb should be an integral part of assessing shoulder complex and arm symptoms.

Inspection

Observe the patient from front, back, and side and systematically note abnormal findings including sternoclavicular joint, the clavicle, acromioclavicular joint, the shoulder, and the scapulothoracic area. Note any swelling, skin break, apparent deformity, asymmetry compared with the uninjured side, and muscle atrophy. A step-off at AC Joint is seen in severe AC joint disruption. Note scapular winging at rest and on performing wall push-up.

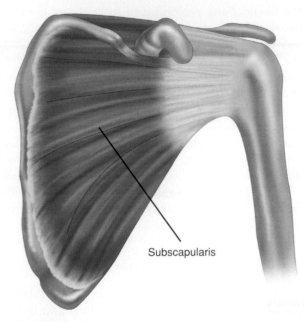

Subscapularis

FIGURE 20-4 ■ Rotator cuff muscles (anterior view).

Palpation

Palpate all areas systematically for tenderness and crepitus.

Movements

Assess active and passive shoulder and scapulothoracic movements. Observe the quality and form of the movements from front, side, and behind. Note the

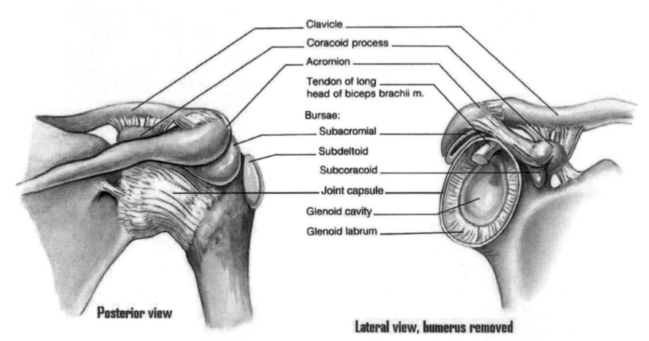

Clavicle
Coracoid process
Acromion
Tendon of long head of biceps brachii m.
Bursae:
Subacromial
Subdeltoid
Subcoracoid
Joint capsule
Glenoid cavity
Glenoid labrum

Posterior view

Lateral view, humerus removed

FIGURE 20-3 ■ Anatomy of shoulder. (*Used with permission from Van De, Graff KM. Human Anatomy, 6th ed. New York:McGraw Hill;2002: Figure 8-25, p 216.*)

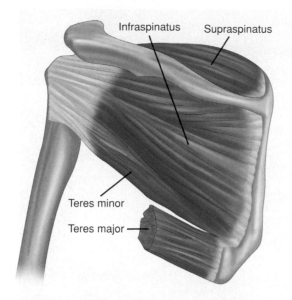

FIGURE 20-5 ■ Rotator cuff muscles (posterior view).

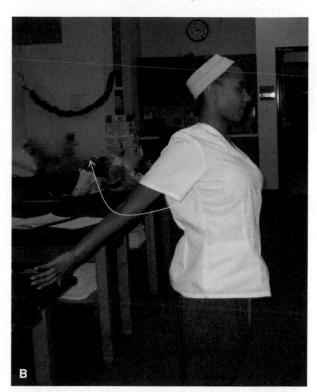

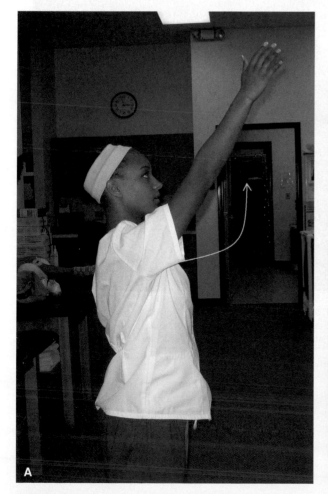

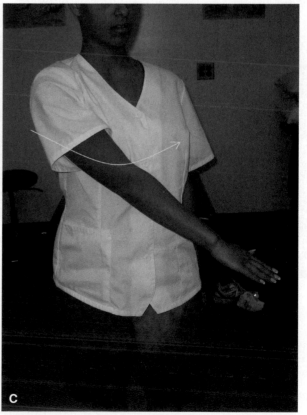

FIGURE 20-6 ■ Movements of shoulder. **(A)** Flexion **(B).** Extension **(C).** Adduction. (*continued*)

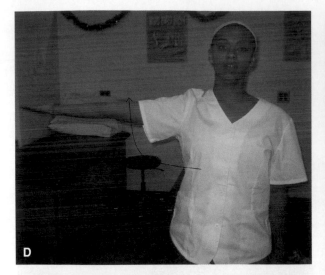

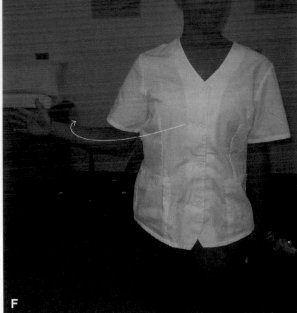

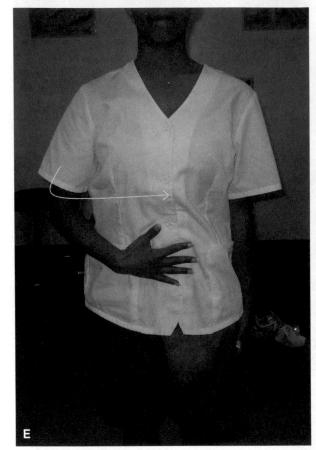

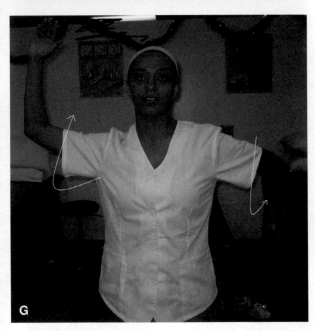

FIGURE 20-6 ■ *(Continued)* **(D).** Abduction **(E).** Internal rotation **(F).** External rotation **(G).** External rotation (right) and internal rotation (left) at 90 degree abduction of shoulder.

Table 20-2.

Major Acute Injuries Around the Shoulder and Proximal Arm

Fractures
Proximal humeral physis
Humeral shaft
Medial clavicular physis
Lateral clavicular physis
Clavicle shaft
Scapular

Dislocations
Glenohumeral
Acromioclavicular
Sternoclavicular

Musculotendinous
Proximal biceps brachii strains
Pectoralis major strains

Other
Glenoid labrum avulsions

scapulothoracic motion. Assess strength by testing movements against manual resistance.

Special Tests are described and depicted in Figures 20-7 to 20-21.

Diagnostic Imaging

Plain films of the shoulder are indicated to assess the presence and nature of fractures and dislocations. Specific views may be needed for certain injuries as discussed in the subsequent sections. For assessment of

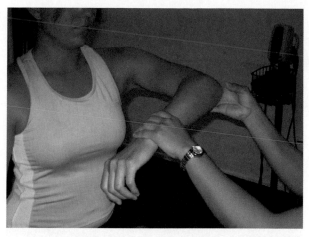

FIGURE 20-8 ■ Hawkins-Kennedy sign. With the athlete standing or sitting on the examination table the arm is forward flexed to 90 degree and forcibly rotated internally. Pain is elicited in injury of the supraspinatus tendon as it impinges against the anterior surface of the coracoacromion ligament and coracoid process.

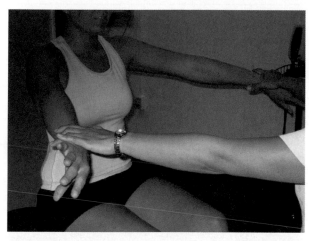

FIGURE 20-9 ■ Supraspinatus test. With the athlete standing or sitting on the examination table the shoulder is abducted to 90 degree, internally rotated (thumbs down) and moved forward to approximately 30 degree. Downward manual resistance is applied while the athlete attempts to hold this position. Pain or weakness is indicative of supraspinatus strain. The test may also be positive in case of suprascapular neuropathy.

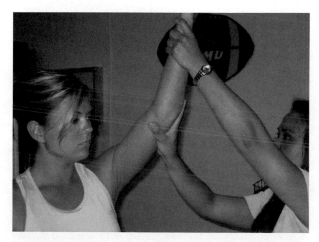

FIGURE 20-7 ■ Neer sign. Sudden and forceful forward flexion of the arm impinges the greater tuberosity against the inferior surface of the acromion. Elicitation of pain is considered a positive Neer impingement sign.

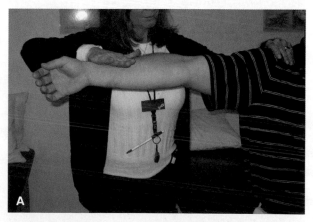

FIGURE 20-10 ■ Drop arm test. The examiner assists the athlete to bring the shoulder to a position of 90-degree abduction **(A)**. Then the athlete is asked to slowly lower the arm to the side *(continued)*

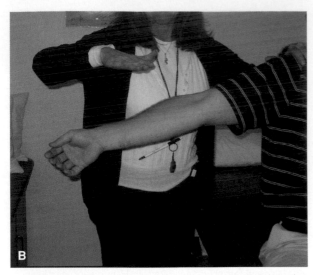

FIGURE 20-10 ■ *(Continued)* **(B)**. In case of rotator cuff tear, pain is elicited as the athlete is lowering the arm or the arm drops suddenly to the side because of weakness.

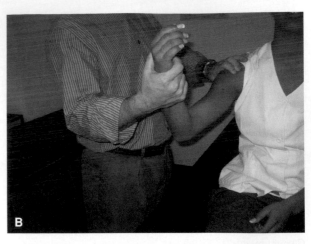

FIGURE 20-12 ■ *(Continued)* **(B)**. Pain and tenderness is elicited in case of biceps tendnitis. Biceps tendon may also be felt to subluxate from the bicipital groove.

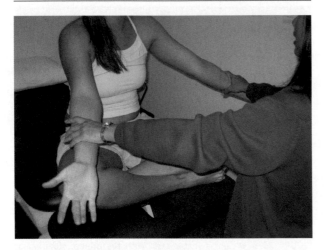

FIGURE 20-11 ■ Speed test. With the arm straight and supinated the athlete is asked to forward flex against manual resistance. Pain and tenderness in the bicipital groove is indicative of biceps brachii tendinitis.

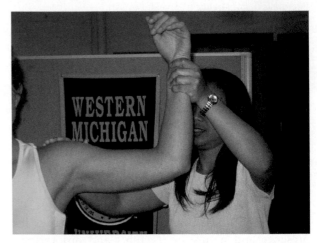

FIGURE 20-13 ■ Apprehension test. With arm abducted at 90 degrees, the shoulder is gently rotated externally. In case of anterior glenohumeral instability the athlete feels a sense of apprehension as if the shoulder is going to dislocate.

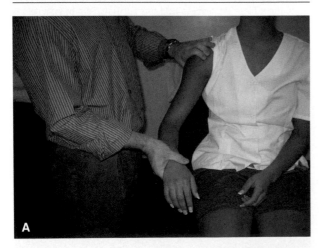

FIGURE 20-12 ■ Yergason test. With the arm by the side, the elbow held at 90 degree, and forearm pronated **(A)**, the athlete is asked to supinate the forearm and flex the elbow against manual resistance, while the examiner is palpating the biceps tendon over the bicipital groove with his other hand

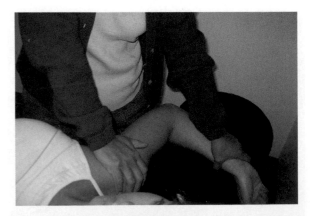

FIGURE 20-14 ■ Jobe relocation test. With the athlete supine and shoulder at the edge of the table the arm is abducted and shoulder gently rotated externally. In case of anterior instability the athlete will feel pain (or a sense of apprehension) during external rotation. At this point a posteriorly directed stress is applied to proximal arm with relief of the pain or apprehension.

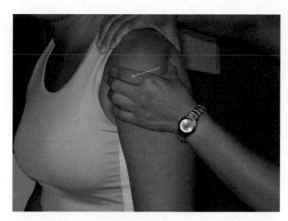

FIGURE 20-15 ■ Load and shift test. With the athlete seated resting arms by the side and palms resting on her thighs (thumbs posterior) the examiner from behind the athlete stabilizes the shoulder with one hand and grasps the head of the humerus with her other hand. The examiner then gently moves the head of the humerus in anterior direction and notes the amount of translation. A relative increase in the movement of the head of the humerus is associated with anterior instability.

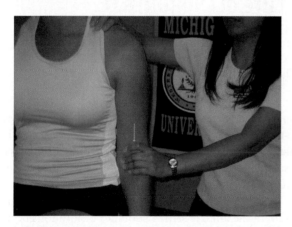

FIGURE 20-16 ■ Sulcus sign. With the athlete seated or standing with the arm by hers side and relaxed, the examiner grasps hers arm and pulls it downward. Appearance of a sulcus below the acromion is indicative of inferior shoulder instability.

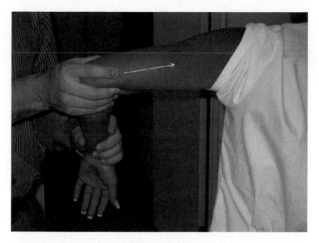

FIGURE 20-18 ■ Crank test. The athlete's shoulder is held at 90-degree abduction, and then axial load is applied as the arm is internally rotated. In case of a SLAP lesion the athlete will feel pain or grinding sensation in the shoulder.

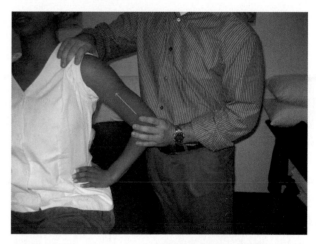

FIGURE 20-19 ■ Anterior slide test. The athlete is sitting resting her hands on the waist. From behind the athlete, the examiner stabilizes the shoulder with one hand and with the other hand over the elbow applies anteroposterior force. In case of a tear of the glenoid labrum a pop or crack is felt as the head of the humerus slides over the labrum.

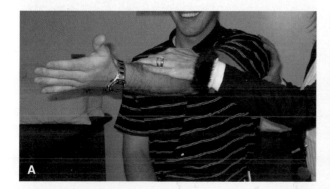
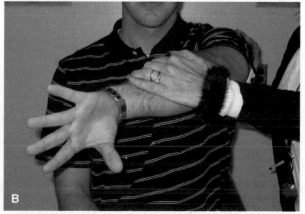

FIGURE 20-17 ■ O'Brien sign. The athlete's shoulder is held in 90 degree of forward flexion, 10 degree of horizontal adduction, and full internal rotation. The examiner applies downward manual resistance to distal forearm while the athlete attempts to hold the position. Pain is elicited in case of glenoid labral tears.

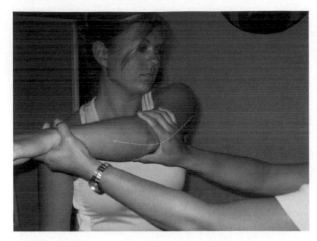

FIGURE 20-20 ■ Cross adduction test. The athlete's arm is held at 90 degree of abduction and then adducted across the chest. Pain is elicited at the acromioclavicular joint area in case of localized pathology.

Box 20-1 When to Refer.

Injuries that Need Orthopedic Consultation

Shoulder dislocations

Superior labral anterior posterior tears with persistent pain and disability

Full thickness acute rotator cuff tears

Displaced fracture of proximal humerus

Type 3, 4, and 5 acromioclavicular joint sprains

Significantly displaced clavicle shaft fractures

Posterior dislocation of the sternoclavicular joint

Complete rupture or avulsion of proximal biceps brachii

Complete tears of the pectoralis muscle

Scapula fractures that are open, displaced, and involving glenoid or neck

Fractures of the acromion

Fractures of the distal clavicle (lateral to the coracoclavicular ligaments)

Any open fracture

Any injury associated with neurovascular compromise

---

soft tissue injuries such as musculotendinous tears, MRI is the study of choice. MR arthrogram may be indicated in the assessment of glenoid labral tears.[2,3] Radiographic findings for specific injuries are described under individual conditions.

Treatment

Immediate treatment depends upon the nature of the injury. In general, in case of fracture with or without neurovascular involvement, the shoulder and arm should be splinted and immobilized in a sling and the athlete should be sent to the emergency department for definitive evaluation and orthopedic consultation as appropriate. Indications for orthopedic consultation are listed in Box 20-1.

ACUTE GLENOHUMERAL DISLOCATION

Definitions and Epidemiology

In a shoulder dislocation the humeral head is at some point completely translated outside the glenoid, and will usually require a reduction to replace the head into the glenoid. Anterior dislocations, in which the humerus is usually dislocated anterior and inferior to the glenoid, are by far the most common.

Shoulder dislocations in general are rare in children. In the athletic setting shoulder dislocations occur in adolescents most often near the time of skeletal maturity, mostly in collision sports. Up to 40% of all primary shoulder dislocations occur in patients younger than 22

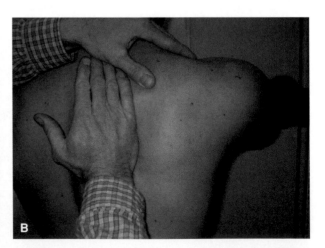

FIGURE 20-21 ■ Scapular retraction test. From behind the athlete the examiner stabilizes the medial border of the scapula as the athlete elevates the arm. A positive test is indicated by relief of rotator cuff impingement pain and suggests a role of the periscapular muscles in the pathophysiology and rehabilitation of the impingement syndrome.

years of age, and the overall incidence of shoulder dislocation is as high as 7% in youth hockey.[1,4]

Mechanism

The mechanism for anterior dislocations is an anteriorly directed force placed on an abducted and externally rotated shoulder, as in being blocked while attempting a throw or similar mechanism. Anterior dislocation can also result from a fall on the externally rotated abducted outstretched arm.

Clinical Presentation

With the more common anterior dislocation the athlete will present acutely on the field or on the sideline with pain, a prominent humeral head anteriorly, with the arm in external rotation, and will not want to move the shoulder. Palpate brachial artery. Test sensation to touch and pin prick over the arm. Loss of sensation over the lateral aspect of the shoulder over the deltoid indicates axillary nerve injury.

Diagnostic Imaging

A true AP, an axillary lateral, and a supraspinatus outlet view plain films should be obtained to assess the dislocation (Figure 20-22) and look for a possible associated Hill-Sach and Bankart lesions or other fractures (Figures 20-23 and 20-24).

Treatment

Many coaches and trainers have reduced the athlete's shoulder on the field or on the sideline before the athlete is seen in the emergency department or in the office.

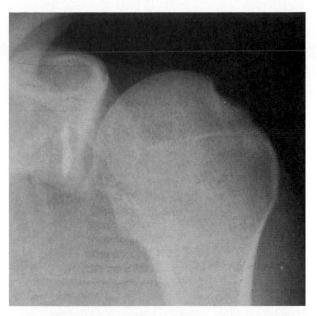

FIGURE 20-23 ■ X-ray of Hill-Sachs' lesion. Hill-Sachs' lesion is characterized by a compression fracture of the head of the humerus where it has impacted on the glenoid rim.

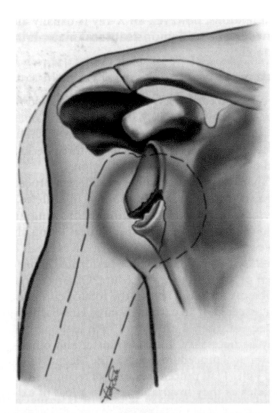

FIGURE 20-24 ■ Bankart lesion. Bankart lesion is characterized by a fracture of the inferior glenoind rim. (*Used with permission from Brukner P, Khan K. Clinical Sports Medicine. 3rd ed. New York:McGraw Hill; 2007:265.*)

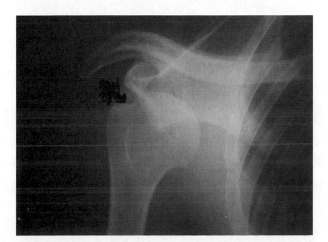

FIGURE 20-22 ■ X-ray of anterior shoulder dislocation.

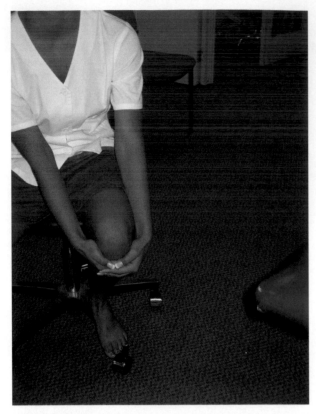

FIGURE 20-25 ■ Technique for self-reduction of anterior shoulder dislocation. With the athlete seated on the table she is asked to grasp the knee (same side as the dislocated shoulder) with her hands around it then gently extend the knee exerting axial traction to the arm until the shoulder is reduced.

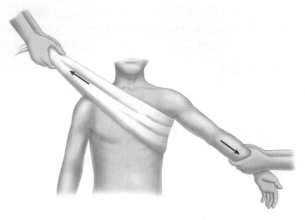

FIGURE 20-26 ■ Traction-counter traction technique. With the athlete supine on the examination table the chest is wrapped in a sheet and pulled by an assistant in the direction opposite to that of the axial traction being applied to the dislocated arm by the treating physician.

prevalent in many centers. Each patient should be evaluated expeditiously and on an individual basis by orthopedic surgeon. Other injuries such as an avulsion of the glenohumeral ligaments or labral tear, will present similarly to a shoulder dislocation and will need surgery.[5,6]

Often the athlete reduces the dislocation himself or herself by placing traction on the arm and rotating the humerus gently until the humeral head reduces, particularly if this is not a first-time dislocation (Figure 20-25). The physician may attempt, depending on his or her personal experience, to reduce the dislocation on the sideline. Ideally, reduction of a dislocated shoulder is best done with conscious sedation and close monitoring of the patient in a controlled setting to minimize the risk of further injury to the shoulder. Postreduction x-rays should be obtained to assess the reduction as well as any associated fractures.[5]

There are a number of effective methods to reduce the dislocated shoulder including traction counter traction (Figure 20-26), modified Stimson technique (Figure 20-27), and the Hennepin technique (Figure 20-28). The shoulder should be reexamined in approximately 1 week. Shoulder and arm should be immobilized in an arm sling for approximately 2 to 3 weeks, followed by range of motion and strengthening rehabilitation exercises. The athlete may expect to return to sports in approximately 8 to 12 weeks' time.

Recurrence rate without surgery in the skeletally immature athlete is between 90% and 100%. Early surgery, either open or arthroscopic, is becoming more

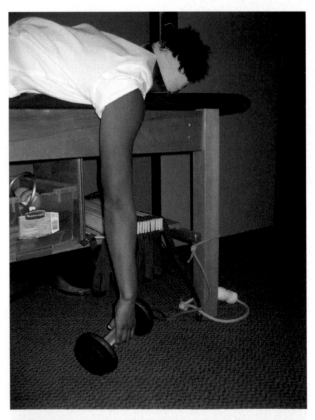

FIGURE 20-27 ■ Stimson technique. The athlete lies prone on the examination table with the dislocated arm hanging over. With a strap around the wrist, a 10 to 15 lbs weight is suspended over a period of 20 to 30 minutes by which time most anterior shoulder dislocations tend to reduce.

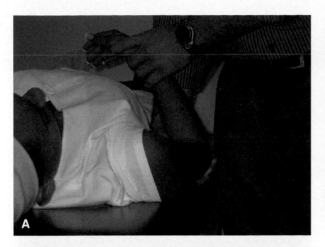

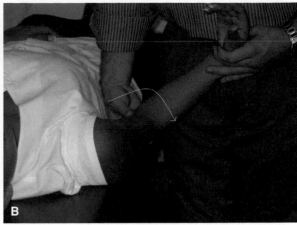

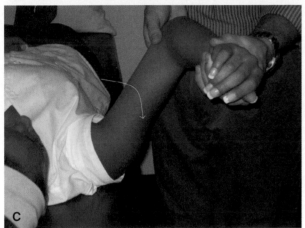

FIGURE 20-28 ■ Hennepin technique. The athlete is seated upright at 45 degree or supine on the examination table **(a)**. The examiner slowly brings the arm to 90 degree of external rotation **(b)**, followed by gentle elevation until the shoulder is reduced **(c)**.

SUPERIOR LABRAL ANTERIOR POSTERIOR TEAR (SLAP)

Definition and Epidemiology

The labrum of the shoulder forms a bumper, which extends and enlarges the contact area between the humeral head and the glenoid. The long head of the biceps tendon blends into the superior labrum and attaches to the glenoid in this region (see Figure 20-3). A tear of the superior labrum is more common in overhead athletes such as baseball players, soccer goalies, and in other throwing sports, as well as weight lifters. The long head of biceps tendon detaches with a portion of the labrum, and different types of tears have been described.[7]

Mechanism

During repeated overhead movements (hyperabduction, external rotation) of the shoulder and arm in baseball, basketball, swimming, and weight lifting as well as other sports, athletes may tear or avulse the superior labrum and the biceps tendon attachment, creating a SLAP.

Clinical Presentation

These injuries lead to pain with overhead use of the shoulder. The athlete may also report that the arm was pulled on or rotated and forced backward while the shoulder was abducted, and will also often describe pain during activities such as incline bench weight lifting. Athletes with SLAP tears may also present with shoulder instability, depending upon the size and the location of the tear, and any associated capsular injury.

O'Brien test (Figure 20-17), crank sign (Figure 20-18), and anterior slide (Figure 20-19) tests are specific for assessing labral tears. O'Brien test (Figure 20-17) consists of the athlete placing the affected arm across the body, with the thumb turned toward the floor, with the examiner applying active resistance as the patient attempts to lift the arm upward. If the athlete has more pain during this maneuver with the thumb and hand turned toward the floor, the examination is consistent with a SLAP tear. This test has a greater than 80% sensitivity and specificity for SLAP tears.[7]

Diagnostic Imaging

Standard x-rays of the shoulder may show Hill-Sach (Figure 20-23) or Bankart lesions, but are not usually helpful in demonstrating the SLAP tear or associated biceps tendon injury. MR arthrogram is the study of choice used in many centers to detect SLAP lesions.[2,3]

Treatment

Athletes with SLAP tears often can and do continue to play, and surgical repair is planned at the end of the season. A short course of NSAIDs, ice, sling, and rest may help alleviate many of the acute symptoms in these athletes, and operative treatment is not indicated in all patients. Persistent pain with activity that limits function is an indication to consider operative treatment.

After a labral repair, most athletes are able to return to sports, once a course of appropriate rehabilitation and sport-specific conditioning is completed. Return to play is expected 4 to 6 months after reconstructive surgery. Short- and long-term results of these repairs are excellent in most athletes, but there are no large series looking at SLAP repairs exclusively in young athletes.

ACUTE TEARS OF THE ROTATOR CUFF

Definition and Epidemiology

Rotator cuff injuries occur often in overhead sports such as baseball, swimming, and tennis as a result of overload of the rotator cuff. Acute rotator cuff tears are rare in children and adolescents, and are usually small and partial thickness.

Mechanism

These injuries are often associated with underlying instability of the shoulder, or with impingement of the shoulder. Acute tear of the rotator cuff can result from sudden forceful elevation of the arm against resistance, sudden heavy lifting, or a direct fall on the shoulder.

Clinical Presentation

The young athlete with an acute rotator cuff tear injury usually presents with sudden onset of anterolateral shoulder pain made worse by continued activity or sports. Often, especially in swimmers and throwers, the posterior capsule is very tight on the injured side, and there is a marked deficit in internal rotation of the affected shoulder. Internal rotation is tested by having the athlete abduct the shoulder to 90 degrees and then internally rotate in a forward arc, or by measuring the vertebral level at which the athlete can place the affected hand behind the back compared to the unaffected side. The athlete also will demonstrate positive Neer (Figure 20-7) and Hawkins-Kennedy (Figure 20-8) impingement signs. Hawkins test is a positive Hawkins sign, which is subsequently relieved by a subacromial injection of local anesthetic. Shoulder abduction is also weak and painful. In large complete tears the athlete may not able to initiate active abduction of the shoulder and the drop arm test may be positive (Figure 20-10).

Diagnostic Imaging

Plain radiographs, AP, outlet, and axillary lateral, are indicated to rule out acute fractures. MRI is indicated to assess acute rotator cuff tears and an MR arthrogram may be needed if a labral tear is suspected.[2,3]

Treatment

The arm should be placed in sling and the athlete should be given analgesics for pain. Generally, the athlete initially should perform exercises below shoulder level, and then progress gradually from there, under the direction of a therapist or athletic trainer. Early self-directed physical therapy is not ideal in a young athlete. Formal rehabilitation will usually allow the athlete to return to competition after 6 to 12 weeks of treatment. The patient should also be maintained on a program of self-directed exercises and conditioning of the shoulders. Surgery is the last resort for rotator cuff problems in a young athlete, and most patients respond well to conservative treatment.[8,9]

ACUTE PROXIMAL HUMERAL PHYSEAL FRACTURES

Definition and Epidemiology

Proximal humeral fractures account for 0.45% of all pediatric fractures and comprise between 4% and 7% of all epiphyseal fractures. This includes sports injuries and those injuries caused by major trauma. Salter-Harris type 1 fractures usually occur in children younger than 5 years, type 2 fractures occur in those between 5 and 11 years of age, and type 3 fractures are most common in children older than 11 years of age.[10,11]

Mechanism

The proximal humeral physis is formed from three secondary centers of ossification at the age of 5 to 7 years. The epiphyseal ossification center appears by 6 months, and the greater and lesser tuberosity centers at 3 and 5 years, respectively. The proximal physis is open in boys until 16 to 18 years of age and in girls until 14 to 17 years of age. The proximal physis contributes to 80% of the longitudinal growth of the humerus.

The mechanism of fracture of the physis is similar to shoulder dislocation in the adult, and occurs in throwing and contact sports, as well as in higher energy sports injuries such as snowboarding, and a fall on the outstretched arm.

Clinical Presentation

The child will present with acute shoulder and upper arm pain, will refuse to move the shoulder, and will usually support the affected internally rotated arm with the other hand. Assess the neurovascular status of the upper extremity. Observe local swelling and deformity over the proximal arm. There will be localized proximal humeral tenderness.

Diagnostic Imaging

Standard x-rays, AP, and a lateral or a transcapular Y view will usually demonstrate the fracture without moving the injured shoulder (Figure 20-29). If there is a high-energy injury with comminution or significant joint involvement, the orthopedist may obtain a CT scan for treatment planning.

Treatment

Most proximal humeral fractures are treated initially with immobilization with a sling, or a sling with an abduction pillow for 3 to 4 weeks. Overall, these injuries are much more benign than they appear on x-ray. The ability of the proximal humerus to remodel is remarkable, and the great mobility of the shoulder enables the athlete to compensate well for any small residual remaining rotational or angulatory deformity.

Surgery or closed reduction is usually not necessary in the majority of these fractures in young children. In adolescents approaching skeletal maturity, it is more likely that a reduction and pinning may be needed. The rare open fracture will require open treatment and debridement. Operative treatment in young children may be complicated by osteomyelitis, loss of fracture reduction, and refracture after hardware removal.

ACROMIOCLAVICULAR JOINT INJURIES

Definition and Epidemiology

True acromioclavicular (AC) joint sprain and separation are uncommon in the skeletally immature athlete before the age of 15 years. AC joint injuries are classified based on the disruption of the AC joint and ligaments (Figure 20-30). Most are type 1 or 2 injuries.

Mechanism

The AC sprains result from a fall on the shoulder, a direct blow to the shoulder, or a fall on outstretched arm.

Clinical Presentation

The athlete with a type 1 or 2 injury will present with localized AC joint pain, tenderness and some swelling. The pain is exacerbated by cross-arm adduction at 90 degree (Figure 20-20). Type 3 to 5 injuries will cause more pain, swelling, and apparent step-off deformity over the AC joint.

Diagnostic Imaging

If pain is significant, and there is a large localized swelling or apparent AC joint and distal clavicular deformity, plain radiographs, AP and cephalic tilt views, are indicated to rule out associated fractures.

Treatment

Type 1 and 2 injuries are treated by local ice, oral analgesics, and relative rest of the arm in a sling for approximately 1 week. The athlete may return to sports when there is no pain and examination is normal. The treatment of type 3 injuries is mostly conservative, although some advocate surgical consideration. Athletes with type 4, 5, and 6 injuries should be referred to orthopedic surgeon.

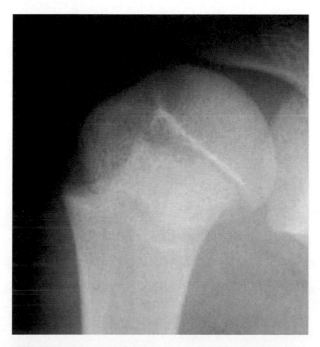

FIGURE 20-29 ■ X-ray of proximal humeral physis fracture.

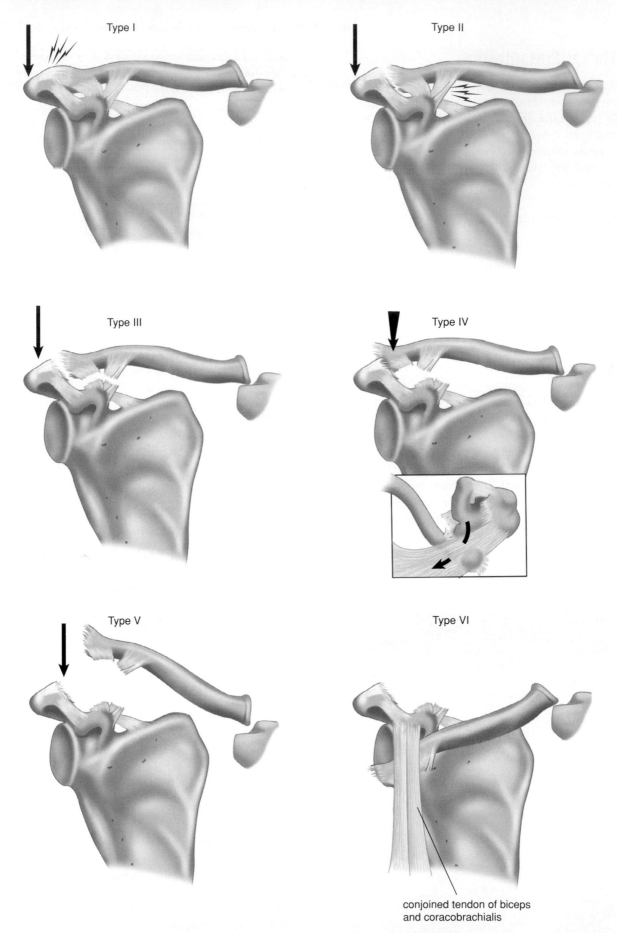

FIGURE 20-30 ■ Rockwood classification of of acromioclavicular injuries in skeletally mature individuals.

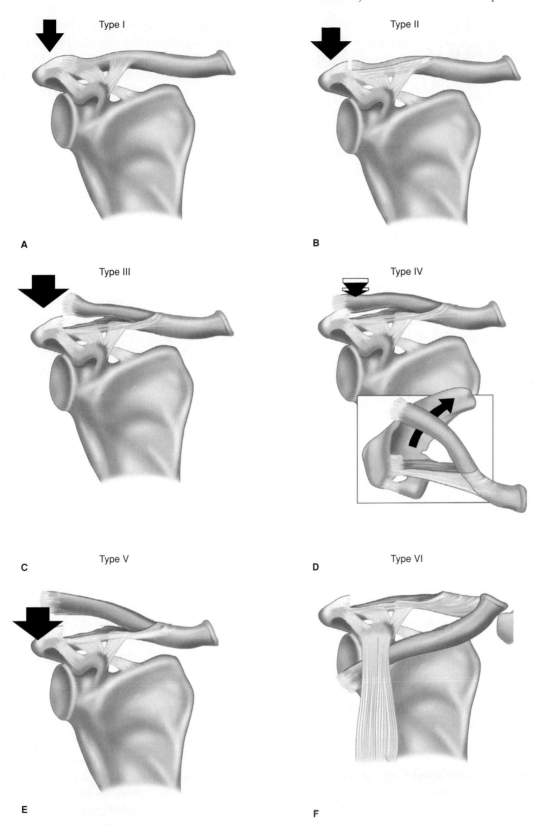

FIGURE 20-31 ■ Dameron and Rockwood classification of distal clavicle and acromioclavicular joint injuries in children. Type I—mild sprain of the AC ligaments without disruption of the periosteal tube. The distal clavicle is normal on examination. Type II—partial disruption of the dorsal periosteal tube. Mild degree of instability of the distal clavicle on examination. Type III—large dorsal, longitudinal split in the periosteal tube with gross instability of the distal clavicle on examination. Type IV—in addition to type III disruption, the clavicle is displaced posteriorly and button-holed through the trapezius. Type V—complete dorsal periosteal split with superior subcutaneous displacement of the clavicle often associated with deltoid and trapezius detachments. Type VI—inferior dislocation of the distal clavicle. The distal clavicle is lodged beneath the coracoid process.

FRACTURES OF THE LATERAL END OF THE CLAVICLE

Definition and Epidemiology

Most injuries to distal end of the clavicle and the AC joint region in the skeletally immature athlete are distal clavicle fractures often through the physis. The distal clavicular epiphysis appears at age 19 years, and quickly unites to the shaft. In the skeletally immature athlete, the clavicle is covered by a periosteal tube that extends the entire length of the clavicle to the AC joint. The injury involves fracture of the lateral end of the clavicle and tears in the dorsal aspect of the periosteal tube. Unlike the injury in the true AC joint separation, the coracoacromial and coracoclavicular ligaments remain intact. Therefore, these injuries are classified based on the position of the distal clavicle and the degree of tear of the dorsal periosteal tube (Figure 20-31).

Mechanism

The mechanism of the injury is similar to that of AC joint injuries (see above).

Clinical Presentation

The young athlete presents with localized pain, swelling, and tenderness. The athlete is reluctant to move the arm because of pain and will hold the arm by the chest supported by the other hand.

Diagnostic Imaging

Plain films of the shoulder and clavicle include an AP, and cephalic tilt view to better demonstrate the distal clavicle and AC joint.

Treatment

These injuries are treated with a sling for comfort, and a few weeks of rest. The athlete may begin gentle pendulum exercises 10 to 14 days after injury, followed by gradually increased range of motion exercises. The athlete may return to full use of the shoulder and competitive play 6 to 12 weeks from the injury.

CLAVICLE SHAFT FRACTURES

Definition and Epidemiology

Fractures of the clavicle shaft are the most common fractures in children and account for 10% to 15% of all children's fractures. Fractures of the clavicle are classified into those involving the medial third, the middle third or the midshaft, and the lateral third. Ninety percent of clavicle fractures are midshaft, with the incidence of lateral fractures increasing as the child grows older. Fractures of the medial or lateral end generally are physeal fractures.

Mechanisms

Clavicles fractures result from a fall on the point of the shoulder, a fall on outstretched hand, or a direct blow to the shoulder or the clavicle.

Clinical Presentation

The child presents with localized pain and swelling over the clavicle. The child will often support the arm and shoulder in an attempt to avoid motion at the site of the fracture. Localized tenderness and crepitus may be felt. Most fractures are closed and nondisplaced or minimally displaced. Significantly displaced closed fracture may be associated with neurovascular injury associated with dysesthesias, marked swelling, or a pulse deficit.

Diagnostic Imaging

Imaging consists of special views of the clavicle with cephalic tilt of the x-ray beam, as well as a true AP of the shoulder.

Treatment

Most clavicle fractures are treated closed, in a sling or with a figure of 8 strap, with excellent long-term results. The sling or strap is discontinued once there is evidence of fracture consolidation by x-ray and by clinical examination, with painless motion of the arm and shoulder. This usually occurs in 4 to 6 weeks. The athlete then undergoes rehabilitation to regain shoulder range of motion, and gradual upper extremity conditioning. Most athletes can expect to return to play in 3 to 4 months.

Most closed midshaft clavicle fractures can be treated conservatively in the primary care setting. Open fractures, significant tenting of the overlying skin and neurovascular signs are indications for orthopedic consultation. Some athletes who develop later residual weakness of shoulder motion, likely because of shortening of the clavicle, should be referred to the orthopedic surgeon.

In a series of 939 pediatric patients who sustained a fracture of the clavicle, 1.6% required surgery. The most common cause of fracture was a fall from a scooter or bicycle, followed by a fall onto the affected shoulder during sports. Most patients who needed surgery were operated on within 1 day of injury. Some of the operative fractures were associated with AC joint or more medial clavicle injuries as well, and these injuries were taken care of at the time of surgery for the clavicle. All operative patients had a good outcome, with full range of motion, and no significant complaints of pain or loss of function at follow-up.

TRAUMATIC STERNOCLAVICULAR JOINT DISLOCATIONS

Definition and Epidemiology

Sternoclavicular joint dislocations involve displacement of the medial end of the clavicle either anteriorly or posteriorly relative to the sternum. Traumatic SC Joint dislocations are rare in the pediatric athlete.

Mechanism

Anterior SC Joint dislocation may be caused by indirect force transmitted to the joint from an impact to the shoulder, clavicle, or the chest wall. Posterior dislocation can result similarly from indirect force or from a direct posteriorly directed force to the clavicle.

Clinical Presentation

There will be localized pain and tenderness over the SC Joint. In anterior dislocations there will be localized swelling or prominence at the SC Joint, whereas in posterior dislocation there will be depression. Potential complications of the posterior dislocation include airway and vascular compromise.

Diagnostic Imaging

A plain film including an AP of the SC joint region and serendipity or tilt views to separate the SC joint from the plane of the sternum help determine anterior or posterior displacement of the SC joint. In some difficult cases a CT scan is indicated.

Treatment

Anterior dislocation: Closed reduction of the SC joint is attempted, with gentle pressure over the area, but the reduction is usually not stable. Most anterior dislocations are treated with a short course of immobilization with a sling. An anterior dislocation may sometimes lead to late SC joint instability and pain, but surgery is usually not required. In some cases a reconstruction or sling procedure of the SC joint is performed.

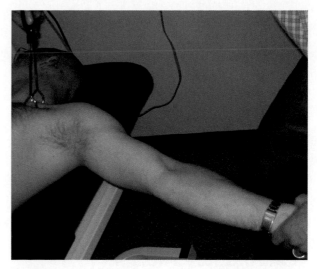

FIGURE 20-32 ■ Simulation demonstrating method of reduction for posterior dislocation of the sternoclavicular joint. With the athlete supine on the examination table the arm is abducted and axial traction is applied. With arm maintained in that position the medial clavicle is pulled forward to reduce the posterior dislocation. While this may be attempted urgently, the athlete with acute traumatic posterior dislocation of SC Joint must be managed emergently in a controlled setting in the hospital by a team of experts.

Posterior dislocation: Posterior dislocation of the SC joint may lead to airway or vascular complications, and should be treated urgently with closed or open reduction by an orthopaedist, with a vascular surgeon standing by. A closed reduction by the abduction-traction technique may be attempted (Figure 20-32). All posterior dislocations must be followed closely by orthopedic surgeon and thoracic surgeon for potential later SC Joint instability and airway, vascular, and esophageal complications that may need further intervention. Significant posterior instability and associated complications may preclude the athlete from returning to contact/collision sports.

FRACTURES OF THE MEDIAL PHYSIS OF THE CLAVICLE

Definition and Epidemiology

Medial clavicular epiphysis appears between 18 and 20 years of age and fuses with the clavicle shaft between 23 and 25 years of age. Most injuries to the medial end of the clavicle and SC Joint region in the skeletally immature athlete affect the medial clavicle physis and are Salter-Harris type fractures. These injuries are relatively rare.

Mechanism and Clinical Presentation

The mechanisms of injury and clinical presentation are similar to that of SC Joint dislocation.

Diagnostic Imaging

X-rays will demonstrate Salter-Harris type fracture patterns of the medial physis.

Treatment

Most medial clavicle physeal fractures heal completely within 4 to 6 weeks. Often the child is first seen several weeks following the fracture because the parent notices a local swelling from callus formation that may persist for 4 to 8 months.

FRACTURES OF THE SHAFT OF THE HUMERUS

Definition and Epidemiology

Fractures of the humeral shaft are commonly associated with throwing sports such as baseball, or with other large torque moments on the bone such as in arm wrestling. These injuries occur in collision sports, skiing, and snowboarding.

Mechanism

Humeral shaft fractures are caused by factors such as overuse, repeated pitching of extra innings in baseball, extra practices, playing through pain, and poor pitching mechanics. There are reports of spiral humeral shaft fractures occurring in Greco-Roman wrestling, and in arm wrestling as well owing to the high torque moment placed on the shaft of the humerus.

These young athletes with humeral shaft fracture may also have an underlying unicameral bone cyst or an aneurysmal bone cyst, which weakens the humerus and predisposes it to fracture with very little stress.

Clinical Presentation

The athlete presents with significant swelling and pain of the arm. A careful examination of the entire upper extremity is conducted to look for any wounds, which indicate an open fracture, and a thorough neurovascular examination is performed. Check the radial nerve in particular distally, assessing sensation of the forearm and hand dorsally, and wrist and finger extension.

Diagnostic Imaging

Once the arm is splinted in a well padded bulky coaptation splint, x-rays including AP and lateral views of the humerus are obtained.

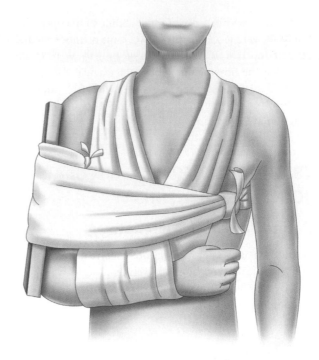

FIGURE 20-33 ■ In case of fracture of the shaft of the humerus, initially the arm is splint immobilized in a well-padded bulky splint while awaiting definitive care.

Treatment

The arm should be immobilized in a well padded bulky coaptation splint (Figure 20-33). Neurovascular status of the upper extremity should be closely monitored clinically. Radial nerve injury or neuropraxia is not an emergent indication for open treatment, and the nerve function is evaluated clinically for a period of few months to assess recovery.

Most fractures through a unicameral bone cyst will heal with simple immobilization. Some unicameral cysts can be more aggressive and problematic, and these athletes often require surgery and bone grafting to heal the defect properly.

STRAINS OF PROXIMAL BICEPS BRACHII

Definition and Epidemiology

Acute strains of the biceps brachii (Figure 20-34) are uncommon in children and adolescents. Proximal biceps tendon injuries often occur in weight lifters, particularly those who lift heavy weights and may abuse anabolic steroids. The injury also occurs in sports such as football and wrestling.

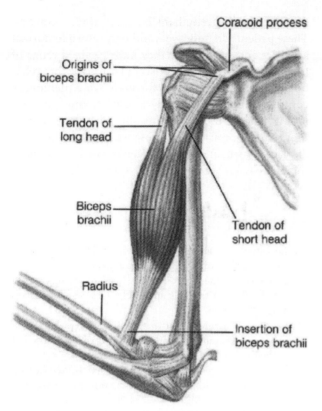

FIGURE 20-34 ■ Biceps brachii muscle anatomy. (*Used with permission from Brukner P, Khan P. Clinical Sports Medicine. 3rd ed. New York: McGraw Hill; 2007.*)

Mechanism

The military press, in particular, stresses the biceps anchor and the superior labrum and leads to injury to the tendon itself or to the labrum and the biceps attachment.

Clinical Presentation

The athlete presents with a history of sudden onset pain associated with a loud pop following forced heavy repetitive weight lifting. These injuries usually occur at the musculotendinous junction in adolescents nearing skeletal maturity. There will be swelling ("Popeye" appearance of arm) and tenderness over the proximal biceps, and some loss of supination strength. The athlete may also have a mild loss of flexion strength, but the majority of flexion power comes from the brachialis muscle.

Diagnostic Imaging

Plain films aid in ruling out bony injury, and MRI scan or MR arthrogram may be needed to assess for other injuries such as a SLAP tear and biceps tendon subluxation or subscapularis muscle tear.

Treatment

Acute grade 1 and 2 strains can be treated conservatively with a period of rest for 1 to 2 weeks for the soft tissue to heal, followed by rehabilitation exercises. Grade 3 or complete tear or avulsion of the long head of biceps brachii should be referred to orthopedic surgeon. Not all proximal biceps tears need to be operatively repaired and the decision is individualized.

Most of these injuries are treated similarly to adult injuries, with tenodesis of the biceps tendon. Return to heavy lifting is delayed for approximately 4 months. Admonitions about weight limits, gradually increasing reps with lighter weights, and avoidance of excessively long workouts with strict elimination of performance-enhancing substances, especially the use of anabolic-androgenic steroids is in order.

PECTORALIS MUSCLE TEARS

Definition and Epidemiology

Pectoralis muscle tears may be complete or incomplete, and are more common in adolescent athletes nearing skeletal maturity, particularly those who engage in body building or power lifting.[12]

Mechanism

The pectoralis muscle tendon unit is overloaded by exercises such as a heavy bench press, and usually the tendon fails catastrophically at the musculotendinous junction.

Clinical Presentation

There will be an immediate pop and severe discomfort in the athlete's chest during heavy bench press lift or free weight work with arm presses. The athlete will usually not be able to lift after the injury because of pain, and presents with pain and swelling over the lateral aspect of the upper chest. The pectoralis major insertions at the sternal and clavicular heads may both be torn, and the muscle retracted, giving obvious asymmetry to the athlete's chest. If the injury is a few days old, there will be marked ecchymosis over the lateral upper chest and arm. If the tear is partial, the contour of the anterior lateral chest may appear normal or near normal, and the primary complaint will be pain and associated weakness in the pectoralis major.

Diagnostic Imaging

No specific imaging is required to diagnose a pectoralis major tear. MRI scan may be indicated to plan definitive treatment after orthopedic evaluation.

Treatment

Initial treatment is RICE, NSAIDs, and a sling for comfort until seen by orthopedic surgeon a few days after injury. Nonoperative treatment is effective for partial pectoralis muscle tears, both in athletes and nonathletes alike, and will give a very acceptable appearance to the chest wall with good function of the pectoralis major.

These athletes want to have the tendon repaired to restore appearance and strength. In most cases the first question from these athletes is how soon they can return to heavy lifting. Pectoralis muscle tears are often repaired acutely with good results. These injuries also do fairly well if repaired late. The athlete is then restricted from lifting, and may return to the weight room once the tendon has healed and motion is restored to the shoulder, 3 to 5 months after surgical repair.

SCAPULAR FRACTURES

Definition and Epidemiology

Fractures of the scapula are rare in children and adolescents. Scapular fractures are also very rare in youth sports.

Mechanism

Scapular fractures typically result from a significant direct impact over the scapula such as seen in motor vehicle accidents or a fall from a bike.

Clinical Presentation

The patient will have pain on shoulder motion and there will be localized tenderness and ecchymosis over the fracture site.

Diagnostic Imaging

X-rays, shoulder AP and scapular Y view, may show the acute fracture. A CT scan may be needed in some cases.

Treatment

Most injuries are nondisplaced scapular body fractures, and are treated closed with a sling and relative rest for a 4 to 6 weeks followed by physical therapy to regain motion and to strengthen the periscapular muscles. These patients do quite well, and may return to normal activities and sports once they have regained range of motion (ROM) and the periscapular muscles are rehabilitated. There is potential for underlying pulmonary contusion in scapular body fractures, and inpatient monitoring of these patients should be considered. More complex fractures or those which are significantly displaced, open, or involve the glenoid or scapular neck should be referred to orthopedic surgeon.[13]

REFERENCES

1. Rockwood CA, Matsen F, Wirth M, eds. The Shoulder. 3rd edition, 2004. Philadelphia PA: Saunders.
2. Potter H, Birchansky S. Magnetic resonance imaging of the shoulder: a tailored approach. *Tech Shoulder Elbow Surg.* 2005;43-56.
3. Sanders T, Miller M. A systematic approach to magnetic resonance imaging interpretation of sports medicine injuries of the shoulder. *Am J Sports Med.* 2005;33: 1088-1105.
4. Deitch J, Mehlman C, Foad S, Obbehat A, Mallory M. Traumatic anterior shoulder dislocation in adolescents. *Am J Sports Med.* 2003;31(5):758-763.
5. Jones K, Wiesel B, Ganley T, Wells L. Functional outcome of early arthroscopic bankhart repair in adolescents aged 11 to 18 years. *J Pediatr Orthop.* 2007;27(2):209-213.
6. Wilk K, Meister K, Andrews J. Current concepts in the rehabilitation of the overhead throwing athlete. *Am J Sports Med.* 2002;30:136-151.
7. Nam E, Synder S. The diagnosis and treatment of superior labrum, anterior and posterior (SLAP) lesions. *Am J Sports Med.* 2003;31(5):798-810.
8. Kibler WB. Rehabilitation of rotator cuff tendinopathy. *Clin Sports Med.* 2003;22:837-847.
9. Millet P, Wilcox R, O'Holleran J, Warner J. Rehabilitation of the rotator cuff: an evaluation-based approach. *J Am Acad Orthop Surg.* 2006;14:599-609.
10. Chee Y, Agorastides I, Garg N, Bass A, Bruce C. Treatment of severely displaced proximal humeral fractures in children with elastic stable intramedullary nailing. *J Pediatr Orthop B* 2006;15:45-50.
11. Ortiz E, Isler M, Navia J, Canosa R. Pathologic fractures in children. *Curr Ortho Related Res.* 2005;432:116-126.
12. Petilon J, Carr D, Sekiya J. Pectoralis muscle injuries: evaluation and management. *J Am Acad Orthop Surg.* 2005;13:59-68.
13. Zlowski M, Bhandari M, Zelle B, Kergor P, Cole P. Treatment of scapula fractures: systematic review of 520 fractures in 22 case series. *J Orthop Trauma.* 2006;20(3):230-233.

CHAPTER 21

Overuse Injuries of the Shoulder

Dilip R. Patel and E. Dennis Lyne

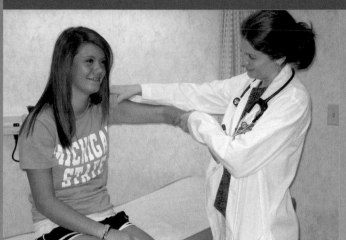

PROXIMAL HUMERUS PHYSEAL STRESS INJURY

Definitions and Epidemiology

Although epiphysiolysis of the proximal humerus occurs primarily in young baseball players, it has also been reported in cricket (fast bowlers), volleyball, swimming, gymnastics, and racquet sports.[1,2] The proximal humeral physis accounts for 80% of the longitudinal growth of the humerus. In sports involving overhead throwing, the physis is subjected to significant amount of stress, leading to microtrauma, throwing-related pain, and characteristic changes seen on the radiographs. This is classically described as the "little leaguer's shoulder," because of its original description in little league pitchers.

Mechanism

It is unclear whether the underlying changes represent inflammation caused by overuse or stress fracture through the physis. The mechanism is believed to be repetitive, high intensity, rotational stress to the physis during throwing, and other overhead activities.

The head of the humerus develops from two ossification centers that fuse into one at 7 years of age. The proximal physis of the humerus closes between 19 and 22 years of age; most close by 17 years of age. This injury pattern is most common during rapid growth, and occurs most often in adolescent boys, between the ages 11 and 16 years, with a peak at 14 years. In baseball pitchers, throwing a curve ball and higher pitch counts have been shown to be associated with a higher rate of stress injury to the proximal humeral physis. Most throwers demonstrate excessive external rotation at shoulder, whereas the internal rotation is relatively restricted, accompanied by acquired contracture of the posterior capsule, a maladaptation referred to as the glenohumeral internal rotation deficit.

Clinical Presentation

The athlete typically presents with a gradual onset of shoulder or proximal arm pain associated with throwing. The average duration of symptoms ranges from 7 to 8 months. Often, the symptoms are mild lasting for several weeks to months, and there is pressure to continue to play, thus, there is a delay in seeking medical help. Tenderness over the lateral aspect of the proximal humerus is the most common finding on examination, and may be present in almost 70% of athletes.[2-4] A few athletes may have weakness of external rotators of shoulder. Usually, the active and passive range of motions of shoulder is normal, until later in the course, when a relative decrease of internal rotation develops.

Diagnostic Imaging

The radiographic findings are characteristic and seen in almost all athletes at the time of presentation. Radiographs with shoulder in external and internal rotation, as well as AP and lateral views should be obtained. Comparison views of the opposite shoulder should also be obtained. The classic finding is a widening of the proximal physis, which may or may not be associated with fragmentation, calcification, sclerosis, and demineralization (Figure 21-1).

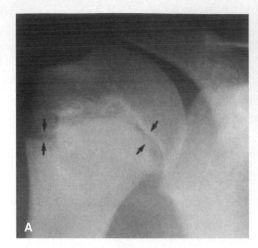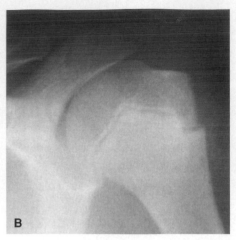

FIGURE 21-1 ■ X-ray of stress injury of proximal humeral physis shows widening of the physis (**A**), compared to the normal side (**A**). (*Used with permission from DeLee JC, Drez D Jr, Miller MD, eds. DeLee and Drez's Orthopedic Sports Medicine. Philadelphia, PA: Saunders Elsevier Imprint; 2003: Figure 21M2-7, p 1136.*)

Treatment

Treatment of proximal humeral physeal stress injury is rest, modification of throwing patterns, and appropriate training and conditioning. Gradual progression to athletic activities is allowed after symptoms abate. The best treatment is advice and counseling to the parents, the child, and the coach to avoid overuse injury in the future. Most of these young athletes will on an average undergo 6 weeks of rest from throwing. Once pain-free, the athlete then undergoes an interval throwing program and returns to competition 3 to 4 months after the injury. All players should be instructed on appropriate limitations on the number and types of pitches, practices, and games they may play in (Table 21-1).[5–10] Current US Baseball Medical and Safety Committee recommendations are summarized in Table 21-2. Similar treatment principles of rest, activity limitations, and training and conditioning are applied for treatment of players participating in other sports who present with proximal physeal injury.

Proximal humeral osteochondrosis

Proximal humeral osteochondrosis is a rare problem in children of unknown etiology, exacerbated by overuse in a throwing athlete with a genetic predisposition. These athletes will present similarly to little leaguer's shoulder. Imaging studies reveal fragmentation of the proximal humeral epiphysis. Treatment of nondisplaced fragments is rest and a reduction of stresses about the shoulder. Throwers should refrain from throwing until completely asymptomatic, and then should undergo appropriate conditioning before return to full time play.

SHOULDER IMPINGEMENT SYNDROME

Definitions and Epidemiology

The rotator cuff muscles (see Figures 20-4 and 20-5 in Chapter 20) (supraspinatus, infraspinatus, teres minor, subscapularis) are predominantly involved in the pathophysiology of this syndrome, hence the condition is also referred to as rotator cuff impingement syndrome. External (anterior) impingement refers to a lesion of the supraspinatus tendon caused by its impingement under the undersurface of the acromion; whereas, internal (posterior) impingement refers to a lesion of the glenoid labrum—specifically superior labrum anterior–posterior or SLAP lesion caused by impingement of the articular surface of the rotator cuff.[5–7] Shoulder impingement syndrome is a common cause of shoulder pain in

Table 21-1.
Recommendations for Pitching Limits

	Recommended Pitching Limits			
	Maximum Number of Pitches Per			
Age Years	**Game**	**Week**	**Season**	**Year**
9–10	50	75	1,000	2,000
11–12	75	100	1,000	3,000
13–14	75	125	1,000	3,000

USA Baseball Medical & Safety Advisory Committee. Position Statement on Youth Baseball Injuries. May 2006.

Table 21-2.

Recommendations of USA Baseball Medical and Safety Committee for Pitching

Recommendations

1 Pitchers who complain or show signs of arm pain during a game should be removed immediately from pitching. Parents should seek medical attention if pain is not relieved within 4 days or if the pain recurs immediately the next time the player pitches. League officials should inform parents about this consideration.

2 Pitch counts should be monitored and regulated in youth baseball. Recommended limits for youth pitchers are shown in Table 21-1. Pitch count limits pertain to pitches thrown in games only. These limits do not include throws from other positions, instructional pitching during practice sessions, and throwing drills, which are important for the development of technique and strength. Backyard pitching practice after a pitched game is strongly discouraged.

3 The risk of throwing breaking pitches until physical maturity requires further research but throwing curves and sliders, particularly with poor mechanics appears to increase the risk of injury.

4 Pitchers should develop proper mechanics as early as possible and include more a year-round physical conditioning as their body develops.

5 Pitchers should be prohibited from returning to the mound in a game once they have been removed as the pitcher.

6 Baseball players—especially pitchers—are discouraged from participating in showcases because of the risk of injury. The importance of "showcases" should be de-emphasized, and at the least, pitchers should be permitted time to appropriately prepare.

7 Baseball pitchers are discouraged from pitching for more than 1 team in a given season.

8 Baseball pitchers should compete in baseball not more than 9 months in any given year, as perioidization is needed to give the pitcher's body time to rest and recover. For at least 3 months a year, a baseball pitcher should not play any baseball, participate in throwing drills, or participate in other stressful overhead activities (javelin throwing, football quarterback, softball, competitive swimming, etc).

swimmers (swimmer's shoulder), tennis players, gymnasts, and most overhead throwing sports.

Mechanism

The rotator cuff muscles help stabilize the head of the humerus in the glenoid. The rotator cuff muscles along with the long head of biceps prevent the head of the humerus from moving upward when the arm is abducted. Impingement occurs when the tendons of long head of biceps and supraspinatus, the subacromial bursa, and the greater tuberosity pass underneath the coraco-acromial arch, when the arm is abducted, elevated, or externally rotated. Glenohumeral instability, tendon overload, muscle weakness, and strength imbalance mainly contribute to impingement in young athletes. Repetitive overuse in overhead activities as seen in pitchers, swimmers, and tennis players, can lead to chronic inflammation of the rotator cuff tendons leading to edema and swelling, which will compromise the subacromial space. On the other hand, in weight lifters and gymnasts the mechanism seems to be sustained isometric muscle contractions leading to tendon overload. Either way with continued activity, a vicious cycle of impingement, edema and swelling, and further impingement sets in. The natural course of untreated condition has been described as a continuum progressing from an acute inflammation and swelling (stage I), to chronic inflammation, scarring, and tendinitis (stage II), eventually leading to rotator cuff tear (stage III). Other factors believed to contribute to the development of impingement, especially in older age group, are decreased vascularity, degeneration, and calcification of the rotator cuff tendons.

Swimmers and other overhead athletes will often have significantly weak scapular stabilizer muscles as well, and many will demonstrate scapular winging on examination, with a weak serratus anterior and other periscapular muscles, as well as poor overall coordination of the periscapular muscle groups.

Clinical Presentation

The athlete presents with progressively worsening, insidious onset shoulder pain of several days or weeks duration, exacerbated with activity. Some athletes will have discomfort at rest as well as nocturnal pain, especially when associated with glenohumeral instability. The pain is usually diffuse in most athletes, described as deep in the shoulder; however, sometimes it is noted predominantly superolaterally or posteriorly. The pain is exaggerated by overhead movements of the arm. Pain is felt specifically upon abduction between 70 and 120 degrees. The athletes notice that their performance has deteriorated.

Initially, the range of motion is not affected; however, later in the course there may be limitation of abduction and internal rotation. Palpation may reveal tenderness under the acromion process and over the long head of biceps tendon as it traverses the bicipital groove anteriorly, if it is also inflamed. Supraspinatus is tested for pain on resisted movement and weakness. Resistance is applied to arm abducted to 90 degrees, forward flexed at 30 degrees, and internally rotated (empty can sign) (Figure 20-9). Pain is also elicited with abduction, internal rotation, flexion of the arm (Figure 20-8), and forward flexion of the internally rotated arm (Figure 20-7) (impingement signs). Glenohumeral stability should be assessed by moving the humeral head in anterior, posterior, and inferior directions in relation to the glenoid (load and shift test, Figure 20-15). With anterior instability, pain, and discomfort can be elicited when the shoulder is abducted and externally rotated, and improves when the humeral head is moved in a posterior direction (relocation test) (Figure 20-14). Laxity in other joints should also be assessed, because generalized laxity is not an uncommon finding in adolescents. Pain can be temporarily relieved by injection of xylocaine into the subacromial bursa.

Diagnostic Imaging

Plain radiographs are normal in most young athletes and magnetic resonance imaging scan is not indicated unless rotator cuff tear, or glenoid labral tear is suspected and surgical intervention is a consideration. Tear of the rotator cuff, especially the supraspinatus, is extremely rare in young athletes. Other conditions to be considered in the differential diagnosis of recurrent or chronic shoulder pain in a young athlete are listed in Table 21-3.

Table 21-3.

Intrinsic Causes of Chronic/Recurrent Shoulder Pain in Young Athletes

Relatively more common
Stress injury of the proximal humeral physis
Glenohumeral joint instability
Rotator cuff tendonitis and impingement
Subacromial bursitis

Relatively less common
Glenoid labral tears
Atraumatic osteolysis of the distal clavicle
Scapular dyskinesis

Relatively rare
Stress fracture of scapula
Long thoracic neuropathy
Suprascapular neuropathy
Scapulothoracic bursitis

Treatment

Treatment consists of pain control, modification of activities, and progressive rehabilitation. Initially, complete rest from offending activities may be necessary for a short period of time. A progressive rehabilitation program will help restore full range of motion, strength, balance, and endurance of the rotator cuff muscles. Rehabilitation is followed by sport-specific training and conditioning. Training errors must be identified and corrected. Prognosis for resolution of symptoms and full return to sports is excellent in young athletes, although, it may take several weeks to months before the athletes may return to their previous level of participation. Surgical treatment is rarely a consideration in young athletes. Surgical release of acromio-clavicular ligament has been shown to be effective in some cases. Failure to respond to the conservative treatment should prompt reevaluation and careful consideration of any other underlying cause for the pain. If a cuff or labral tear is suspected orthopedic consultation should be obtained (Box 21-1).

GLENOHUMERAL JOINT INSTABILITY

Definitions and Epidemiology

Glenohumeral instability refers to excessive motion of the glenohumeral joint associated with relatively greater laxity of the joint stabilizers that result in either acute (traumatic) or chronic (nontraumatic) clinical symptoms and signs.[11] The spectrum of instability can range from microinstability to subluxation to dislocation of the glenohumeral joint. Although shoulder instability has been described based on the degree, frequency, acuity, etiology, and direction, for practical purposes, it is useful to consider two broad clinical presentations, namely acute traumatic dislocation (anterior, posterior, inferior) and chronic nontraumatic symptomatic instability (anterior, posterior, inferior, and multidirectional). Acute traumatic shoulder dislocation is covered in Chapter 20. Atraumatic instability is reviewed here.

Mechanism

The main static stabilizers of the glenohumeral joint are the head of the humerus and the glenoid, the glenohumeral ligaments, and the glenoid labrum, whereas the main dynamic stabilizers are the rotator cuff muscles. The role of the long head of the biceps brachii muscle in shoulder function has not been fully elucidated. The major mechanisms underlying the chronic atraumatic shoulder instability are described in Table 21-4. Shoulder laxity can be part of various genetic syndromes (e.g., Marfan, Ehler-Danlos) and systemic disorders.

Clinical Presentation

Multidirectional instability itself is a common problem, particularly in young female athletes, and can be one cause of rotator cuff tendonitis. Psychologic factors should be explored in the history. Most athletes with atraumatic instability are asymptomatic. The athlete with symptomatic instability will present with shoulder pain associated with overhead movements, a sense of weakness, and deterioration in sport performance. There may be a positive family history of the shoulder laxity.

On examination, the shoulder often will be unstable in several planes, with the athlete able to demonstrate multiple lax joints. On load and shift test, the athlete will demonstrate relatively greater than normal motion of the humeral head anteriorly and posteriorly on the glenoid (Figure 20-15). It is graded from I to IV, with grade I being translation of the humeral head within the glenoid, grade II translation of the humeral head to the rim, grade III translation of the humeral head up onto the rim of the glenoid and labrum, and grade IV translation of the humeral head beyond the glenoid and labrum. The most accurate way to assess this is to have the patient supine, with the arm in neutral rotation and grasp the proximal humerus, translating it anteriorly on the glenoid.

The sulcus sign is also positive with inferior instability (Figure 20-16). In a normal shoulder, this may be

Table 21-4.

Mechanisms of Instability

1. Repetitive overhead arm and shoulder movements such as seen in throwing sports, swimming, volleyball, and tennis.
2. Repetitive impingement of the rotator cuff complex underneath the coracoacromial arch during overhead activities.
3. Excessive motion of the head of the humerus mostly because of stretching and increased laxity of the ligaments and capsule.

present as well but usually will disappear with the arm in external rotation, which will tighten the rotator interval and eliminate the sulcus sign. Patients with multidirectional instability often can and will spontaneously and voluntarily subluxate or dislocate their shoulder(s). The relocation test is also positive (Figure 20-14) indicating anterior instability.

There is often associated capsular laxity and shoulder instability demonstrated in the asymptomatic shoulder as well. Laxity of the shoulder does not always correlate with symptoms.

Treatment

Athletes with symptomatic atraumatic instability must undergo a prolonged course of monitored comprehensive rehabilitation, followed by long-term home physical therapy for up to a year or more. Most athletes are not candidates for any surgical reconstruction or intervention other than rehabilitation, unless they prove to have a labral tear or other similar problems such as a significant capsular injury, which in a few cases will require an open or arthroscopic reconstruction. It takes a great deal of patience on the part of the young athlete, the family, and the surgeon to allow prolonged course of rehabilitation therapy to work.

DISORDERS OF LONG HEAD OF BICEPS BRACHII

Definitions and Epidemiology

The long head of the biceps brachii muscle (Figure 21-2) can be injured or inflamed resulting in pain or dysfunction. Disorders of the long head are uncommon in adolescent athletes but have been reported with acute trauma or repetitive overhead activities.[12]

Mechanism

The tendon originates from the posterosuperior labrum and the supraglenoid tubercle in the glenohumeral joint. It traverses out of the joint encased within the synovial sheath of the joint. It occupies the bicipital groove and is mainly restrained in position during shoulder movements by the surrounding soft tissue. The biceps brachii traverses both the shoulder and the elbow joints. It acts as a flexor and supinator of the elbow joint, but its role in shoulder movements has not been clearly elucidated. Biceps tendonitis may occur generally associated with rotator cuff tendonitis. Acute trauma is associated with glenoid labral injuries. The tendon may also subluxate or dislocate from the bicipital groove.

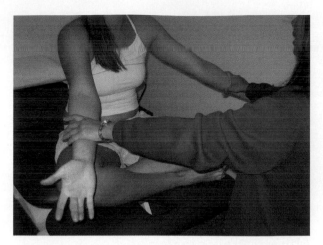

FIGURE 21-3 ■ Speed test. With the arm straight and supinated the athlete is asked to forward flex against manual resistance. Pain and tenderness in the bicipital groove are indicative of biceps brachii tendinitis.

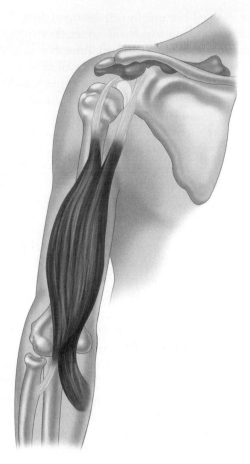

FIGURE 21-2 ■ Long head of biceps brachii tendon originates from the posterosuperior labrum and the supraglenoid tubercle in the glenohumeral joint.

Clinical Presentation

In case of an acute rupture or dislocation, the athlete will present with acute pain, localized tenderness, and soft tissue swelling. Injury can occur during activities such as throwing or heavy weight lifting. Biceps tendonitis is generally associated with rotator cuff tendonitis and impingement sings. The pain is exacerbated with arm in abduction, extension, and internal rotation. There will be localized tenderness over the bicipital groove and the speed test (Figure 21-3) may be positive.

Diagnostic Imaging

Generally no imaging is indicated. Evaluation of the tendon can be done with ultrasound or MRI scan, if indicated.

Treatment

Acute or chronic inflammation is treated with rest, ice, and NSAIDs. Rupture generally do not affect function and is treated conservatively with rehabilitation exercises. Surgical treatment has been reported for dislocating tendon.

ATRAUMATIC OSTEOLYSIS OF THE DISTAL CLAVICLE (AODC)

Definition and Epidemiology

AODC is characterized by chronic changes seen in the lateral end of the clavicle. It is seen most commonly in those engaged in body building and competitive weight lifting. Less commonly such lesions have been reported in tennis players, baseball pitchers, and football players. Most cases occur in boys, but the condition has been described in girls.

Mechanism

AODC is believed to be because of repetitive excess load and associated microtrauma to the distal end of the clavicle.

Clinical Presentation

The pain is of gradual onset, dull aching, unilateral or bilateral, over distal clavicle, and acromioclavicular area, experienced soon after exercise. Pain is elicited or exacerbated by adduction of the arm across the chest at horizontal flexion at 90 degrees (Figure 20-20). There may be localized tenderness over the acromioclavicuar joint area.

Diagnostic Imaging

The diagnostic features on plain films include microcysts, loss of subchondral bone detail, and osteolysis of distal clavicle (Figure 21-4). An increased uptake on

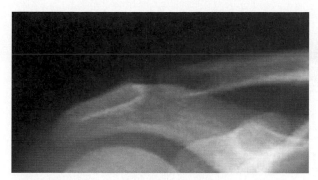

FIGURE 21-4 ■ X-ray characteristics of atraumatic osteolysis of distal clavicle.

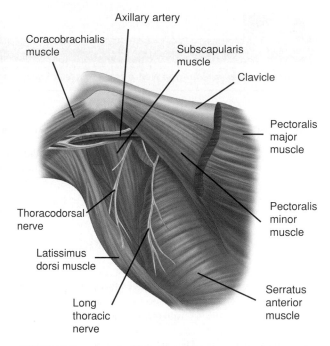

FIGURE 21-5 ■ Course of long thoracic nerve.

Technetium-99-m labeled phosphate scintigraphy is considered diagnostic by some experts.

Treatment

The athlete must make the difficult and often personally unacceptable decision to give up the weight lifting or other inciting activity. In these cases, surgical resection of distal clavicle has been shown to be quite effective.

LONG THORACIC NERVE NEUROPATHY

Definition and Epidemiology

Compression or direct injury of the long thoracic nerve can result in serratus anterior paralysis. Long thoracic nerve injury has been reported in many sports including basketball, bowling, discus throwing, football, gymnastics, hockey, tennis, weight lifting, wrestling, and soccer.[13]

Mechanism

The course of the long thoracic nerve is shown in Figure 21-5. In sports, long thoracic neuropathy can result from direct blow or repetitive trauma.

Clinical Presentation

The patient may present with diminished forward elevation of the shoulder, pain in the posterior shoulder, and the trapezius, with apparent winging or winging with attempted wall pushups or similar exercises. Differentiating features of common neurologic causes of scapular winging are summarized in Table 21-5. There also is often spasm of the trapezius and trigger point pain over the posterior superior scapula related to overuse of the trapezius muscle in an attempt to stabilize the scapula and elevate the shoulder.

Diagnostic Studies

Electromyography and nerve conduction studies are diagnostic.

Treatment

Many younger and adult athletes will regain full shoulder function after a several weeks course of scapular muscle and rotator cuff closed chain exercises and focused rehabilitation. Others will benefit from a longer term physical therapy, some up to 2 years for full recovery.

SUPRASCAPULAR NEUROPATHY

Definitions and Epidemiology

Compression or direct blow to the suprascapular nerve can result in partial or complete paralysis of either infraspinatus and/or supraspinatus muscles. Suprascapular neuropathy has been reported in throwing sports, volleyball, tennis, weight lifting, and swimming.

Table 21–5.

Clinical Features of Common Neurogenic Causes of Scapular Winging

Clinical Feature	Serratus Anterior Palsy (Long Thoracic Nerve)	Trapezius Palsy (Spinal Accessory Nerve)	Weakness of the Rhomboids (Dorsal Scapular or C5 Root)
Pain	Minimal; localized to scapular region	Mild to moderately severe, involving suprascapular fossa and shoulder	Pain usually major complaint; most marked along medial border of scapula
Winging at rest	Minimal; slight winging of lower part of scapula; lower part of medial border is closer to spine	Minimal; inferior angle is closer to spine	Minimal
Winging during activity	Accentuated by forward elevation and pushing with outstretched arms	Accentuated by arm abduction at shoulder level	Best demonstrated by having patient slowly lower arms from forward elevated position
Deformity at rest	Minimal, especially in frontal view	Trapezius wasting, suprascapular fossa appears deeper on affected side, shoulder droops	Minimal; rhomboidal atrophy if symptoms are long-standing
Scapular displacement during activity	Inferior angle farther from midline	Inferior angle moved toward midline	Shifted laterally and dorsally, especially lower portion

From Saeed, MA, Gatens PF Jr, Singh S: Winging of scapula. Am Fam Physician 24:139, 1981, with permission.

Mechanism

Repetitive trauma, direct blow, traction, or compression can result in suprascapular neuropathy in athletes. Suprascapular nerve compression is commonly associated with backpack straps or other straps or protective devices, which place pressure on the nerve as it exits above the scapula through the suprascapular notch. Compression of the nerve can also result from a ganglion or cyst. The course of the suprascapular nerve is shown in Figure 21-6.

Clinical Presentation

The compression may cause infraspinatus and supraspinatus muscle atrophy and weakness, and insidious onset shoulder pain, limited range of motion, and overall shoulder dysfunction. There is weakness of external rotation and abduction of the shoulder. Asymptomatic muscle wasting may be the only initial presentation (Figure 21-7). The clinical characteristics of various neuropathies about the shoulder are summarized in Table 21-6.

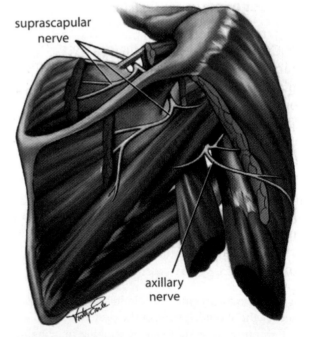

FIGURE 21-6 ■ Course of suprascapular nerve. (*Used with permission from Brukner P, Khan K. Clinical Sports Medicine. 3rd ed. New York: McGraw Hill; 2007:Figure 17-27, p 273.*)

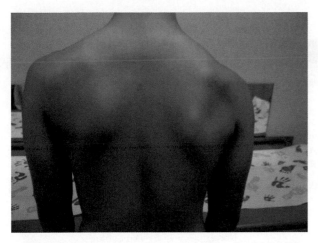

FIGURE 21-7 ■ Asymptomatic muscle wasting in suprascapular neuropathy.

Diagnostic Studies

EMG and nerve conduction studies are diagnostic. MRI scan may be indicated to evaluate the specific cause of compression such as a ganglion or a cyst in some cases.

Treatment

A simple compression or traction injury often will resolve with simple cessation of the irritating device, such as discontinuing use of a backpack for several weeks. Injuries which are persistent, may require an arthroscopic or open release of the suprascapular nerve, which is very effective in relieving pain, and may allow return of muscle mass and strength depending upon the

Table 21–6.

Peripheral Neuropathies About the Shoulder

Involved Nerve Root	Muscle Weakness	Sensory Alteration	Reflexes Involved	Mechanism
Suprascapular nerve (C5–C6)	Supraspinatus, infraspinatus (external rotation)	Superior aspect of shoulder from the clavicle to spine of scapula. Pain in posterior aspect of shoulder radiating into arm	None	Compression. Traction (scapular protraction plus horizontal adduction). Direct blow. Space-occupying lesion
Axillary (circumflex) nerve (posterior cord; C5–C6)	Deltoid, teres minor (abduction)	Deltoid area. Anterior shoulder pain	None	Anterior glenohumeral dislocation. Fracture of surgical neck of humerus. Forced abduction
Radial nerve (C5–C8, T1)	Triceps, wrist extensors, finger extensors (shoulder, wrist, and hand extension)	Dorsum of hand	Triceps	Fracture of humeral shaft. Direct pressure (e.g. crutch palsy)
Long thoracic nerve (C5–C6, C7)	Serratus anterior (scapular control)			Direct blow. Traction. Compression against internal chest wall (backpack injury). Heavy effort above shoulder height. Repetitive strain
Musculocutaneous nerve (C5–C7)	Coracobrachialis, biceps, brachialis (elbow flexion)	Lateral aspect of forearm	Biceps	Compression. Muscle hypertrophy. Direct blow. Fracture (clavicle and humerus). Dislocation (anterior). Shoulder surgery

(continued)

Table 21–6. (Continued)

Peripheral Neuropathies About the Shoulder

Involved Nerve Root	Muscle Weakness	Sensory Alteration	Reflexes Involved	Mechanism
Spinal accessory nerve (cranial nerve XI: C3–C4)	Trapezius (shoulder elevation)	Brachial plexus symptoms possible because of drooping of shoulder Shoulder aching	None	Direct blow Traction (shoulder depression and neck rotation to opposite side)
Subscapular nerve (posterior cord; C5–C6)	Subscapularis, teres major (internal rotation)	None	None	Direct blow Traction
Dorsal scapular nerve (C5)	Levator scapulae, rhomboid major, rhomboid minor (scapular retraction and elevation)	None	None	Direct blow Compression
Lateral pectoral nerve (C5–C6)	Pectoralis major, pectoralis minor	None	None	Direct blow
Thoracodorsal nerve (C6–C7, C8)	Latissimus dorsi	None	None	Direct blow
Supraclavicular nerve	—	Mild clavicular pain Sensory loss over anterior shoulder		Compression

Used with permission from Dutton M. Orthopaedic examination, evaluation, and intervention. 1st ed. New York: McGraw Hill; 2004:490.

length of time the injury has been present. The athlete may also present with primarily pain in the suprascapular region, with EMG showing delayed conduction in the suprascapular nerve, but not necessarily demonstrate any muscle wasting. These cases usually will require open or arthroscopic release of the ligament, which is compressing the nerve in the suprascapular notch.

SCAPULAR DYSKINESIS

Definition and Epidemiology

Scapular dyskinesis is characterized by abnormal alterations in the position of the scapula and its movements in relation to thoracic cage.[14]

Mechanism

Abnormalities of coordination and activation of scapulothoracic and shoulder complex muscles resulting from various causes are thought to be the most common underlying mechanisms of scapular dyskinesis. Deficiencies of scapular retraction, protraction, and elevation have been described in athletes with scapular dyskinesis. Shoulder and scapulothoracic overuse in sports requiring overhead activities such as pitching and tennis can result in altered scapulothoracic muscle function. Some of the conditions resulting in altered muscle function include direct trauma to the scapular area, injury to the long thoracic nerve or spinal accessory nerve, shoulder pathology, acromioclavicular joint pathology, or abnormal posture.

Clinical Presentation

The athlete presents with deterioration in sport performance and shoulder or scapular pain with movements. The intensity of overall activity should be assessed as overuse is a contributing factor for dyskinesis. Examination should include evaluation of the overall posture. With the patient standing both arms resting by sides observe for scapular prominence, asymmetry, or winging. Tenderness may be elicited over the scapula, the medial border, or superiorly. Abnormalities of scapular position and motion are assessed by scapular assistance test (Figure 21-8), scapular retraction test (Figure 21-9), and lateral scapular slide test (Figure 21-10).

Diagnostic Imaging

No specific imaging is indicated.

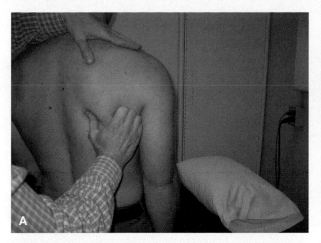
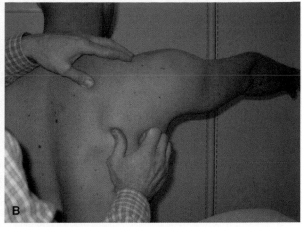

FIGURE 21-8 ■ Scapular assistance test. From behind the athlete, the examiner assists the scapula, with the hand positions as shown (**A**) in the figure, during rotation as the arm is elevated (**B**). This will assist the activities of the lower trapezius and serratus anterior during scapular elevation. Elimination or reduction of shoulder impingement pain with scapular assistance is a positive test and indicates the role of trapezius and serratus anterior muscles in impingement and need for their rehabilitation.

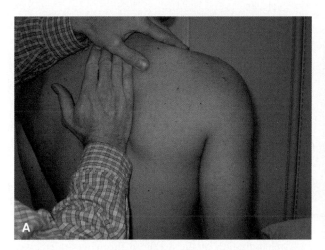
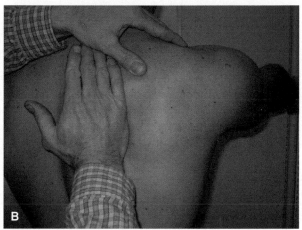

FIGURE 21-9 ■ Scapular retraction test. From behind the athlete, the examiner stabilizes the medial border of the scapula (**A**) as the athlete elevates the arm (**B**). A positive test is indicated by relief of rotator cuff impingement pain and is indicative of the role of scapular instability in the impingement symptoms.

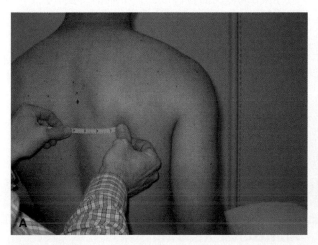
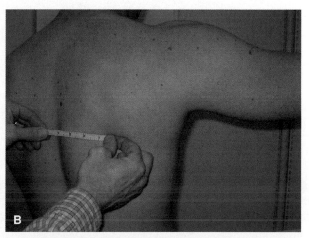

FIGURE 21-10 ■ Lateral scapular slide test. This test provides a means for quantitative measurement of scapular stabilizer muscles strength. With the athlete standing with arms by the side (**A**), locate and mark the inferior angles of the scapulae on both sides. A reference point is marked on the nearest spinous process at the same level. Measure the distance between the two points on both sides. Then the athlete is asked to place palms over the hips with thumbs posterior and shoulder slightly extended. Measure the distance between the two points (the spinous process and the inferior angle of the scapula) on both sides. Then ask the athlete to elevate the arms to 90 degrees (**B**). Again mark the inferior angle of the scapula and measure its distance to the reference point on the spinous process. Normally, the distance measured should not vary by more than 1.5 cm from the original measurement in each position. Greater variation is indicative of scapular instability during the glenohumeral movements.

Treatment

Any underlying condition such as shoulder or AC joint pathology should be treated by appropriate specific treatment. The mainstay of treatment of dyskinesis is physical therapy to correct the muscle imbalance, improve strength and coordination, improve sport technique, and improve flexibility. Athlete should be referred to physical therapy knowledgeable with the rehabilitation of this condition. Most young athletes will respond well to 8 to 12 weeks of specific rehabilitation program.

SCAPULOTHORACIC BURSITIS AND CREPITUS

Bursae around the scapula are shown in Figure 21-11. Although rare in adolescents, scapulothoracic bursitis can be a cause of recurrent or chronic scapulothoracic pain in athletes engaged in sports requiring a high intensity, repetitive overhead arm, and shoulder movements.[15] On examination, there will be localized tenderness and soft tissue swelling may be present. Treatment is conservative in most cases with rest from offending activity and rarely requiring excision of the bursa.

Scapulothoracic crepitus is generally normal in most individuals. Crepitus associated with pain may be because of bursitis or other rare causes such as osteochondroma of the rib or scapula, a rib fracture, or elastofibroma. Most will respond to conservative treatment with few requiring surgical treatment for specific underlying condition.

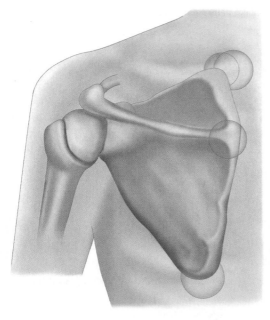

FIGURE 21-11 ■ Various scapulothoracic bursae locations. Symptomatic bursitis may affect the infraserratus bursae at the inferior angle of the scapula as well as the superomedial angle. A small bursa over the base of the spine of the scapula, called the trapezoid bursa may also be affected.

REFERENCES

1. Hutchinson MR, Ireland ML. Overuse and throwing injuries in the skeletally immature athlete. *AAOS Instructional Course Lectures* 2003;52:25-36.
2. Meister K. Injuries to the shoulder in the throwing athlete: biomechanics, pathophysiology, classification of injury. *Am J Sports Med.* 2000;28(2):265-275.
3. Meister K. Injuries to the shoulder in the throwing athlete: evaluation and treatment. *Am J Sports Med.* 2000;28(4): 587-601.
4. Altchek DW, Levinson M. The painful shoulder in the throwing athlete. *Orthop Clin North Am.* 2000;31(2): 241-245.
5. Ryu RKN, Dunbar WH, Kuhn JE, McFarland EG, Chronopoulos E, Kim TK. Comprehensive evaluation and treatment of the shoulder in the throwing athlete. *J Arhroscopy Relat Surg.* 2002;18(9):70-89.
6. Lyman S, Fleisig GS, Waterbor JW et al: Longitudinal study of elbow and shoulder pain in youth baseball pitchers. *Med Sci Sports Exerc.* 2001;33:1803-1810.
7. Sciascia A, Kibler WB. The pediatric overhead athlete: what is the real problem? *Clin J Sports Med.* 2006;16 (6): 471-477.
8. Lyman S, Fleisig GS, Andrews JR et al. Effect of pitch type, pitch count and pitching mechanics on risk of elbow and shoulder pain in youth baseball pitcher. *Am J Sports Med.* 2002;30:463-468.
9. Wilk KE, Meister K, Andrews JR. Current concepts in the rehabilitation of the overhead throwing athlete. *Am J Sports Med. 2002*;30(1):136-151.
10. McFarland EG, Ireland ML. Rehabilitation programs and prevention strategies in adolescent throwing athletes. *AAOS Instructional Course Lectures* 2003;52:37-42.
11. Walton J, Paxinos A, Tzannes A, Callanan M, Hayde K, Murrell AC. The unstable shoulder in the adolescent athlete. *Am J Sports Med.* 2002;30(5):758-767.
12. Sethi N, Wright R, Yamaguchi K. Disorders of the long head of the biceps tendon. *J Shoulder Elbow Surg.* 1999;8: 644-654.
13. Patel DR, Nelson TL. Winging of the scapula in a young athlete. *Adolesc Med.* 1996;7(3):433-438.
14. Kibler WB, McMullen J. Scapular dyskinesis and its relation to shoulder pain. *J Am Acad Orthop Surg.* 2003;11: 142-151.
15. Kuhn JE, Plancher KD, Hawkins RJ. Symptomatic scapulothoracic crepitus and bursitis. *J Am Acad Orthop Surg.* 1998;6:267-273.

Additional Reading

American Academy of Pediatrics Committee on Sports Medicine and Fitness. Risk of injury from baseball and softball in children. *Pediatric.* 2001;107(4):782-784.

Safran MR. Nerve injury about the shoulder in athletes, part 1, suprascapular nerve and axillary nerve. *Am J Sports Med.* 2004;32(3):803-819.

Safran MR, Nerve injury about the shoulder in athletes, part 2. Long thoracic nerve, spinal accessory nerve, burners. stingers, thoracic outlet syndrome. *Am J Sports Med.* 2004;32(4):1063-1076.

Bruckner P, Khan K, Kibler WB, Murrell. Shoulder pain. In: Bruckner P, Khan K, eds. *Clinical Sports Medicine.* 3rd ed. New York: McGraw Hill Professional; 2007:243-288.

Kibler WB. Shoulder rehabilitation: principles and practice. *Med Sci Sports Exerc.* 1998;30:S40-S50.

Reid DC. *Sports Injury Assessment and Rehabilitation.* New York: Churchill Livingstone; 1992:895-998.

CHAPTER 22

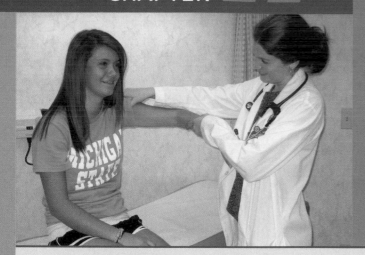

Acute Injuries of Elbow, Forearm, Wrist, and Hand

Steven Cline

ELBOW ANATOMY

The elbow joint (Figures 22-1–22-6) is a compound synovial joint and consists of the radiohumeral (radio-capetellar), ulnohumeral (trochlear), and proximal radioulnar articulations. The movements of elbow flexion and extension occur at the ulnohumeral joint and range between 150 and 160 degrees, with between 0 and 10 degrees of hyperextension. The main flexor muscles are biceps brachii and brachialis, whereas the main extensor muscle is triceps. The movements of supination and pronation occur at the proximal radioulnar joint and the radiohumeral joint. Biceps brachii muscle and supinator muscles are the primary supinators, whereas the pronator teres is the primary pronator. The ulnar or medial collateral ligament is the major stabilizer of the elbow joint during the throwing motion. The timing of appearance of secondary ossification centers around the elbow is listed in Table 22-1. All fuse to form

Table 22-1.	
Appearance of Elbow Ossification Centers	
Secondary Ossification Center	Age at Appearance (y)
Capitellum	1–2
Radial head	4–5
Inner (medial) epicondyle	5–7
Trochlea	9–10
Outer (lateral) epicondyle	10–12
Common fused elbow epiphysis	14–17

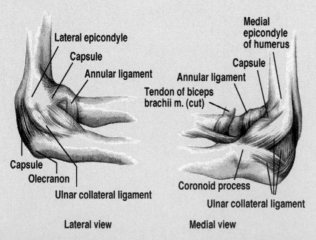

FIGURE 22-1 ■ Elbow anatomy. (*Used with permission from Van De, Graaff KM. Human Anatomy. 6th ed. New York: McGraw Hill; 2002: Figure 8-27, p 218.*)

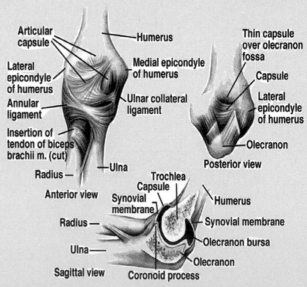

FIGURE 22-2 ■ Elbow anatomy. (*Used with permission from Van De, Graaff KM. Human Anatomy. 6th ed. New York: McGraw Hill; 2002: Figure 8-27, p 218.*)

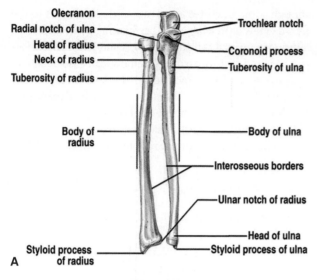

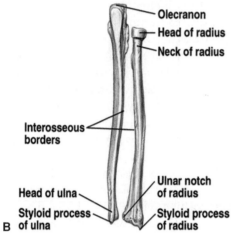

FIGURE 22-3a, 22-3b ■ Forearm anatomy. (*Used with permission from Van De, Graaff KM. Human Anatomy. 6th ed. New York:McGraw Hill; 2002:Figure 7-6, 7-7, p 177.*)

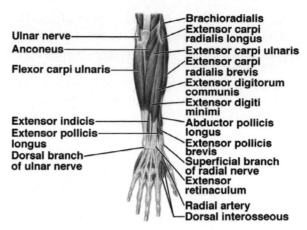

FIGURE 22-5 ■ Forearm anatomy. (*Used with permission from Van De, Graaff KM. Human Anatomy. 6th edition. New York:McGraw Hill; 2002: Figure 9-32, p 271.*)

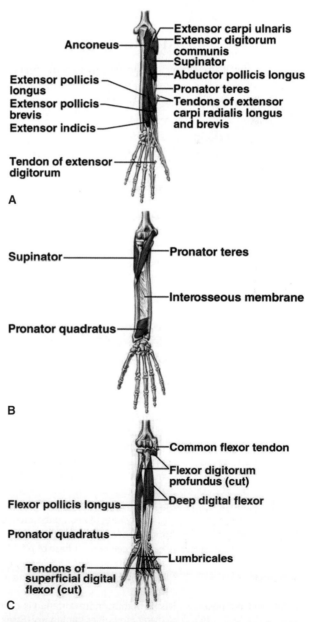

FIGURE 22-6 ■ Forearm anatomy. (*Used with permission from Van De, Graaff KM. Human Anatomy. 6th ed. New York:McGraw Hill; 2002: Figure 9-38, p 272.*)

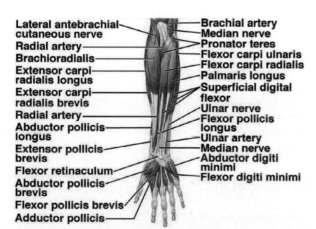

FIGURE 22-4 ■ Forearm anatomy. (*Used with permission from Van De, Graaff KM. Human Anatomy. 6th ed. New York:McGraw Hill; 2002: Figure 9-32, p 271.*)

a singe epiphysis between 14 and 17 years of age. The distal humeral physis contributes approximately 20% to final length of humerus.

The elbow itself is richly supplied with blood, and has a robust collateral circulation, except for the lateral condyle which has an end arterial blood supply without significant arterial collateral supply. This leads to an increased susceptibility to osteonecrosis with lateral condyle fractures. The ligaments about the elbow are closely associated with growth plates, and this can lead to avulsion or displacement injury of the apophyses during periods of rapid growth, as the ligaments themselves are stronger than the physes at this time in development.

FRACTURES ABOUT THE ELBOW

Definitions and Epidemiology

Fractures about the elbow can occur through the metaphysis (torus, buckle, or complete), physis (Salter-Harris type), or apophyses (avulsions). Eighty percent of all sport-related acute fractures in children and adolescents are of upper extremities and between 7% and 9% of these are about the elbow. Fractures about the elbow are relatively more common in boys and peak incidence is between 5 and 10 year of age.

Mechanisms

Most elbow fractures are owing to a fall on an outstretched arm in various positions (extension type),

though some fractures are owing to direct impact to the flexed elbow as in a fall while performing gymnastics and landing incorrectly (flexion type). A sudden varus or valgus force to the forearm and elbow can also result in apophyseal avulsion fractures of the lateral side or the medial side respectively. The type of fracture depends on the direction of force, the amount of energy imparted to the elbow, and the level of skeletal maturity of the athlete. Major elbow fractures are listed in Table 22-2.[1-6]

Clinical Presentation

The athlete presents with a history of a fall on outstretched arm or a sudden, forceful impact to the elbow. The elbow with an acute fracture is painful, swollen, and tender. The athlete is reluctant to move the elbow and typically will hold the injured arm supported by the other hand. In displaced fractures, there will be apparent deformity, whereas nondisplaced fractures will only have mild swelling and can be initially difficult to recognize clinically and often by x-ray as well. Given the history that can result in elbow fractures, the physician's assessment should be guided by a high index of suspicion, in cases in which findings of examination are minimal. Always assess perfusion, arterial pulses, and sensation to touch distally. Assess wrist and finger movements and strength. If a fracture is apparent or suspected, the elbow and the arm should be placed in a well-padded splint in neutral position (elbow at 90-degree flexion) with an arm sling (Figure 22-7) and the standard x-rays should be obtained before further manipulation of the elbow.

Table 22-2.

Summary List of Elbow Fractures

Fracture	Comments
Supracondylar	Break above condyles of humerus. Increased risk with elbow recurvatum. Most are extension type from FOOSH. Peak at 5–8 y. Rare after age 15 y. High risk for neurovascular complications
T-condylar	Codyles split by intra-articular extension of the T-component Caused by direct impact to flexed elbow by a fall. Peak at 12–13 y.
Lateral condyle physis	Fracture caused by forced varus movement, as in push-off with sudden extension of elbow. Increase risk with cubitus varus elbow. High risk for avascular necrosis of lateral condyle, delayed ulnar nerve palsy.
Lateral epicondyle	Apophyseal avulsion. Similar mechanism as lateral condyle fracture. Extremely rare.
Medial condyle physis	Caused by direct fall on outstretched arm. Rare before age 8 y.
Medial epicondyle	Apophyseal avulsion fracture. Seen with throwing, sudden forceful valgus stress during late cocking, early acceleration phase of pitching in baseball. Peak at 11–12 y. High association with elbow dislocations. Fractures epicondyle may get trapped in the joint.
Olecranon	Caused by overload of triceps. Rarely seen as an isolated fracture. Most are associated with other elbow fractures.
Radial head and neck	Neck fractures more common in children. Caused by direct impact or FOOSH. Check for associated distal radioulnar joint injury–Essex–Lopresti injury in which the athlete presents with pain at elbow and wrist.

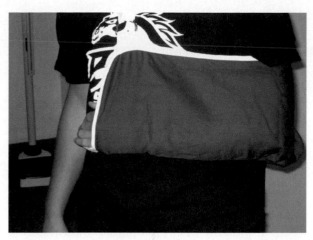

FIGURE 22-7 ■ Elbow splint immobilization. If a fracture is of elbow is suspected, the elbow and the arm should be placed in a well-padded splint in neutral position and supported by an arm sling.

Box 22-1 When to Refer to Specialist.*

Fractures about the elbow
Elbow dislocations
Forearm bone fractures
Complete tear of ulnar collateral ligament of thumb metacarpophalangeal joint
Displaced fracture of scaphoid
Nonunion of scaphoid fracture
Fractures of other carpal bones
Scapholunate dissociation
Closed flexor digitorum profundus avulsions
All open fractures of the hand bones
Displaced and angulated fractures of the metacarpals and phalanges
Thumb metacarpal fractures
Failure of closed reduction of dislocated metacarpophalaeal and interphalangeal joints

*Orthopedic or hand surgeon as applicable

Diagnostic Imaging

Standard x-rays of the elbow include AP view with elbow in extension, and a lateral view with the elbow at 90-degree flexion in neutral position. In the skeletally immature athlete, always obtain comparison views of the uninjured side. On the AP view, look for metaphyseal or epiphyseal fractures. Look for any asymmetry of the ossification center of the lateral condyle. On the lateral view, look for the normally well-defined teardrop appearance just above the capitellum, and posterior fat pad sign (Figure 22-8). For adequate evaluation of condyle fractures, varus or valgus stress views may be indicated.

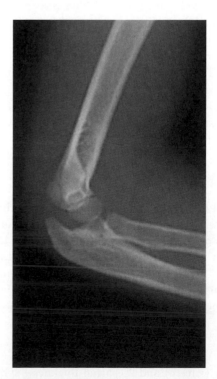

FIGURE 22-8 ■ Posterior fat pad sign.

Treatment

Initial treatment consists of immobilization in a well-padded posterior splint, a sling, ice, and elevation, with repeat neurovascular checks and orthopedic referral (Box 22-1). All displaced fractures, open fractures, and those associated with any neurovascular signs must be seen by orthopedic surgeon emergently. The athletes can expect to return to sports in approximately 8 to 12 weeks in most cases when they have no elbow pain, and have full range of pain free elbow movements.

POSTERIOR DISLOCATION OF THE ELBOW

Definitions and Epidemiology

Elbow dislocations are relatively rare in childhood, most are posterior, and account for <6% of pediatric elbow injuries. Most pediatric age elbow dislocations are seen in adolescent boys (70%) at 13 to 14 years of age. Up to 50% of elbow dislocations are associated with fractures of the medial epicondyle. *Monteggia fractures* are a variant of elbow dislocations and include a fracture of the ulna with a radial head dislocation.

Mechanism

Posterior dislocations occur with hyperextension of the elbow as in a fall on an extended outstretched arm.

Clinical Presentation

The athlete presents with a history of fall on outstretched arm and a sudden onset of severe pain and

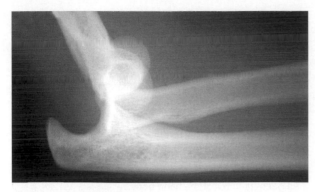

FIGURE 22-9 ■ X-ray of posterior dislocation of elbow.

swelling of the elbow. The deformity is apparent on examination. The olecranon will be prominent, the elbow is held in flexion, and the injury is usually closed. The adolescent is reluctant to move the arm. A meticulous neurovascular assessment must be done. Clinical differentiation of posterior elbow dislocation from supracondylar fracture may be difficult.

Diagnostic Imaging

AP and lateral x-rays will demonstrate the dislocation and any associated fractures (Figure 22-9).

Treatment

The athlete should be seen immediately in the emergency department and orthopedic consultation should be obtained. After x-rays have confirmed that there are no associated fractures, closed reduction is attempted under appropriate analgesia (Figure 22-10). The elbow

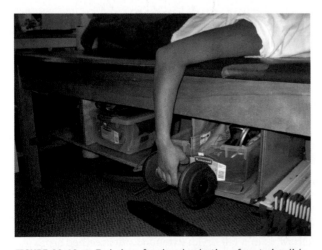

FIGURE 22-10 ■ Technique for closed reduction of posterior dislocation of the elbow. With the athlete lying prone on the examination table and the arm with dislocated elbow hanging over the edge of the table as shown, weight (5–10 lbs) is suspended with a strap around the wrist for approximately a period of 5 to 10 minutes by which most posterior dislocations tend to reduce.

usually is easily reducible and stable. Postreduction x-rays should be obtained. The arm is immobilized in a splint for 3 weeks with orthopedic follow-up.

ACUTE SPRAINS OF THE ULNAR COLLATERAL LIGAMENT (UCL) OF ELBOW

Definitions and Epidemiology

UCL sprains may result in partial-thickness or full-thickness complete tear. A full-thickness tear results in elbow instability. Acute sprains of UCL are rare in young children and most are seen in adolescents nearing skeletal maturity.

Mechanism

The ulnar or medial collateral ligament, particularly the anterior band provides stability to the elbow in conjunction with the bony anatomy, and it acts as a restraint to valgus stress of the elbow, especially during overhead throwing motion. Ulnar collateral ligament injury is most commonly associated with valgus extension overload during the pitching or throwing motion.

Clinical Presentation

The athlete will present with sudden onset medial elbow pain and tenderness, and in some cases may have paresthesias, pain, or weakness in the ulnar nerve distribution, over the ulnar border of the hand, ring, and little fingers. The elbow is best examined in slight flexion, with a small valgus load applies to the forearm (Figure 22-11). There will be discomfort with this maneuver and with a milking maneuver (Figure 22-12), which will localize the posterior band of the UCL.

Diagnostic Imaging

Look for osteophytes, loose bodies, and osteochondritis dissecans on standard x-rays. Instability is not always obvious on physical examination, or by static imaging, and may require stress films. MRI or MR arthrogram may be indicated to delineate the degree and nature of the ulnar collateral ligament injury, and associated soft tissue and cartilage injuries about the elbow.

Treatment

Grade 1 (stretch) and 2 (partial-thickness) sprains are initially treated conservatively. The usual treatment is

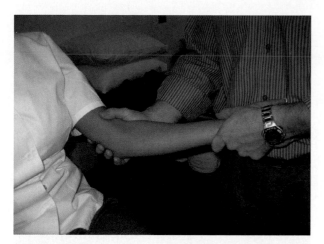

FIGURE 22-11 ■ Elbow ulnar collateral ligament stress test. With forearm in pronation elbow flexed approximately 30 degrees, a valgus stress is applied to the forearm. Pain or increased laxity is indicative of sprained medial or ulnar collateral ligament of the elbow.

rest, ice, a short period of sling use, and NSAIDs. Once the athlete has no pain in the elbow, range of motion, and progressive strengthening exercises are started. Six weeks after injury, the stability of the elbow is reassessed.

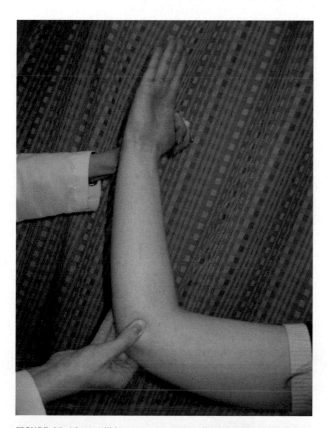

FIGURE 22-12 ■ Milking maneuver. The elbow is held at 90-degree flexion with shoulder in 90-degree abduction. The examiner places one hand over the medial elbow and with the other hand grasps the athlete's hand and thumb. The arm is supinated and externally rotated while maintaining a valgus stress at the elbow. Assess for pain or instability of the medial elbow.

If a grade 3 (full-thickness) sprain is diagnosed, and the athlete wishes to return to competitive throwing, a surgical reconstruction is often recommended. In those with a partial-thickness tear but persistent pain and dysfunction despite 3 months of conservative care, surgical reconstruction may be considered. Many young athletes will undergo collateral ligament reconstruction to improve function in the elbow, and at the same time address other coexisting elbow pathology through the arthroscope, such as loose bodies, cartilage injury, and posterior osteophytes.[7–9]

FOREARM BONE FRACTURES

Definition and Epidemiology

Fractures of the forearm can involve radius, ulna, or both. Most are distal radius or ulnar physeal or metaphyseal fractures. Physeal fractures are classified based on the Salter-Harris classification of acute growth plate fractures (see Chapter 19). Metaphyseal fractures can be incomplete (torus or greenstick) or complete fractures.

Distal radius fractures comprise 8% to 15% of pediatric fractures. Distal radius fractures can occur with either a fall on outstretched arm or a direct blow to the distal forearm and are seen in such activities as roller skating, *skate boarding, and inline skating*. The incidence of *fractures of the distal metaphysis* of the radius peaks in adolescents during peak growth velocity. Distal metaphyseal fractures can be torus, buckle, or complete fractures. Fractures of the distal radius physis are the most common physeal injury with a peak incidence at 13 to 14 years in boys and 9 to 10 years in girls.

Most distal ulnar fractures are metaphyseal fractures, distal ulna physeal fractures are rare. Distal ulnar fractures are most common in ice hockey and other stick sports such as lacrosse and field hockey. Metalphyseal fractures of both the radius and ulna peak at 11 to 12 year of age in girls and 13 to 14 years in boys. Galleazi fractures are forearm fractures with displacement or instability of the distal radioulnar joint.

Mechanism

Most are because of a fall on an outstretched extended hand, and rarely are because of a direct impact to the arm or wrist.

Clinical Presentation

The young athlete will present with pain around wrist and distal forearm after a fall, usually with a swollen tender wrist and limited motion of the wrist caused by pain. Nondisplaced, torus, and greenstick fractures may go unrecognized for days until the athlete is seen because of continued wrist pain and x-ray is obtained. Deformity of the distal forearm and wrist will be apparent with significantly displaced fractures.

Diagnostic Imaging

A pronator fat pad sign on lateral x-rays is an indication of occult fracture of the distal radius metaphysis or physis. Carefully look for torus or greenstick fractures.

Treatment

The forearm and wrist should be immobilized in a splint and a sling. Most are nondisplaced, closed injuries and can be treated in a long arm cast for 2 to 4 weeks. Most heal within 6 to 8 weeks.

SCAPHOID FRACTURES

Definitions and Epidemiology

Fractures of the scaphoid are classified into midwaist, distal pole, and proximal pole fractures (Figure 22-14).[10–12] Scaphoid fractures are the most common (60%) carpal bone fractures in children accounting for 0.45% of upper extremity fractures and 2.9% of hand and wrist fractures in children. The ossific nucleus of the scaphoid appears by age 5 to 6 years and is fully ossified between the ages of 13 and 14 years. The peak incidence of scaphoid fractures in the skeletally immature adolescent is at 15 years of age and most are distal pole fractures.

Mechanism

The classic mechanism of injury for a scaphoid fracture is a fall on an outstretched hand with large tensile forces acting across the scaphoid.

Clinical Presentation

The athlete presents with a history of fall on an outstretched hand and wrist pain exacerbated with movements. The athlete often presents late, a few weeks after the injury with complaints of an aching and stiff as well as a somewhat painful and swollen wrist. Such injuries are more common in gymnastics, as the gymnast's wrist is repeatedly placed under a heavy load. On examination,

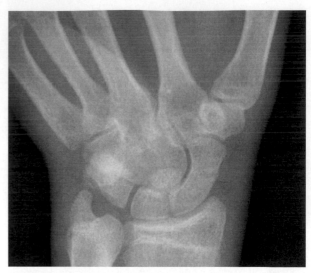

FIGURE 22-13 ■ X-ray of fracture of the waist of the scaphoid. (*Used with permission from Rakel RE, ed. Rakel Textbook of Family Medicine. 7th ed. Philadelphia, PA:Saunders Elsevier; 2007: Figure 42-35.*)

there may be tenderness over the snuff box and over the distal pole of the scaphoid.

Diagnostic Imaging

Plain x-rays may not demonstrate a nondisplaced scaphoid fracture for up to 2 weeks after initial injury. Special views, including clenched fist, and radial and ulnar deviation views may better delineate the fracture (Figure 22-13). MRI scan is sometimes indicated to diagnose these injuries in high-performance athletes.

Treatment

If a scaphoid fracture is suspected clinically, place the athlete in a long arm thumb spica splint or cast (see

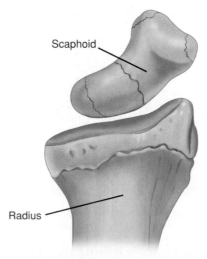

Scaphoid

Radius

FIGURE 22-14 ■ Line diagram showing scaphoid fracture sites.

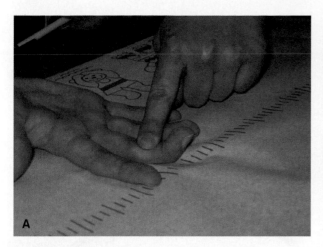
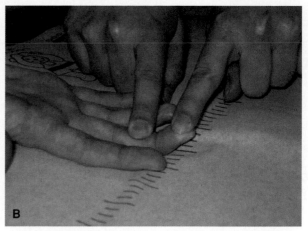

FIGURE 22-19 ■ Flexor digitorum profundus test. With the proximal interphalangeal joint held in extension, the athlete is asked to flex the distal interphalageal joint. Pain or weakness on DIP joint flexion will be present with FDP injury.

jersey at the player is pulling away. The ring finger is the most commonly affected.

Clinical Presentation

The athlete will usually recall the injury, describe a pop in the digit, and is unable to actively flex the distal interphalangeal joint (DIPJ) with proximal interphalangeal joint (PIPJ) and metacarpophalangeal joint (MCPJ) held in extension (Figure 22-19).

Diagnostic Imaging

AP and lateral x-rays of the finger(s) may sometimes show a small fleck of bone avulsed with the tendon from the base of the distal phalanx.

Treatment

The finger should be splinted in a slightly flexed position with immediate referral to a hand surgeon. There are various levels of retraction of the FDP after injury, and those tendons, which have retracted to the palm must be repaired within 7 to 10 days. If FDP ruptures are not repaired early and the athlete requires fine use of the hand, tendon grafts may be needed, otherwise the DIP joint may be fused. After tendon repair, a program of passive flexion and active extension for several weeks is employed. Athletes may return to competition in some cases at 2 weeks, if wearing a protective splint. Those athletes with flexor tendon repairs in sports which require a power grip, are kept from competition requiring gripping for up to 12 weeks.

FINGER EXTENSOR TENDON INJURY (MALLET FINGER)

Definition and Epidemiology

Mallet finger (dropped finger) represents a larger proportion of tendon injuries in children than in adults. Mallet finger is defined an avulsion of the terminal finger extensor tendon from its insertion at the dorsal aspect of the base of the distal phalanx.

Mechanism

Usually, the injury is from a direct blow to an extended finger in soccer, football, and more commonly basketball (Figure 22-20).

Clinical Presentation

The affected athlete cannot actively extend the DIPJ, and the joint and finger will be swollen and tender.

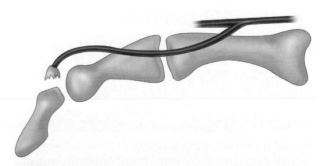

FIGURE 22-20 ■ Mechanism of mallet finger injury.

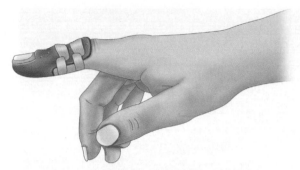

FIGURE 22-21 ■ Mallet splint. The finger is splinted with distal interphalageal joint held in extension.

Diagnostic Imaging

Plain film AP and lateral images of the finger will rule out other injuries and in those with open growth plates will help identify Salter-Harris type fractures.

Treatment

Treatment is closed in most cases, utilizing a splint which holds the DIP extended and allows motion of the PIP joint (Figure 22-21). Splinting is 6 weeks full time, then 4 weeks at night for a soft tissue injury.[11,12,14,15] Overall outcome is generally good, but some athletes will develop a few degrees of extensor lag and occasionally a mild flexion deficit of the DIP joint. Open injuries and those associated with fractures are sometimes repaired, with similar outcome, but less extensor lag. Those who undergo surgical repair may have more stiffness of the DIP joint.

There is also a special type of mallet finger in children, a type IV epiphyseal fracture in those with open physes. These are usually treated with closed reduction and splinting with the DIP extended for 3 to 4 weeks. The main problem with this injury is a possible interposition of periosteum or other soft tissues, which requires open reduction and fixation of the fracture as well as treatment of any nail bed injury.

EXTENSOR TENDON CENTRAL SLIP INJURY (BOUTONNIÈRE DEFORMITY)

Definition and Epidemiology

This is a disruption of the central slip of the extensor tendon from its insertion on the dorsal aspect of the base of the proximal phalanx (Figure 22-22). The injury usually does not present with typical deformity initially, as this will develop over the subsequent few weeks time if the injury is not treated early. Boutonnière deformity

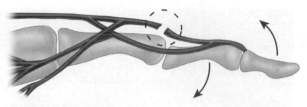

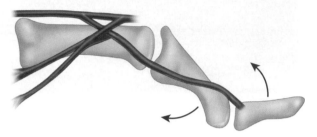

FIGURE 22-22 ■ Central slip disruption.

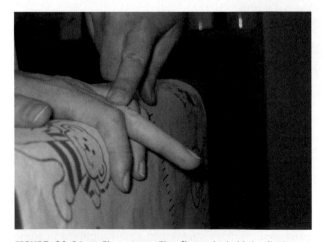

FIGURE 22-23 ■ Boutonnière deformity.

refers to the finger flexed at PIPJ and hyperextended at the DIPJ (Figure 23-23).

Mechanism

The injury results from a direct blow over the dorsum of the middle phalanx that causes forced flexion, while attempting to extend the finger. In some cases, there may be associated palmar dislocation of the PIPJ that may go unrecognized initially.

Clinical Presentation

The athlete will present with pain and tenderness over the dorsal PIPJ. To perform Elson test (Figure 22-24),

FIGURE 22-24 ■ Elson test. The finger is held in flexion at 90 dgreee at the PIP joint over the edge of the table. The athlete is then asked to extend the PIP joint. Normally, there is active extension at PIP joint. In case of central slip disruption, there will be no extension at the PIP joint; instead the extension occurs only at the DIP joint because of the action of the intact lateral extensions.

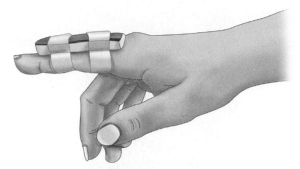

FIGURE 22-25 ■ Boutonnière splint. The finger is splinted with the proximal interphalageal joint held in extension.

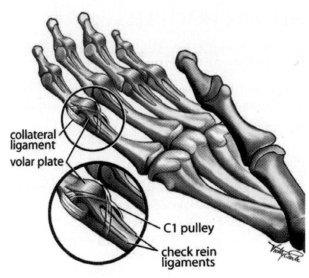

FIGURE 22-26 ■ Volar plate anatomy. (*Used with permission from Brukner P, Khan K. Clinical Sports Medicine. 3rd ed. New York:McGraw Hill; 2007:327.*)

hold the PIPJ at 90-degree flexion and ask the athlete to extend the finger. Inability to actively extend at PIPJ indicates rupture of the central slip. An injury that presents 10 days later or longer will often demonstrate flexion contracture of the PIPJ and hyperextension of the DIPJ, as the lateral bands of the extensor mechanism have subluxed volarly.

Diagnostic Imaging

Plain films of the digit will show any associated fracture or subluxation.

Treatment

If the injury is acute, the PIPJ is splinted in extension for 8 to 12 weeks while allowing motion of the adjacent joints (Figure 22-25). If diagnosed within several weeks, the patient will begin to develop the boutonniere deformity, and a splint to extend the PIPJ, and occupational therapy may correct the subsequent deformity and preserve PIPJ motion. Later on with a fixed deformity, correction may require more complex surgeries to the extensor mechanism and other procedures. Early protected active motion of the PIPJ with the injury stabilized is the preferred treatment for most PIPJ injuries. There are significantly more long-term problems with late stiffness of the PIPJ than with instability of the joint.

VOLAR PLATE DISRUPTION

Definition and Epidemiology

Volar plate is a thick fibrocartilagenous structure on the volar aspect of the PIPJ (Figure 22-26). Injury to the volar plate most commonly involves avulsion of the volar plate from its attachments to the phalanx.

Mechanism

Hyperextension of the PIPJ with a "jamming" injury in basketball or volleyball, for example, a direct hit with a ball on the finger is the most common mechanism of injury. The volar plate is tough but rigid, and will avulse with significant direct impact.

Clinical Presentation

The athlete will present with a painful and stiff PIPJ. There will be tenderness over the volar (palmar) aspect of the PIPJ and the joint may be boggy and quite swollen. If there is an associated avulsion fracture at the base of middle phalanx, the PIPJ may be subluxated dorsally. Sprain of collateral ligaments is often associated with instability of the PIPJ.

Diagnostic Imaging

AP and lateral x-rays should be obtained to rule out associate fracture and dislocation.

Treatment

The finger should be splinted for 6 to 8 weeks with the PIPJ at 20-degree flexion. Avulsion fractures and dislocation or subluxations of the PIPJ are indications for orthopedic consult. In the skeletally immature athlete with open growth plates, this is the most frequent articular injury, and is a Salter-Harris type III fracture of the growth plate at the base of the middle phalanx. The fracture is usually stable and only requires immobilization and buddy taping of the finger after a few days in a hand splint.

PHALANX FRACTURES

Definition and Epidemiology

Fractures of the phalanx are categorized as proximal, middle, and distal. These are extremely common injuries in ball and contact sports.

Mechanism

In a phalangeal fracture, the flexor and extensor tendons and muscle tendon units about the finger as well as the intrinsic muscles of the hand shorten and deform the fracture as the injury occurs. These injuries are usually closed, with intact neurovascular status, and an obviously deformed digit if there is significant displacement.

Clinical Presentation

The athlete will present with a painful and swollen digit. Angulation and deformity may be apparent in displaced fractures.

Diagnostic Imaging

X-rays, AP and lateral, as well as obliques will readily demonstrate the fracture.

Treatment

First ensure that there are no open wounds, that the fracture is closed, then assess motor, pin prick, and perfusion of the digit. Nondisplaced fractures are treated closed, with splinting and buddy taping. Digits which demonstrate angulation, rotation, shortening, or instability of the fracture often require closed reduction and pinning. Intra-articular or displaced condylar fractures may require open reduction internal fixation (ORIF). It is important to restore rotation and axial alignment to these fractures to restore hand function. Final angulation of phalangeal fractures should be less than 10 degrees.

METACARPAL FRACTURES OF 2nd TO 5th DIGITS

Definition and Epidemiology

Metacarpal fractures are categorized as fractures of the head, neck, shaft, or base of the metacarpal. Metacarpal fractures comprise up to 36% of all hand fractures. The boxer's or fifth metacarpal fracture accounts for 20% of all hand fractures.

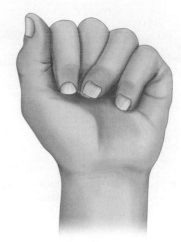

FIGURE 22-27 ■ Metacarpal fracture with angular deformity resulting in overriding of the finger.

Mechanism

Most metacarpal fractures result from an axial force directed to the metacarpal usually with closed fist striking an object of other person. Rarely a fracture can result from direct blow to the metacarpal.

Clinical Presentation

The athlete presents with localized pain, tenderness, and swelling over the fracture site. Depending upon the displacement, there may be deformity. The finger range of motion is limited because of pain. With the fingers flexed, note dropped knuckle and relative shortening of the injured finger. Over-riding fingers suggest rotational deformity (Figure 22-27). Note any abrasions or open wounds.

Treatment

All open injuries should be treated immediately emergently with hand surgery consultation. All closed fractures should be immobilized in ulnar (for ring and little finger fractures) or radial (for index and middle finger fractures) gutter splint and referred to a hand surgeon for definitive management. Metacarpal fractures are not universally benign, and a study in adult patients demonstrated loss of grip, loss of range of motion, and chronic pain after healing of minimally angulated and rotated metacarpal fractures.

EPIPHYSIOLYSIS

Definition and Epidemiology

Epiphysiolysis refers to acute Salter-Harris type epiphyseal fractures of the fingers and thumb. The epiphyses are located at the base of the phalanges, and the heads of the metacarpals, with the exception of the thumb metacarpal whose epiphysis is located at the base. The most common injury in the skeletally immature athlete is a Salter-Harris Type II fracture of the base of the fifth proximal phalanx.

Mechanism

Injuries are often caused by a torquing and abduction injury as the digit is caught or grasped and pulled by another child.

Clinical Presentation

The digit will be swollen and tender. In displaced fractures, the digit may display obvious deformity, usually in valgus, and may be rotated as well.

Diagnostic Imaging

X-rays of the digit in AP and lateral views will be diagnostic.

Treatment

All physeal fractures of the fingers should be managed in consultation with orthopedic or hand surgeon. With a type II fracture, the usual treatment is closed casting for 3 weeks with the MCP joint in 90 degrees of flexion. In a type III or IV or displaced fracture, one would reduce the fracture and open and fix the fracture if displacement is more than 2 mm. Type I injuries can be treated with simple immobilization and type V or crush injuries should be followed closely as there is a high risk of growth abnormalities.

FRACTURES OF THE THUMB METACARPAL

Definition and Epidemiology

Most fractures of the first metacarpal involve the base. The fracture can be extraarticular or intraarticular; and in the skeletally immature athlete can be epiphyseal.

Mechanism

These fractures result from direct impact to a flexed thumb as occurs with punching an object with a closed fist. Less commonly, fractures can result from forced abduction or flexion of the thumb.

Clinical Presentation

The athlete will present with localized pain and tenderness over the base of the thumb and limitation of movements.

Diagnostic Imaging

AP, lateral, and oblique view of the thumb should be obtained.

Treatment

The thumb should be immobilized in a thumb spica splint and the athlete referred to an orthopedic surgeon for definitive management. These fractures heal within 4 to 6 weeks, and the athlete may return to sports in 6 to 8 weeks.

THUMB ULNAR COLLATERAL LIGAMENT SPRAIN

Definition and Epidemiology

The ulnar collateral ligament (UCL) spans the medial or ulnar side of the metacarpophalangeal (MCP) joint. UCL sprains are common in hockey, skiing (skier's thumb), and lacrosse. Sprain of the thumb UCL is also called gamekeeper's thumb.

Mechanism

Sprain of the ulnar collateral ligament occurs with forced abduction of the hyperextended MCPJ of the thumb (Figure 22-28). In the skeletally immature patient, there is also a Salter-Harris type III epiphysiolysis

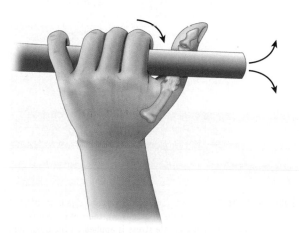

FIGURE 22-28 ■ Mechanism of sprain of the ulnar collateral ligament of the thumb metacarpophalngeal joint.

phalanx fractures is allowed once the wound and the fracture is healed, 6 to 8 weeks after initial injury. After injury, a short course of splinting for 2 to 3 weeks is done, then simple padding and buddy taping with protected use of the hand usually suffices. If there is a significant crush injury to the fingertip, parents and children need to be warned that there may be chronic pain in the digit, along with altered sensation, and some loss of range of motion of the DIP joint, as well as an altered appearance of the nail, or failure of a new nail to grow.

REFERENCES

1. Snead D, Rettig A. Hand and wrist fractures in athletes. *Curr Opin Ortho.* 2001;12:160-166.
2. Twee D, Herrera-Soto J. Elbow injuries in children. *Curr Opin Pediatr.* 2003;15:68-73.
3. Milbrandt T, Copley L. Common elbow injuries in children: evaluation, treatment, and clinical outcomes. *Curr Opin Orthop.* 2004;15:286-294.
4. Lee S, Mahar A, Miesen D, Newton P. Displaced pediatric supracondylar humerus fractures: biomechanical analysis of percutaneous pinning techniques. *JPO.* 2002;22:440-443.
5. Leet A, Young C, Hoffer M. Medial condyle fractures of the humerus in children. *JPO.* 2002;22:2-7.443.
6. Pirjol A. Isolated distal radial fractures in children-a word of caution. *JBJS.* 1999;81-B(suppl3):313.
7. Dodson C, Thomas A, Dines J, Nho S,Williams R, Altchek D. Medial ulnar collateral ligament reconstruction of the elbow in throwing athletes. *Am. J. Sports Med.* 2006; 34(12):1926-1932.
8. Kocher M, Anderson J. MCL Reconstruction in the pediatric athlete's elbow. *Tech in Orthop.* 2006;21(4):299-310.
9. Wilk K, Reinold M, Andrews J. Rehabilitation of the thrower's elbow. *Tech in hand and upper extr surg.* 2003; 7(4):197-216.
10. Goddard N. Carpal fractures in children. *CORR.* 2005; 432:73-76.
11. Vadivelu R, Dias J, Burke F, Stanton J. Hand injuries in children: a prospective study. *JPO.* 2006;26(1):29-35.
12. Valencia J, Leyva F, Gomez-Bajo G. Pediatric hand trauma. *CORR.* 2005;432:77-86
13. Alt V, Gasnier J, Sicre G. Injuries of the scapholunate ligament in children. *JPO-B.* 2004;13:326-329.
14. Rohrbough J, Judge K, Schilling R. Overuse injuries in the elite rock climber. *Med Sci Sports Exer.* 2000;32:981369-981372.
15. Frelberg A, Pollard B, Macdonald M, Duncan MJ. Management of proximal interphalangeal joint injuries. *JOT.* 1999;46(3):523-528.
16. Ardouin T, Poirier P, Rogez JM. Fingertips and nailbed injuries in children: a series of 241 cases. *JBJS.* 1999;81-B(suppl 3:350.
17. Fetter-Zarzeka A, Joseph MM. Hand and fingertip injuries in children. *Pediatr Emer Care.* 2002;18(5):341-345.

Additional Readings

Brukner P, Khan K, eds. *Clinical Sports Medicine.* New York:Mcgraw Hill Professional;2007:308-339.

Brukner P, Khan K, Garnham A, Ashe M, Gropper P. Wrist, hand, and finger injuries. In: Rettig AC, ed. Athletic injuries of the wrist and hand, part 1: traumatic injuries of the wrist. *Am J Sports Med.* 2003;31:1038-1048.

Chen F, Diaz V, Loehenberg M, Rosen J. Shoulder and elbow injuries in the skeletally immature athlete. *J Am Acad Orthop Surg.* 2005;13:172-185.

DiFiori J, Puffer J, Aish B, Dorey F. Wrist pain in young gymnasts: frequency and effects upon training over 1 year. *Clin J Sports Med.* 2002;12:348-353.

Kobayashi K, Burton K, Rodner C, Smith B, Caputo A. Lateral compression injuries in the pediatric elbow: Panner's disease and osteochonditis dissecans of the capitellum. *J Am Acad Orthop Surg.* 2004;12:246-254.

Morgan W, Schulz Slowman L. Acute hand and wrist injuries in athletes: evaluation and management. *J Am Acad Orthop Surg.* 2001;9:389-400.

Rettig AC. Athletic injuries of the wrist and hand, part 2: overuse injuries of the wrist and traumatic injuries to the hand. *Am J Sport Med.* 2004;32:262-273.

Strickland JW, Rettig AC. *Hand Injuries in Athletes.* Philadelphia, PA: WB Saunders: 1992.

Zlotolow D. Proximal ulnar fractures and dislocations. *Curr Opin in Orthop.* 2006;17:355-363.

Overuse Injuries of Elbow, Forearm, Wrist, and Hand

Dilip R. Patel and E. Dennis Lyne

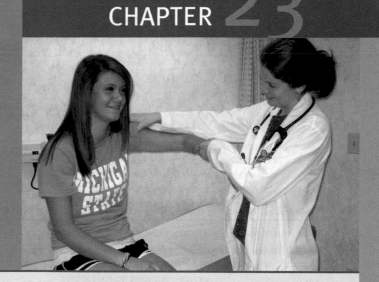

An estimated 20% of injuries to upper extremities involve the elbow, and approximately 10% involve the wrist; the majority of these injuries are overuse type of injuries.[1–4] Sports in which overuse injuries of the elbow and wrist in an adolescent occur are listed in Table 23-1. Also, in racquet sports (such as tennis or badminton) and in gymnastics, the elbow is subject to significant stress resulting in overuse injuries.

Table 23-1.
Sports in Which Overuse Injuries of Elbow and Wrist Are Seen

Relatively more common
Gymnastics
Racquet sports (e.g., tennis, badminton)
Throwing sports (e.g., baseball, softball)

Relatively less common
Archery
Basketball
Bowling
Canoeing
Golf
Handball
Kayaking
Martial arts
Rowing
Volleyball
Water-skiing
Weight lifting/training

ELBOW OVERUSE INJURIES IN THROWING ATHLETES

Definitions and Epidemiology

Repetitive throwing action can result in multiple injuries of elbow and are summarized in the Table 23-2.[5–11] Collectively, varying degrees of these injuries represent the "little leaguer elbow," which is a less preferred and nonspecific term.

Mechanisms

The secondary ossification centers around the elbow include the capitellum, radial head, medial epicondyle

Table 23-2.
Elbow Injuries Associated with Throwing

Medial epicondyle apophysitis
Medial epicondyle avulsion
Ulnar collateral ligament sprain
Ulnar neuritis
Elbow flexion contractures
Flexor-pronator syndrome
Olecranon osteophytes
Olecranon stress fracture
Osteochondritis dissecans of the capitellum
Intra-articular loose bodies
Triceps tendonitis

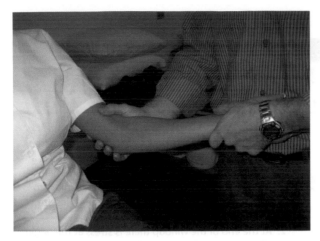

FIGURE 23-3 ■ Elbow ulnar collateral ligament stress test. With forearm in pronation elbow flexed approximately 30 degree a valgus stress is applied to the forearm. Pain or increased laxity is indicative of sprained medial or ulnar collateral ligament of the elbow.

common in throwing athletes, hyperextension should be considered abnormal.

Localize bony or soft tissue tenderness by systematic palpation. Localization of tenderness will suggest the anatomic etiology of elbow pain. The two major ligaments are the medial (ulnar) and lateral (radial) collateral ligaments. The medial or ulnar collateral ligament is the major stabilizer of the elbow during throwing motion.

Palpate the medial or ulnar collateral ligament with elbow at 50 degree of flexion. Valgus stress test is performed with elbow at approximately 20 to 30 degrees flexion (Figure 23-3) to assess ligament and elbow joint stability. Next perform valgus extension overload test in which the elbow is repeatedly extended from slight flexion while applying a valgus stress at the same time (Figure 23-4).

Palpate the ulnar nerve as it courses posterior to the medial epicondyle. Tenderness is elicited in neuritis. In

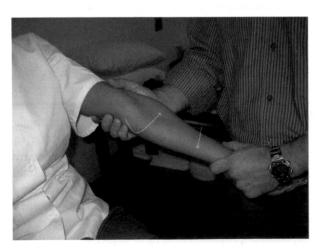

FIGURE 23-4 ■ Valgus extension overload test. The elbow is repeatedly extended from slight flexion while applying a valgus stress at the same time.

compressive neuropathy of the ulnar nerve at elbow Tinel sign will be positive with paresthesia felt in the ulnar nerve distribution. Assess pin-prick sensation in the upper extremity, palpate brachial and radial arterial pulses. Strength of entire upper extremity muscles should be assessed and compared to the asymptomatic side.

A number of conditions associated with chronic or recurrent activity-related elbow pain should be considered in the differential diagnosis (Table 23-4).[8–11]

Diagnostic Imaging

AP, lateral, oblique, and axial view x-rays with comparative views of the opposite side should be obtained in a young athlete with chronic or recurrent episodes of elbow pain. The x-rays are normal early in the course. The findings depend on the major underlying pathology and include hypertrophy and fragmentation of the medial epicondyle, widening of the medial epicondyle physis, olecranon osteophytes, or osteochondritis dissecans of the capitellum. More advanced imaging such as CT scan or MRI scan should be considered in consultation with the radiologist.

Treatment

With early recognition and rest from throwing, the clinical syndrome of medial elbow pain in throwing young athletes generally resolves completely. Nonsteroidal anti-inflammatory medications and local

Table 23-4.

Intrinsic Causes of Chronic Elbow Pain in Young Athletes

Lateral
Lateral epicondylitis
Osteochondritis dessicans of the capitellum or radial head
Posterior interosseus nerve entrapment

Medial
Flexor-pronator syndrome
Medial collateral ligament sprain or insufficiency
Ulnar neuritis or compression neuropathy
Medial epicondyle aphophysitis
Medial epicondylitis
Medial epicondyle avulsion

Posterior
Olecranon bursitis
Triceps insertional tendinitis
Stress fracture of the olecranon
Intra-articular loose bodies

Anterior
Biceps strain
Flexor-pronator exertional compartment syndrome
Anterior capsulitis

application of ice help alleviate inflammation and pain. With improvement of pain, the athlete can do progressive strengthening exercises for the upper extremity and gradually return to increasing levels of activity. Depending upon the severity, it may take from 6 weeks to 6 months for the athlete to return to full level of activity.

Measures to prevent throwing-related injuries in young athletes include proper preseason conditioning and limitation of the overall pitching or throwing activity. The age of the player and the type and velocity of the throwing techniques are also important factors to be addressed in an effective prevention program. If not recognized and treated early, further complications can occur. These include osteochondritis dissecans of the radial head or the capitellum, ulnar neuropathy, intra-articular loose bodies, flexion contracture at elbow, and early arthritis.

MEDIAL EPICONDYLE APOPHYSITIS

Definition and Epidemiology

Medial epicondyle is affected by repetitive stress during throwing and other overhead activities. This results in inflammation and painful apophysitis. Medial epiconyle apophysitis and avulsion are the most common injuries reported in young baseball pitchers. Similar lesions have also been reported in tennis, softball, football, and track and field, in which overhead arm movements are required.

Mechanism

The etiology is repeated tension stress over the attachment of the ulnar (medial) collateral ligament of the elbow on the medial epicondyle, from valgus movements and repetitive forceful contractions of the flexor-pronator muscle mass, which is attached to the epicondyle. Repetitive valgus stresses may lead to ultimate stress failure of the medial epicondylar apophysis and avulsion.

Clinical Presentation

Medial epicondyle apophysitis is characterized by the insidious onset of medial elbow pain with throwing. There is diminished ability to throw, medial elbow pain, and loss of pitch velocity or distance. Pain is usually most severe in late cocking and early acceleration. Examination often demonstrates pain with valgus stress of the elbow, point tenderness over the medial epicondyle, and a flexion contracture of the elbow may be present.

Diagnostic Imaging

AP and lateral x-rays of the elbow with comparison views of the uninvolved elbow are indicated. In the early stage,

x-ray may be normal, later, a widening of the apophysis is seen. Avulsion of the medial epicondyle apophysis can be confirmed on the basis of x-ray. X-rays may show subtle widening of the aphophysis, and this is confirmed by comparison views of the opposite elbow. Hypertrophy and fragmentation of the epicondyle may be present.

Treatment

Treatment is to stop throwing for a minimum of 6 weeks, initial ice and NSAIDs, and a short course of 1 to 2 weeks of immobilization in a sling. If there is a flexion contracture present, rehabilitation to regain motion is instituted, and a course of stretching and strengthening is started. A graduated course of throwing on a strict schedule is begun once the athlete is completely asymptomatic and nontender. Medial apophysitis responds well to nonsurgical treatment without long-term functional deficits. Athletes with medial epicondyle avulsion should be referred to orthopedics (Box 23-1).

ELBOW ULNAR COLLATERAL LIGAMENT SPRAINS

Acute sprains of the ulnar collateral ligament of the elbow are rare in young children and adolescents who are more likely to sustain medial epicondylar injury. Ligament sprains are more common in skeletally mature or near mature athletes and are reviewed in Chapter 22.

ULNAR NEURITIS

Definition

Ulnar neuritis is characterized by painful inflammation of the ulnar nerve as passes along the medial side of the elbow.

Mechanism

Traction owing to repetitive valgus stress, compression of the nerve from flexor muscle hypertrophy or osteophytes, or friction owing to subluxation, can also lead to ulnar neuritis in the throwing athletes. Elbow valgus instability is found in many throwing athletes who develop ulnar neuritis.

Box 23-1. When to Refer to Orthopedics.

Osteochondritis dissecans of the capitellum
Osteochondritis dissecans of the radial head
Flexion contractures of elbow in the throwing athlete
Triangular fibrocartilage complex tears*
Entrapment neuropathies at elbow and wrist*

*Hand surgeon

Clinical Presentation

Athletes present with medial side elbow pain worse during throwing or other overhead activities. There will be numbness or tingling radiating to the small and ring fingers of the affected side. Tinel sign is positive. There will be localized tenderness medially over the elbow and increased laxity on valgus stress may be elicited. Major features of nerve injuries about the elbow are summarized in Table 23-5.

Diagnostic Studies

Diagnosis is generally apparent clinically and can be confirmed by EMG or nerve conduction studies.

Treatment

Initial treatment is cessation of all throwing and overhead activities until symptoms subside. This may take up to 6 weeks on an average. During this period local ice and NSAIDs also help. This is followed by physical therapy and gradual return to sports. Athletes who fail to respond to conservative treatment should be referred to orthopedics.

OSTEOCHONDRITIS DISSECANS OF CAPITELLUM

Definition

Osteochondritis dissecans of the capitellum is caused by overuse of the elbow, particularly pitching in baseball. This is more common in male athletes, who form a larger proportion of young pitchers and baseball players. OCD of capitellum is also seen in young competitive gymnasts. Highest incident is between ages 11 and 15 years.

Mechanism

The articular cartilage overt the capitellum and the subchondral bone are subject to repetitive compression stress during the accleration and follow-through phases of pitching leading to localized necrosis and OCD lesion.

Clinical Presentation

The athlete presents with a painful, often swollen elbow, with lateral tenderness along the radiocapitellar (lateral elbow) joint, and decreased game and practice performance. By the time the athlete seeks medical attention he or she has been pitching for 3 to 5 years with elbow pain present for several months. Joint catching or locking indicate intra-articular loose body. Elbow pain is exacerbated with active radiocapitellar compression test in which the athlete is asked to supinate and pronate the forearm with elbow in full extension. There is often flexion contracture of the elbow.

Diagnostic Imaging

AP, lateral, and oblique x-rays are indicated. OCD lesion can be seen as localized radiolucency (Figure 23-5). In advanced cases there may be loose bodies and associated fragmentation of the capitellum.

Treatment

Early treatment would consist of rest from throwing, ice and NSAIDs, which may alleviate the symptoms in the elbow in the short-term. The elbow should be immobilized in a splint until athlete is asymptomatic, which may take several days to weeks. Presence of locking or catching is a sign of intra-articular loose bodies. These athletes and those who fail to respond to conservative treatment may need operative treatment and should be referred to orthopedics (Box 23-1).

PANNER DISEASE

Definition and Epidemiology

Panner disease is an osteochondrosis characterized by degeneration or necrosis of the ossification center of the capitellum followed by regeneration and recalcification. Panner disease is most common between 7 and 10 years of age.

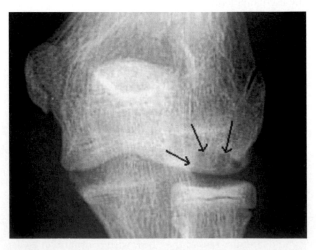

FIGURE 23-5 ◼ X-ray of osteochondritis dissecans of the capitellum.

Table 23–5.

Nerve Injuries About the Elbow

Nerve	Motor Loss	Sensory Loss	Functional Loss
Median nerve (C6–C8, T1)	Pronator teres Flexor carpi radialis Palmaris longus Flexor digitorum superficialis Flexor pollicis longus Lateral half of flexor digitorum profundus Pronator quadratus Thenar eminence Lateral two lumbricals	Palmar aspect of hand with thumb, index, middle, and lateral half of ring finger	Pronation weakness Wrist flexion and abduction weakness Loss of radial deviation at wrist Inability to oppose or flex thumb Thumb abduction weakness Weak grip Weak or no pinch (ape hand deformity)
Anterior interosseous nerve (branch of median nerve)	Flexor pollicis longus Lateral half of flexor digitorum profundus Pronator quadratus Thenar eminence muscles Lateral two lumbricals	None	Pronation weakness, especially at 90 degree elbow flexion Weakness of opposition and thumb flexion Weak finger flexion Weak pinch (no tip-to-tip)
Ulnar nerve (C7–C8, T1)	Flexor carpi ulnaris Medial half of flexor digitorum profundus Palmaris brevis Hypothenar eminence Adductor pollicis Medial two lumbricals All interossei	Dorsal and palmar aspect of little and medial half of ring finger	Weak wrist flexion Loss of ulnar deviation at wrist Loss of distal flexion of little finger Loss of abduction and adduction of fingers Inability to extend second and third phalanges of little and ring fingers (benediction hand deformity) Loss of thumb adduction
Radial nerve (C5–C8, T1)	Anconeus Brachioradialis Extensor carpi radialis longus and brevis Extensor digitorum Extensor pollicis longus and brevis Abductor pollicis longus Extensor carpi ulnaris Extensor indicis Extensor digiti minimi	Dorsum of hand (lateral two thirds) Dorsum and lateral aspect of thumb Proximal two thirds of dorsum of index, middle, and half of ring finger	Loss of supination Loss of wrist extension (wrist drop) Inability to grasp Inability to stabilize wrist Loss of finger extension Inability to abduct thumb
Posterior interosseous nerve (branch of radial nerve)	Extensor carpi radialis and brevis Extensor digitorum Extensor pollicis longus and brevis Abductor pollicis longus Extensor carpi ulnaris Extensor indicis Extensor digiti minimi	None	Weak wrist extension Weak finger extension Difficulty stabilizing wrist Difficulty with grasp Inability to abduct thumb

From Dutton M. Orthopaedic Examination, Evaluation, and Intervention. New York: McGraw Hill Medial; 2004:558.

Mechanism

Exact etiology is not known. Degeneration and necrosis of the capitellum are the main pathologic features.

Clinical Presentation

The child presents with dull, aching, lateral elbow pain, worse with throwing. There will be localized tenderness, swelling, and decreased range of motion. Examination findings are similar to those of osteochondritis dissecans. Panner disease is the most common cause of activity-related lateral elbow pain in a young child whereas osteochondritis dissecans is the most common cause in the adolescent.

Diagnostic Imaging

There are few radiographic changes of the capitellum, and usually no loose bodies or significant fragmentation are seen on elbow plain films.

Treatment

It is usually treated with rest, NSAIDs, activity modifications, and graded return to play over several months. In these children one must pay careful attention to pitch counts, innings played, and avoid overuse and inappropriate pitching styles. There are few long-term sequelae from Panner disease, as the younger athlete has more ability to heal the injured cartilage, and doesn't subject his elbow to the higher levels of impact and shear loading, or the long-term repetitive trauma that older and stronger athletes do.

TENNIS ELBOW

Definition and Epidemiology

Lateral epicondylitis or tennis elbow refers to microtears and inflammation of the lateral collateral ligament and common extensor origin, especially extensor carpi radialis brevis (ECRB) tendon, and extensor of the wrist and middle finger. The condition is less common in adolescents, however, reported with increased frequency in highly competitive young tennis players. Lateral epicondylitis is more common in a novice tennis player with poor stroke technique.

Mechanism

Inflammation and microtears of the common extensor origin, especially ECRB owing to repetitive overuse with incorrect technique is the main underlying mechanism of lateral epicondylitis.

Clinical Presentation

The athlete will complain of lateral discomfort just distal to the lateral epicondyle, and pain on resisted grip, and with wrist and middle finger extension against manual resistance. The player will describe an overload injury, commonly occurring with a one-handed backstroke, and with multiple games and hours of play. There is localized pain and tenderness over the lateral epicondyle. With athlete's elbow flexed at 90 degree, resisted extension at wrist elicits sharp pain over the lateral aspect of the elbow (Figure 23-6).

Treatment

Treatment consists of avoiding tennis till pain resolves, correcting wrong stroke techniques, local ice application, and nonsteroidal anti-inflammatory medication. A forearm counterforce brace may help as the athlete returns to tennis. The athlete should perform forearm strengthening exercises on a regular basis as an essential aspect of a prevention program. Conservative treatment may have to be continued for several weeks, and prognosis is very good in young athletes. Some athletes with chronic pain may benefit from local corticosteroid injection, however, great caution is advised in young athletes. If pain is not resolved with conservative treatment, orthopedic consultation should be obtained. Unrelenting tennis elbow unresponsive to conservative care and nearing skeletal maturity may be considered for an open or arthroscopic surgery to debride the ECRB tendon.

WRIST OVERUSE INJURIES

The articulation of the distal end of the radius with the scaphoid and lunate constitutes the radiocarpal or wrist

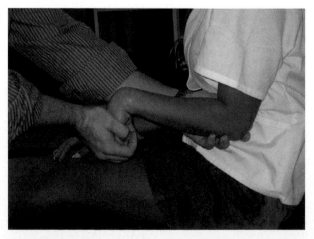

FIGURE 23-6 ■ Test for lateral epicondylitis. With the athlete's elbow held at 90 degree, resisted extension of wrist elicits sharp pain over the lateral aspect of the elbow.

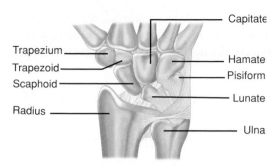

FIGURE 23-7 ■ Schematic diagram of wrist joint.

joint (Figure 23-7). The triangular fibrocartilagenous disk extends from the medial aspect of the distal radius to the lateral surface of the base of the ulnar styloid process. There is a compound articulation between the proximal and distal rows of carpal bones, constituting the midcarpal joints. There is also an articulation between the distal radius and ulna, called the distal or inferior radioulnar joint (Figure 23-8). Flexion, extension, radial deviation, and ulnar deviation are the major movements about the wrist. Extension at the wrist predominantly involves the radiocarpal articulation, while flexion involves the midcarpal articulations. Supination and pronation occur at the distal radioulnar joint.

STRESS INJURY OF THE DISTAL RADIAL PHYSIS

Definition and Epidemiology

Injury to the distal radial physis is more common in female gymnasts, between ages 12 and 14 years, engaged

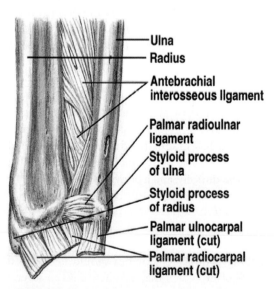

FIGURE 23-8 ■ Inferior radioulnar articulation. (*Used with permission from Van De Graaff KM: Human Anatomy. 6th ed. New York: McGraw Hill; 2003.*)

in high-level competitive gymnastics, affecting 25% to 80% of gymnasts.[12–15]

Mechanism

In the young gymnast the growth plate of the distal radius is particularly susceptible to stress injury. The distal radial physis is closed by 15 years in females and 17 years in males. In gymnastics, the wrist joint becomes a weight bearing joint, subject to excessive, repetitive loading activity, especially in a dorsiflexed position. This may result in a number of injuries causing wrist pain. Practice or game time that exceeds 35 h/wk has been shown to be a strong predisposing factor. Three stages of progression have been described, namely, (1) preradiographic, (2) radial physeal radiographic changes, and (3) radial physeal radiographic changes plus secondary ulnar positive variance.[12–15]

Clinical Presentation

The gymnast presents with recurrent or chronic wrist pain. The pain is aggravated by movements, especially stressing the wrist in dorsiflexion. Bilateral wrist pain has been reported in up to 30% of gymnasts. Associated discomfort and forearm pain are also common. In female gymnasts floor exercises and vault are most often associated with wrist pain whereas in male gymnasts floor exercises and pommel horse are most often associated. There may be localized tenderness and prominence of the distal radial physis. This and other causes of chronic wrist pain are listed in Table 23-6.[2,7,12–15]

Diagnostic Imaging

AP and lateral x-rays of the wrist are indicated. X-ray may be normal in the early stages. Characteristic changes seen on x-ray include widening of the distal radial physis, beaking of the physis, cystic changes in the metaphysis, and indistinct appearance of the physis (Table 23-7).

Ulnar variance on the AP view of the wrist refers to the length of distal ulna relative to that of the distal radius. In positive ulnar variance, the length of distal ulna exceeds by more than 1 mm, to that of distal radius; whereas it is the opposite in negative ulnar variance. Normally ulnar variance is negative before skeletal maturity, when it is generally neutral. In mature gymnasts a higher prevalence of positive ulnar variance has been reported, attributed to various factors such as overgrowth of the distal ulnar physis, growth arrest of the distal radial physis, or genetic predisposition. Chronic wrist pain has been reported to be more prevalent in those with positive ulnar variance.

MRI imaging in these athletes demonstrated damage to the physis and to the distal bony metaphysis as

Table 23-6.

Intrinsic Causes of Chronic Wrist Pain in Young Athletes

Relatively more common
Distal radial physis stress injury
Triangular fibrocartilage complex injury
De Quervain tenosynovitis
Dorsal soft tissue impingement syndrome

Relatively less common
Carpal instabilities
Distal radioulnar instability
Extensor tendinitis
Flexor tendinitis
Median nerve entrapment neuropathy
Ulnar nerve entrapment neuropathy
Intersection syndrome
Kienbock's disease
Ganglion cysts
Wrist capsulitis
Stress fracture of scaphoid
Scapholunate dissociation

well. There was relative lengthening of the ulna in these cases owing to the shortening of the radius.

Treatment

A period of avoiding wrist loading from 2 to 4 weeks duration generally results in significant symptomatic improvement. The return to activity should be gradual, and carefully monitored for recurrence of pain. Prevention measures include correcting the techniques and using a dorsiflexion block. In more chronic and severe cases, prolonged wrist immobilization may be needed. In some cases long-term complications include premature fusion of the distal radial physis and radial shortening. Orthopedic consultation should be obtained in these cases.

If a physeal injury is suspected, the athlete is withdrawn from training and competition until

Table 23-7.

Roy et al. Radiographic Criteria for Stress Injury of Distal Radial Physis

One or more of the following
1. Widening of the distal radial growth plate
2. Cystic changes of the metaphyseal aspect of the epiphysis
3. A beaked effect of the distal aspect of epiphysis
4. Hazziness within the usually radiolucent area of the growth plate

asymptomatic. It needs to be emphasized that further participation may lead to permanent growth arrest, functional problems, chronic pain, and future arthritis.

DORSAL IMPINGEMENT SYNDROME

Definition and Epidemiology

Dorsal impingement syndrome in gymnasts is characterized by wrist joint capulitis or synovitis and thickening. Impingement syndromes are common in gymnastics, in which the wrist is used as a weightbearing joint. More than 50% of young beginner to midlevel gymnasts have wrist pain. Furthermore, the pain is persistent with 89% of competitive gymnasts in one study experiencing pain 1 year after the initial onset of wrist pain. The most commonly diagnosed problem in gymnasts with persistent wrist pain is dorsal wrist capsulitis from repetitive hyperextension.

Mechanism

The constant vaulting and tumbling with frequent rapid loading of the wrist in gymnastics causes a variety of injuries ranging from distal radial physeal stress reaction and scaphoid impaction, to dorsal wrist impingement with capsulitis. These athletes may develop a bony dorsal exostosis on x-ray, with impingement and loss of wrist extension.

Diagnostic Imaging

X-rays may be negative in many cases. MRI scan with high field magnets may make it easier to differentiate scaphoid and physeal injuries from capsulitis and other causes of wrist pain. Plain AP, lateral and oblique films of the wrist may demonstrate an exostosis, and occasionally a CT scan is needed to better define the injury.

Clinical Presentation

The gymnast with wrist pain usually presents for care because of the loss of ability to perform at his or her usual level, and has gradually adapted to the limited motion in the wrist. The wrist joint is sometimes swollen with tenderness dorsally, and a bony prominence may be felt on the dorsal aspect primarily over the radius.

Treatment

The offending gymnastic activities should be stopped until pain resolves, which may take few days to several weeks. Splint immobilization and NSAIDs for short period will alleviate the pain. If the pain persists intra-articular corticosteroid injection may be considered.

The athlete with persistent pain may later require a cheilectomy to remove the coexisting osteophyte.

TRIANGULAR FIBROCARTILAGE COMPLEX INJURY

Definition and Epidemiology

Triangular fibrocartilage complex (TFCC) is an intra-articular fibrocartilagenous disk in the wrist joint (Figure 23-9) subject to both acute and overuse injuries. Injury to TFCC can occur in many sports including racquet sports, hockey, and gymnastics, and may be caused by acute trauma or chronic stress.

Mechanism

The TFCC has wrist stabilizing and cushioning functions. The fibrocartilagenous disk is an intra-articular structure, and is susceptible to injury from repetitive loading, supination, and pronation movements especially with ulnar deviaton. This can lead to perforation or tear of the disk.

Clinical Presentation

There is recurrent or chronic wrist pain, generally located on the ulnar side of the joint, particularly aggravated by supination and pronation. Movements at wrist may be associated with a clicking sensation. Swelling is uncommon, and usually there is no significant limitation of motion. Localized tenderness can be elicited over the ulnar side of the wrist joint line.

Diagnostic Imaging

Plain x-rays are usually normal; in some cases there may be a positive ulnar variance. MRI scan is the study of choice for detecting a tear or perforation of the TFCC, although in some cases it may fail to detect the tear or perforation and arthroscopy may be indicated.

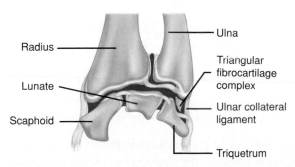

FIGURE 23-9 ■ Schematic showing triangular fibrocartilage complex.

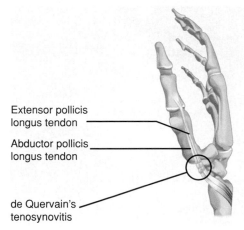

FIGURE 23-10 ■ Tendons affected in de Quervain tendonitis. (*Used with permission from Brukner P, Khan K. Clinical Sports Medicine. 3rd ed. New York: McGraw Hill; 2007322.*)

Treatment

The offending activity should be stopped and wrist immobilized initially for 4 to 6 week duration (sometimes longer). TFCC injuries are often difficult to heal and an orthopedic or hand surgery consultation should be considered.

De QUERVAIN TENDINITIS

Definition and Epidemiology

This is a stenosing tenosynovitis involving the tendons of the abductor pollicis longus and extensor pollicis brevis (the first dorsal compartment of the wrist) (Figure 23-10). In sports, it has been most commonly reported in golf, squash, and racquet sports especially badminiton.

Mechanism

Repetitive gliding of the dorsal compartment tendons over the radial styloid leads microtrauma and inflammation. Forceful grasping with the hand associated with ulnar deviation or repetitive use of the thumb predispose to tenosynovitis.

Clinical Presentation

There is pain and tenderness along the course of the tendons over the thumb and wrist. Occasionally creptitus may be felt. The pain is aggravated by movements of the thumb. With the thumb placed in palm to make a fist, ulnar deviation of the wrist elicits pain along the tendons (Finkelstein's test) (Figure 23-11).

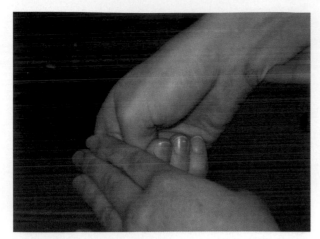

FIGURE 23-11 ■ Finkelstein test. With the thumb placed in palm to make a fist, ulnar deviation of the wrist elicits pain along the thumb extensor and abductor tendons.

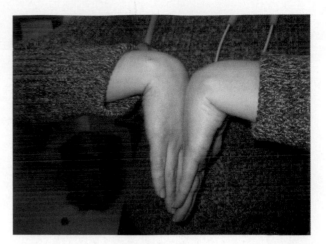

FIGURE 23-12 ■ Phalen test. With the wrist in full flexion for at least 1 minute, tingling or numbness may be elicited in the thumb, index or middle finger in positive Phalen test.

Diagnostic Imaging

No specific studies are indicated.

Treatment

Treatment consists of control of pain and inflammation, along with modification of any identified precipitating activity. Occasionally, splint immobilization in a thumb spica for few days to several weeks may be needed. Local corticosteroid injection may be beneficial for severe pain with great caution in the young athlete.

CARPAL TUNNEL SYNDROME

Definition and Epidemiology

Carpal tunnel syndrome is entrapment neuropathy of the median nerve at wrist as it traverses the carpal tunnel. Carpal tunnel syndrome has been reported in weight trainers, rowers, skiers, pitchers, and catchers, and in wheelchair athletes from repetitive local pressure.

Mechanism

Median nerve entrapment can occur in the carpal tunnel at wrist in athletes as a result of overuse. Since flexor tendons acccompany the median nerve in the canal, flexor tendinitis is also often associated.

Clinical Presentation

The initial symptom is wrist pain, which may be associated with an activity or may occur at night waking up the athlete. Also, there may be stiffness associated with the

pain; paresthesia and numbness are present in the median nerve distribution—thumb, index, and middle fingers. The motor function is tested by having the patient touch the tips of thumb and little finger. With the wrist in complete flexion for at least 1 minute, tingling or numbness may be produced in the thumb, index, or middle finger (Phalen's test) (Figure 23-12). Percussion of the median nerve over the carpal tunnel may also produce a tingling sensation distally (Tinel's sign). Other causes associated with carpal tunnel syndrome (such as local trauma, hypothyroidism, and diabetes mellitus) should be considered in the differential diagnosis.

Diagnostic Studies

EMG and NCV studies are diagnostic.

Treatment

Conservative treatment consists of rest, wrist immobilization in a splint for several weeks (depending upon the severity of the condition), and nonsteroidal anti-inflammatory medications. Most young athletes respond well to this conservative treatment. In a few cases, however, failure of conservative treatment is an indication to obtain surgical consultation for further management.

ULNAR NERVE ENTRAPMENT AT WRIST (CYCLISTS "PALSY")

Definition and Epidemiology

Ulnar nerve neuropathy is an entrapment neuropathy as the nerve traverses the Guyon canal and is seen most commonly in cyclists.

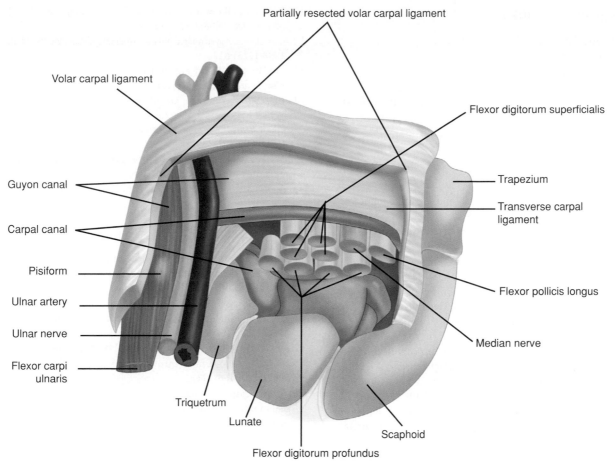

FIGURE 23-13 ■ Guyon canal.

Mechanism

The ulnar nerve passes into the hand through Guyon's canal (Figure 23-13). It is susceptible to repetitive injuries and entrapment from local trauma (as catching ball) or chronic pressure (from handle bar in cycling).

Clinical Presentation

The athlete presents with a complaint of having an altered sensation in the little finger; atrophy of the hypothenar eminence can be seen in chronic cases. Thumb adduction is tested by having the patient pinch a piece of paper between thumb and index finger. When the adductors are weak, the thumb interphalangeal joint flexes trying to hold on to the paper (Froment's sign) (Figure 23-14). The interossei are tested by asking the patient to abduct and adduct the fingers against manual resistance. The hypothenar muscles are tested by asking the patient to move the little finger away from other fingers against manual resistance.

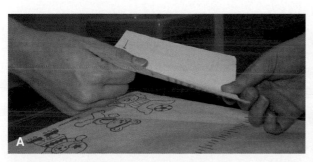
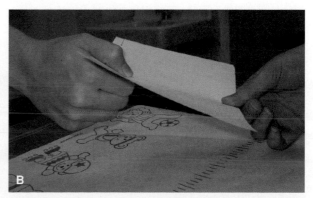

FIGURE 23-14 ■ Froment sign. When the adductors of the thumb are weak, the thumb interphalageal joint flexes trying to hold on to the paper as shown.

Diagnostic Studies

EMG and NCV studies are diagnostic.

Treatment

Conservative treatment consists of avoiding the offending activity, and a period of rest. Failure of symptoms to resolve is an indication for surgical consultation.

REFERENCES

1. DiFiori JP. Overuse injuries in children and adolescents. *Phys Sportsmed*. 1999;27(1):10-18
2. Strickland JW, Rettig AC. *Hand Injuries in Athletes*. Philadelphia,PA: WB Saunders; 1992.
3. Micheli LJ. Overuse injuries in children's sports : the growth factor. *Orthop Clin North Am*. 1983;14:337.
4. Andrish JT. Upper extremity injuries in the skeletally immature athlete. In: Nicholas JA, Hershman EB, eds. *The Upper Extremity in Sports Medicine*. Philadelphia, PA: Mosby; 1990:675.
5. DaSilva M, Williams JS, Fadale PD, et al. Pediatric throwing injuries about the elbow. *Am J Orthop*. February 1998:90.
6. Whiteside JA, Andrews JR, Fleisig GS : Elbow injuries in young baseball players. *Phys Sportsmed*. 1999;27(6):87.
7. Reid DC. Forearm, wrist, and hand. In: Reid DC *Sports Injury Assessment and Rehabilitation*. New York: Churchill Livingstone; 1992:1053-1130.
8. Gill TJ 4th, Micheli LJ. The immature athlete: common injuries and overuse syndromes of the elbow and wrist. *Clin Sports Med*. 1996;15:401.
9. Kelly AM, Pappas AM. Shoulder and elbow injuries and painful syndromes. *Adolesc Med State Art Rev*. 1998;9(3):569.
10. Field LD, Savoie FH. Common elbow injuries in sport. *Sports Med*. 1998;26(3):193.
11. Retig AC. Elbow, forearm and wrist injuries in the athlete. *Sports Med*. 1998;25(2):115.
12. Gabel GT. Gymnastic wrist injuries. *Clin Sports Med*. 1998;17(3):612.
13. Weiker GG. Hand and wrist problems in the gymnast. *Clin Sports Med*. 1992;11(1):189.
14. Brukner P, Khan K, Garnham A, Ashe M, Gropper P. Wrist, hand and finger injuries. In: Brukner P, Khan K, eds. *Clinical Sports Medicine*. Sydney, Australia: McGraw-Hill; 2007:308-339.
15. Weiker GG. Upper extremity gymnastic injuries. In: Nicholas JA, Hershman EB, eds. *The Upper Extremity in Sports Medicine*. Philadelphia, PA: Mosby; 1990:861.

Additional Readings

Brukner P, Khan K, Bell S. Elbow and forearm pain. In: Brukner P, Khan K, eds. *Clinical Sports Medicine*. Sydney, Australia: McGraw-Hill Professional;2007:289-307.

Cain EL, Dugas J, Wolf RS, Andrews JR. Elbow injuries in throwing athletes: a current concepts review. *Am J Sports Med*. 2003;31(4):621-635.

Chen AL, Youm T, Ong BC, Rafii M, Rokito AS. Imaging of the elbow in the overhead throwing athlete. *Am J Sports Med*. 2003;31(3):466-473.

DiFiori JP, Caine DJ, Malina RM. Wrist pain, distal radial physeal injury and ulnar variance in the yound gymnast. *Am J Sports Med*. 2006;34(5):840-849.

Gerbino PG. Elbow disorders in throwing athletes. *Orthop Clin North Am*. 2003;34:417-426.

Nirschl RP. Elbow tendinosis/Tennis elbow. *Clin Sports Med*. 1992;11(4):851.

Reid DC. *Sports Injury Assessment and Rehabilitation*. Philadelphia, PA: Churchill Livingston; 1992:999-1130.

Rettig AC. Athletic injuries of the wrist and hand, part 2: overuse injuries of the wrist and traumatic inuries of the hand. *Am J Sports Med*. 2004;32(1):262-273.

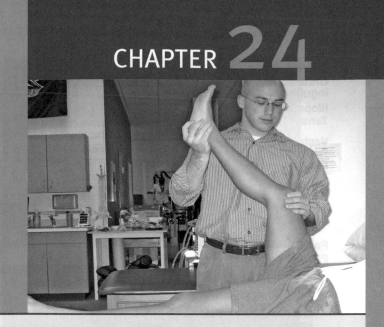

CHAPTER 24

Acute Injuries of the Hip, Pelvis, and Thigh

Steven Cline

ANATOMY

Anatomy, relevant to the present discussion, is depicted and described in Figures 24-1 to 24-4.

Definitions and Epidemiology

One study reported that 2.5% of all sports injuries were hip injuries, and in high school athletes, hip injuries were 5% to 9% of all athletic injuries. Apophyseal avulsions and musculotendinous strains are the most common acute injuries of hip, pelvis, and groin seen in youth sports.[1–9]

Mechanisms

Mechanisms are discussed below under specific injuries. Common mechanisms of injury include waterskiing and hurdling for hamstrings tears or avulsions, direct trauma to the anterior pelvis for iliac crest avulsions, and skiing and snowboarding falls with associated hip dislocations, and acetabular fractures.

Clinical Presentation

The athlete may present with a history of direct or indirect injury to the hip and pelvis from a fall, collision, or injury from "noncontact" sports. The young athlete may also present with chronic hip pain after overuse, such as distance running, which may be associated with a stress fracture of the femoral neck, or other associated injuries.[4,5]

The main symptom in many cases is the sudden onset of groin or hip pain, or pain along the iliac crest with avulsion injuries, as well as thigh or buttock pain with hamstring tears or apophyseal injuries. The patient may be reluctant to bear weight on the limb with a proximal femur or acetabular fracture, or an injury to the femoral

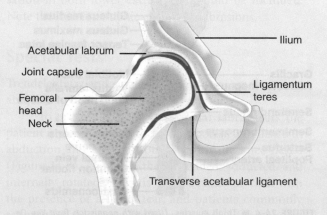

FIGURE 24-1 ■ Pelvis. (*Used with permission from Van De Graaff KM. Human Anatomy. 6th ed. New York: McGraw Hill;2002.*)

FIGURE 24-2 ■ Schematic drawing of the hip joint.

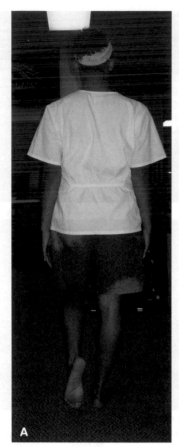

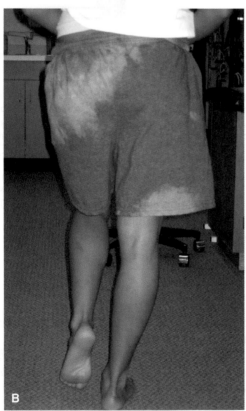

FIGURE 24-6 ■ Trendelenburg test. The athlete is asked to stand on one leg. Normally the pelvis does not sag or remains level (**A**). If the pelvis on the non-weight bearing leg sags (**B**), it is an indication of gluteus medius muscle weakness of the weight bearing leg.

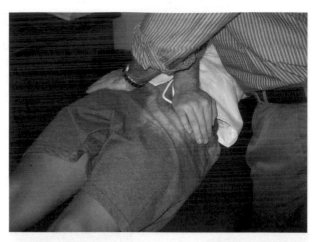

FIGURE 24-7 ■ Pelvic compression test (gapping or transverse anterior stress test.) With the athlete supine on the examination table, the examiner stresses the pelvis by pressure over the iliac bones pushing down and out. In case of sprain of sacroiliac ligaments pain in the buttock or posterior thigh is elicited on the injured side.

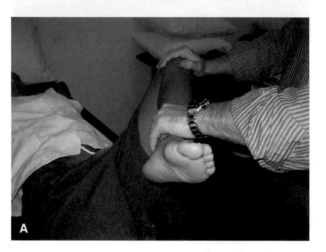

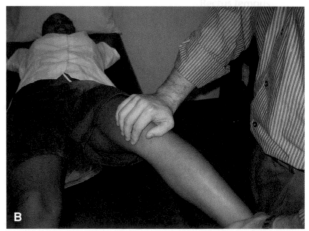

FIGURE 24-8 ■ Labral test. To test for posterior acetabular labral tears the athlete is placed supine, the hip supported and flexed in abduction and external rotation with knee flexed (**A**). The hip is then extended, adducted, and internally rotated (**B**). There is often a clunk or click with the presence of a labral tear.

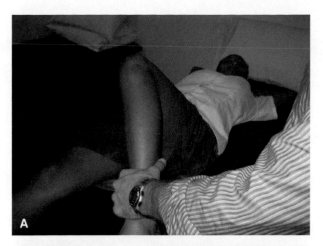

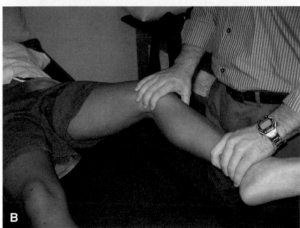

FIGURE 24-9 ■ Test for snapping hip. To test for external snapping hip the hip is flexed and adducted in internal rotation (**A**), then extended, abducted, and externally rotated (**B**). This often produces a click or snapping over the anterior proximal thigh.

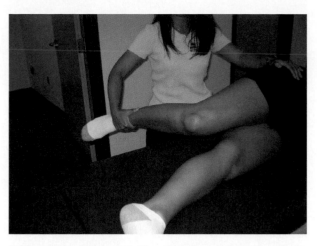

FIGURE 24-10 ■ Ober test. The athlete lies on the side with the affected side up. The examiner grasps the leg with one hand and flexes the knee, circumducts the hip moving it into abducted and extended position. Normally the knee falls back to neutral in adduction. Failure of the knee to fall back to neutral is indicative of tight iliotibial band.

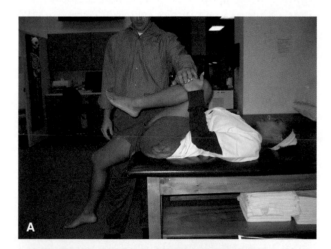

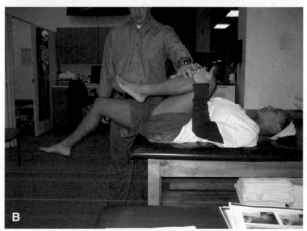

FIGURE 24-11 ■ Modified Thomas test. With the athlete supine on the table and back flat flex the hip and knee fully of one leg at a time. Normally the contralateral hip should remain extended and the back should remain straight (**A**). With tight rectus femoris and hip contracture of the contralateral side, there will be flexion of the hip and knee (**B**).

hip is flexed and adducted in internal rotation then extended, abducted, and externally rotated (Figure 24-9). This often produces a click, or snapping over the anterior proximal thigh, and very often reproduces the patient's pain.

For a tight iliotibial band the patient is placed on the unaffected side facing away from the examiner at the edge of the table, and the hip is extended and the affected leg lowered below the table's edge to perform an Ober test (Figure 24-10). This will often reproduce the athlete's discomfort, and also will demonstrate limited flexibility in those with a tight iliotibial band.

The athlete should also be assessed for tightness in the quadriceps (Figure 24-11). Hamstrings flexibility is assessed with the hip at 90 degrees, while extending the knee with the calf supported.

One should also check for Achilles tendon tightness, with the knee bent at 90 degrees and the patient sitting up by measuring dorsiflexion of the ankle.[6–8,11,12] Measure the leg length (Figure 24-12).

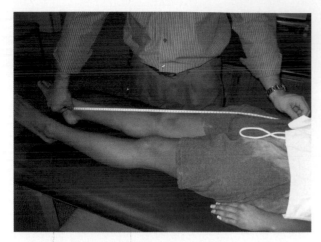

FIGURE 24-12 ■ Measuring lower limb length. With the athlete supine and legs extended measure the distance between anterior superior iliac spine and medial malleolus.

Diagnostic Imaging

Injuries to the apophyses may be best seen on plain films. Other imaging studies such as CT scan or MRI scan may be needed if it is difficult to visualize the injury on plain films. Bone scan is useful for stress fractures and other injuries about the pelvis, but will not be positive for approximately 3 days after an acute injury, and may not show the level of detail needed for some injuries. MRI is usually positive within 24 hours of injury because of the bone edema associated with an acute injury. MRI is also useful to demonstrate associated muscle, tendon, chondral, and labral injuries.

In a suspected labral tear of the hip, an MR arthrogram is indicated. Ultrasound may helpful in some cases to demonstrate soft tissue or tendon injuries, bursal fluid, and hip effusions, but requires a technically adept operator who performs these tests frequently to obtain the best results. CT imaging is useful to look at suspected femoral head fractures, acetabular fractures, and also to delineate occult fractures about the hip. In many level I trauma centers, a patient presenting with significant pelvic or abdominal trauma will undergo CT scanning in the emergency department by the trauma service prior to the patient being seen by or referred to other physicians. Current high-definition, high-speed spiral CT scan has supplanted plain film Judet views for acetabular fractures in many centers. There are no specific indications at this time for the performance of PET scans on acute musculoskeletal injuries in young athletes.[13–15]

Treatment

In the acutely injured hip, the first priority is to assess the patient's vascular as well as neurologic status, and quickly ascertain whether the hip joint itself is injured or dislocated. In a patient with marked discomfort in the groin and hip, who is reluctant to move the hip, the best course of action is to obtain plain films of the affected hip and pelvis immediately and then treat based on the findings of these films and other imaging studies, which may then be needed to further delineate the injury and plan treatment. Treatment for specific injuries is described in following sections.

ACUTE TRAUMATIC HIP DISLOCATIONS

Definition and Epidemiology

Overall, most athletic hip dislocations are posterior. Hip dislocations occur in freestyle skiing and snowboarding, as well as in motocross and other high-energy and impact sports. In addition to hip dislocation, athletes in high-impact or jumping sports may also sustain chondral injuries and fractures of the femoral head, which can predispose the patient to significant long-term disability, early arthritis, loss of ROM of the hip, and chronic hip pain. Hip dislocation with a femoral head or pipkin fracture was present in 30% of snowboarders with a hip dislocation and 12.5% of skiers with a hip dislocation[2,16]

Mechanism

Most hip dislocations are posterior and commonly occur from an anterior blow to a flexed knee, and may be associated with a fracture of the posterior wall of the acetabulum. Anterior dislocations are less common.[16]

Clinical Presentation

Patients commonly present with a history of a fall or other significant trauma, and are unable to move the hip or bear weight. Following acute traumatic event, an athlete presents with a history of acute, severe hip pain, decreased range of motion, and does not want to move the leg or bear weight. The mechanism of injury may help determine whether the dislocation is anterior or posterior. The posteriorly dislocated hip is held in flexion, adduction, and internal rotation, and the patient will complain of marked pain in the hip. The athelete will not be able to range the hip, or bear weight. The anteriorly dislocated hip is held in flexion, abduction, and external rotation.[16]

Diagnostic Imaging

Standard x-rays will show the dislocated hip. CT scan or MRI scan may be indicated to assess associated fractures or labral injuries.

Treatment

A hip dislocation is an emergency and must be seen and reduced within a few hours of injury. On field reduction can be attempted but is neither uniformly practiced nor recommended. Initial treatment following reduction is non-weight bearing for 6 weeks, often followed by repeat MRI scan. Some patients will develop chondrolysis or avascular necrosis of the femoral head following a dislocation, particularly a posterior dislocation. Return to sports can be allowed in 6 to 12 weeks if imaging, including MRI, is negative and there is no pain with ROM of the hip or with ambulation.

Method of closed reduction

Posterior: With the patient supine on the examination table, properly sedated or under general anesthesia and the knee flexed, the thigh is pulled anteriorly as the hip is gently externally rotated.[16]

Anterior: These are reduced with inline traction, adduction and internal rotation of the hip, once appropriate sedation or anesthesia is in place.

HIP SUBLUXATION

Hip subluxation is a more recently recognized problem and presents in a more subtle fashion. A simple fall onto a flexed knee with the hip adducted, forces the femoral head up onto the rim of the acetabulum. This may occur with a sudden stop as the athlete halts and quickly pivots over the extremity in sports such as basketball, gymnastics, or soccer. There is frequently an associated fracture of the posterior acetabulum present.[9,17] These patients will have hip or groin pain, and may limit weight bearing on the affected limb. Plain films, AP and lateral, of the hip may be normal or show malposition of the hip or an associated fracture. Judet views of the pelvis or a CT scan of the pelvis will better demonstrate any associated fractures. MRI will demonstrate associated labral and chondral injuries.[13–15]

APOPHYSEAL AVULSIONS

Definition and Epzidemiology

Apophyseal avulsion fractures often occur in the adolescent athlete. These injuries are seen most often between

Table 24-2.		
Appearance and Fusion of Apophyses		
Apophysis	Age at Appearance (yr)	Age at Fusion (yr)
Iliac crest	13–15	21–25
Anterior superior iliac spine	13–15	21–25
Anterior inferior iliac spine	13–25	16–18
Ischial tuberosity	13–15	20–25
Lesser trochanter	9–13	15–17
Greater trochanter	2–3	16–17

the ages of 14 and 25. The age of appearance and fusion of the apophyses are presented in Table 24-2.

Mechanism

The mechanism of injury is usually a violent contraction of a muscle against its attachment through the apophysis, which is the weakest point in the muscle tendon unit in the growing child. The apophysis usually fails through the zone of provisional calcification.[9,18–22] The apophyses, respective muscle group attached, muscle actions, and mechanisms are summarized in Table 24-3.

Clinical Presentation

The patient will present with marked pain of sudden onset, with tenderness on palpation over the area of the origin or insertion of the musculotendinous unit through the apophysis. There will be localized swelling over the site of the apophysis. Pain is elicited on movement of the attached muscle group against manual resistance (Table 24-3).

Diagnostic Imaging

Standard x-rays of the pelvis will be useful in detecting the avulsed apophysis in most cases (Figure 24-13). In some cases, these avulsions are difficult to visualize on standard x-rays, and CT scan may show small avulsions not well seen on x-ray and may be needed to help plan treatment. MRI scan will better demonstrate associated soft tissue injuries such as muscle and tendon tears, and may show partial avulsions better, as well as demonstrating signal change early on at approximately 24 hours after the avulsion injury.[9,13–15,22]

Treatment

The overall treatment of apophyseal injuries is a short course of relative rest for 2 to 3 weeks, and then early

Table 24-3.

Apophyses, Muscle Attachments, Actions, Mechanisms of Injuries, and Test that Elicit Pain

Apophysis	Attached Muscle	Action of the Muscle	Mechanism of Avulsion Fracture	Test that Elicit Pain
Iliac crest	Abdominal obliques	Flexion and rotation of trunk	Direct impact, as in lacrosse or hockey, or caused by forceful trunk rotation	Resisted hip flexion, trunk flexion or rotation
ASIS	Sartorius, tensor fascia lata	Flexion of hip and knee	Sudden hip extension and knee flexion during running or sprinting	Active or resisted adduction or flexion of the hip
AIIS	Straight head of rectus femoris	Flexion of hip, extension of knee	Kicking, overloading the straight head of rectus femoris, or sprinting in which case it may be bilateral	Resisted hip flexion with extended knee. Passive extension of hip
Ischial tuberosity	Hamstrings	Flexion of knee, extension of hip	Maximal hamstring contraction with the knee extended and the hip flexed; as in pulling up out of the water while waterskiing or in hurdling or gymnastics	Passive knee extension with flexed hip. Resisted hip extension
Lesser trochanter	Iliopsoas	Flexion of hip	Sudden, forceful hip flexion such as may occur in football, gymnastics and track	Resisted flexion of the hip with knee in flexion
Greater trochanter	Gluteus maximus	Adduction of hip		Resisted hip abduction

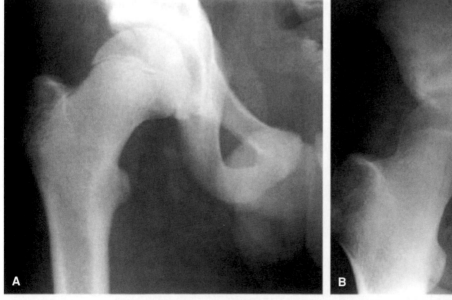
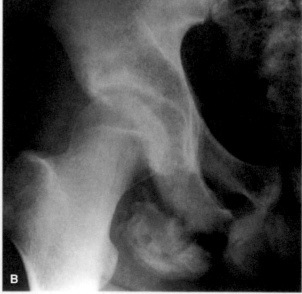

FIGURE 24-13 ■ X-ray showing avulsed ischial tuberosity apophysis. Large avulsion of the ischial tuberosity (**A**), large area of ossification 6 months later (**B**), and unuited ischial tuberosity 3 years later (*Continued*)

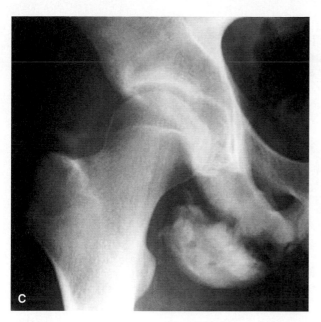

FIGURE 24-13 ■ *(Continued)*(**C**). (*Used with permission from Green. Skeletal Trauma in Children. 3rd ed. Philadelphia,PA: Saunders Elsevier Imprint; 2006, Figure 2-11*).

physical therapy with the intent of first regaining pain-free range of motion. Next a course of gradual strengthening is instituted, and at approximately 6 weeks the athlete will work through sport-specific therapy such as plyometrics or pilates. Return to sport is often possible 6 to 8 weeks after the initial injury, depending upon the severity of the injury and the athlete's progress in therapy.

Before allowing a return to sports the athlete should have no pain, ROM should be restored, and strength should be 80% of the uninjured side. Should the athlete demonstrate a completely displaced apophyseal injury such as a severe hamstring tear from the ischial tuberosity, or similarly a fracture of the ASIS with displacement of the origin of the sartorius, surgical consult is indicated.[9,22]

More recent literature shows that significantly displaced injuries to the apophysis do less well with nonoperative care. However, there is no large series in the orthopedic literature, which demonstrates surgery as clearly superior to nonoperative treatment in any specific case. Initial x-ray displacement of the apophysis greater than 2 cm usually warrants surgical treatment. Further imaging including MRI is sometimes helpful in these cases as well to delineate associated muscle and soft tissue injury associated with the apophyseal injury itself.

HIP POINTER

Definition and Epidemiology

Hip pointers are contusions over the greater trochanter or iliac crest, and are more common in adolescent athletes near or at skeletal maturity.

Mechanism

The cause is a direct blow to the iliac crest such as in a tackle or being checked into a wall during hockey, or a fall onto a hard surface or landing badly while stealing a base.[6]

Clinical Presentation

The athlete will have localized pain, bruising, and tenderness over the iliac crest or greater trochanter. There is increased pain with trunk bending or rotation, and there may be a hematoma over the iliac crest or lateral thigh and hip. Increasing or unrelenting pain may be caused by an arterial injury or a developing compartment syndrome in rare cases.

Diagnostic Imaging

Generally no routine imaging is indicated.

Treatment

The initial treatment consists of rest, ice, elevation, and compression. Crutches are used to rest the area. When pain abates, range of motion, followed by gradual stretching and strengthening exercises are begun. The use of NSAIDs early on may exacerbate the hematoma. Return to sports can be expected by 2 to 8 weeks depending upon the severity of the injury and the time needed for recovery. Complications include lateral femoral cutaneous nerve palsy, shortening of the muscles owing to scar, bursitis, or myositis ossificans. Early physical therapy with assisted active motion may reduce the incidence of complications. Aggressive passive stretching is not recommended and is likely to increase the risk of myositis ossificans.[6]

ACUTE ADDUCTOR STRAINS

Definition and Epidemiology

The adductor muscles (Figure 24-14) are frequently involved in muscle strain injuries, particularly in sports such as hockey, football, and soccer.[9] These injuries

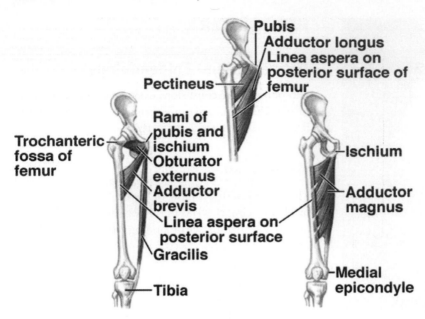

FIGURE 24-14 ■ Adductor and other major muscles. (*Used with permission from Van De Graaff KM. Human Anatomy. 6th ed. New York: McGraw Hill;2002.*)

often occur early in the season of play, when athletes are not well conditioned.

Mechanism

The mechanism of injury is usually an eccentric contraction of a loaded muscle, and the injury commonly occurs at the muscle tendon junction in adolescents near skeletal maturity, rather than at the apophysis as occurs in younger athletes. Muscle strains occur in the same locations as apophyseal injuries, with similar presenting symptoms, but in older adolescents with closing apophyses.

Clinical Presentation

Groin or medial thigh pain is the most common complaint from the athlete, and there is pain when the patient adducts the leg against resistance. Localized tenderness in the groin is present, and with grade 3 strains (full-thickness tears) a defect in the muscle or tendon may be palpable.

Diagnostic Imaging

X-rays and sometimes MRI are needed to image the area and to ascertain the degree of associated muscle and soft tissue injury as well as any bony injury present.[13–15]

Treatment

Initial treatment is relative rest, ice, compression, and elevation of the limb for first few days, gradual mobilization, followed by stretching and strengthening exercises. The athlete can return to play when asymptomatic and conditioned adequately. Associated injuries, which may also occur in adolescent athletes near skeletal maturity as well as in younger athletes, include hip and thigh contusions and nerve irritation.[9]

ACUTE STRAIN OF HAMSTRINGS

Definition and Epidemiology

Hamstring muscle strains usually occur near the musculotendinous junction near their proximal attachment over the ischial tuberosity (Figure 24-15). Midsubstance and distal strains are uncommon. Hamstring strains are uncommon in youth sports where apophyseal avulsions of the ischial tuberosity are more common.

Mechanism

Eccentric loading of the hamstrings muscle, often in a rapid manner, as in a waterskiier overloading the hamstrings while trying to get up on the skiis, or a sprinter, hurdler, or football player repeatedly hyperflexing the hip and overstretching the loaded hamstrings muscles during a hard driving run.

Clinical Presentation

The athlete presents with acute, severe pain, often at the origin of the hamstrings at the ischial tuberosity.

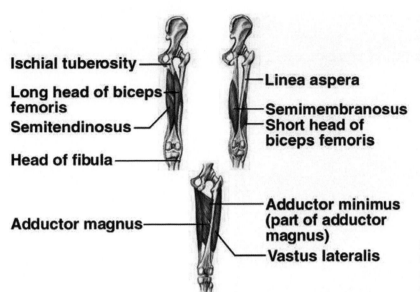

FIGURE 24-15 ■ Hamstring and other major muscles. (*Used with permission from Van De Graaff KM. Human Anatomy. 6th ed. New York: McGraw Hill;2002.*)

There may be significant spasm, swelling, or even defect present if the hamstrings are partially or completely avulsed.

Diagnostic Imaging

X-rays are not indicated routinely. If an avulsion or full-thickness tear is suspected, and surgical treatment is being considered, MRI scan is indicated to define the extent of the injury.

Treatment

In most cases treatment consists of RICE (rest, ice, compression, elevation), stretches, crutches, and a short rest from play. In adult professional football players hamstring injuries are routinely injected with corticosteroids, with early return to play and little reported long-term sequelae. However, this course of treatment is not recommended in adolescents. In some cases repair or reattachment of the muscles or the apophysis is performed. Most hamstrings tears, however, are of partial thickness, and in both the adult and younger athletes, are treated conservatively with good long-term results, with return to play after a course or rest, stretching and strengthening.[9]

QUADRICEPS CONTUSIONS

Definition and Epidemiology

Direct blow to the quadriceps can result in a muscle contusion. There is usually a partial tear of the muscle fibers and in some cases a very large hematoma in the muscle.

Mechanism

A direct blow to the front of the thigh in contact and collision sports is the usual mechanism for quadriceps contusion.

Clinical Presentation

The athlete will present with pain, swelling over the affected anterior thigh, and possibly weakness with active knee extension. If the patient clinically has firm compartments (thigh) and pain, which is not controlled with appropriate pain medications, or if there are neurologic changes or clinical suspicion of a compartment syndrome, such as paresthesias or pain with passive flexion of the knee, compartment syndrome should be suspected.

Diagnostic Imaging

In a large hematoma MRI scan is indicated to define the extent of muscle injury.

Treatment

Immediate treatment is the application of ice over the injured muscle. It can be held in place with the athlete's hip at 90 degree flexion and knee fully flexed with a bag of crushed ice tied to the thigh with a ACE wraps (Figure 24-16). Partial weight bearing is allowed within few days depending upon the severity of the initial injury

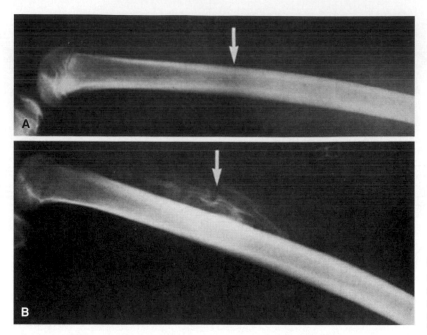

FIGURE 24-16 ■ X-ray of myositis ossificans. (*Used with permission from DeLee JC, Drez D, Miller MD, eds. DeLee and Drez's Orthopedic Sports Medicine. 2nd ed. Philadelphia,PA: Saunders Elsevier Imprint; 2003, Figure 26A-13.*)

and patient comfort. This is followed by very gentle active stretching of the quadriceps. Early and forceful stretching and passive stretching must be avoided. The athlete can return to play when he has or she no pain, no tenderness, and full ROM and strength of the quadriceps. This may take several weeks.

MYOSITIS OSSIFICANS TRAUMATICA

Definition and Epidemiology

Myositis ossificans traumatica is characterized by calcification or ossification occurring in the soft tissues, usually in damaged muscle owing to the muscle injury itself, and the associated hematoma after a fracture or significant soft tissue trauma. These injuries are more common in high-energy trauma, with femur fractures, acetabular or pelvic fractures or other similar injuries. One of the more common locations is in the distal one third of the thigh in the vastus intermedius muscle.

Mechanism

A hematoma often exists within the injured muscle and other soft tissues, and may go on to ossify, with calcification, with mature bone forming trabeculae at the periphery of the lesion. These lesions will continue to mature for up to a year or more after trauma, and can become quite large and symptomatic. There will be elevated alkaline phosphatase levels present and often elevated calcium levels as the mass grows and matures.

Clinical Presentation

The athlete presents with a history of prior trauma, and usually notes that the mass has gotten larger over the preceding months and is very firm. The mass may limit ROM, tendon gliding, and the use of adjacent joints, and is sometimes painful. It is not common to have isolated significant night pain with this entity, which is more common with benign bone tumors such as osteoid osteomas, as well as with malignant bony and soft tissue tumors.

Diagnostic Imaging

A firm mass can be palpated, which on x-ray will demonstrate calcification; usually separate from the bone, with more mature bony architecture at the periphery (Figure 24-16).

Treatment

If myositis ossificans develops, it is first treated with physical therapy and mobilization to try to enable the tissue to heal and the mass to remodel or resorb. In most cases the myositis will resolve. However, if a refractory large mass develops and continues to interfere with function of the limb, it is sometimes excised. Excision is usually done 6 to 12 months after injury once the mass is mature by clinical examination and once there is normal serum alkaline phosphatase and calcium levels present in serum.

ACETABULAR LABRAL TEARS

Definition and Epidemiology

Acute tears of the acetabular labrum are associated with hip pain and can result from any significant acute hip trauma such as hip dislocations. It has been reported in such activities as dancing, skiing, and gymnastics.

Mechanisms

Isolated acetabular labral tears of the hip occur more often anteriorly. Pediatric and adolescent athletes who repeatedly flex, flex and abduct, or extend and externally rotate their hips may be at higher risk for anterior tears. There is also evidence that many labral tears are related to subluxation of the hip and underlying preexisting acetabular dysplasia.[7–9,13–15]

Clinical Presentation

The athlete will complain of locking, grinding sensation and groin pain, as well as pain with hip flexion and adduction. Younger athletes in particular may complain of a catching type of pain in their hip, and a click. To examine hip for an anterior labral tear the examiner places the hip in flexion, external rotation, and abduction, followed by extension with internal rotation and adduction (Figure 24-8). These maneuvers usually produce discomfort and a catch or click in the hip. Those with a posterior labral tear will have discomfort with the hip passively flexed, internally rotated, and loaded in a posterior direction.[7–9]

Diagnostic Imaging

X-rays, AP, lateral, and frog leg views of the hip and pelvis will help detect fractures, old developmental dys-

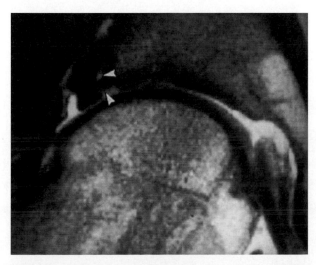

FIGURE 24-17 ■ MRI of acetabular labral tear.

Box 24–1 When to Refer to Orthopedics.

Fractures of hip, pelvis, femur
Acute traumatic dislocations of hip
Acetabular labral tears
Complete rupture of quadriceps
Slipped capital femoral epiphysis

plasia of hip, slipped capital femoral epiphysis, or avascular necrosis of hip. An MR arthrogram will usually demonstrate the labral tear, with leakage of dye beneath the labrum, or the displaced labrum will be seen on the images[27–20](Figure 24-17). The MR arthrogram will also often demonstrate related chondral pathology, loose bodies, and other problems, which may benefit from arthroscopic or open hip surgery.[13–15]

Treatment

Treatment of labral tears begins with partial weightbearing for a month, and in some patient's local anesthetic hip injection for diagnostic and therapeutic purposes. Some investigators have reported substantial symptomatic improvement after arthroscopic debridement of labral tears in children and adolescents.[7–9]

FRACTURES OF HIP, PELVIS, AND PROXIMAL FEMUR

Slipped capital femoral epiphysis and various apophyseal avulsion fractures are the main fractures seen in young athletes. All other fractures, such as femoral head, acetabulum, femoral shaft, or pelvic, are rare in youth sports and usually occur in severe high-energy trauma such as motor vehicle accidents and need emergent evaluation and orthopedic care (Box 24-1).[21–27]

REFERENCES

1. Torjussen J, Bahr R. Injuries among competitive snowboarders at the national elite level. *Am J Sports Med.* 2005;33:370-377.
2. Matsumoto K, Sumi H, Sumi Y, Shimizu K. An analysis of hip dislocation among snowboarders and skiers: a 10-year prospective study from 1992-2002. *J Ortho Trauma.* 2003; 55:946-948.
3. Silber J, Flynn J. Changing patterns of pelvic fractures with skeletal maturation: implications for classification and management. *J Pediatr Ortho.* 2002;22:22-26.
4. Paluska S. An overview of hip injuries in running. *Sports Med.* 2005;35(11):991-1014.
5. Lehman R, Shah S. Tension-sided femoral neck stress fracture in a skeletally immature patient. *J Bone Joint Surg.* 2004;86-A(6):1292-1295.

6. Melamed H, Hutchinson M. Soft tissue problems of the hip in athletes. *Sports Med Arthroscopy Rev.* 2002;10: 168-175.

7. Kocher M, Kim Young-Jo, Millis M, et al. Hip arthroscopy in children and adolescents. *J Pediatr Ortho.* 25(5):680-686.

8. Kelly B, Williams Riley J III, Phillopon M. Hip arthroscopy: current indications, treatment options, and management issues. *Am J Sport Med.* 2003;31(6):1020-1037.

9. Anderson K, Strickland S, Warren R. Hip and groin injuries in athletes. *Am J Sport Med.* 2001;29:521-533.

10. Darin L, Ireland ML, Willson J, Ballantyne B, Davis IM. Core stability measures as risk factors for lower extremity injury in athletes. *Med Sci Sports Exerc.* 2004;36(6): 926-934.

11. Gruen g, Scioscia T, Lowenstein J. The surgical treatment of internal snapping hip. *Am J Sports Med.* 2002;30: 607-613.

12. Fredericson M, Weir A. Practical management of iliotibial band friction syndrome in runners. *Clin J Sports Med.* 2006;16(3):261-268.

13. Potter H, Steven S, Adler RS. Imaging of the hip in athletes. *Sports Med Arthroscopy Rev.* 2002;10(2):115-122.

14. Lattin G, Gould F, Ly J, Beall D, Tall M. MR Imaging of hip trauma: clinical implications and posttraumatic findings of the osseous structures, articular cartilage, and acetabular labrum. *Contemp Diagn Radiol.* 2006;29(7):1-6.

15. Bencardino J, Kasarjian A, Palner W. Magnetic resonance imaging of the hip: sports-related injuries. *Top Magn Reson Imaging.* 2003;14(2):145-160.

16. Chudik S, Allen A, Lopez V, Warren R. Hip dislocations in athletes. *Sports Med Arthroscopy Rev.* 2002;10:123-133.

17. Moorman C, Warren R, Hershman E, et al. Traumatic posterior hip subluxation in American football. *J Bone Joint Surg-A.* 2003;85-A:1190-1196.

18. Skaggs D, Tolo V. Legg-Calve'-Perthes disease. *J Am Aced Ortho Surg.* 1996;4(1):9-16.

19. Nickey J, Lemons D, Waber P, Seikaly M. Bisphosphonate use in children with bone disease. *J Am Acad Ortho Surg.* 2006;14:638-644.

20. Aronsson D, Loder R, Breus G, Weinstein S. Slipped capital femoral epiphysis: current concepts. *J Am Acad Ortho Surg.* 2006;14:666-679.

21. Iwinski H. Slipped capital femoral epiphysis. *Curr Opin Orthop.* 2006;17:511-516.

22. Amendola A, Wolcott M. Bony Injuries around the hip. *Sports Med Arthroscopy Rev.* 2002;10:163-167.

23. Karunakar M, Goulet J, Mueller K, Bedi A, Le Theodore T. Operative treatment of unstable pediatric pelvis and acetabular fractures. *J Pediatr Ortho.* 2005;25(1):34-38.

24. McDonnel M, Schachter, Phillips D, Liporace F. Acetabular fracture through the triradiate cartilage after low energy trauma. *J Orthop Trauma.* 2007;21(7):495-498.

25. Lee, Soon-Hyuck, Baek Jong-Ryoon, Han Seung-Bum, Park Sang-Won. Stress fractures of the femoral diaphysis in children. *JPO.* 2005;25(6):734-738.

26. Ahfeld SK, Makley JT, Derosa GP, Fisher DA, Mitchell JQ. Osteoid osteoma of the femoral neck in the young athlete. *Am J Sports Med.* 1990;271-276.

27. Moroz L, Launay F, Kocher M, et al. Titanium elastic nailing of fracture of the femur in children. *J Bone Joint Surg.* 2006;88-B:1361-1366.

Additional Readings:

Frank JB, Jarit G, Bravman JT, Rosen JE. Lower extremity injuries in the skeletally immature athlete. *J Am Acad Orthop Surg.* 2007;15:356-366.

Millis MB, Kocher M. Hip and pelvis inuries in the young athlete. In: DeLee JC, Drez D, Miller MD, eds. *Orthopaedic Sports Medicine.* Philadelphia, PA: Saunders Elsevier; 2003:1463-1480.

CHAPTER 25

Overuse Injuries of the Hip, Pelvis, and Thigh

Dilip R. Patel, E. Dennis Lyne, and Sarah Bancroft

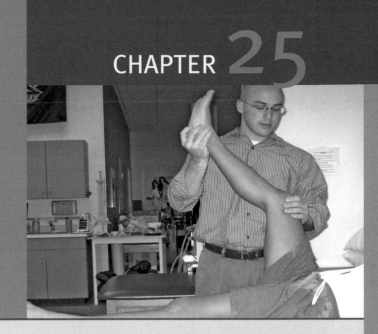

ILIAC APOPHYSITIS

Definition and Epidemiology

Iliac apophysitis is an overuse related traction injury affecting the iliac crest apophysis. The iliac apophysis closes on an average round 17 years of age. It is most commonly seen in long-distance runners and skaters. It has been reported in hockey, lacrosse, and football players. The exact incidence in not known.

Mechanism

The mechanism of injury is the repetitive microtrauma because of overuse.

Clinical Presentation

The athlete presents with a history of gradual onset of pain over the iliac crest while running. In contrast, the athlete with an acute traumatic avulsion injury of the iliac crest or the anterior superior iliac spine will present with a sudden onset of severe pain. In athletes with iliac apophysitis, there is no history of direct impact trauma to the iliac crest. Pain is exaggerated by abduction of the hip against resistance. Tenderness is localized over the iliac crest.

Diagnostic Imaging

X-ray is not indicated and is normal, unless an avulsion is suspected.

Treatment

Treatment is symptomatic with local ice, pain medication if needed, and modification or rarely complete cessation of the offending activity in some athletes. Resolution of symptoms gradually occurs typically over a period of 4 to 6 weeks. Once pain-free and normal examination, the athlete can resume unrestricted sport participation.

OSTEITIS PUBIS

Definition and Epidemiology

Osteitis pubis is characterized by symphysis pubis pain, and chronic stress related changes in the subchondral bone, reported most commonly in athletes participating in soccer, ice hockey, basketball, and running. The condition has also been reported in fencing, Australian rules football, and cricket.

Mechanism

Overuse related stress affecting the symphysis pubis is believed to be the cause for development of osteitis pubis. The exact mechanism is not known; however, it is believed that repetitive shearing forces accompanying side to side and up and down movement at the pubic symphysis predisposes to osteitis pubis. These types of movements can occur in sports requiring sudden change in direction, running, kicking, acceleration, or deceleration. Forceful contractions of hip adductors can also pull on the pubic symphysis.

Table 25-1.

Causes of Groin Pain in Young Athletes

Musculotendinous strains—adductor strain, iliopsoas strain
Bursitis—iliopectineal bursitis, ischial bursitis
Stress fractures—femoral neck, proximal femur, pubis ramus
Hip disorder—SCFE, septic arthritis, inflammatory arthritis
Apophyseal avulsion fractures—ASIS, AIIS, ischial tuberosity
Entrapment neuropathies—ilioinguinal N, obturator N,
    genitofemoral N
Snapping hip syndrome
Osteitis pubis
Osteomyelitis of symphysis pubis
Sports hernia
Intra-articular pathology—acetabular tears, loose bodies
Referred pain—lumbar spine and cord, abdominal, pelvic,
    genitourinary disease

Clinical Presentation

There is an insidious onset of pain over the symphysis pubis area or groin exaggerated by continued activity, and there is localized tenderness over the symphysis pubis. Athletes may also report pain in the thigh, hip, or perineum. Pain is aggravated by running, kicking, pivoting, sudden acceleration, and deceleration. Soccer players adapt to avoid certain kicks that cause the most pain. Pain can be reproduced or exacerbated on examination by having the athlete adduct the hip against manual resistance or passively abduct the hip. Osteomyelitis affecting the pubis symphysis must be considered in the differential diagnosis. Other causes of groin pain in young athletes are noted in Table 25-1. [1-4] Differentiating features of some hip conditions are summarized in Table 25-2. [1-6]

Table 25-2.

Clinical Features of Some Hip Conditions*

Diagnosis	History	Physical Findings	Differential Diagnosis
Legg-Calvé-Perthes disease	Insidious onset (1–3 mo) of limp with hip or knee pain	Limited hip abduction, flexion, and internal rotation	Juvenile arthritis, other inflammatory conditions of the hip. Muscle strain, avulsion fracture
Slipped capital femoral epiphysis	Acute (<1 mo) or chronic (up to 6 mo) presentation, pain may be referred to knee or anterior thigh	Pain and limited internal rotation, leg more comfortable in external rotation; chronic presentation may have leg length discrepancy	
Avulsion fracture	Sudden, violent muscle contraction; may hear or feel a "pop"	Pain on passive stretch and active contraction of involved muscle; pain on palpation of involved apophysis	Muscle strain, slipped capital femoral epiphysis
Hip pointer	Direct trauma to iliac crest	Tenderness over iliac crest, may have pain on ambulation and active abduction of hip	Contusion, fracture
Contusion	Direct trauma to soft tissue	Pain on palpation and motion, ecchymosis	Hip pointer, fracture, myositis ossificans
Myositis ossificans	Contusion with hematoma approximately 2–4 wks earlier	Pain on palpation, firm mass may be palpable	Contusion, soft tissue tumors, callus formation from prior fracture
Femoral neck stress fracture	Persistent groin discomfort increasing with activity, history of endurance exercise, female athlete triad (eating disorder, amenorrhea, osteoporosis)	ROM may be painful, pain on palpation of greater trochanter	Trochanteric bursitis, osteoid osteoma, muscle strain
Osteoid osteoma	Vague hip pain present at night and increased with activities	Restricted motion, quadriceps atrophy	Femoral neck stress fracture, trochanteric bursitis
Iliotibial band syndrome	Lateral hip, thigh, or knee pain, snapping as iliotibial band passes over the greater trochanter	Positive Ober's test	Trochanteric bursitis

(continued)

Table 25-2. (Continued)

Clinical Features of Some Hip Conditions*

Diagnosis	History	Physical Findings	Differential Diagnosis
Trochanteric bursitis	Pain over greater trochanter on palpation, pain during transitions from standing to lying down to standing	Pain on palpation of greater trochanter	Iliotibial band syndrome; femoral neck stress fracture
Avascular necrosis of the femoral head	Dull ache or throbbing pain in groin, lateral hip or buttock, history of prolonged steroid use, prior fracture, slipped femoral capital epiphysis	Pain on ambulation, abduction, internal, and external rotation	Early degenerative joint disease
Piriformis syndrome	Dull posterior pain, may radiate down the leg mimicking radicular symptoms, history of track competition, or prolonged sitting	Pain on active external rotation, passive internal rotation of hip, and palpation of sciatic notch	Nerve root compression, stress fractures
Iliopsoas bursitis	Pain and snapping in medial groin or thigh	Reproduce symptoms with active and passive flexion/extension of hip	Avulsion fracture
Meralgia paresthetica	Pain or paresthesia of anterior or lateral groin and thigh	Abnormal distribution of lateral femoral cutaneous nerve on sensory examination	Other causes of peripheral neuropathy
Degenerative arthritis	Progressive pain and stiffness	Reduction in internal rotation early, in all motion later, pain on ambulation	Inflammatory arthritis

*Adapted from: Dutton M. Orthopaedic Examination, Evaluation, and Intervention. New York: McGraw Hill Medical; 2004:689-680.

Diagnostic Imaging

Early in the course, the x-rays are normal. X-ray may show local sclerosis 2 to 3 weeks after the onset of the pain, while a bone scan is positive early in the course. Other x-ray changes include subchondral microcysts, osteolytic lesions, joint widening, or narrowing (Figure 25-1). Instability at pubic symphysis may be detected with x-ray taken with athlete standing on one leg (Flamingo view). MRI scan is highly sensitive for early diagnosis.

Treatment

The condition is self-limited with an excellent prognosis in young athletes for resolution of pain and return to full sports. A period of complete rest and judicious use of NSAIDs help alleviate the pain. Once pain is resolved, a program of stretching and strengthening of hip rotators, flexors, and adductors is initiated and maintained.[1,5,7,8] Most young athletes on an average are pain-free within 6 months (ranging 3–12 months). Rarely, those with significant instability need orthopedic consultation and may need symphysiodesis (Box 25-1).

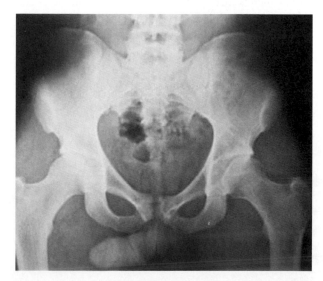

FIGURE 25-1 ■ X-ray of osteitis pubis. (*Used with permission from DeLee JC, Drez D Jr, Miller MD, eds. DeLee and Drez's Orthopaedic Sports Medicine. 2nd ed. Philadelphia, PA: Saunders Elsevier Imprint;. 2003: Figure 25A-4, p 1448.*)

FEMORAL NECK STRESS FRACTURES

Definition and Epidemiology

Stress fractures of the proximal femur occur more often in young military recruits subjected to repetitive overuse and excessive conditioning. In athletes, femoral stress fractures have been reported most commonly in competitive runners. Other sports with similar stress can also lead to stress fractures. Female athletes with pathogenic weight control behaviors and amenorrhea are at a higher risk.

Mechanism

Two types of femoral neck stress fractures are described, one affecting the inferior or medial side of the femoral neck or the compression type, and the other type affecting the tension or lateral side of the femoral neck or the distraction type. [1,9–12] The underlying mechanism that results in stress fracture is repetitive microtrauma.

Clinical Presentation

The young athlete will present with thigh, knee, or groin pain, which is worse with weight-bearing, and decreases with rest. Athlete may avoid weight-bearing on the affected side and have an antalgic gait. On examination, there is tenderness over the proximal femur and the groin. There may be limitation of hip flexion and internal rotation. There is an increased risk for similar stress fracture on the opposite side.

Diagnostic Imaging

Initial x-rays may be normal, up to 2 weeks. Later sclerosis or a fracture may be noted on repeat films (Figure 25-2). MRI scan is the study of choice for early diagnosis and characterization of the fracture type (Figure 25-3). The opposite side should also be evaluated as there is a higher risk for bilateral fractures.

Treatment

Treatment is started based on clinical diagnosis not awaiting radiographic confirmation. The athlete should

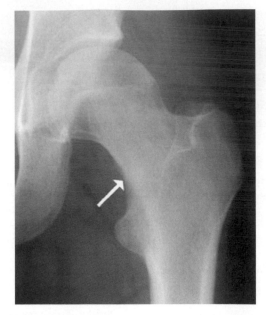

FIGURE 25-2 ■ X-ray of femoral neck fracture. (*Used with permission from DeLee JC, Drez D Jr, Miller MD. eds. DeLee and Drez's Orthopaedic Sports Medicine. 2nd ed. Philadelphia, PA: Saunders Elsevier Imprint; 2003: Figure 16A-21.*)

be nonweight-bearing and referred to orthopedics. Compression side femoral neck fractures are not at risk for displacement and the treatment is nonoperative, with several weeks of modified weight-bearing, but must be followed closely with frequent repeat films and physical examination. Tension sided fractures are at high risk for displacement and will need internal fixation and must be

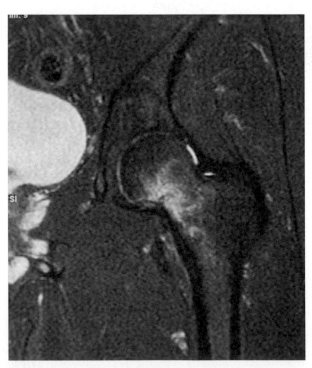

FIGURE 25-3 ■ MRI scan of femoral neck fracture on the compression side

referred to orthopedics expeditiously. Complications of delayed treatment and displaced fractures include nonunion, avascular necrosis of the femoral head, early onset of arthritis, and later varus deformity. Return to sports is considered after the athlete is pain-free, has normal findings on examination, and has radiographic evidence of complete healing of the fracture. Return to sport should be gradual over a period of several months.

SNAPPING HIP SYNDROME

Definition and Epidemiology

Snapping hip is characterized by popping or audible or palpable snapping of the hip, that may or may not be accompanied by pain, associated with certain movements of the hip as specific tendons traverse over bony landmarks. Snapping hips are commonly seen in distance runners, but have also been reported in other athletes including dancers and hurdlers.

Mechanism

Snapping of the hip can be external, internal, or intra-articular. External snapping hip is more common, and is owing to the iliotibial band snapping over the greater trochanter with hip flexion and extension (Figure 25-4). Adduction of the hip with knee extension tightens the iliotibial band and will accentuate the snapping. There may be associated trochanteric bursitis in these athletes as the bursa lies between the iliotibial band and the greater trochanter.

    Internal snapping of the hip is owing to the iliopsoas tendon catching on the pelvic brim or on the femoral head, the iliopectineal eminence or the lesser trochanter as the hip moves from a flexed, abducted and externally rotated position to extended, adducted, and internally rotated position (Figure 25-5).

    Intra-articular snapping is associated with hip joint pathology such as acetabular tears or loose body.

Clinical Presentation

Athlete usually presents with insidious onset pain localized over the greater trochanter area in case of external snapping or deep in the groin in case of internal or intra-articular snapping. Most have snapping without any pain. There is localized tenderness. Swelling is usually not present. With external snapping, one can elicit an audible or palpable snap with passive flexion of the extended hip, whereas with internal snapping a similar snapping can be elicited with passive extension, internal rotation, abduction of the flexed, externally rotated, and adducted hip. Differentiating features of snapping hips are summarized in Table 25-3.

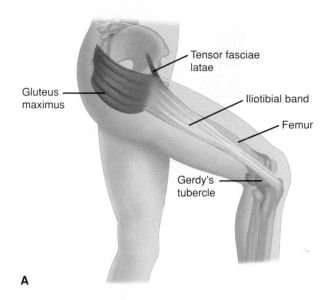

A

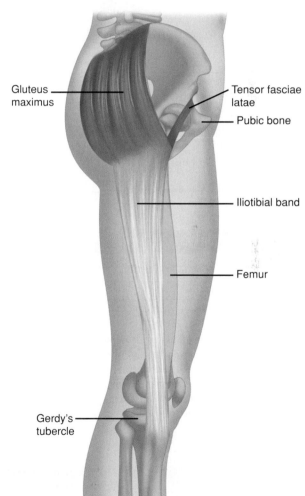

B

FIGURE 25-4 ■ Iliotibial band causing snapping hip.

Diagnostic Imaging

X-ray may be indicated to exclude fractures and hip ultrasound and MRI scan may be indicated to evaluate hip joint pathology.

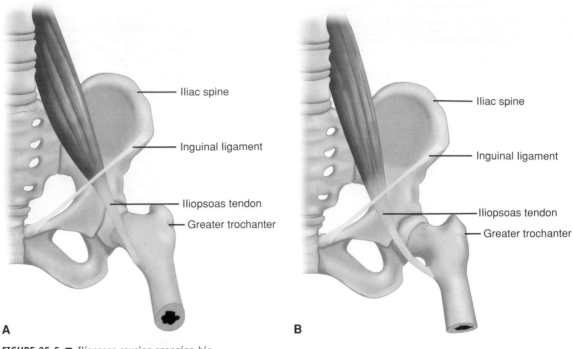

A   **B**

FIGURE 25-5 ■ Iliopsoas causing snapping hip.

Treatment

Most young athletes respond well to a short period of rest and physical therapy that includes appropriate stretching and strengthening exercises. Pain can be managed with a short course of NSAIDs. Orthopedic consultation is indicated, if the athlete fails to improve or intra-articular pathology is suspected.

Table 25-3.

Types of Snapping Hip Syndrome*

Type	Cause	Diagnostic Test	Imaging	Treatment
External	Thickened posterior aspect of the ITB or anterior gluteus maximus rubs over greater trochanter as hip is extended	Passive flexion of an extended hip may elicit a palpable and audible snap with pain over the greater trochanter	Dynamic ultrasonography	Activity modification, ITB stretching, pain medication (e.g., NSAIDs), steroid injection, surgery
Internal	Iliopsoas tendon rubs over anterior hip capsule or iliopectineal eminence	Passive extension, internal rotation, and adduction of a flexed, externally rotated, and abducted hip may elicit a palpable and audible snap with pain in the anterior hip or groin	Static and dynamic ultrasonography, tenography, CT scan, bursography	Activity modification, hip flexor stretching and strengthening, pelvic mobilization, alignment exercises, pain medication (e.g., NSAIDs), steroid injection, surgery
Intra-articular	Loose bodies, torn acetabular labrum, recurrent subluxation, habitual hip dislocation in children, or synovial chondromatosis	Depends on the cause	Plain x-rays, ultrasonography, MRI, or CT scan	Depends on the cause

ITB = iliotibial band; NSAIDs = nonsteroidal anti-inflammatory drugs; CT scan = computed tomography;
MRI = magnetic resonance imaging
Adapted from: Idjadi J, Meislin R. Symptomatic snapping hip: targeted treatment for maximum pain relief. Physician Sports Med. 2004;32(1):25–32.

PIRIFORMIS SYNDROME

Definition and Epidemiology

Piriformis syndrome is characterized by deep buttock pain often associated with sciatic nerve compression symptoms and signs caused by pressure from the piriformis muscle. Sports such as skiing, ice skating, gymnastics, and dance are associated with this syndrome.

Mechanism

The piriformis muscle originates from the anterior surface of the sacrum and is inserted into the greater trochanter. Sciatic nerve passes underneath the piriformis muscle and it exists through the sciatic notch (Figure 25-6). Piriformis syndrome may be caused by myositis ossificans of the piriformis caused by trauma, excessive exercise, infection, blunt trauma to the buttock and hip, hypertrophy or inflammation or spasm in the piriformis, as well as pseudoaneurysm of the inferior gluteal artery.

Clinical Presentation

The athlete will present with sciatica, tenderness at the sciatic notch, and sometimes with a positive straight leg raise, and usually has improvement with rest. Pain is felt in the buttock or posterior thigh, may radiate into the leg, can be burning or aching, and is aggravated when the athlete stoops forward.

Examination may demonstrate local muscle spasm and buttock tenderness over the greater sciatic notch. A palpable, tender soft tissue swelling deep in the buttock is considered a characteristic finding. In chronic cases, there may be atrophy of the gluteus maximus. Pain is frequently made worse by placing the hip in internal rotation, flexion, and adduction (Figure 25-7).

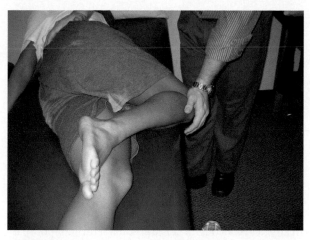

FIGURE 25-7 ■ Piriformis test. The athlete lies on the side with affected leg up. The hip is flexed to 60 degrees with knee flexed. The examiner stabilizes the hip with one hand while applying downward stress to the knee. Pain deep in the buttock or sciatica type symptoms will be elicited in piriformis syndrome.

Diagnostic Imaging

Generally, the diagnosis is clinical. Plain x-rays are generally not helpful and MRI scan may be indicated to evaluate underlying etiology.

Treatment

Most young athletes respond to nonoperative measures with rest and appropriate physical therapy, that addresses any biomechanical problems, such as a leg length discrepancy, pelvic obliquity, and postural and foot and ankle problems. Physical therapy should include stretching the piriformis and hip abductor strengthening. Modalities such as ultrasound and TENS (transcutaneous electrical nerve stimulator), NSAIDs help alleviate pain. In athletes who do not respond local injection with corticosteroid and anesthetic may be tried. Surgery is considered only if conservative treatment is unsuccessful. In refractory cases, surgery with resection of piriformis has demonstrated good success.

LEGG-CALVE-PERTHES DISEASE

Legg-Calve-Perthes disease or avascular necrosis, the hip is always in the differential of hip pain, though not specifically associated with athletics. It is well described in standard pediatric literature. Competitive or high-impact sport participation is generally restricted in these athletes until complete healing has occurred. In some cases with the disease affecting less than 50% of the femoral head, earlier sport participation may be allowed as healing progresses. Residual deformation can be mild or significant collapse of the femoral head associated with hip joint

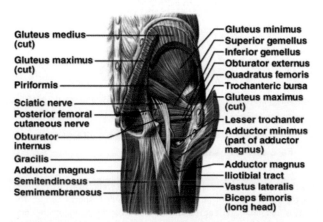

Gluteus medius (cut)
Gluteus maximus (cut)
Piriformis
Sciatic nerve
Posterior femoral cutaneous nerve
Obturator internus
Gracilis
Adductor magnus
Semitendinosus
Semimembranosus

Gluteus minimus
Superior gemellus
Inferior gemellus
Obturator externus
Quadratus femoris
Trochanteric bursa
Gluteus maximus (cut)
Lesser trochanter
Adductor minimus (part of adductor magnus)
Adductor magnus
Iliotibial tract
Vastus lateralis
Biceps femoris (long head)

FIGURE 25-6 ■ Piriformis anatomy. (*Used with permission from Van De Graaff KM. Human Anatomy. 6th ed. New York:McGraw Hill; 2002.*)

incongruity may occur. These athletes are at a higher risk for injuries. Generally, younger patients have better healing potential because of longer time for the bone to remodel. Overall, the level and timing of sport participation in patients with Legg-Calve-Perthes disease should be determined in consultation with treating orthopedic surgeon and is guided by the age of the patient, progression of healing, and residual deformation.

SLIPPED CAPITAL FEMORAL EPIPHYSIS

In athletes treated for SCFE, a gradual return to sport participation is considered once the growth plate fusion is evident. A fracture around the hardware used for internal fixation can still occur. Generally, the hardware is not removed from all patients, but in athletes some orthopedic surgeons remove the hardware after growth plate has fused. A period of several months, usually at least 3 months, is allowed for healing to occur after removal of the hardware, before a gradual return to sports is begun.

SPORTS HERNIA*

Definition and Epidemiology

A sports hernia is defined as a defect in the posterior wall of the inguinal canal. The term "hernia" is actually not an accurate description of this problem because nothing actually herniates through the posterior wall, but this nomenclature has remained the most common despite new findings on the injury. Other names for this injury include: sportsman's hernia, athletic hernia, incipient hernia, and athletic pubalgia. [13] Sports hernias represent up to 50% of groin injuries in patients with chronic groin pain of all ages. [14] It is hypothesized that patients with this diagnosis are not younger than age 12 because growth plates of the pelvis and hip are still open in younger individuals. Injuries can be to either one or both sides of the groin and males are affected more commonly than females. [13]

Mechanism

Cause for this injury has been thought to be from the adductor muscle pulling against the pubic tubercle leading to a tearing of the transversalis fascia of the posterior inguinal wall (Figure 25-8). [1,15,17]

Clinical Presentation

The patient will present with pain around the insertion of the abdominal muscles at the pubic bone and may or may not have tenderness over the insertion of the adductor muscles. [16] History of pain may be present for as little as a few weeks or for as long as years and is usually alleviated partially at rest. The most common sports affected include soccer, hockey, and football. [13]

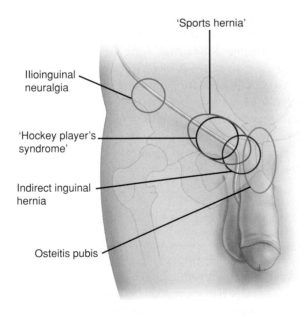

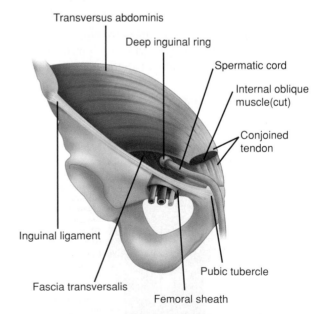

FIGURE 25-8 ■ Sports hernia schematic. Patients who have sports hernia will often point to the proximal adductors (green oval) as the area of maximal tenderness. The conjoined tendon, inguinal ligament, and fascia transversalis are often injured or disrupted in sports hernia. The external oblique and the internal oblique muscles run anterior to the transversus abdominis. Strengthening exercises for the obliques are common first-line treatment for sports hernia.

*Written in personal communication with Joseph Congeni, M.D. and Daniel McMahon, M.D. of Akron Children's Medical Center in Akron, OH

On physical examination, there may be no distinct physical findings. However, the physician should assess for other types of hernias including direct, indirect and femoral hernias, as well as assessing the hips and pelvis for other abnormalities. There may be a more prominent external inguinal ring, pain over the pubic tubercle or adjacent to it where the abdominal muscles and adductors insert. Pain may also be present with flexion of the abdominal muscles, internal rotation of the hip, with hip flexion against resistance, or hip adduction against resistance.[15,16]

Treatment

The diagnosis of sports hernia is something that cannot be made until other causes of groin pain have been ruled out.[13] Imaging may be used to help exclude other causes and should begin with x-rays of the hips and pelvis. Other imaging may also include bone scan, ultrasound, or MRI depending on other findings from history and physical examination. Bone scan may be positive up to 75% of the time with increased uptake at the pubic symphysis in sports hernia.[18]

Preliminary evidence suggests that patients in the pediatric population ranging from 13 to 21- year-old, presenting with a diagnosis of sports hernia, should be referred to a sports medicine physician and undergo 4 to 6 weeks of physical therapy. If after a trial of physical therapy, their symptoms do not improve, they should be referred to an experienced surgeon for possible surgical repair. Patients with unilateral disease who underwent surgical repair had overall positive outcomes versus poor outcomes in patients who had bilateral sports hernia with surgical repair.[19,20]

ENTRAPMENT NEUROPATHIES

Entrapment neuropathies around the hip area can be a cause of groin pain and represent overuse injuries. Obturator nerve entrapment (Figure 25-9) in athletes is generally caused by a fascial band at the distal end of the obturator canal. The athlete presents with an activity related groin and medial thigh pain, and paresthesia. There may be relative weakness of hip abduction. Pain may be elicited with hip external rotation and abduction with the patient standing on one leg. Accurate diagnosis requires use of EMG and nerve conduction studies. Treatment of obturator entrapment caused by fascial band requires surgery.

Lateral femoral cutaneous nerve entrapment (meralgia paresthetica) can occur as the nerve passes over the iliac crest near the anterior superior iliac spine (Figure 25-10). The athlete presents with anterolateral thigh pain and paresthesia. Treatment is nonoperative, with rest and physical therapy.

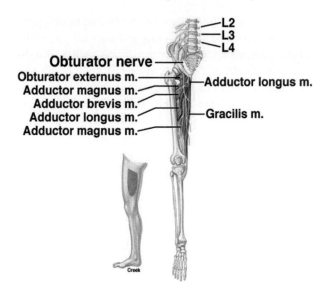

FIGURE 25-9 ■ Obturaror nerve. (*Used with permission from Van De Graaff. Human Anatomy. 6th ed. New York: McGraw Hill; 2002.*)

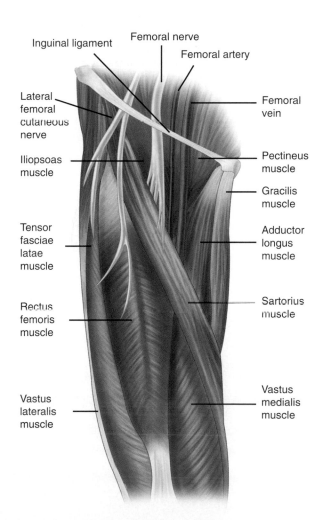

FIGURE 25-10 ■ Lateral femoral cutaneous nerve. Compression often occurs between the inguinal ligament and the sartorius muscle.

Ilioinguinal nerve entrapment can occur as it traverses the superficial inguinal ring and inguinal canal. The athlete presents with sensory symptoms such as numbness, paresthesia, and pain in groin, scrotum, or labium. In athletes, the predisposing factor is believed to be abdominal muscle hypertrophy caused by excessive exercise. Treatment is rest from activities and physical therapy.

REFERENCES

1. Anderson K, Strickland SM, Warren, R. Hip and groin injuries in athletes. *Am J Sports Med.* 2001;29:521-533.
2. Roos HP. Hip pain in sport. *Sports Med Arthroscopy Rev.* 1997;5:292-300.
3. Mens J, Inklaar H, Koes BW, Stam HJ. A new view on adduction-related groin pain. *Clin J Sports Med.* 2006;16:15-19.
4. Morelli V, Espinoza L. Groin injuries and groin pain in athletes: part 1. *Prim Care Clin.* 2005;32:163-183.
5. Morelli V, Espinoza L. Groin injuries and groin pain in athletes: part 2. *Prim Care Clin.* 2005;32:185-200.
6. Dutton M. *Orthopaedic Examination, Evaluation, and Intervention.* New York: McGraw Hill Medical; 2004: 667-733.
7. Johnson RJ. Osteitis pubis. *Curr Sports Med Rep.* 2003;2: 98-102.
8. Lovell G, Galloway H, Hopkins W, Harvey A. Osteitis pubis and assessment of bone marrow edema at the pubic symphysis with MRI in and elite male junior soccer squad. *Clin J Sports Med.* 2006;16:117-122.
9. Kaeding CC, Yu JR, Wright R, et al. Management and return to play of stress fractures. *Clin J Sport Med.* 2005;15:442-447.
10. Dobbs MB, Gordon JE, Luhmann SJ, et al. Surgical correction of the snapping iliopsoas tendon in adolescents. *J Bone Joint Surg Am.* 2002;84-A:420-424.
11. Crawford JR, Villar RN. Current concepts in the management of femoroacetabular impingement. *J Bone Joint Surg Br.* 2005;87-B:1459-1462.
12. Joesting DR. Diagnosis and treatment of sportsman's hernia. *Curr Sports Med Rep.* 2002;1:121-124.
13. Moeller JL. Sportsman's hernia. *Curr Sports Med Rep.* 2007;6:111-114.
14. Lovell, G. The diagnosis of chronic groin pain in athletes: a review of 189 cases. *Aust J Sci Med Sport.* 1995;27:76-79.
15. Meyers WC, et al. Management if severe lower abdominal or inguinal pain in high-performance athletes. *Am J Sports Med.* 2000;28:2-8.
16. Ahumada LA, et al. Athletic pubalgia. *Ann Plast Surg.* 2005;55:393-396.
17. Swan KG, et al. The Athletic hernia: a systematic review. *Clin Orthop.* 2007;455:78-87.
18. Steele P, et al. Surgery for posterior wall inguinal deficiency in athletes. *J Sci Med Sport.* 2004;7:415-421.
19. Author: "Sports Hernia in the Pediatric Patient." *Unpublished data* [personnel communication: Sarah Beneroft, Joseph Congeni].
20. McCrory P, Bell S. Nerve entrapment syndromes as a cause of pain in the hip, groin and buttock. *Sports Med.* 1999;27:261-274.

CHAPTER 26

Acute Injuries of the Knee

Steven Cline

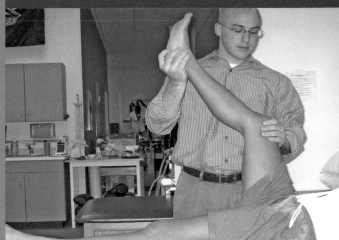

ANATOMY

The anatomical structures of the knee relevant to the present discussion are shown in Figures 26-1 and 26-2.

DEFINITIONS AND EPIDEMIOLOGY

Acute injuries of the knee can cause sprains, dislocations, or fractures (Table 26-1). The anterior cruciate ligament (ACL) itself is injured most often in youth sports such as football and soccer, although this injury can happen in any sport, which involves running, cutting, or jumping. ACL injuries are more common in older adolescent athletes nearing skeletal maturity. There are also gender differences in ACL injury in adolescent athletes. One Norwegian study demonstrated a 5.4 fold increased risk of ACL injury in female athletes in matched soccer cohorts aged 15 to 18 years. In addition, the female athletes had a much lower rate of return to play following treatment than males.[1] Isolated posterior cruciate ligament injuries are uncommon in skeletally immature athletes, and may occur in sports such as football. The medial collateral ligament is one of the most commonly injured structures in the knee. Meniscal tears are not common in children and adolescents. Meniscal tears are more common in sports such as soccer, football, and wrestling, but have been reported in may other sports. There is greater variability in the types of meniscus tears in the young athlete, but horizontal tears are relatively uncommon.[2–4]

Lateral view

Bursae:
- Suprapatellar
- Subcutaneous prepatellar
- Cutaneous prepatellar
- Deep infrapatellar

Femur
Patellar area on condyles
Lateral condyle of femur
Fibular collateral ligament
Lateral meniscus
Fibula
Tibia
Anterior view

Medial condyle of femur
Posterior cruciate ligament
Anterior cruciate ligament
Medial meniscus
Tibial collateral ligament
Transverse ligament
Patellar ligament (cut)
Posterior view

FIGURE 26-1 ■ Knee anatomy. (*Used with permission from Van De Graaff KM. Human Anatomy. 6th ed. New York: McGraw Hill; 2002.*)

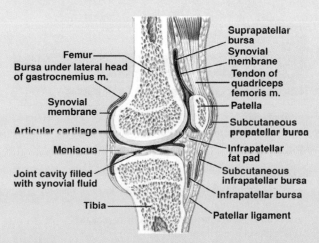

Femur
Bursa under lateral head of gastrocnemius m.
Synovial membrane
Articular cartilage
Meniscus
Joint cavity filled with synovial fluid
Tibia

Suprapatellar bursa
Synovial membrane
Tendon of quadriceps femoris m.
Patella
Subcutaneous prepatellar bursa
Infrapatellar fat pad
Subcutaneous infrapatellar bursa
Infrapatellar bursa
Patellar ligament

FIGURE 26-2 ■ Knee anatomy. (*Used with permission from Van De Graaff KM. Human Anatomy. 6th ed. New York: McGraw Hill; 2002.*)

Table 26-1.

Major Acute Injuries of the Knee

Soft tissue contusions—quadriceps, hamstrings
Musculotendinous—quad tear, patellar tendon avulsion
Patellar dislocation or subluxation
Ligament tears—cruciate and collateral ligaments
Posterolateral corner
Meniscal tears
Fractures (see Table 26-6)

MECHANISMS

The mechanisms of injuries are reviewed below under discussion of specific injuries.

CLINICAL PRESENTATION

The athlete may be seen by the pediatrician on the field or the sideline or later in the office. On the field, the athlete may present with a history of an injury to the knee or the leg following a fall, sudden twisting of the leg, or collision with another player. Rapid onset swelling, radiation of the pain, numbness, paresthesias, and sensation of cold, distal to knee may suggest neurovascular involvement, typically associated with displaced fractures or dislocations, that need urgent appropriate surgical consultation and treatment.

Most cases are seen by pediatricians in the office setting when the athlete is seen either for a follow-up after seen on the field or the emergency department, or for initial visit following the injury. Key elements of the history are listed in Table 26-2. Causes of locking and giving away are listed in Table 26-3.

Table 26-2.

Key Elements of History in Acute Knee Trauma

Onset of injury
Duration, severity, and progression of pain or swelling
Locking
Pain
Paresthesias in leg
Sense of instability or giving away of the knee or the leg
Degree of functional impairment
Type of sport, sport surface, conditions of playing
Athlete's level of participation
Use of protective equipment
Mechanism of injury

Table 26-3.

Causes of Locking and Giving Away

Locking
Meniscal tear
Osteochondral fracture
Intraarticular loose body
Pseudolocking—muscle spasm—e.g., hamstring
Plica

Giving away
ACL tear
Quadriceps tear or weakness
Chondromalaciae patellae
Chronic instability
Uncommon—meniscal tear

History should ascertain the mechanism of the injury. Ask the athlete how the injury occurred. Determine if the athlete was running, changing direction, or stopped suddenly, and the position of the leg and the knee at the time. Sudden change in direction, especially with foot planted can result in sprain of the ACL and injury to meniscus. Landing off balance may also result in anterior cruciate sprain. Collateral ligaments are typically injured as a result of a direct impact to the medial or lateral aspect of the knee. A direct impact against tibia when the knee is flexed is associated with isolated sprain of the posterior cruciate ligament.[2,5]

The athlete feels immediate pain at the time of a ligamentous injury, dislocation, or fracture.[2,5] The key findings on examination of acutely injured knee include swelling, tenderness, deformity, and instability. Details of examination of the knee are reviewed above.

PHYSICAL EXAMINATION

In the setting of acute trauma to the knee encountered on the field, the initial assessment should be directed toward identifying injuries that may need immediate treatment. In the presence of gross deformity of the knee, pallor and diminished arterial pulse distally, and decreased sensation or weakness distal to the knee, a neurovascular injury, dislocation, or fracture should be suspected, that require emergent orthopedic consultation and treatment. The leg should be splinted and the athlete transported to the local hospital emergency department for further evaluation and treatment. Always examine the entire lower limb from hip to toe with the athlete in shorts or gown and not wearing socks or shoes, and compare findings to that of the uninjured limb.

Table 26-4.

Causes of Acute Post-Traumatic Hemarthrosis

ACL tear
Osteochondral fracture
Other fractures
Peripheral meniscal tear
Patellar dislocation
Quadriceps tear
Patellar tendon tear

INSPECTION

Note swelling, deformity, skin break, and ecchymoses. Intra-articular effusion usually first obliterates the hollow medial to the patella, later extending superiorly, and the laterally. Causes of acute posttraumatic hemarthrosis are listed in Table 26-4.

RANGE OF MOTION

Assess active, passive, and against manual resistance: knee flexion and extension.

PALPATION

Crepitus associated with anterior knee pain suggests chondromalacia patellae. Localization of tenderness may provide clue to the injured structures. Perform patellar ballottement test to assess intra-articular effusion (Figure 26-3).

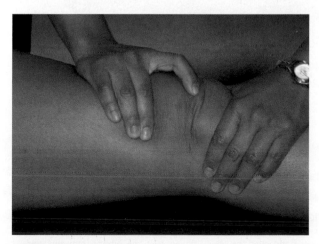

FIGURE 26-3 ■ Ballotment test. With the knee extended grasp the knee just below the patella and push upward. With the fingers of the other hand, gently tap the patella to see if it is ballotable. With knee effusion the patella will be ballotable.

SPECIAL TESTS

Lachman

Check anterior translation of the tibia on the femur by stabilizing the femur with one hand and at 30 degrees of flexion pulling the tibia forward. This is the most sensitive and specific test for an ACL tear (Figure 26-4).

Posterior Drawer

This assesses the PCL. At 90 degrees of flexion, grasp the tibia with both hands and attempt to translate the tibia posteriorly relative to the femur (Figure 26-5).

McMurray

This test places a load and a shear force on the menisci, and is the most sensitive for assessing meniscal tears. A + McMurray is described as demonstrating popping or

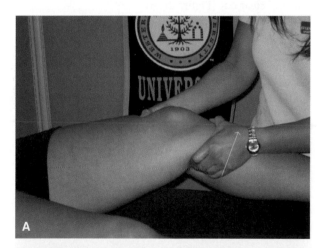

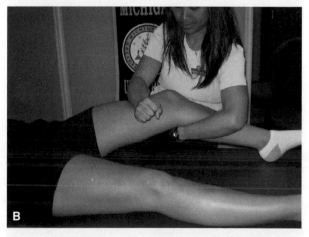

FIGURE 26-4 ■ Lachman test. Check the anterior translation of the tibia on the femur by stabilizing the femur with one hand and at 30 degrees of knee flexion pulling the tibia forward with the other hand. Soft end point is positive Lachman test indicative of anterior cruciate ligament injury.

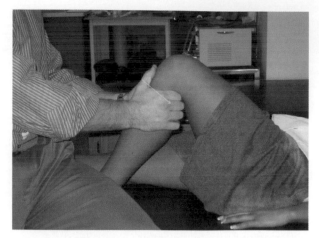

FIGURE 26-5 ■ Posterior drawer test. With the athlete supine and knee at 90-degree flexion stabilize the leg and gently push of tibia the tibia posteriorly. Soft end point and increased translation indicate posterior cruciate ligament injury.

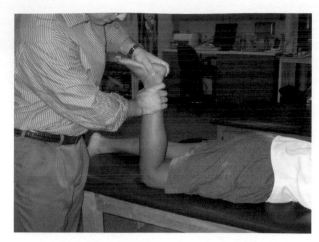

FIGURE 26-7 ■ Appley test. With the athlete lying prone on the table and the knee flexed to 90 degrees, rotate the knee externally and internally while maintaining axial pressure. Pain is often elicited with meniscus tear.

palpable motion of the meniscus on examination, which is likely to occur with a displaced bucket handle tear, however with many meniscal injuries the findings are not that clear cut (Figure 26-6).[5]

loaded and rotated to check the menisci. This examination is uncomfortable in many patients who do not have a meniscal tear, but this examination does reliably demonstrate focal tenderness in many patients who have a torn meniscus (Figure 26-7).

Appley

With the patient prone, the tibia and ankle are held gently, the tibia is flexed to 90 degrees and the tibia is then

Valgus and Varus Stress

These tests assess the medial and lateral collateral ligaments respectively and are performed at 30 degrees

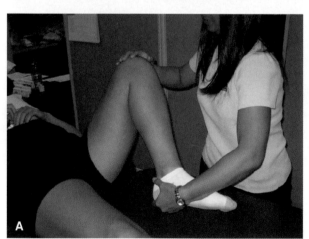

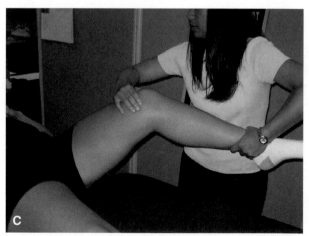

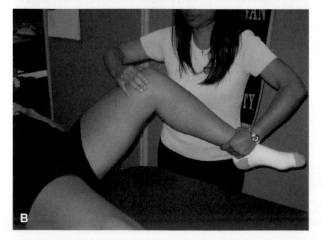

FIGURE 26-6 ■ McMurray test. With the athlete supine on the table grasp the leg with one hand and flex the hip and knee fully, with the other hand over the knee (thumb over the lateral joint line and fingers over the medial joint line) (**A**), followed by extension and external rotation of the knee (**B,C**) to assess the medial meniscus and extension and internal rotation to assess lateral meniscus. Pain (sometimes accompanied by a click or snap) is elicited with a meniscus tear.

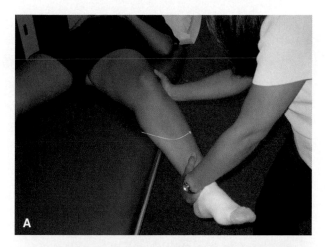

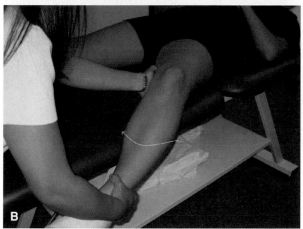

FIGURE 26-8 ■ Varus and valgus stress test. With the athlete supine hold the knee at 30-degree flexion and apply valgus stress to assess medial collateral ligament (a) and varus stress to assess lateral collateral ligament (b). Pain or increased laxity indicates sprain of the ligament.

of flexion with a gentle varus and valgus stress placed across the knee (Figure 26-8).

Patellar Apprehension

This test is performed with the patient supine and the leg extended. Gentle pressure is used to translate the patella laterally, which usually elicits discomfort in patients with retropatellar pain or subluxation. If there has been an acute dislocation, this maneuver should not be performed (Figure 26-9).

Patellar Tilt

This test is done by placing the examiners thumb beneath the lateral patella with the knee extended and using the fingers to control the patella as it is tilted up. In those with a tight lateral retinaculum or lateral patellar compression syndrome, the patella will not usually tilt above neutral. Patellar mobility measured from the

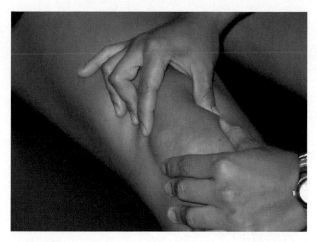

FIGURE 26-9 ■ Patellar apprehension test. With the athlete supine gently attempt to push the patella laterally. In case of subluxation or dislocation of the patella, the athlete will be apprehensive and may have pain.

center of the knee in quadrants should also be checked with gentle medial and lateral translation. Superior inferior mobility of the patella should also be assessed in the same manner.

DIAGNOSTIC IMAGING

Generally in most cases of acute knee trauma, AP, lateral, notch, and sunrise view x-rays are indicated (Table 26-5). MRI scan is indicated in some cases to assess ligament sprains, osteochondral fractures, or meniscal tears.

TREATMENT

Based on the initial assessment, a decision is made as to the urgency of treatment as noted above when a neurovascular injury or a fracture or dislocation is identified

Table 26-5.

Indications for X-Ray in Acute Knee Trauma

A history of significant direct impact to the knee
Difficulty to bear weight
Rapid onset of swelling
Instability
Localized bony tenderness
Gradual onset of pain which is recurrent or chronic
A history of loose body sensation
Recurrent locking
Deformity
Decreased range of motion

Box 26-1. When to Refer.

Indications for Orthopedic Referral and Consultation

Complete tear of anterior or posterior cruciate ligaments
Complete tear of medial or lateral collateral ligaments
Torn meniscus
Patellar dislocation
Knee dislocation
Fractures in and around knee
Ruptured or avulsed quadriceps or patellar tendon
Intra-articular loose body
Osteochondritis dissecans
Posterolateral corner injuries
Osteomyelitis
Pyogenic arthritis
Suspect neurovascular injury

---

or suspected. In nonurgent cases, the athlete should be removed from further sport participation, the knee placed in an immobilizer, and the athlete advised not to weight bear until definitive evaluation later. Treatment for specific injuries is reviewed below. Conditions that indicate orthopedic referral and consultation are listed in Box 26-1.

ANTERIOR CRUCIATE LIGAMENT SPRAINS

Definition and Epidemiology

Acute sprains of the ACL can be partial-thickness or full-thickness tears. Midsubstance tears of the ACL are uncommon before age 12. Young children are more likely to avulse the femoral attachment of the ACL (tibial spine avulsion). ACL sprains are seen most commonly in basketball, soccer, hockey, and American football.

Mechanism

In most cases, ACL sprain is a noncontact injury resulting from sudden deceleration and pivoting (external rotation) of knee (Figure 26-10). Statistically, ACL injuries are more prevalent in female than male athletes, and this may have to do with firing patterns of the quadriceps and hamstrings, overall conditioning and training, as well as leg position with the feet wider than the toes when landing from a jump.

Clinical Presentation

After an ACL sprain (or avulsion of the tibial spine), there is a rapid onset (usually within 4 hours) swelling of the knee (traumatic hemarthrosis). The athlete will also often describe feeling a large pop, or snap in the

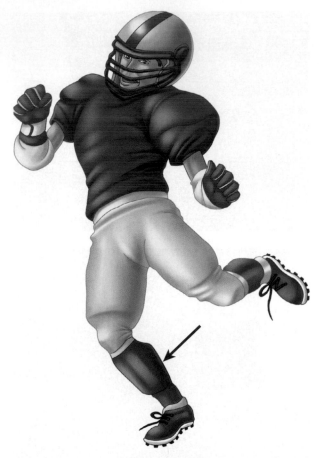

FIGURE 26-10 ■ Mechanism of injury for ACL sprain.

knee with immediate instability (a sense of giving away of the knee or the leg) of the knee at the time of injury. Acutely, it may be difficult to obtain a meaningful ligament examination due to swelling, pain, and muscle spasm. It is essential to perform a neurovascular examination as the young athlete may have sustained a knee dislocation rather than a simple ACL injury.

In a few days to a week, once the athlete has been placed in an immobilizer, and has iced the knee and rested it, thoroughly examine all the knee ligaments and menisci again. Lachman test is positive in ACL sprains and avulsion of the tibial spine. If there are associated injuries to the collateral ligaments the varus or valgus stress will be positive. McMurray test will be positive if the meniscus is torn. Ninety percent of the ACL sprains can be diagnosed bases on findings of history and examination. A tense hemarthrosis, may need to be aspirated to alleviate the athlete's pain and to obtain a more meaningful examination.[2,3,4,6]

Diagnostic Imaging

X-rays are indicated to rule out associated fractures. MRI is diagnostic (Figure 26-11 and 26-12).[7]

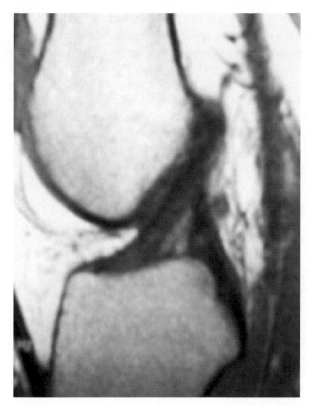

FIGURE 26-11 ■ MRI with normal ACL.

Treatment

The leg is placed in a knee immobilizer. The athlete is recommended, nonweight-bearing crutch walking, with rest, local application of ice and elevation of the leg, and referred to orthopedic surgeon. The treatment of ACL injury in the skeletally immature athlete is the subject of intense debate between those surgeons who

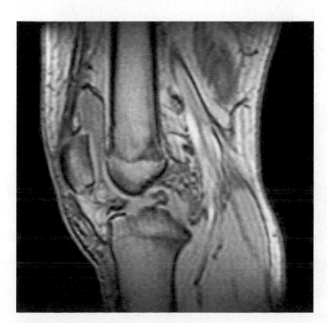

FIGURE 26-12 ■ MRI with torn ACL.

advocate rehabilitation and waiting until skeletal maturity before reconstruction of the ACL, and those who advocate early reconstruction.

The ACL is reconstructed in many young athletes to avoid ongoing instability and further chondral and meniscal injuries. ACL is reconstructed in most cased the, arthroscopically followed by intensive rehabilitation. Accelerated ACL rehabilitation protocols do return some athletes to competition at 4 months postop, but many surgeons will hold the athlete out from competition for 6 months after an ACL reconstruction.

The results of ACL reconstruction in the skeletally immature athlete are good, but are difficult to compare across studies as multiple techniques are used, with small numbers of patients in each study, and the patients are of different ages and skeletal maturity levels. There is a risk of physeal arrest with ACL reconstruction in skeletally immature patients, but specific techniques to avoid the physis, and soft tissue grafts fixed away from the physis are utilized to minimize these risks. Current results demonstrate generally good success with a stable ACL graft, and minimal length or angular deformity of the leg in these young athletes. The overall goal of reconstruction is to give the athlete a stable knee and to avoid further chondral and meniscal injury.[2]

AVULSION FRACTURES OF THE TIBIAL SPINE (INTERCONDYLAR EMINENCE)

Definition and Epidemiology

Knee injuries in skeletally immature athletes often involve avulsion of the ACL insertion on the tibial spine itself, rather than a classic midsubstance ACL ligament injury as in older adolescents and adults. The ACL itself is usually injured to a degree with avulsion of the tibial spine. Tibial spine or intercondylar eminence fractures are seen most commonly between 8 and 15 years of age.

Mechanism

Tibial spine avulsion fractures are caused by the same mechanisms as ACL injuries in older athletes and adults.[3] A classification scheme of tibial spine avulsion fractures is depicted in Figure 26-13.

Clinical Presentation

The athlete presents with a history of a fall on the knee or a sudden deceleration and pivoting of the knee followed by immediate pain, pain on weight-bearing, rapid onset of swelling, and a sense of the knee or the leg giving away.

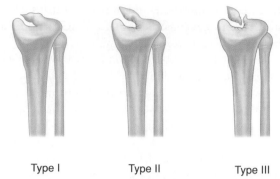

Type I   Type II   Type III

FIGURE 26-13 ■ Meyers and McKeever classification of tibial spine fractures. Type I Minimal displacement of fractured fragment. Type II Partial displacement (typically anterior one third to one-half) of the fractured fragment that remains hinged posteriorly. Type III Complete separation of the fractured fragment.

There is localized knee tenderness and Lachman test is positive. A tense hemarthrosis may need to be aspirated. The aspirate will be positive for fat droplets seen of the surface.

Diagnostic Imaging

The avulsed fracture fragment will be seen best on the notch view or AP view (Figure 26-14).

Treatment

Initial treatment of these injuries is often closed, placing the athlete in a long leg cast with the knee slightly flexed,

as long as x-rays in the cast demonstrate good reduction of the tibial spine. Type III or type IV, a more complex displaced fracture, will require surgery for reduction and fixation. The outcome of tibial spine avulsion fractures treated either closed or with surgery is not uniformly benign, and some young athletes will go on to have residual instability of the knee with a lax ACL, once the fracture is healed. This places the athlete at a higher risk for subsequent meniscal tear and chondral injury. These athletes may need to undergo an ACL reconstruction in the long term.[3]

POSTERIOR CRUCIATE LIGAMENT (PCL) SPRAINS

Definition and Epidemiology

The injury usually includes an avulsion of the PCL, most often from its tibial attachment. Femoral sided injuries are usually soft tissue in nature. PCL sprains are uncommon in youth sports.

Mechanism

The PCL limits posterior translation of the tibia on the femur and knee rotation, and is often injured in adolescent football lineman. The injury commonly occurs because of a direct blow to the anterior knee or tibia with the knee flexed (Figure 26-15).

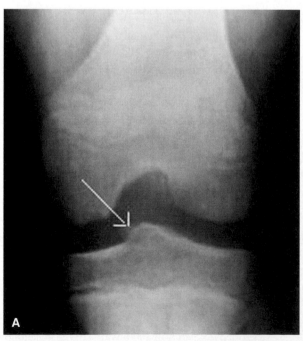
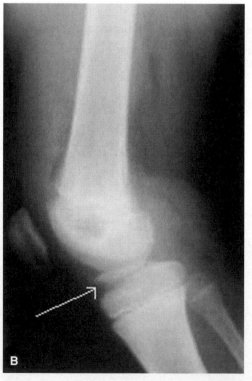

FIGURE 26-14 ■ X-ray of avulsed tibial spine. (*Used with permission from Zionts LF. Chapter 14, in Green's Skeletal Trauma in Children. 3rd ed. Philadelphia, PA: Saunders Elsevier Imprint; Figure 14-15.*)

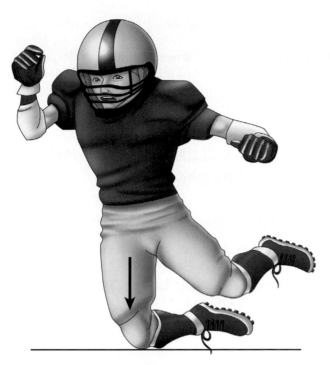

FIGURE 26-15 ■ Mechanism of PCL sprain.

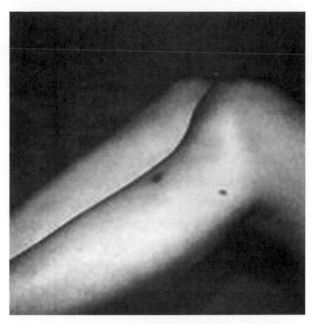

FIGURE 26-16 ■ Drop sign for posterior cruciate ligament sprain. With the athlete supine on the examination table and knee at 90-degree flexion, observation from the side will reveal a drop just distal to the knee of the affected side (left leg) relative to the unaffected side (right leg).

Clinical Presentation

The athlete will usually report a more subtle feeling of instability in the knee than that of the ACL injured patient, and may have felt a pop with contact, but usually will not have a marked or immediate hemarthrosis. Posterior drawer (Figure 26-6) and drop signs (Figure 26-16) are positive. There may be an effusion present as well, and there may be associated chondral or meniscal injury.

Diagnostic Imaging

MRI will demonstrate redundancy of the posterior cruciate ligament (PCL), or loss of tension in the ligament, and will also reliably demonstrate any other ligamentous, meniscal, or cartilage injuries which are present.[7]

Treatment

Orthopedic consultation is indicated for definitive treatment of PCL sprains. Multiple factors influence the decision to reconstruct the PCL and not all athletes need surgery. If there is significant displacement of a bony avulsion, repair is indicated either with sutures or with a screw that does not violate the physis. Soft tissue avulsions of the PCL may be fixed with sutures. Minimally displaced avulsions can be treated closed, with a long leg cast. There is often residual laxity after bony healing because of interstitial injury to the PCL itself. Rehabilitation for the PCL focuses on quadriceps exercises and avoiding active hamstrings exercises for several months. Return to play timeline is similar to those following ACL reconstruction.

MEDIAL COLLATERAL LIGAMENT (MCL) SPRAINS

Definition and Epidemiology

Like all ligament sprains, MCL sprains are also graded I, II , and III, with a grade I injury demonstrating tenderness but no true instability, a grade II injury demonstrating less than 1 cm of laxity, and a grade III injury showing more than 1 cm of opening with soft end point with a valgus stress.

Mechanism

The medial collateral ligament is commonly injured by a medially directed blow to the lateral side of the knee, overloading the medial side as seen in soccer, football, and other related sports (Figure 26-17). There may be associated injuries to the menisci and the ACL present as well.

Clinical Presentation

The athlete presents with medial side knee pain and tenderness. In isolated sprains swelling is minimal. The

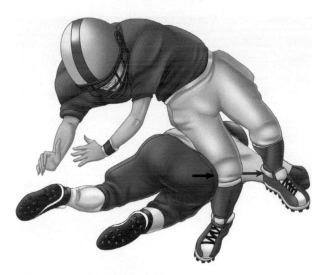

FIGURE 26-17 ■ Mechanism of injury for MCL sprain.

valgus stress test will be positive for pain or increased laxity (Figure 26-9).

Diagnostic Imaging

X-rays are done to detect bony avulsion associated with grade III sprains.

Treatment

Grade I and II sprains are treated in a hinged brace (Figure 26-18) for protection for 4 to 6 weeks, with early

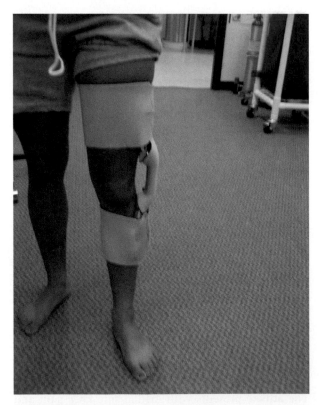

FIGURE 26-18 ■ Hinged brace for MCL sprain.

range of motion and strengthening exercises. Most grade III sprains are treated similarly over a longer period of time. Surgical treatment of grade III sprains is controversial. If there are other associated injuries to the knee which require surgery, the MCL is sometimes repaired at that time.[8]

LATERAL COLLATERAL LIGAMENT (LCL) SPRAINS

Definition and Epidemiology

Sprains of the lateral collateral ligament can result in either partial-thickness or full-thickness tears of the ligament. More likely, LCL sprains are associated with other significant posterolateral corner injuries of the knee.

Mechanism

Lateral collateral ligament tears may occur when a sudden, forceful varus stress is placed across the knee with a blow to the medial side of the knee. The lateral aspect of the knee has a very complex anatomy, and these injuries do not always occur in isolation.

Clinical Presentation

There is pain and tenderness over the lateral aspect of the knee. Swelling may be minimal. There may be increased laxity of the lateral collateral at 30 degrees of flexion and tenderness along the course of the ligament or over its bony origin or insertion at the fibular head. One should be sure to rule out other injuries such as a posterolateral corner injury and assess the ACL, MCL, and PCL as well.

Diagnostic Imaging

X-rays may show a small avulsion fragment from the femur or the fibula, or may be negative.

Treatment

A grade I injury with <5 mm of laxity on examination may be treated in a hinged brace for 2 to 4 weeks with close follow-up. Grade II or III injuries with 5 to 10 mm of laxity or >1 cm of laxity should be braced and referred to orthopedics. Significant laxity of the LCL may lead to chronic knee instability and long-term knee problems. In those athletes with gross instability requiring repair, primary repair is the preferred treatment.[8]

MEDIAL MENISCUS TEARS

Definition and Epidemiology

Medial meniscus tears are the most common meniscal injuries, and are more common in the posterior horn of the medial meniscus. There are rare medial discoid menisci which are more prone to tear than a normal meniscus, but the reported rate of occurrence is 0.25%.[4]

Mechanism

A shearing injury (twisting motion of the planted leg) across the knee joint with the knee somewhat flexed is a common mechanism of injury. This occurs in sports such as soccer, lacrosse, gymnastics, and football, but can occur in any sport. The meniscus is a C-shaped fibrocartilaginous wedge that develops prenatally. The menisci distribute joint load between the femur and tibia, aid in lubrication of the knee, and contribute secondarily to knee stability, specifically the medial meniscus, which helps provide stability in conjunction with the ACL. Both menisci are tethered by meniscotibial ligaments, but the medial meniscus has half the excursion of the lateral meniscus. Additionally, the medial meniscus serves as a secondary stop to anterior and posterior translation of the knee, and this makes it more susceptible to injury.

Clinical Presentation

The athlete often reports a twisting injury to the knee or a fall in deep flexion. One-third of athletes report no injury at all. The knee may not swell much initially, but the athlete usually complains of catching, locking, clicking, and feelings of instability in the knee. On examination, there may be a small effusion and discrete tenderness along the joint line over the affected meniscus. McMurray, Appley, and Thessaly (Figure 26-19) tests may be positive. Physical examination is >90% sensitive and specific for meniscal tears.

Diagnostic Imaging

It is useful to obtain AP, lateral, notch views, and a sunrise view of the knee to look for associated avulsion of the collaterals, possible tibial spine avulsion, osteochondral injuries, as well as physeal injuries. If a meniscal injury is suspected, MRI may prove helpful, but normal increased signal in a skeletally immature athlete often resembles a tear. The sensitivity and specificity of MRI for mensical tears in young patients is much lower than that of physical examination. Physical examination is reported to be 93.3% sensitive and 92.3% specific vs.

MRI which was 50% sensitive and had a 37.5% accuracy rate for pediatric meniscal tears in one study. MRI should be used as an adjunct to the history and physical examination, if needed.[4]

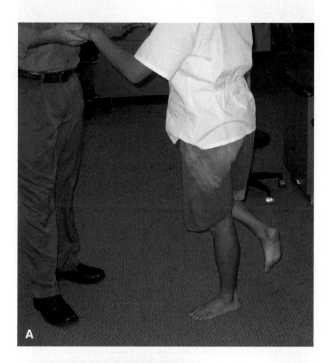

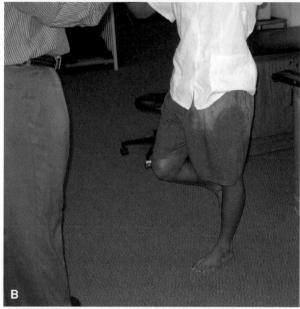

FIGURE 26-19 ■ Thessaly test. Thessaly test reproduces the load transmission in the knee. The athlete is standing on the injured leg with foot flat on the ground and knee flexed at 5 degrees. She then rotates the knee and body internally and externally 3times. Repeat the same at 20 degrees of knee flexion. In case of a meniscus tear, the athlete will experience joint line pain and a sense of knee locking or catching. The reported diagnostic accuracy of Thessaly test at 20 degrees of knee flexion in detecting meniscal tears exceeds 90%. (Karachalios T, Hantes M, Zibis AH, Zachos V, Karantanas AH, Malizos KN. Diagnostic accuracy of a new clinical test (The Thessaly Test for early detection of meniscal tears. *J Bone Joint Surg.* 2005;87A(5): 955-962.) *(continued)*

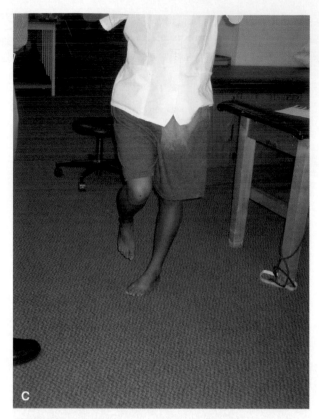

FIGURE 26-19 ■ *(Continued).*

Treatment

In suspected meniscal tears in skeletally immature athletes orthopedic consultation is indicated. Small meniscal tears found at arthroscopy, less than 1 cm in length, stable, and vertical in nature, may be treated with a short course of modified weight-bearing, refraining from running, cutting, and jumping, followed by a short period of rehabilitation.

Larger tears, in particular vertical peripheral tears which displace more than 3 mm, are usually repairable and do well with surgery. Most flap and radial tears are not repairable, and a small portion of the meniscus is excised at arthroscopy. The results of meniscus repair depend on the type and location of the tear, the technique used for repair, and the age of the tear. Vertical tears in the peripheral one-third heal in 80% to 90% of patients if properly repaired. More central vertical tears in young athletes have a better healing rate than those in adults, and therefore these tears are most often fixed in young athletes.[4]

Resection of even a small portion of the meniscus increases loading of the tibial and femoral cartilage in that particular compartment, thereby increasing the later risk of osteoarthritis. It is best to preserve as much meniscal tissue as possible at surgery. If a simple resection of a portion of meniscus is performed, there is usually a short period of time, a few days to a week of crutch use, and then limitation of impact or running and jumping activities for a few weeks. Allograft menisci are not utilized nor well studied in skeletally immature patients. There should be a low threshold to perform early arthroscopy in a young patient with meniscal symptoms, thereby protecting the remainder of the meniscus and the cartilage surfaces of the knee from further injury.

DISCOID LATERAL MENISCUS

Definition and Epidemiology

The discoid meniscus is an anatomic variant, which exists in roughly 3% to 5% of the US population, and up to 15% to 20% of the population in Japan. The discoid meniscus is more prone to tear because of its altered anatomy and collagen structure vs. a normal meniscus.[4]

Mechanism

Sudden deceleration and twisting of the planted extended leg is a common mechanism of lateral meniscal tear. Twisting of the legs upon landing from a height can also cause lateral meniscal tears.

Clinical Presentation

An athlete with a tear of a discoid meniscus may report a sudden locking of the joint near full extension after a twisting fall, or upon landing from a jump. An unstable discoid meniscus variant may also lock or catch in the joint. These injuries are often reported in young military parachutists, on landing from a hard jump, with a report of immediate pain, a snap, and then transient locking of the knee, which may be difficult to unlock. There may be a localized swelling over the lateral joint line. The patient may be able to voluntarily demonstrate locking, unlocking, or catching of the knee to the examiner. It is not recommended that you ask or encourage the patient to do this.

Diagnostic Imaging

X-rays will often demonstrate squaring of the lateral femoral condyle, cupping of the lateral tibial plateau, hypoplasia of the lateral tibial spine, and a slightly increased lateral joint space (Figure 26-20). MRI is best to demonstrate the discoid meniscus and any tears, as well as associated chondral or ligamentous injuries (Figure 26-21).[4,7,9,10]

Treatment

These young athletes may require partial resection of the discoid meniscus, including some of the uninjured

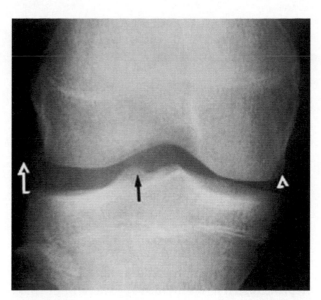

FIGURE 26-20 ■ X-ray of discoid meniscus. (*Used with permission from DeLee JC, Drez Jr, D, Miller MD. DeLee and Drez's Orthopedic Sports Medicine. 2nd ed. Philadelphia, PA: Saunders Elsevier Imprint; 2003:Figure 28D 2-17.*)

as well as the torn portion, and sometimes reattachment of the meniscus to the capsule. Discoid menisci are more prone to retear than normal lateral menisci. After any meniscal repair, the patient is placed at limited weight-bearing in an immobilizer or in a range of motion brace, with specific motion limitations for 4 to 6 weeks, based on the location and type of the tear. Return to sports varies based on the type of tear and the repair needed, and can be up to 4 to 6 months. Meniscal allografts are not an effective treatment option in the skeletally immature patient.[4,9,10]

POSTEROLATERAL CORNER INJURIES

Definition and Epidemiology

Posterolateral corner of the knee injuries also occur in the young athlete and the adolescent. In the developing knee, the ligaments and tendons are often stronger than the physes or apophyses, and this can lead to avulsion injuries of the collaterals or of the posterolateral corner, which consists of multiple structures and is critical for varus and rotatory stability of the knee.

Mechanism

The mechanism of injury may be a lateral varus stress in running and ball sports or a twisting injury on a partially flexed knee. These injuries may tear the posterolateral corner, and also often injure the ACL and/or the PCL, leading to a very unstable knee. There must be heightened suspicion in these cases for a knee dislocation and neurovascular (popliteal vessels and the peroneal nerve) injury.

Clinical Presentation

There will be immediate lateral and posterior knee pain and swelling. The more complex injuries of the postero-lateral corner may demonstrate instability in rotation, varus, and valgus and often a positive anterior or posterior drawer. Increased external rotation of the foot, compared to uninjured knee, with the patient prone and the knee flexed 30 degrees is consistent with a posterolateral corner injury (Figure 26-22).

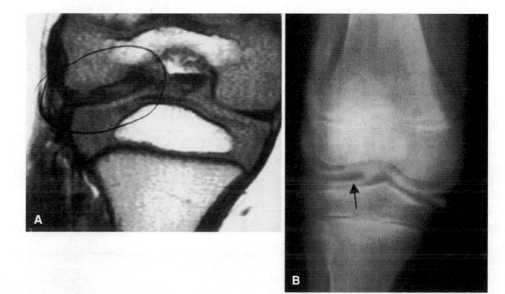

FIGURE 26-21 ■ MRI of discoid meniscus. (*Used with permission from DeLee JC, Drez Jr, D, Miller MD. DeLee and Drez's Orthopedic Sports Medicine. 2nd ed. Philadelphia, PA: Saunders Elsevier Imprint; 2003, Figure 28 12-15.*)

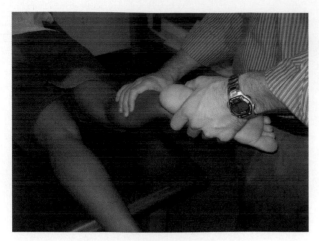

FIGURE 26-22 ■ Test for posterolateral corner injury of the knee. Increased external rotation of the foot with the athlete prone and the knee flexed at 30 degrees is indicative of a posterolateral corner injury.

Diagnostic Imaging

In some cases, an angiogram and other imaging studies including MRI in addition to plain films are warranted.

Treatment

The lateral collateral ligament and other posterolateral structures can cause chronic long-term knee instability and dysfunction, and these patients should be placed in a brace or immobilizer, on crutches, iced, and referred immediately to an orthopedist. The lateral structures and the posterolateral corner should be reconstructed early, usually within 2 weeks of injury, for the best outcome for the patient; but can be reconstructed later with allograft, with good long-term results as well. Most of these injuries occur in the adolescent who is nearing skeletal maturity. These injuries are often high energy, just as knee dislocations are, and bear close observation and follow-up.

PATELLAR SUBLUXATION AND DISLOCATION

Definition and Epidemiology

Patella normally slides up and down during knee flexion and extension along the femoral groove. When the patella suddenly slides out of its normal path and the femoral groove, usually laterally, a dislocation or a subluxation results. Postulated risk factors for recurrent dislocations are hypermobility of the patella, congenital ligamentous laxity, a dysplastic vastus medialis obliquus, patella alta, tibial and femoral rotational malalignment, a dysplastic trochlea, or a combination

of these problems. In patients who first dislocated patella as teenagers, recurrent subluxation or dislocation is much more common.

Mechanism

A direct impact to the patella or a forceful quadriceps contraction during a cutting motion can result in *acute patellar dislocation.* In the vast majority of cases, the patella is dislocated laterally (Figure 26-23).[6,11,12]

Clinical Presentation

Patellar dislocation is associated with immediate severe pain, rapid onset of knee swelling, obvious deformity, restriction of knee motion, and significant tenderness. Apprehension test is performed by gently trying to push the patella laterally. The patient immediately feels discomfort or a sense of the patella subluxing or dislocating. The patient will often have a significant effusion in the knee, and may have increased lateral translation of the patella versus the uninjured side. This examination may not be comfortable acutely, and the patient should

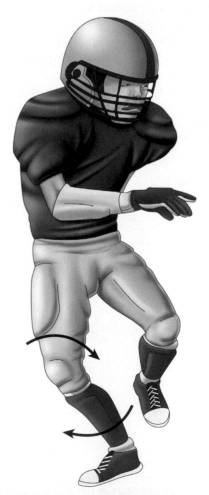

FIGURE 26-23 ■ Mechanism of patellar dislocation.

then be placed in a knee immobilizer, iced, and placed on crutches and referred or examined again in 5 to 7 days. It is not necessary to forcibly translate the patella laterally or medially on examination, but it is useful to get an idea of its mobility relative to the unaffected knee.[6,11,12]

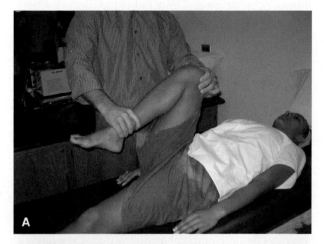

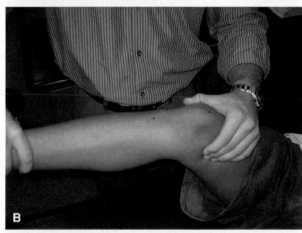

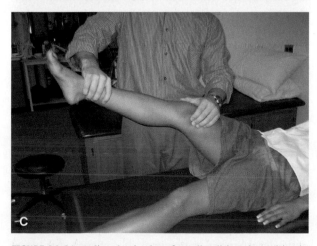

FIGURE 26-24 ■ Closed reduction of patellar dislocation. With athlete relaxed and supine the leg is flexed at the hip and knee (**A**). The knee is then gently extended with pressure maintained over the patella directed from lateral to medial direction (**B,C**).

Diagnostic Imaging

Diagnosis is apparent clinically. Standard x-rays, AP, lateral, and sunrise views are confirmatory.

Treatment

If the patella is still subluxated or dislocated at presentation, the treatment is immediate reduction and a short period of immobilization followed by quadriceps strengthening exercises. Reduction can be achieved, if the quadriceps and hamstrings are relaxed. Closed reduction may be performed with athlete relaxed and supine, with the leg flexed at the hip and knee (Figure 26-24). The knee is then gently extended with pressure over the patella from lateral to medial direction. One should carefully rule out associated fracture or rupture of the quadriceps. In certain cases, particularly with associated bony injuries or chronic patellar instability, soft tissue or bony reconstructive procedures may be needed to restore stability and function.

PATELLOFEMORAL OSTEOCHONDRAL FRACTURES

Definition and Epidemiology

Fracture of the patellofemoral articular cartilage and the underlying subchondral bone constitute osteochondral fracture.

Mechanism

Osteochondral fractures of the patella and femur are usually caused by direct trauma or related to shearing injuries with a patellar dislocation. Patellar dislocations in children are associated with osteochondral fractures in 5% to 71% of patients in various studies, with the greatest number of these injuries documented when the articular surfaces were examined with an arthroscope.[6,12]

Clinical Presentation

The patient will present with a painful, swollen knee joint, and is reluctant to place weight on the leg. There is often a large hemarthrosis present. If the hemarthrosis is aspirated, there is likely to be fat present, suggesting an osteochondral injury somewhere in the knee. There may be tenderness over the portion of the joint which is injured, and the athlete will also often demonstrate apprehension and a gap over the medial patellar retinaculum, indicating a tear of the retinaculum and capsule as well as possibly the medial patellofemoral ligament.

Diagnostic Imaging

Standard x-rays often may not demonstrate the injury well and a CT scan or MRI scan may be indicated.

Treatment

Athletes with osteochondral fractures should be referred to orthopedic surgeon. Treatment is primarily surgical, with replacement of larger fragments from the weight-bearing surfaces if possible, and drilling of small lesions. After the surgery, the athlete is kept from full weight-bearing until radiographs or CT scan images show complete healing. Outcome after fixation of large weight-bearing fragments is not always good. The patient may experience stiffness and adhesions of the knee, quadriceps weakness, and anterior knee pain. Redislocation of the patella may also occur and may require further surgery, repair of the medial patellofemoral ligament (MPFL), medial capsular plication, patellar realignment, or other procedures, depending upon the skeletal maturity of the athlete. In the skeletally immature, procedures such as a soft tissue graft to the MPFL and soft tissue realignment procedures may be helpful.[6,11,12]

DISLOCATION OF THE KNEE

Definition and Epidemiology

These are usually higher-energy injuries and may occur in sports such as skiing and snowboarding. There are often multiple ligaments injured, including the ACL and/or PCL as well as the collateral ligaments and the posterolateral corner of the knee.

Mechanism

Mechanisms are multiple and ligament injuries vary based on the direction of applied forces to the knee at the time of the injury. There is further concern with a high-energy injury for significant meniscal and chondral injury, as well as vascular and neurologic injuries to the knee.

Clinical Presentation

The athlete presents with a painful, swollen knee, and may demonstrate obvious deformity of the leg, with the tibia translated relative to the femur. Pulses and sensation may be diminished. There should be a very low threshold to order a vascular consult and studies, and all these patients should be admitted, once the knee joint is reduced, with repeat neurovascular examinations and close follow-up.

The patient if able will usually give a history of fall from a height while skiing, or a high energy injury in motocross or similar mechanism. Gentle examination of the knee may reveal instability of the knee to gentle stress. One always needs to uncover the knee and be certain there are no open injuries or fractures, as well as assess the leg for signs of compartment syndrome, such as pain with passive stretch, paresthesias, altered sensation, or other findings. The threshold to check compartment pressures in any higher-energy limb injury should be very low. Additionally with a high-energy injury to the knee, the patient is often distracted by pain, and will be unable to give a reliable examination early on when checking for compartment syndrome. Any pain out of proportion to the injuries seen should heighten suspicion of a compartment syndrome of the leg. Advanced imaging, particularly MRI, may demonstrate the extent of ligamentous, bony, and cartilage injury of the knee.

Diagnostic Imaging

X-rays of the knee may show the dislocation, but these injuries often are partially or fully reduced at presentation, and do not demonstrate the true magnitude of injury or displacement at time of injury. MRI is done to assess for associated ligamentous, meniscal, and cartilage injury and to plan surgical reconstruction.

Treatment

Treatment is early closed reduction, with open reduction in some cases. Once reduced, the knee is immobilized and the patient is hospitalized and kept under orthopedic and vascular surgery care. There is a significant risk of popliteal artery and peroneal nerve injury with knee dislocations, which can lead to serious sequelae including early compartment syndrome with permanent muscle damage, foot drop or muscle weakness, as well as long-term gait problems with significant loss of function of the limb. Reconstruction is best performed early if lateral or posterolateral structures are injured, before 3 weeks. There is a significant risk of knee stiffness, with loss of range of motion and possible arthrofibrosis especially after multiple ligament reconstruction.

ACUTE FRACTURES ABOUT THE KNEE

Fractures about the knee (Table 26-6) in the skeletally immature athlete can be Salter-Harris type acute fractures of the distal femoral or proximal tibial physes , apophyseal avulsions, or metaphyseal fractures (buckle, torus, or complete).[13–17] Sports-related acute fractures about the knee in children and adolescents are uncommon.

Table 26-6.

Acute Fractures About the Knee

Intra-articular fractures
Osteochondral fractures
Fractures of the tibial spine (intercondylar eminence)

Extra-articular fractures
Distal femoral epiphyseal fractures
Proximal tibial epiphyeal fractures
Avulsion of the tibial tubercle
Patellar fractures

All fractures about the knee in skeletally immature patients need expert orthopedic evaluation and definitive immediate care and long-term follow-up. In the presence of neurovascular signs, obvious deformity, rapid onset swelling, and severe pain the patient must be evaluated and treated urgently. The knee should be placed in an immobilizer; patient not allowed to move the leg or bear weight and immediately referred for orthopedic care.

REFERENCES

1. Loud K, Micheli L. Common athletic injuries in adolescent girls. *Curr Opin Pediatr.* 2001;13:317-327.
2. Beasley L, Chudik S. Anterior cruciate ligament injury in children: update of current treatment options. *Curr Opin Pediatr.* 2003;15:45-52.
3. Kocher M, Mandiga R, Klingele K, Bley L, Micheli L. Anterior cruciate ligament injury versus tibial spine fracture in the skeletally immature knee. *J Pediatr Ortho.* 2004;24(2): 185-188.
4. Moti A, Micheli L. Meniscal and articular cartilage injury in the skeletally immature knee. In: Mary Lloyd Ireland, ed. *Sports Medicine Instructional Course Lectures American Academy of Orthopedic Surgeons;* 2005:363-370.
5. Cosgarea A, Jay P. Posterior cruciate ligament injuries: evaluation and management. *J Am Acad Orthop Surg.* 2001;9:297-307.
6. Frank J, Jarit G, Bravman J, Rosen, J. Lower extremity fractures in the skeletally immature athlete. *J Am Acad Surg.* 2007;15:356-366.
7. Strouse P, Koujok Khaldoun. Magnetic resonance imaging of the pediatric knee. *Top MRI.* 2002;13(4):277-294.
8. Larson R, Ulmer T. Ligament injuries in children. In: Mary Lloyd Ireland, ed. *Sports Medicine Instructional Course Lectures AAOS.* 2005; 38:357-361.
9. Andrisani D, Miller L, Rubenstein D. Surgical management of discoid meniscus. *Tech Knee Surg.* 2006;5(2): 128-133.
10. Klingele K, Kocher M, Hresko T, Gerbino P, Michele L. Discoid lateral meniscus prevalence of peripheral rim instability. *J Pediatr Ortho.* 2004;24(1):79-82.
11. Fulkerson J. Diagnosis and treatment of patients with patellofemoral pain. *Am J Sports Med.* 2002;30:447-456.
12. Boden B, Pearsall A, Garrett W, Feagin J. Patellofemoral instability: evaluation and management. *J Am Acad Ortho Surg.* 1997;5:47-57.
13. Zionts L. Fractures around the knee in children. *J Am Acad Ortho Surg.* 2002;10(5):345-355.
14. Flynn J, Skaggs D, Sponseller P, Ganley T, Kay R, Leitch K. The operative management of pediatric fractures of the lower extremity. *J Bone Joint Surg.* 2002;84-A:2288-2300.
15. Shindle M, Foo L, Kelly R, et al. Magnetic resonance imaging of cartilage in the athlete: current techniques and spectrum of disease. *J Bone Joint Surg.* 2006;88-A:27-46.
16. Setter K, Palomino K. Pediatric tibia fractures: current concepts. *Curr Opin Pediatr.* 2006;18(30):30-35.
17. Ortiz E, Isler M, Navia J, Canosa R. Pathologic fractures in children. *Curr Ortho Related Res.* 2005;432:116-126.

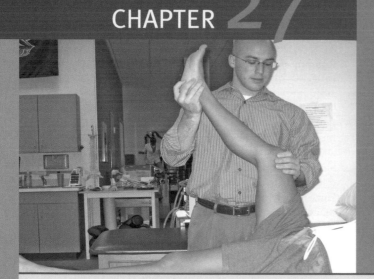

CHAPTER 27

Overuse Injuries of the Knee

Dilip R. Patel and E. Dennis Lyne

IDIOPATHIC ANTERIOR KNEE PAIN

Definition and Epidemiology

Idiopathic anterior knee pain has been described by various other terms (Table 27-1). It refers to nonspecific, vague, mostly activity-related anterior knee pain and is the most common cause of knee pain in adolescents. Anterior knee pain has been reported in half of adolescent athletes at some time.

Mechanism

Many factors have been postulated to contribute to the development of anterior knee pain in adolescents (Table 27-2).[1-4] Intense physical activity overloading the patellofemoral mechanism (Figure 27-1) appears to be the most consistent factor leading to the development of anterior knee pain. The patellofemoral unit provides the mechanism for knee extension and deceleration. The stability of the patella in the femoral groove is provided by the surrounding soft tissue attachments and the bony supporting structures (Figure 27-2). Malalignment and abnormal tracking of the patella have been postulated to contribute to anterior knee pain. Vastus medialis obliquus plays an important role in stabilizing the patella in the femoral groove and its proper tracking. A chondromalacia patella is a pathologic diagnosis indicating softening and erosion of the cartilage of the patellofemoral joint; in some athletes, it is a cause of severe anterior knee pain.[2]

Clinical Presentation

The young active athlete presents with either acute or gradual onset anterior knee pain affecting one or both knees, usually seen following a recent increase in physical activity. The pain is increased after prolonged sitting (theater sign), ascending or descending stairs, and

Table 27-1.

Synonyms for Anterior Knee Pain

Patellofemoral pain syndrome
Patellalgia
Gonalgia paresthetica
Retropatellar arthralgia
Peripatellar syndrome
Patellar maltracking syndrome
Chondromalacia patella

Table 27-2.

Factors Postulated to Contribute to Anterior Knee Pain

Overuse
Patella alta
Patellar maltracking
Abnormal Q angle
Knee extensor and flexor muscle strength imbalance
Knee and patellar ligamentous laxity
Exaggerated lumbar lordosis
Genu varus
Genu valgus
Hyperpronated feet
Tight Achilles
Patellar chondromalacia

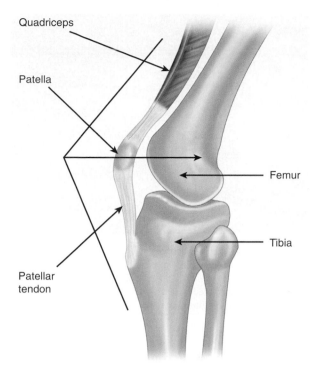

FIGURE 27-1 ■ Patellofemoral mechanism. Patellofemoral mechanism provides the basis for effective knee extension. During the movement of the knee from flexion to extension there is increasing patellofemoral compression force.

repeated squatting exercises. Usually, the pain has been present for few weeks with intermittent activity-related exacerbations and improvement with a period of rest. Deterioration of sports performance because of increased frequency and worsening of the pain, leads the athlete to seek medical attention. The athlete may give a history of the knee catching, pseudolocking, or giving away.

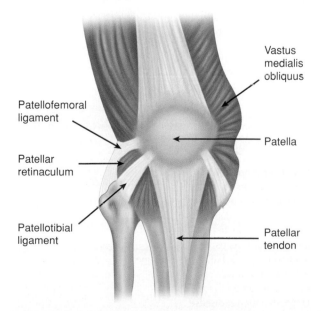

FIGURE 27-2 ■ Soft tissue patellofemoral stabilizers.

On examination, look for abnormal gait, increased lumbar lordosis, and any asymmetry of hips or lower extremities; also observe for atrophy and weakness of the quadriceps muscles by comparing it to the normal side. A decrease in flexibility of the hamstrings and quadriceps is a common finding (Figure 27-3). Isometric quadriceps contraction with the leg extended, may reveal a subtle lateral patellar deviation.

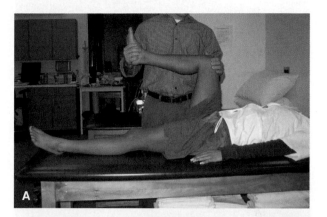

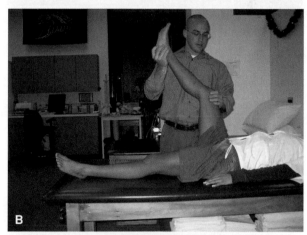

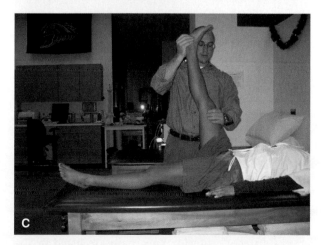

FIGURE 27-3 ■ Test for hamstring flexibility. With the athlete supine on the table first flex the hip and knee (A). This is followed by bringing the hip to 90-degree flexion and gently extending the knee (B). Normally the knee should extend close to 180 degrees (C). Lack of extension is a measure of hamstring tightness.

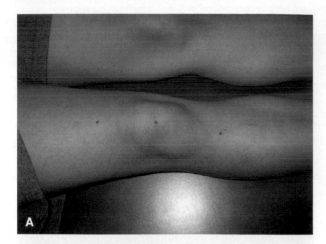

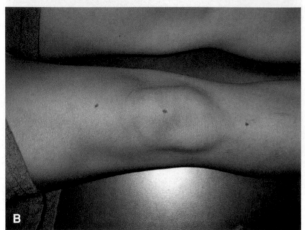

FIGURE 27-4 ■ Test for patellar tracking. Isometric quadriceps contraction with the leg extended may reveal a subtle lateral patellar deviation. This can be assessed by placing a row of three dots in a straight line while the knee is relaxed **(A)**. One dot is placed several inches above the knee in the midline, one several inches below, and one at mid patellar point. Look for lateral displacement of the patellar dot on isometric quadriceps contraction **(B)**. No significant lateral deviation of the patella is noted here.

This can be assessed by placing a row of three dots in a straight line while the knee is relaxed (one several inches above the knee in the midline, one several inches below, and one at midpatellar point); then look for lateral displacement of the patellar dot on isometric quadriceps contraction (Figure 27-4). Knee effusion or soft tissue swelling is an uncommon finding. A full range of motion is maintained. In some athletes, tenderness may be elicited by palpating and exerting pressure on the articular margins of the patella while displacing it medially or laterally. A crepitus may be felt in some athletes. Pain is elicited with patellar inhibition or compression test (Figure 27-5).

Causes of anterior knee pain are listed in Table 27-3.[1,5-7] Knee pain can be referred pain from the hip or lumbar spine pathology. Hip conditions to be considered include slipped capital femoral epiphysis, Legg-Calve-Perthes disease, and femoral neck stress

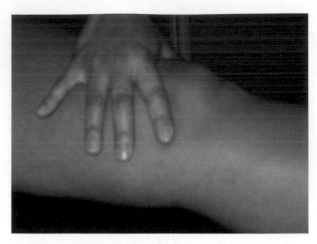

FIGURE 27-5 ■ Patellofemoral compression test. With the athlete supine and knee in extension, have the athlete contract the quadriceps to assess if pain is elicited because of patellar compression. This can be further exacerbated by placing a hand just proximal to patella and not allowing it to glide upward with quadriceps contraction.

fracture, whereas spine conditions to be considered include tumors of the spine or the cord, herniated disk, or spinal stenosis. Pain around the knee joint can also occur in osteosarcoma, Ewing sarcoma, synovial tumors, or osteoid osteoma. Systemic causes of knee pain include chronic juvenile arthritis, sickle cell arthropathy, and leukemia.

Diagnostic Imaging

Plain x-ray films may help rule out other conditions causing anterior knee pain such as osteochondritis dissecans of the patella or knee, or stress fracture of the patella. Radiographs are not indicated routinely. Abnormal tilt of the patella may indicate maltracking, best seen on a tangential view at 45 degrees of flexion of the knee (Figure 27-6).

 Table 27-3.

Causes of Anterior Knee Pain

Quadriceps tendonitis
Prepatellar bursitis
Patellar stress fracture
Osteochondritis dissecans of the patella
Multipartite patella
Infrapatellar bursitis
Sinding-Larsen-Johansson syndrome
Patellar tendonitis
Hoffa syndrome
Osgood-Schlatter disease
Idiopathic anterior knee pain

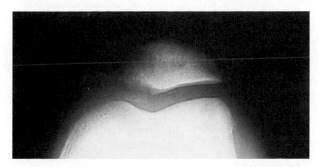

FIGURE 27-6 ■ Tangential view x-ray of patella.

Treatment

In adolescent athletes, the prognosis for resolution of pain and continued sports participation is excellent with conservative treatment. It is a benign, self-limited condition with gradual resolution over a period of few weeks; rarely in some athletes, it may take up to 2 years for complete resolution of symptoms.

Conservative treatment consists of relative rest with modification of activities, local ice, and a short-term use of anti-inflammatory medications (Appendix D) to help control the pain. Complete rest and cessation of all activities are generally not necessary, and the athlete should be allowed to continue all activities as tolerated. Prolonged sitting, squatting, climbing up or going downstairs, and full arc knee extension exercises should be avoided. Alternative activities such as cycling with a proper fit, swimming, and walking are encouraged as tolerated. The effectiveness of different kinds of taping techniques and knee braces varies considerably; their use should be individualized.

Rehabilitation exercises focus on increasing the flexibility, strength, endurance, and neuromuscular retraining of the quadriceps, hamstrings, gastrocnemius, and soleus muscles (Appendix C).[8] Closed kinetic chain exercises are found to be most effective. Knee immobilization is not recommended, except in rare instances when pain is severely affecting daily activities.

OSGOOD-SCHLATTER DISEASE

Definition and Epidemiology

Osgood-Schlatter disease is an overuse injury, a traction apophysitis, affecting the tibial tubercle apophysis. Osgood-Schlatter disease is commonly seen during Tanner stage 2 or 3. It is more common in adolescent boys. The incidence is higher in athletes compared to nonathletes, 21% in athletes compared to 4.5% in nonathletes in one study.

Mechanism

Rapid growth and increased physical activity predisposes to the development of this condition during early adolescence. The immature patellar tendon-tibial tubercle junction is highly susceptible to submaximal, repetitive tensile stress resulting from high-intensity sport activity. The underlying pathology is suggestive of minor avulsions at the site and subsequent inflammatory reaction.

Clinical Presentation

Osgood-Schlatter disease is most commonly seen between 11 and 13 years of age in girls and between 12 and 15 years in boys. Adolescent presents with pain over the tibial tubercle just below the knee. The pain is bilateral in 20% to 30% of patients. The pain is aggravated by sports involving jumping, squatting, and kneeling, and is relieved by a period of rest. Localized tenderness and sometimes swelling over the tibial tubercle are noted on examination.

Diagnostic Imaging

X-ray may show fragmentation of tibial tubercle and sometimes an ossicle in the patellar tendon (Figure 27-7).

Treatment

Treatment is conservative. Decreased activity and rest will result in significant improvement in pain. In some

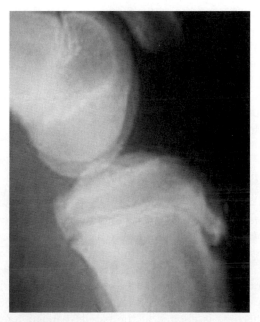

FIGURE 27-7 ■ X-ray of Osgood-Schlatter disease.

athletes, it is not uncommon for recurrent pain to last up to 2 years before complete resolution. Osgood-Schlatter disease is a benign, self-limited condition and overtreatment should be avoided. The adolescent should be allowed to participate in all sports as tolerated. Hamstrings and quadriceps stretches should be done on a regular basis to improve and maintain flexibility. The most common complication is a persistent localized swelling, which may only be of cosmetic concern.

Ossicle formation in the patellar tendon may be a source of chronic pain in some athletes and removal of such an ossicle may be indicated. Presence of Osgood-Schlatter disease does not necessarily predispose the athlete for complete avulsion of the patellar tendon from the tibial tuberosity. This is only a potential concern during rapid growth phase just prior to fusion of the tublercle to tibia.

SINDING-LARSEN-JOHANSSON SYNDROME

Definition and Epidemiology

This overuse injury affects the junction of the inferior pole of the patella and the insertion of the patellar tendon characterized by tendonitis, tendon avulsion and later localized calcification.[9,10] The condition is most commonly seen in 10 to 13 year age group.

Mechanism

Repetitive traction at the inferior pole of the patella leads to Sinding-Larsen-Johansson syndrome. During early adolescence the inferior pole of the patella is immature and chronic excessive traction leads to tendonitis, microavulsions at the proximal attachment of the patellar tendon, and de novo calcification and ossification at the junction of the inferior pole and patellar tendon.

Clinical Presentation

The athlete presents with intermittent activity-related anterior knee pain of gradual onset of several weeks or months duration. Pain is aggravated by jumping and running activities. It is localized over the inferior pole of the patella and proximal attachment of the patellar tendon. Usually, there is no history of direct trauma to the area. On palpation point tenderness is elicited at the patella-patellar tendon junction.

Diagnostic Imaging

Calcification and ossification at the patella-patellar tendon junction is seen on plain films (Figure 27-8). This should be differentiated from a bipartite patella or a patellar sleeve fracture (Figure 27-9). Medlar and Lyne roentgenographic stages are summarized in Table 27-4.[9]

Treatment

This is a benign condition and results in no long-term complications. The athlete should be allowed to participate in sports as tolerated. Because the pain is activity related, some modification in activity level may be needed. In some cases the recurrent pain may persist for 12 to 18 months before spontaneous resolution occurs. Because decreased flexibility of hamstrings is a common finding in many athletes, regular hamstrings stretches should be done. Acute painful episodes respond well to decreased activity, local ice massage, and short-term use of NSAIDs. Local injection of corticosteroid into and around the patellar tendon is contraindicated, and may predispose to tendon weakness and rupture.

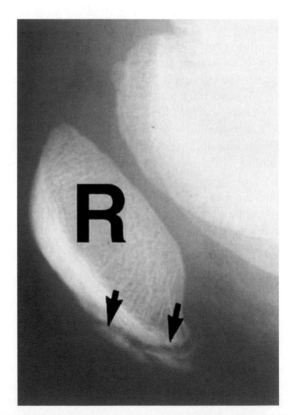

FIGURE 27-8 ■ X-ray of Sinding-Larsen-Johansson disease. (*Used with permission from DeLee JC, Drez D Jr, Miller MD, eds. DeLee and Drez's Orthopaedic Sports Medicine. 2nd ed. Philadelphia, PA: Saunders Elsevier; 2003, Figure 28E7-38.*)

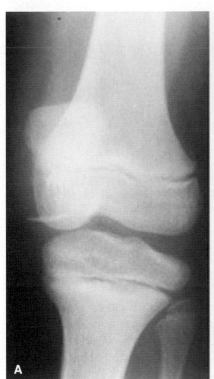
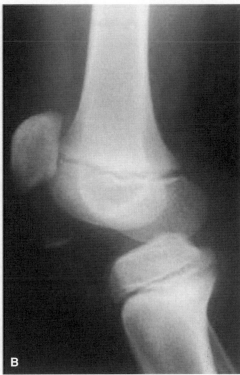

FIGURE 27-9 ■ X-ray of patellar sleeve fracture. (*Used with permission from DeLee JC, Drez D Jr, Miller MD, eds. DeLee and Drez's Orthopaedic Sports Medicine. 2nd ed. Philadelphia, PA: Saunders Elsevier, 2003.*)

JUVENILE OSTEOCHONDRITIS DISSECANS

Definition and Epidemiology

Juvenile osteochondritis dissecans (JOCD) is a significant cause of knee pain in adolescents, both athletes and the nonathletes. JOCD is characterized by delamination and localized necrosis of the subchondral bone, with or without the involvement of the overlying articular cartilage.[10–13] Lateral aspect of the medial condyle of the femur is the most common site of JOCD, accounting for 75% of JODC lesions.

Mechanism

The exact etiology or mechanism leading to the JOCD lesion is not known. Repetitive microtrauma is considered

Table 27-4.

Medlar and Lyne Roentgenographic Stages of Sinding-Larsen-Johansson Disease

1. Normal finding
2. Irregular calcifications at the inferior pole of patella
3. Coalescence of the calcification
4A. Incorporation of the calcification into the patella to yield a normal roentgenographic configuration of the area
4B. Coalesced calcification mass separate from patella

to be a significant factor leading to JOCD. Local bone vascular insufficiency is also postulated to contribute to JOCD. The lesion of JOCD can be either closed or open and either stable or unstable as shown in Figure 27-10.

Clinical Presentation

JOCD is four times more common in males than in females and the lesion is bilateral in 10% to 20% of the cases. The highly active athlete presents with a history of aching and gradual onset of knee pain of several days to weeks' duration typically located over anterior knee, worse during activity. There may be a history of intermittent knee swelling following a practice or game session.

Examination may or may not reveal mild effusion or limitation of motion of the knee. Findings may also vary depending on the stage of the disease. In early stages with the articular cartilage over the femoral condyle still intact, the signs are nonspecific. In late stages when the articular cartilage is eroded, the fragment may separate and become an intra-articular loose body. This can cause pain, effusion, and locking. When the athlete flexes internally rotated leg, from full extension to approximately 30 degrees, pain is elicited, that is relieved upon external rotation (Wilson sign). This is typical only for the lesion on the medial femoral condyle.

Diagnostic Imaging

X-rays are indicated when JOCD is suspected. In addition to the AP and lateral views, a tunnel view is useful to see the lesion, which appears as a well-demarcated

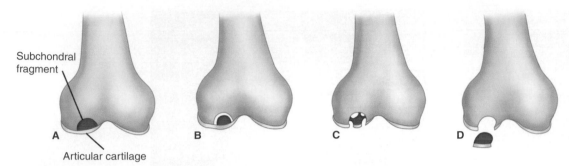

FIGURE 27-10 ■ Schematic diagram showing classification of osteochondritis dissecans lesions. The articular cartilage is intact in closed lesions. The subchondral fragment may be intact **(A)** or begin to separate **(B)**. In open lesions the articular cartilage continuity is lost. The subchondral fragment may remain attached **(C)** or detach **(D)** and become an intra-articular loose body.

radiolucent area (Figure 27-11). In those who demonstrate significant edema or hemarthrosis as well as marked discomfort and inability to bear weight without pain, an MRI is often obtained.

Treatment

Early diagnosis followed by restriction of activities and symptomatic treatment of pain generally allows for healing of lesions over a period of 8 to 12 weeks. Spontaneous healing of the lesion is the usual outcome in children and adolescents with open distal femoral physis. Full sport participation can be resumed once the athlete is pain free and there is roentgenogrphic evidence

of healed lesion. Prognosis is excellent in younger patients (Table 27-5).

In more advanced cases when there is separation of the osteochondral fragment, knee immobilization may be needed. All such cases should be referred to an orthopedic surgeon as surgical intervention may be necessary for further management (Box 27-1). Treatment is based on the stability of the lesion and the status of the overlying cartilage. In some cases the lesion may be unstable or loose, and these cases as well as athletes with large effusions or with marked symptoms, which do not improve with conservative care, may opt surgery for drilling, reattachment, or excision of the osteochondral lesion.

JOCD may also be treated with osteochondral autografts of the knee in those who are skeletally

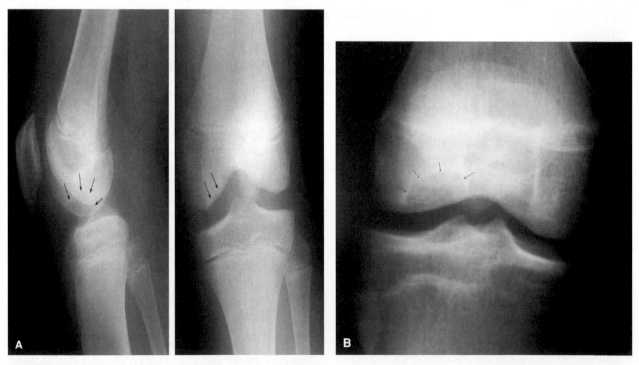

FIGURE 27-11 ■ X-ray showing lesion of JOCD.

Table 27-5.

Pappas Classification of Juvenile Osteochondritis Dissecans

	Skeletal Age (y)		
Category	Girls	Boys	Prognosis
I	11	13	Excellent
II	12–20	14–20	Less certain
III	20	20	Poor; increased need for surgical intervention

mature. At arthroscopy or arthrotomy of the knee, other lesions such as meniscal tears can also be repaired. Currently patients with JODC are treated with partial weight bearing for approximately 3 months and often allowed a slightly earlier return to usual activities. Weight bearing and activity modifications are continued in all cases until imaging and clinical confirmation of healing has occurred and the athlete is completely asymptomatic.

BIPARTITE OR MULTIPARTITE PATELLA

Definition and Epidemiology

Patella generally develops from a single ossification center.[13] Sometimes it develops from two (bipartite) or more (multipartite) ossification centers and the segments are united by fibrous union. Acute or chronic repetitive trauma to the patella can result in painful bipartite or multipartite patella. Reported incidence of bipartite patella is between 0.2% and 6%, most are unilateral, and the male to female ratio is 9:1.

Mechanism

Patella begins to ossify at 3 years of age and by 6 years of age ossification has progressed enough so that the patella is visible on x-ray. The sites of fibrous union between segments of patella are subject of either acute or chronic injury resulting in pain. Acute direct blow to

the patella can result in fracture through the junction between the segments of patella.

Clinical Presentation

Most athletes with symptomatic bipartite or multipartite patella present with insidious onset of anterior knee pain aggravated by jumping, running, squatting, or kneeling. There is localized patellar tenderness and mild swelling. In cases of patellar fracture there may be hemarthrosis and restricted knee motion.

Diagnostic Imaging

X-rays of the patella are diagnostic (Figure 27-12).

Treatment

Most athletes will respond to a 3 to 4 weeks of rest from activity. In cases of fracture a knee immobilizer or long leg cast may be used for 6 weeks. If there is a displaced fracture, fixation may be indicated. Knee arthroscopy and percutaneous lag screw fixation is a common method of treatment for displaced fractures. In some injuries with small avulsions, particularly those seen on a chronic basis or presenting late, a lateral release of the patella to unload the fragment and improve patellar tracking has proven successful.

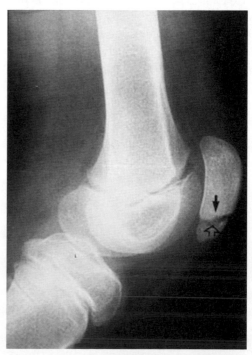

FIGURE 27-12 ■ X-ray bipartite patella. (*Used with permission from DeLee JC, Drez D Jr, Miller MD, eds. DeLee and Drez's Orthopaedic Sports Medicine. 2nd ed. Philadelphia, PA: Saunders Elsevier; 2003, Figure 28E7-41.*)

Box 27-1 When to Refer to Orthopedics.
■ Juvenile osteochondritis dissecans
■ Severe symptomatic plica
■ Severe symptomatic iliotibial band friction syndrome

PLICA SYNDROME

Definition and Epidemiology

Embryologically the knee develops from three separate compartments, namely, medial, lateral, and suprapatellar.[5,13] Synovial plicae are believed to be the remnants of these synovial compartments. Suprapatellar, infrapatellar, medial (most common), and lateral plicae are normally found in the knee (Figure 27-13). Pain related to plica is related to the inflammation of the medial plica. This syndrome though rare in young children is not uncommon in adolescent athletes. The exact incidence and prevalence in adolescent athletes is not known.

Mechanism

Three types of mechanisms are related to symptomatic plica in young athletes, direct trauma to the medial aspect of the knee and patella, injury to the plica as it is entrapped between the medial patellar facet and the medial condyle, and overuse injuries with the knee in flexion and with repeated external rotation of the tibia.

Clinical Presentation

Most plicae are asymptomatic. In symptomatic medial plica, the athlete will present with medial knee pain that is activity related. Pain may be present intermittently for weeks to months before the athlete is seen. There may be a history of feeling pop or snap during flexion of the knee. Athlete may also describe a sense of knee locking. On examination, there will be localized tenderness over the anteromedial aspect of the patella and there may be

Table 27-6.

Causes of Medial Knee Pain

Medial meniscus tear
Pathologic medial plica
Pes anserine bursitis
Pes anserine tendonitis
Semimembranosus bursitis
Semimembranosus tendonitis
Osteochondritis dissecans of the knee

some soft tissue swelling. The plica may also be palpated in some patients as they flex and extend the knee.

The active knee extension test, in which the patient quickly extends the knee from 90-degree flexion as in a soccer kick, will elicit pain with stretching of the plica. A flexion block test is also described in which the patient takes the knee from full extension into 30 to 60 degrees of flexion and the knee is stopped in that position, again stretching the plica. The pain is anterior and above the medial joint line (Table 27-6).

Diagnostic Imaging

Imaging is generally neither indicated nor useful. X-rays or MRI scan may be indicated to exclude other significant causes of medial knee pain based on history and examination findings.

Treatment

Treatment of symptomatic plica is a short period of rest, NSAIDs, and return to usual activities and sports in a period of a few weeks. Some plicae remain symptomatic and require excision at arthroscopy with a thorough examination of the knee and treatment of any associated chondral or meniscal injuries which are found.

ILIOTIBIAL BAND FRICTION SYNDROME

Definition and Epidemiology

On the lateral aspect of the knee, the iliotibial band (ITB) passes over the lateral femoral condyle and is inserted into the Gerdy's tubercle on the lateral aspect of proximal tibia just distal to knee joint line. ITB syndrome refers to overuse injury affecting the tendon as it passes over the lateral femoral condyle. It is the most common cause of lateral knee pain in runners. ITB syndrome has also been reported in cycling, tennis, skiing, football, soccer, and weight lifting.

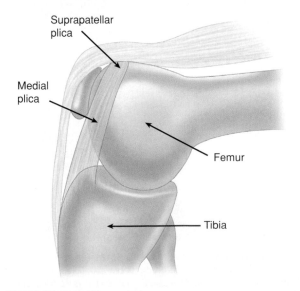

Suprapatellar plica
Medial plica
Femur
Tibia

FIGURE 27-13 ■ Plica anatomy.

Mechanism

With the knee in full extension the ITB lies anterior to the lateral femoral condyle and as the knee is flexed it passes over the femoral condyle at approximately 30 degrees of flexion, and lies posterior to the femoral condyle with further flexion of the knee past 30 degrees (Figure 27-14). Repeated friction between the ITB and the lateral femoral condyle leads to chronic inflammation and activity-related pain. Predisposing factors include overuse, ITB tightness, hamstring tightness, genu varum, internal tibial torsion, and hyperpronated feet.

Clinical Presentation

Athletes present with activity-related lateral knee pain. Pain is characteristically felt only during the activity and

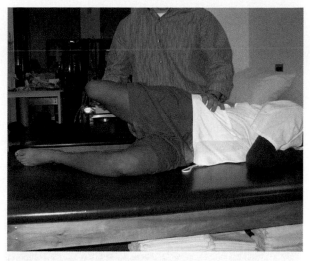

FIGURE 27-15 ■ Ober test. With the athlete on her side with affected side uppermost, grasp at the ankle. Flex and circumduct the hip bringing it into full abduction and extension. In the absence of ITB tightness the knee falls past neutral into adduction. If the ITB is tight the knee fails to fall past the neutral as seen here.

there is no pain at rest either before or after the activity such as running. During running it is more intense than during downhill running on banked surfaces. There is localized tenderness over the lateral femoral epicondyle approximately 3 cm proximal to the lateral knee joint line. Ober (Figure 27-15) and Noble tests (Figure 27-16) are helpful in clinical diagnosis.

Diagnostic Imaging

No specific test or diagnostic imaging is indicated unless to exclude other significant cause of lateral knee pain is suspected.

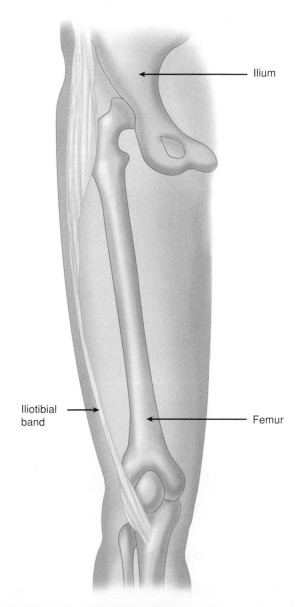

Ilium

Iliotibial band

Femur

FIGURE 27-14 ■ Iliotibial band anatomy.

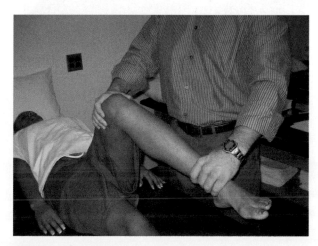

FIGURE 27-16 ■ Noble test. With the athlete supine on the table with knee flexed at 90 degrees and hip at 45 degrees, apply direct pressure over the lateral femoral condyle with the thumb of one hand and passively extend the knee. In case of iliotibial band friction syndrome pain is elicited at 30 degrees of knee flexion.

Table 27-7.

Causes of Lateral Knee Pain

Lateral meniscus tear
Discoid lateral meniscus
Popliteus tendonitis
Iliotibial band friction syndrome
Saphenous nerve entrapment neuropathy
Femoral entrapment neuropathy

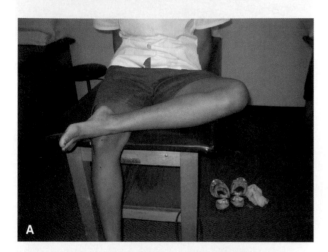

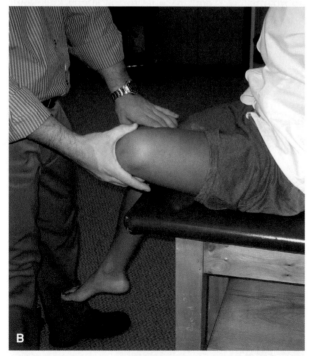

FIGURE 27-17 ■ Popliteus palpation with knee in figure of four position.

Treatment

Most young athletes will respond very well with a short period of rest, modification of activity, local application of ice, and NSAIDs. A referral for physical therapy is indicated if there is no resolution with initial simple measures. Physical therapy will include assessment treatment for any predisposing biomechanical factors such as hamstring and ITB tightness as well as consideration for orthotics for hyperpronated feet. Additionally heat and electrical modalities may be used to control pain and inflammation. Very rarely surgery may be considered in chronic recalcitrant cases.

QUADRICEPS TENDONITIS

Quadriceps tendon strains and tendonitis, usually at the insertion of the quadriceps at the proximal pole of patella, occur with chronic overuse and overloading in the jumping and running activities. The patient will present with pain and tenderness at the superior pole of the patella, sometimes weakness on resisted quadriceps extension. Treatment is rest, local ice application, NSAIDs, and quadriceps stretching.

POPLITEUS TENDONITIS

Popliteus muscle originates from the lateral femoral condyle and is inserted on the posterior tibia. The main functions of the politeus muscle are to initiate and maintain the internal rotation of the tibia in relation to the femur, to assist the posterior cruciate ligament in preventing the posterior motion of the tibia in relation to the femur, and to derotate the knee at the initiation of the flexion. Politeus tendonitis can result from overuse and the athlete presents with activity-related lateral knee pain (Table 27-7). Tenderness is localized on the lateral aspect of the knee and is best elicited with the patient sitting in figure of four position (Figure 27-17). Treatment is conservative with rest and pain management.

REFERENCES

1. Fulkerson JP. Diagnosis and treatment of patients with patellofemoral pain. *Am J Sports Med.* 2002;30(3): 447-456.
2. Stanitski CL. Patellofemoral mechanism, p. In: DeLee JC, Drez D, Miller MD, eds. *Orhtopaedic Sports Medicine.* Philadelphia, PA: Saunders Elsevier; 2003:1815-1839.
3. Stanitski CL. Patellar instability in the skeletally immature patient. In: DeLee JC, Drez D, Miller MD, eds. *Orhtopaedic Sports Medicine.* Philadelphia, PA: Saunders Elsevier; 2003:1749-1759.
4. Stanitski CL. Pediatric and adolescent sports injuries. *Clin Sports Med.* 1997;16:613.
5. Reid DC. Bursitis and knee extensor mechanism pain syndrome. In: Reid DC, ed. *Sports Injury Assessment and*

Rehabilitation. New York: Churchill Livingstone; 1992: 399-436.

6. Muscolo DL, Ayerza MA, Makino A, et al. Tumors about the knee misdiagnosed as athletic injuries. *J Bone Joint Surg.* 2003;85-A:1209.

7. Safran MR, Fu F. Uncommon causes of knee pain in the athlete. *Orthop Clin North Am.* 1995;26:547.

8. Crossley K, Bennell K, Green S, McConnell J. A systemic review of physical interventions for patellofemoral pain syndrome. *Clin J Sports Med.* 2001;11:103-110.

9. Medlar RC, Lyne ED. Sinding-Larsen-Johansson disease. *J Bone Joint Surg.* 1978;60A(8):1113-1116.

10. Smith AD. The skeletally immature knee: what's new in overuse inuries. *AAOS Instructional Course Lectures.* 2003;52:691–697.

11. Kocher MS, Tucker R, Ganley TJ, Flynn JM. Management of osteochondritis dissecans of the knee. *Am J Sports Med.* 2006;34(7):1181-1191.

12. Peters TA, McLean ID. Osteochondritis dissecans of the patellofemoral joint. *Am J Sports Med.* 2000;28: 63-67.

13. Herring JA. Disorders of the knee. In: Herring JA, ed. *Tachdjian's Pediatric Orhtopaedics.* 3rd ed. Philadelphia, PA: Saunders Elsevier; 2002:789-838.

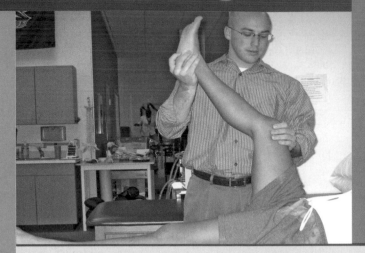

CHAPTER 28

Acute Injuries of the Leg, Ankle, and Foot

Steven Cline and Dilip R. Patel

Tibia and fibula are connected by proximal and distal tibiofibular articulations and by an interosseous membrane between the bones through the entire length. The relevant anatomy of the leg is depicted in Figures 28-1 through 28-4. One head of gastrocnemius muscle arises from the medial and the other from the lateral condyle of the femur. Distally gastrocnemius inserts into the tendon of the Achilles. Achilles tendon is a common tendon formed by the gastrocnemius and soleus muscles which inserts into the posterior calcaneus. Peroneus longus arises from the lateral surface of the fibula and is inserted into the base of the first metatarsal and medial cuneiform. The peroneus brevis originates from the lower two-thirds of the lateral surface of the fibula and is inserted into the base of the fifth metatarsal.

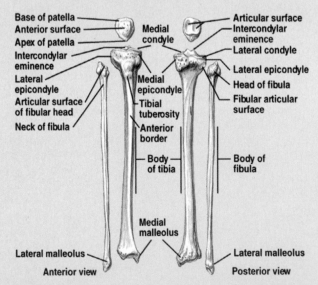

FIGURE 28-1 ■ Anatomy of the leg. (*Used with permission from Van De Graaff KM. Human Anatomy, 6th ed. New York: McGraw Hill; 2002.*)

ACUTE STRAINS OF GASTROCNEMIUS

Definitions and Epidemiology

Acute strains are defined as stretching, partial thickness tears, or full thickness tears of the gastrocnemius muscle, usually of the musculotendinous portion, seen most commonly in adult (older adults) tennis players. It is less common in young athletes but can occur in highly competitive adolescent tennis players.[1–3]

Mechanism

Strains occur after prolonged play, in fatigued muscle, with forceful and sudden eccentric contraction as in a tennis player running toward the net and then forcefully decelerating to a stop to hit a tough shot. It occurs more commonly in poorly conditioned athletes, and those who play an excessive number of sets.

Clinical Presentation

The athlete will complain of considerable pain over the proximal, usually medial calf extending up to the knee and down the leg. There may be considerable swelling over the medial posterior knee, muscle spasm, tenderness, and the muscle is often firm. If the pain in progressively increasing despite ceasing play and rest with firm muscle, immediate evaluation for acute compartment syndrome should be considered. Pain in the calf is elicited or exaggerated by passive stretch produced by dorsiflexion of ankle.

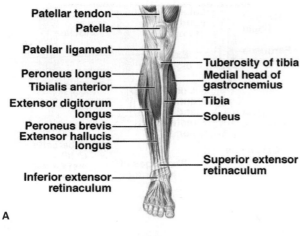

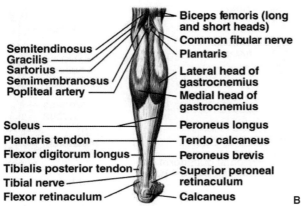

FIGURE 28-2 ■ Anatomy of the leg. (*Used with permission from Van De Graaff KM. Human Anatomy, 6th ed. New York: McGraw Hill; 2002.*)

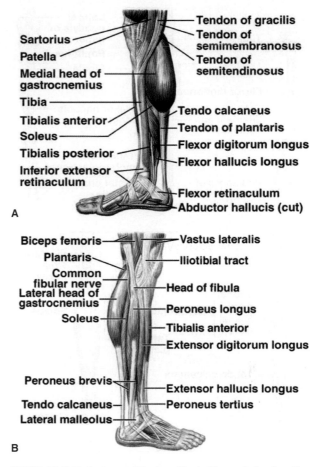

FIGURE 28-3 ■ Anatomy of the leg. (*Used with permission from Van De Graaff KM. Human Anatomy, 6th ed. New York: McGraw Hill; 2002.*)

Diagnostic Imaging

AP, lateral, and sunrise x-ray views of the knee, and with more distal leg findings, an AP and lateral of the tibia and fibula should be obtained to rule out acute fractures. MRI scan will define the extent of the muscle tear and related hematoma, and can reliably differentiate between muscle tears and other masses or injuries about the knee.

Treatment

Immediate treatment for the initial 3 to 5 days for acute strain consists of analgesics, local ice application, elevation of the limb, and nonweight-bearing on the injured limb. Treatment then progresses to gentle stretching of the gastrocnemius muscle in 1 to 3 weeks, once the initial swelling and pain have resolved. Some practitioners are reluctant to give NSAIDs early, because of concern of exacerbating bleeding into the muscle and increasing the zone of injury. Most athletes return to full sports participation within a few weeks.

ACHILLES TENDON RUPTURE

Definition and Epidemiology

Achilles tendon rupture is rare in youth sports. In skeletally immature athletes avulsion of the posterior calcaneal apophysis (site of insertion of Achilles tendon) is a more likely injury seen most commonly in jumping sports.[2–4]

Mechanisms

The injury is caused by eccentric overload of the Achilles tendon, often on landing from a jump in sports such as basketball, or from sudden forceful push off as at the start of a run.

Clinical Presentation

The athlete feels as if he were shot in the heel. There may be a loud pop and the athlete will have sudden and severe posterior ankle or distal calf pain. There is localized tenderness, swelling, and ecchymosis. There

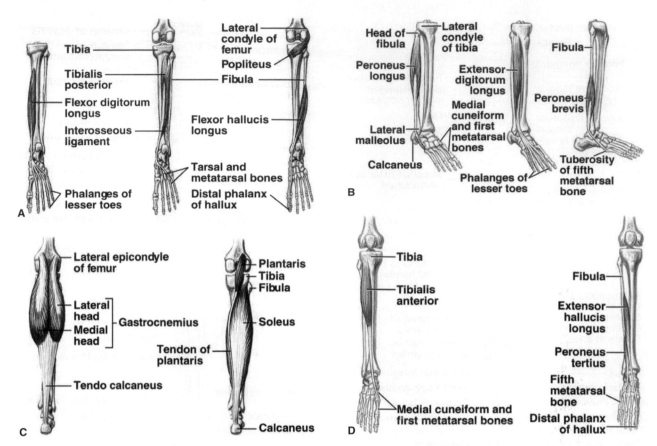

FIGURE 28-4 ■ Anatomy of the leg. (*Used with permission from Van De Graaff KM. Human Anatomy, 6th ed. New York: McGraw Hill; 2002.*)

may be some weak plantar flexion present from the flexor hallucis longus, the plantaris muscle, or the posterior tibialis, but a definite marked decrease in plantar flexion strength is present. Thompson test (Figure 28-5) is positive in complete tears or avulsions. A palpable defect or discontinuity of the tendon can be palpated.

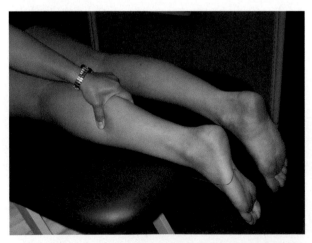

FIGURE 28-5 ■ Thompson test. With the athlete prone on the table with the foot over the edge, gently squeeze the calf. Normally there is plantar flexion of the foot. Absence of plantar flexion indicates rupture of the Achilles.

Diagnostic Imaging

AP, lateral, and mortise views of the ankle are indicated to rule out associated ankle fractures and identify calcaneal apophyseal avulsion. Ultrasound is useful to delineate the tendon defect, is inexpensive, and readily available. MRI scan is rarely indicated, except in cases where other significant soft tissue or osteochondral injuries are suspected.

Treatment

Immediate treatment consists of analgesics, local application of ice, compression dressing, nonweight-bearing on the injured leg, and applying a posterior splint with the foot and ankle in slight plantar flexion. The athlete is referred to orthopedic surgeon for further management.

Definitive treatment consists of closed casting or repair, though in a young athlete it would be unusual to treat the injury closed. Surgical repair is best performed within a day or so of injury. Recovery takes 3 to 4 months for the tendon to heal, and to recondition the leg and regain plantar flexion of the ankle. Athletes may return to play 4 to 6 months after injury, based on the sport, the degree of the injury and the repair, whether the injury was acute or chronic, and their progress in therapy.

SUBLUXATION OR DISLOCATION OF THE PERONEAL TENDONS

Definition and Epidemiology

The peroneal tendons pass from behind and below the lateral malleolus as they enter the foot. The tendons are anchored by the retinaculum in the peroneal groove. When there is disruption of the retinaculum, the tendons slip out of the groove either subluxing or completely dislocating over the lateral malleolus from the groove. Peroneal tendon subluxation is frequently overlooked in the athlete with persistent lateral ankle pain. Most cases are seen in snow skiing, ice skating, running, basketball, soccer, and football.

Mechanism

In some young athletes there may be a shallow groove for these tendons or a lax or absent peroneal retinaculum. Flat hyperpronated feet may also predispose to the injury. The retinaculum also may tear during forced ankle dorsiflexion. The tendon can subluxate or dislocate with sudden, forced eversion dorsiflexion.

Clinical Presentation

The athlete may present as an acute lateral ankle sprain initially with posterolateral ankle pain and tenderness. More often they will show up weeks to months after the initial injury, with a history of recurrent inversion sprains, lateral instability, and snapping of the ankle. Examination may show tendon subluxation with forceful ankle eversion and dorsiflexion.

Diagnostic Imaging

X-rays of ankle may show a small bony avulsion off the posterolateral lateral malleolus in approximately 50% of these injuries.

Treatment

If seen acutely, the athlete's ankle is placed in a cast in slight inversion and plantar flexion for 6 weeks. High demand athletes usually will need surgery once their tendons begin to subluxate or dislocate. The fibular groove is deepened by advancing a shelf of bone off the fibula in those who are skeletally mature. Skeletally immature athletes sometimes require a reconstruction of the area, such as a Chrisman-Snook or other soft tissue procedure.

FRACTURES OF THE SHAFT OF THE TIBIA AND FIBULA

Definitions and Epidemiology

Fractures of the shaft of the tibia in skeletally immature athletes can be either incomplete (torus or greenstick) or complete: 70% are isolated fractures, 50% involve distal third of the tibia, and 39% involve the midshaft. Proximal shaft fractures are uncommon. Fractures of the tibia and fibula are the third most common fractures in children and adolescents and peak incidence is around 8 years of age.[5–7]

Mechanism

The most common mechanism of isolated tibial fracture is rotational stress, particularly with the distal 1/3 tibia fractures seen in younger children. Injuries to the midshaft and proximal tibia also occur with direct blows or heavy axial loading. Rotational stress causes an oblique or spiral fracture whereas a direct impact causes a transverse or comminuted fracture. Fracture of the proximal fibular shaft around the junction of the proximal and middle third can result from indirect force transmitted to fibula in ankle eversion external rotation sprain (Maisonneuve fracture) (Figure 28-6).

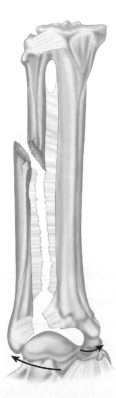

FIGURE 28-6 ■ Maisonneuve fracture. Schematic showing the proximal fibular fracture with ankle external rotation injuries.

Clinical Presentation

The child will present with a history of leg trauma, and sudden pain and swelling of the leg. The child will not bear weight on the affected limb. The leg will be tender at the fracture site, and with displaced fractures there will be an obvious deformity of the leg. Carefully look for lacerations as the tibia is subcutaneous, and a wound usually indicates an open fracture. Perform neurovascular and soft tissue examination of the entire lower limb and be alert for compartment syndrome.

Diagnostic Imaging

AP and lateral x-rays of the tibia and fibula with the knee and ankle included and comparison views of the uninjured leg are indicated.

Treatment

For most closed fractures, the limb is placed in a well-padded long leg splint, with the knee flexed, and the patient nonweight-bearing with crutches. The leg is then iced, elevated, and patient referred to orthopedic surgeon. Because of the risk of compartment syndrome a thorough examination should be conducted, looking for pain with passive motion of the foot and toes, paresthesias, pain out of proportion to the apparent injury, and possible altered sensation in the limb. Late signs of compartment syndrome such as pallor, pulselessness, and inability to move the foot and ankle, usually indicate the muscles are already compromised and compartment releases may not restore function to the limb.

Isolated nondisplaced fracture of the fibula is treated in a short leg walking cast or cast boot for 3 to 4 weeks. Weight bearing is allowed as tolerated. These typically heal in 6 weeks. Nondisplaced or incomplete fractures of the tibia can be treated with a non-weight-bearing long leg cast immobilization for approximately 6 to 8 weeks.

ANATOMY OF THE ANKLE JOINT COMPLEX

Talocrural (or ankle joint) is formed by the articulation of distal tibia and fibula with proximal surface of the talus (Figures 28-7 through 28-11). Dorsiflexion and plantar flexion occur at the talocrural joint (Figure 28-12). Normal range of active dorsiflexion is between 15 and 25 degrees and that of plantar flexion is between 40 and 55 degrees.[2,7] Dorsiflexion is primarily a function of

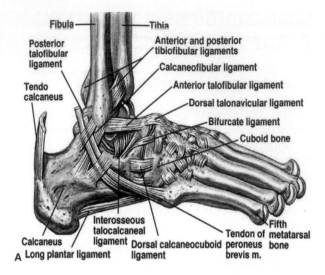

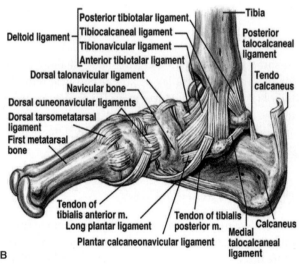

FIGURE 28-7 ■ Ankle anatomy. (*Used with permission from Van De Graaff KM. Human Anatomy, 6th ed. New York: McGraw Hill; 2002.*)

tibialis anterior muscle while plantar flexion is a primarily function of gastrocnemius and soleus muscles.[8,9]

Subtalar joint is formed by articulation of talus proximally with calcaneus and tarsal navicular distally; thus forming the talocalcaneal and talocalcaneonavicular joints. The movements of inversion and eversion occur at the subtalar joint; inversion is primarily a function of tibialis anterior and posterior muscles while eversion is a function of peroneus longus and peroneus brevis.[2,8] Normal range of active nonweight-bearing inversion is between 40 and 60 degrees; that of eversion between 15 degrees and 30 degrees.[2,8] Inversion is associated with supination (combined motion of inversion, adduction, plantar flexion) of the foot and eversion is associated with pronation (combined motion of eversion, abduction, and dorsiflexion) of the foot.[8,9]

Anterior margin of the talar dome is wider than its posterior margin; thus the ankle is most stable in a fully dorsiflexed position (closed-packed position) while

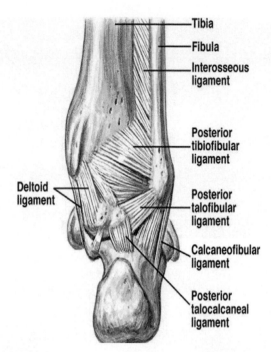

FIGURE 28-8 ■ Ankle anatomy. (*Used with permission from Van De Graaff KM. Human Anatomy, 6th ed. New York: McGraw Hill; 2002.*)

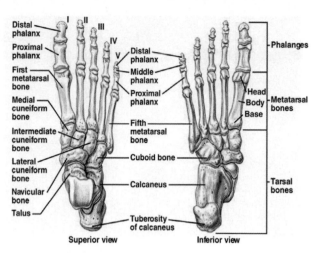

FIGURE 28-10 ■ Foot anatomy. (*Used with permission from Van De Graaff KM. Human Anatomy, 6th ed. New York: McGraw Hill; 2002.*)

relatively more mobile and unstable in plantar flexed position.[2,8] This bony congruity provides stability in the closed packed position. Peronei muscles and the anterior talofibular ligament are the main soft tissue stabilizers of the ankle.

The lateral ligament complex consists of the anterior talofibular ligament (ATFL), calcaneofibular ligament (CFL), and the posterior talofibular ligament (PTFL). The ATFL restrains anterior displacement of the talus and is the most commonly sprained ligament.[1,2,5] Medially, the deltoid ligament is a very strong

ligament consisting of superficial and deep components. Deltoid ligament restrains eversion-pronation and anterior displacement of the talus. The distal tibia and fibula are connected by the anterior and posterior inferior tibiofibular ligaments, and distal interosseous ligament which form part of the tibiofibular syndesmosis; the tibia and fibula being connected the entire length by the interosseous membrane.

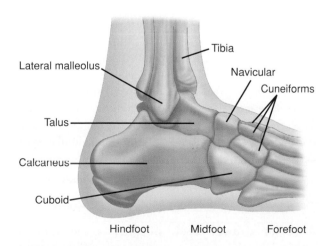

FIGURE 28-9 ■ Ankle anatomy. Schematic showing hindfoot, midfoot, and forefoot.

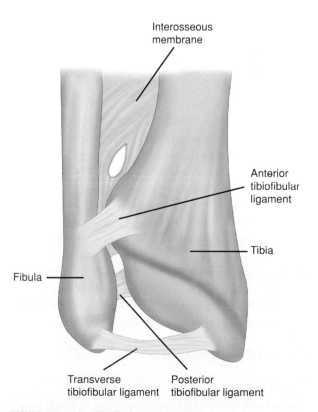

FIGURE 28-11 ■ Tibiofibular syndesmosis.

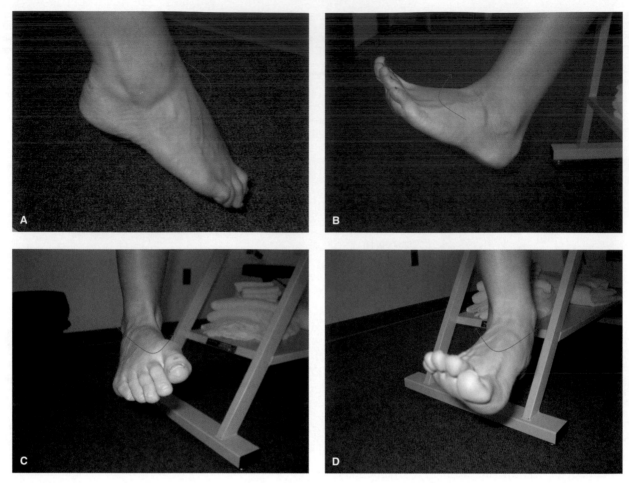

FIGURE 28-12 ■ Movements of ankle. Plantar flexion (**A**), dorsiflexion (**B**), inversion (**C**), and eversion (**D**).

Ankle Physical Examination

Observation

Observe the gait and ability to bear weight. Inability to bear weight correlates with more severe injury. Ankle is best examined with the patient seated on the examination table with knee flexed at 90 degrees. The injured and uninjured ankle should be compared. Initial assessment of an acute injury should rule out any neurovascular injury. Obvious deformity, rapid development of a large joint effusion, and significant limitation of movements may be associated with fracture or complete tear of one or more ligaments. Most inversion ankle sprains are uncomplicated, not associated with other injuries. In case of joint effusion the soft tissue landmarks around the ankle joint cannot be delineated while in case of just soft tissue swelling with no joint effusion, the anatomical configuration can generally be delineated.

Movements

Assess both active and passive range of motion: inversion, eversion, dorsiflexion, and plantar flexion.

Palpation

Localize tenderness by systematic palpation of malleoli, ligaments, tibio-fibular syndesmosis, talus, calcaneus, tarsal navicular, and base of 5th metatarsal.[2,7] Inspect and palpate the Achilles tendon, peroneal tendons around the lateral malleolus, and any swelling or tenderness over the medial aspect of the ankle. In children and adolescents with open distal fibular physis the tenderness is localized approximately 2 cm to 3 cm proximal to the tip of the lateral malleolus, in case of Salter Harris type of fracture of the distal fibular physis. Anterolateral tenderness is typical with sprained ATFL. Tenderness localized over the front of the ankle along the interosseous membrane suggests tibio-fibular syndesmosis injury.[7,8,10]

Special tests

Anterior drawer test. Integrity of the ATFL is assessed by the anterior drawer test.[8] With patient seated, knee flexed at 90 degrees, the distal leg is stabilized with one hand just above the ankle. With the other

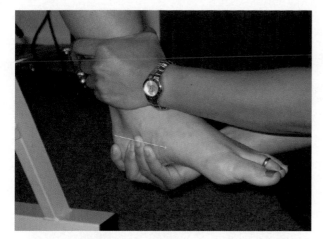

FIGURE 28-13 ■ Anterior drawer test.

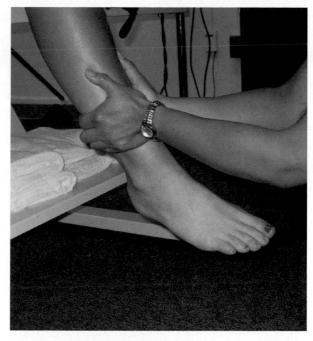

FIGURE 28-15 ■ Squeeze test.

hand around the heel, and the foot, in approximately 20-degree plantar flexed position, is moved forward (Figure 28-13). The uninjured ankle is similarly assessed for comparison. Relative increase in anterior motion and a soft end point to the movement are associated with sprained ATFL.

Talar tilt test. The CFL sprain is rarely an isolated injury; it is typically associated with sprained ATFL. The CFL is assessed by comparison of talar tilt of the injured with the uninjured ankle. Both feet in neutral position are inverted from the front; in case of moderate to severe sprain of CFL there is relatively increased talar tilt (Figure 28-14). In inversion-plantar flexion sprains the ATFL is the first to be sprained followed by the CFL and PTFL in that order.[1-3,5]

Squeeze test. With the patient seated on the examination table with knee at 90 degree flexion, squeeze test is performed by gentle squeeze of the leg at midcalf; pain in the ankle joint is associated with high ankle sprain (Figure 28-15).[8,10]

External rotation test. External rotation test is performed with the patient seated on the examination table, stabilize the leg with one hand and with the other hand gently externally rotate the foot (Figure 28-16); pain in leg and ankle is associated with injury to the syndemosis).[8,10]

ACUTE ANKLE SPRAINS

Definitions and Epidemiology

Ankle sprains refer to acute injuries of ligaments around the ankle joint. Three types of ankle sprains are generally recognized based on the predominant mechanism

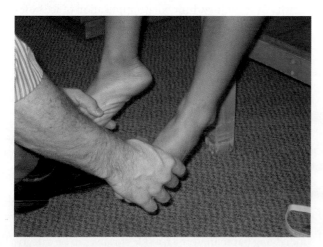

FIGURE 28-14 ■ Talar tilt test.

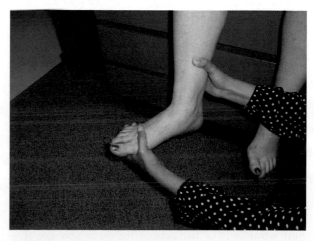

FIGURE 28-16 ■ External rotation test.

of injury and the ligaments involved, namely, lateral or inversion sprains, medial or eversion sprains and syndesmotic or "high" ankle sprains.[9–18]

Overall the ankle is the most commonly injured area in sports and ankle sprains account for 20% to 30% of all musculoskeletal injuries in sports, including high-school and collegiate athletes.[1,2] Eighty-five percent of all ankle injuries are sprains. Ankle sprains can affect lateral ligaments, medial ligaments, or the tibiofibular syndesmosis. Eighty five percent of all ankle sprains are lateral or inversion sprains without any associated injuries.[2,3] Medial ankle sprains are uncommon and account for less than 15% of all ankle sprains.

True ligament sprains are rare in children and uncommon in adolescents before age 15. The exact incidence of ankle ligament sprains in young children is not known, and children are more likely to have injury to the relatively weaker growth plates around ankle, the distal fibular and tibial physes in case of the inversion injury, than to have a ligament sprain.[4] The incidence of ankle injuries is higher in sports involving jumping, running, and sudden change in direction. The highest incidence of ankle injuries has been reported in basketball, followed by volleyball, soccer, and gymnastics.[2,5] A history of previous ankle sprain has been shown to be the most important risk factor for a subsequent sprain. Other potential risk factors include tarsal coalition, tight Achilles, ankle ligamentous laxity, weak peronei, low profile boots, and narrow, long cleats.[2,5,6]

Mechanisms

Inversion sprains

Typical mechanisms of injury include landing from a jump, stepping or landing on one foot, sudden change in direction while running, sudden deceleration or stopping, or loss of balance on uneven surface with a twist of the foot.[1,2,6] Inversion or lateral ankle sprain results from plantar flexion inversion of the foot (Figure 28-17).

Eversion sprains

Sprains of the deltoid ligament are associated with other significant injuries. Sprain of the deltoid ligament can occur with a sudden and forceful dorsiflexion-eversion (pronation external rotation) injury to the ankle.

Syndesmotic sprains

The tibiofibular syndesmosis is injured with a severe eversion external rotation injury of the ankle. This will injure portions of the deltoid ligament and the syndesmosis itself.[19]

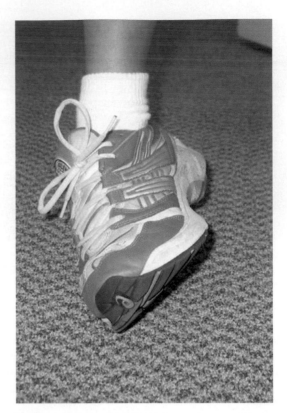

FIGURE 28-17 ■ Mechanism of inversion sprain.

Clinical Presentation

Lateral or inversion sprains

The athlete presents with ankle pain and swelling following the injury. Ascertain the position of the foot at the time of injury. The injury to lateral ligaments occurs when the foot is forced into plantar flexion and inversion. The athlete may give a history of sudden pain or "pop" and with moderate or severe sprains is unable to continue to play and will have pain on weight bearing. Acuity and magnitude of the swelling correlate with the severity of the injury. Immediate application of ice however may reduce the swelling even in severe injury. History of previous sprains to the same ankle is an important risk factor for subsequent sprain.[1,2,5] A sensation of locking may be caused by a loose body in the joint, fracture, or severe muscle spasm.

On examination, there may be ankle swelling, tenderness, decreased range of motion, and pain on weight bearing. In grade 2 or 3 sprains there may be some instability. Anterior drawer test is positive in grade 3 sprains. Pain is elicited on talar tilt with CFL sprains. Tenderness over the fibular physis indicates Salter–Harris type fracture.

Based on the history, examination findings, and underlying pathoanatomy a ankle sprains can be categorized as mild, moderate, and severe (Table 28-1). Typically

Table 28-1.

West Point Grading of Ankle Sprains

Criterion	Grade 1	Grade 2	Grade 3
Location of tenderness	ATFL	ATFL, CFL	ATFL, CFL, PTFL
Edema, ecchymosis	Slight, local	Moderate, local	Significant, diffuse
Weight-bearing ability	Full or partial	Difficult without crutches	Impossible without significant pain
Ligament damage	Stretched	Partial tear	Complete tear
Instability	None	None or slight	Definite

most lateral ankle sprains are not associated with other significant injuries or fractures; however, fractures and other significant soft tissue trauma may be associated with severe lateral sprains and medial or syndesmosis sprains; or these injuries may be the primary injuries, and should be included in the differential diagnosis of ankle sprain (Table 28-2).[2,5,10–20]

Medial sprains or eversion sprains

The young athlete will complain of medial discomfort after a pronation eversion injury to the ankle, and may be significantly swollen over the medial malleolus and the deltoid ligament. There will be tenderness to palpation

Table 28-2.

Potential Associated Injuries/Differential Diagnosis

Ligament/tendon injury
Peroneal tendon strain/dislocation/subluxation
Achilles tendon strain
Posterior tibial tendon strain
Bifurcate ligament sprain

Fractures
Lateral/medial malleolus
Tibial plafond
Distal physes of tibia/fibula
Fibula—shaft
Talus—lateral/posterolateral process
Calcaneus—anterior process
Tarsal navicular
Base of fifth metatarsal
Osteochondral fracture of talus

Nerve injuries
Superficial peroneal nerve
Tibial nerve

directly over the deltoid ligament itself. With a history suggestive of possible medial sprain, based on the mechanism of injury, it is important to look for associated injuries such as medial malleolar fracture, fracture of the fibula, fracture of talar dome, and diastasis of the tibiofibular syndesmosis.[2,3,5,7] Talar tilt with eversion of the foot is associated with increased pain and laxity compared to the uninjured ankle.

Syndesmotic sprains

In severe injuries, it is important to assess for any injury to the tibiofibular syndesmosis (high ankle sprain), which if not recognized and treated appropriately can lead to later complications.[10,11] Localized tenderness at the midway point of the intermalleolar line in the front of the ankle is suggestive of syndesmosis sprain. Squeeze and external rotation tests are positive.

Diagnostic Imaging

X-ray of the ankle is indicated in acute severe injuries when the history and examination indicate possibility of fracture/dislocation.[2] Plain film radiographs may also be useful in the assessment of chronic pain when a stress fracture or missed occult fracture is suspected. Radiographs are also indicated in cases of history of locking and pain on extreme plantar or dorsiflexion. In children and adolescents, the distal physes of fibula and tibia are open and comparison views of the uninjured ankle should be done to aid in the interpretation of the films of the injured ankle. Typical ankle series should include an anteroposterior, lateral, and mortise views.

In adults (ages 18 and above) the applicability and validity of Ottawa Ankle Rules (Table 28-3) is well established with a 100% sensitivity and fairly high specificity, and can reduce the number of unnecessary radiographs by 30% in excluding fractures of the ankle and mid-foot.[21–31] The applicability and validity of Ottawa Ankle rules is less well established in children and adolescents with acute ankle injuries; however, a

Table 28-3.

Ottawa Ankle Rules

An ankle radiographic series is indicated if the patient has pain in the malleolar zone and any of these findings:
(a) Bone tenderness at posterior edge or tip of the lateral malleolus (6 cm in length).
(b) Bone tenderness at the posterior edge or tip of the medial malleolus (6 cm in length).
(c) Inability to bear weight (4 steps) immediately and in the emergency department (or physician's office).

few studies that have looked at their application in children and adolescents suggest that Ottawa Ankle rules in conjunction with clinical judgment can be equally useful in avoiding unnecessary radiography.[16–21] In general these rules can be safely applied in adolescents; however, in younger children their role is not established and the threshold to image the ankle should be lower in the younger patient.

Stress radiographs are not routinely indicated in acute trauma; however, in some cases stress films may aid in confirming severe ligamentous injuries and associated instability. Arthrograms, computed tomography (CT) magnetic resonance imaging, and bone scan are typically not indicated in most cases of acute ankle sprain. CT scan is useful in detecting occult fracture or stress fracture; MRI is useful in detecting and delineating ligament and tendon injuries, as well as syndesmosis sprains.[22]

Initial imaging should include AP, lateral, and mortise views of the ankle, and a full length x-ray of the tibia and fibula to look for an associated fibular fracture. If there is no widening of the syndesmosis or translation of the talus on plain films, and the patient remains symptomatic, weight-bearing films and stress views should be performed. If there is any widening of the syndesmosis (Figure 28-18) noted this should be treated surgically, usually with syndesmosis screw fixation within 2 weeks of injury to avoid late syndesmosis instability and long-term ankle arthritis.

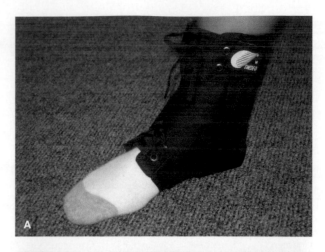

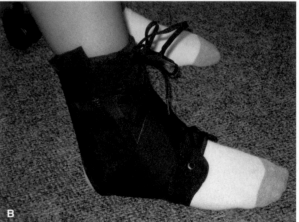

FIGURE 28-19 ■ Lace up braces.

Treatment

Immediate care for an uncomplicated ankle sprain should include protection, rest, ice, compression, and elevation (PRICE).[2,6,23,24] Bracing, taping, or crutches

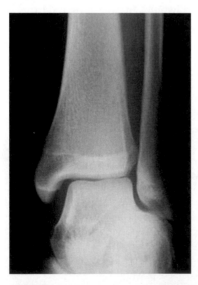

FIGURE 28-18 ■ X-ray of syndesmotic injury. Note widening of the tibiofibular syndesmosis.

aid in immobilization and ambulation. Either a lace up brace or an airstirrup brace can be used (Figures 28-19 and 28-20). A brief period of rest is recommended and the athlete is advised not to bear weight for the first few days until the swelling and pain have subsided. Early mobilization of the joint has been shown to decrease pain and swelling, and is favored over prolonged immobilization for an earlier and more successful return to activity.[32,33]

Ice is used for the first 48 to 72 hours as it decreases edema and pain. Crushed ice bags should be used during at least the first 48 hours, in combination with elevation, for 20 to 30 minutes per session and with a minimum rest period of 1 to 2 hours in between sessions. After the first 48 to 72 hours, cold water immersion in a whirlpool or bath may be used, in conjunction with simple range-of-motion (ROM) exercises. In addition, contrast baths may be introduced in which the affected limb is alternately immersed in cold and warm water at a ratio of 1 minute cold immersion to 3 minutes warm immersion (1:3). Contrast baths are thought to induce a pumping mechanism in the circulatory system to aid in decreasing edema.

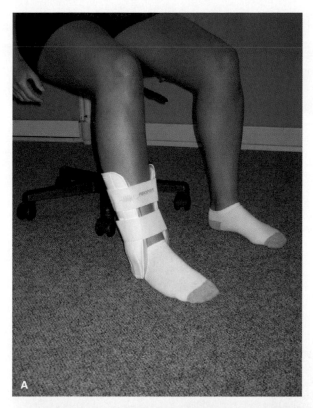

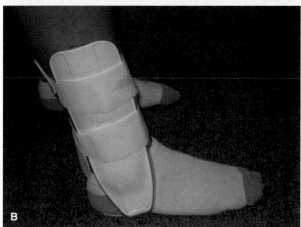

FIGURE 28-20 ■ Air stirrup.

Compression with an open-basket weave ankle taping or simple elastic wrap will increase the athlete's comfort level and serve to limit edema as well. The addition of a felt horseshoe-shaped pad, placed around the lateral malleolus and extending superiorly toward the knee will increase the effectiveness of an elastic wrap in controlling edema.

Elevation of the affected limb above the level of the heart will increase the effectiveness of venous return in eliminating excess fluid from the area. Because of the importance of elevation in the immediate care of an ankle sprain, it is important to wait at least 48 hours before integrating the use of cold whirlpool/bath treatments into the rehabilitation program.

Once the immediate care based on PRICE principles is initiated, the athlete should be seen again in approximately 3 to 7 days. Because of reduced swelling, muscle spasms, and pain, a better examination can be performed at this time, and the severity of the sprain can be better assessed. Mild or grade 1 sprains may not need further specific rehabilitation other than instructions in range of motion exercises followed by strengthening exercises. Rehabilitation has been shown to lead to faster recovery and return to sports as well as to reduce the risk of recurrence of ankle injuries.[1,6,28]

All moderate or grade 2 sprains need specific monitored rehabilitation and the young competitive athlete should be referred to a certified athletic trainer or sports physical therapist.[32,33] Rehabilitation can take from 2–3 weeks to 6–8 weeks before return to full sports activity. Many high schools have certified athletic trainers with whom the athlete can work out the rehabilitation schedule and regular follow-up.

Severe or grade 3 sprains are associated with complete disruption of ligaments and ankle joint instability. Treatment options for grade 3 or severe sprains include surgical repair, immobilization in a short leg cast for 3 to 6 weeks followed by rehabilitation, or early controlled mobilization and rehabilitation (functional treatment).[1,2,4,6] Most evidence suggests that early controlled mobilization and rehabilitation leads to faster recovery and return to sports. Delayed surgical repair for any residual instability has been shown to be equally effective as early repair.

Tibiofibular syndesmosis sprains (high ankle sprains) are often treated with a nonweight-bearing cast for 10 days to 2 weeks. The pitfall is that a "high ankle sprain" may completely tear the syndesmosis, with or without a proximal fibula or Maisonneuve fracture (Figure 28.6) present on plain films, and these will require stabilization of the syndesmosis itself. In those with a syndesmosis separation, the syndesmosis must be fixed and weight kept off the ankle for 6 weeks, with subsequent removal of the screws or other fixation at approximately 10 to 12 weeks from surgery. The ankle is then rehabilitated much as a lateral ankle injury.

Ankle Sprains: Treatment Failure and Delayed Recovery

A small percentage of young athletes will continue to have activity associated pain, recurrent swelling, a sense of instability, and decreased sport performance even after appropriate rehabilitation; some may not be able to progress and complete all phases of rehabilitation. These athletes are considered to have failed treatment and must be reassessed in terms of initial diagnosis and any associated injuries (Figure 28-21). Possible causes of persistent pain and disability are listed in Table 28-4.[1,2,6,10,11]

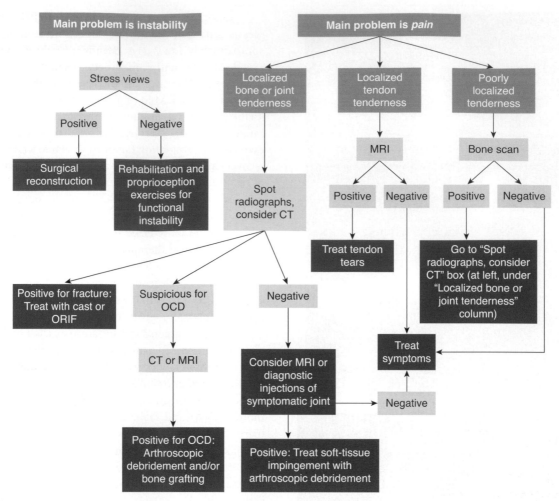

FIGURE 28-21 ■ Algorithm for chronic ankle pain and instability. (*Used with permission from Hockenbury RT, Sammarco JG. Evaluation and treatment of ankle sprains. Phys. Sport. Med. 2001;29(2):62. New York: McGraw Hill.*)

In most uncomplicated lateral ankle sprains the subjective recovery is rapid, and after 5 to 7 days the ankle "looks good," there is no pain or swelling, and

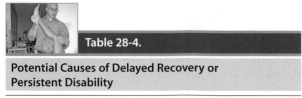

Table 28-4.

Potential Causes of Delayed Recovery or Persistent Disability

Inadequate rehabilitation
Anterior talar impingement
Impingement spurs
Soft tissue impingement
Peroneal subluxation or dislocation
Osteochondral fracture of talus
Syndesmosis sprain
Instability—functional/mechanical
Nerve traction injury—superficial peroneal, sural, tibial
Sinus tarsi syndrome
Unrecognized fracture
Nonunion of fracture
Reflex sympathetic dystrophy

the athlete feels he or she has recovered fully and may not fully appreciate the importance of full rehabilitation. It is important to recognize this and educate the athlete that even though the ankle looks and feels good, full functional recovery takes time and requires completing the full rehabilitation program. It takes 6 to 8 weeks for ankle ligaments to regain the ability to take normal stress and up to 6 to 12 months following the sprain to fully mature and remodel.[1]

The most important prevention strategy for ankle sprains is ongoing long-term appropriate sport-specific training and conditioning of the athlete; to a lesser extent other measures that have been shown to reduce the likelihood of ankle sprains include lace-up ankle brace, taping, and high-top shoes.[2,6,28,29]

Ankle Sprains: Orthopedic Consultation

Most simple ankle sprains should be managed conservatively for 6 months before operative intervention is considered. Chronic pain and swelling in the ankle after appropriate rest, activity modification, and rehabilitation are usually related to continued instability, soft tissue impingement, or osteochondritis dissecans. These patients may benefit from further imaging including MRI and, in some, CT. Those with chronic ankle pain and instability may require arthroscopy, debridement or repair of OCD lesions, and possible ligament reconstruction to improve the function of the ankle and allow return to play and usual activities. Orthopedic consultation is indicated for all severe sprains associated with instability, syndesmotic diastasis, or fractures.

FRACTURES OF THE DISTAL TIBIAL AND FIBULAR PHYSES

Definitions and Epidemiology

Salter–Harris type distal physeal fractures of the tibia and fibula are the second most common physeal fractures; almost 60% of these are related to sport-participation, and they account for between 10% and 40% of all acute musculoskeletal injuries in skeletally immature athletes.[6,34,35]

Mechanism

Because the ankle ligaments are attached distal to the physes and the physes are the weak link around ankle, any significant force directed to the ankle joint complex usually results in physeal fractures rather than a true ankle joint disruption, in skeletally immature athletes. Ankle fractures in skeletally immature children and adolescents are classified based on the anatomical configuration and mechanism of injury. Ankle fractures in sports result from cutting, jumping, sudden deceleration, and twisting the leg on a planted foot. Fibular physis fracture can result from an inversion dorsiflexion injury.

The distal tibial physis closes at age 15 years in girls and 17 years in boys. The physis begins to fuse sequentially beginning in the center, next proceeding medially, and finally laterally, over a period of approximately 18 months. This results in a "transitional" pattern of the distal tibial physis fractures during this period. Two well-described fracture patterns are the juvenile Tillaux (Salter–Harris type IV) and the triplane (Salter–Harris type III) fractures (Figure 28-22).

Clinical Presentation

The athlete with distal tibia fracture will present with an acutely painful and swollen ankle. There may be apparent deformity in severe displaced fractures. The athlete may give a history of sudden twisting or rotational

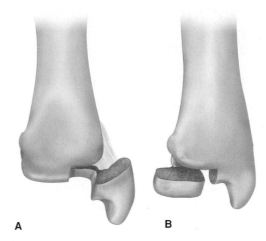

FIGURE 28-22 ■ Schematic of triplane (**A**) and Tillaux fractures (**B**).

injury. There is pain on weight bearing and tenderness over the site.

With distal fibular physis fractures, there will be tenderness over the distal fibula, often at the level of the growth plate, and the child may describe an inversion type injury to the ankle. Symptoms and signs of inversion ankle sprain are noted.

Diagnostic Imaging

X-ray, AP, lateral, and mortise views should be obtained with comparison views of the uninjured ankle. Some fractures such as those of the tibial plafond may be difficult to detect on x-rays and a CT scan may be indicated for further treatment planning.

Treatment

In case of distal tibial physis fracture the ankle should be splinted in a posterior splint, local ice applied, and referred expeditiously for definitive orthopedic evaluation and care. Both the *Triplane* as well as *the juvenile Tillaux fractures* with 2 mm of step off, or greater than 2 to 4 mm of widening usually requires surgery. The primary concern is to maintain a congruent joint. There is little concern over growth arrest, but more concern to avoid chronic ankle pain, stiffness and early arthrosis. Outcome of treatment is excellent provided a congruent reduction is obtained. The athlete should have no limitations once the fracture is healed in approximately 6 weeks. Most nondisplaced distal fibular physeal fractures heal with conservative care over a period of 4 to 6 weeks. Displaced *distal fibular physeal fractures* are usually reduced closed and treated in a cast, though some displaced fractures may rarely require fixation.

OSTEOCHONDRITIS DISSECANS OF THE TALUS

Definition and Epidemiology

Osteochondritis dissecans (OCD) is an injury of the articular cartilage and underlying subchondral bone. These occur in association with ankle sprains and direct impact injuries to the foot and ankle. Based on the Berndt and Harty classification a type I OCD is a small area of compression of subchondral bone. A type II injury is a partially detached osteochondral fragment. Type III injuries are completely detached fragments without displacement from the fragment bed. A type IV injury is a displaced osteochondral fragment.

Inversion injuries of the ankle are more commonly associated with anterolateral cartilage injuries, constituting 44% of OCD lesions. Posteromedial lesions are associated more often with repetitive microtrauma, and constitute 56% of OCD lesions.

Mechanisms

Osteochondritis dissecans of the talus can result from acute direct impact, ankle inversion dorsiflexion injuries, or from repetitive trauma with overloading of the cartilage of the ankle joint.

Clinical Presentation

Most often the onset of pain is insidious, and there may be a history of preceding macrotrauma such as a severe inversion sprain. There may be a history of a recent increase in chronic ankle pain after a recent new ankle sprain. Athletes will report recurrent ankle swelling, and often "weakness" of the ankle. The athlete will complain of chronic aching in the ankle, and occasionally catching or clicking. Pain on motion, tenderness over the anterolateral, or posteromedial talus, and often a small effusion are present.

Diagnosis

X-ray findings are shown in Figure 28-23. In some cases a bone scan or MRI may be needed to confirm the diagnosis and to aid in treatment planning.

Treatment

Initial treatment of types I and II OCD lesions is casting and orthotics in young patients. Type III lesions on the medial side are initially treated in the same way. All type IV lesions and the lateral type III lesions will require

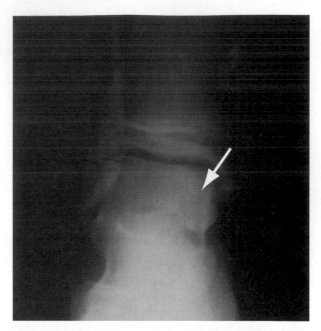

FIGURE 28-23 ■ X-ray osteochondritis dissecans of talus.

arthroscopic drilling, removal, or pinning to best enhance healing potential. In some cases larger OCD lesions may undergo cartilage transfer or grafting procedures.

TURF TOE

Definition and Epidemiology

Turf toe is a first metatarsophalangeal (MTP) joint capsular and ligamentous sprain. This occurs more commonly in football, soccer, and basketball.

Mechanism

The classic mechanism for turf toe is a sudden, forceful hyperextension of the great toe. This is more likely on artificial turf. It is sometimes also seen following hyperflexion injury.

Clinical Presentation

A grade I injury is a stretch or tear of the plantar capsule and ligaments. There is some localized tenderness over the plantar surface of the toe, minimal soft tissue swelling, and no bruising, with no loss of joint motion. A grade II sprain is a partial tear with more swelling, tenderness, ecchymosis, moderate loss of active ROM, and a limp secondary to pain with weight bearing, with symptoms worsening over 24 hours. Grade III sprains are complete tears of the capsule from the metatarsal head, with severe pain, swelling, bruising, and tenderness.

Diagnostic Imaging

In grade III injuries x-rays are obtained to rule out a sesamoid fracture, or disruption of the plantar structures.

Treatment

The adolescent athlete with grade I injury can usually continue to play, with the toe taped. Athletes with grade II injury will require a period of relative rest, and cannot perform at their usual level of play. They should be held out for 3 to 14 days until their symptoms abate.

Athletes with grade III injuries are placed on crutches for 1 to 3 days, and taken out of play for 2 to 6 weeks. Initial treatment of grade III injuries is RICE, adding a shank or steel plate to increase shoe rigidity, and early joint mobilization. Return to play is allowed when the toe can be dorsiflexed to 90 degrees without pain. More recently foot and ankle surgeons are more aggressive about fixing grade III turf toe injuries which demonstrate displacement of the sesamoids on lateral extension views of the first ray (toe).

Turf toe injuries can be functionally disabling. Long-term, there is often decreased first MTP joint motion, impaired push off, and later a hallux rigidus deformity may develop. At 5 years post injury, 50% of these athletes still had persistent symptoms of stiffness and pain in their first MTP joint.

LIS FRANC INJURIES

Definition and Epidemiology

Lis Franc injuries refer to fracture dislocations or dissociations of the tarsometatarsal joints.

Mechanism

Lis Franc injuries are associated with an axial load to the plantar flexed foot (Figure 28-24), and occur in a variety of sports. The weakest point in the midfoot is the ligament which extends from the base of the second metatarsal to the medial cuneiform, the most common type of Lis Franc injury.

Clinical Presentation

The athlete presents with a history of fall on the foot in plantar flexed position. There is sudden pain and localized soft tissue swelling and tenderness. Deformity is apparent with a fracture and dislocation.

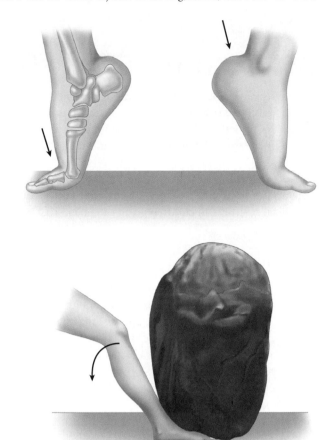

FIGURE 28-24 ■ Mechanism of Lis Franc injury. Indirect or direct force applied to the heel, with the foot in tip-toe position; or when the foot is moved forcibly backward, with the load on the forefoot.

Diagnostic Imaging

X-rays include a weight-bearing AP, lateral and oblique views of the foot. With a Lis Franc injury there is often a nutcracker fracture to the cuboid seen on the x-ray. Normally the metatarsals should line up with their respective cuneiforms on all views. Nonweight-bearing films may not demonstrate the injury. In some cases a CT scan is indicated for planning surgical treatment.

Treatment

If there is less than 2 mm of displacement between the metatarsals at the base on x-ray, the foot is placed in a fracture boot, and the athlete followed up in 1 week. X-rays, including weight-bearing views at the initial examination or at follow-up in 1 week may demonstrate an occult Lis Franc fracture that will need surgery. Full recovery and return to sports may take several months. Some athetes may not be able to return to their pre-injury level of play.

METATARSAL FRACTURES

Definition and Epidemiology

The physes of the metatarsals are at the distal end except for the first metatarsal which is at the proximal end and are subject to Salter–Harris type of acute physeal fractures. Other types of fractures are the metatarsal shaft fractures.

Fifth metatarsal fractures are the most common metatarsal fractures in children. They comprise 90% of metatarsal fractures in children greater than age 10.

Mechanism

In addition to the shaft and physeal fractures, the fifth metatarsal is subject to fracture of the styloid and the fracture of the junction of metaphysis and diaphysis (Jones fracture). Jones fracture occurs at a later age, ranging from 15 to 21 years, in athletes such as basketball players, and track athletes who repeatedly place excessive landing forces across the fifth metatarsal. There is a high rate of nonunion with this particular injury.

Clinical Presentation

The athlete with metatarsal fractures presents with a history of direct trauma to the foot or repeated jumping and landing on the foot. There is localized pain, swelling, and tenderness. Deformity may be noted if there is a displaced fracture. Tenderness is localized over the fracture site.

Diagnostic Imaging

X-rays of the foot are diagnostic of acute fractures (Figures 28-25 and 28-26).

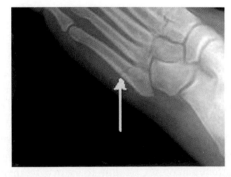

FIGURE 28-25 ■ X-ray of Jones fracture.

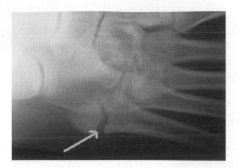

FIGURE 28-26 ■ X-ray of displaced 5th metatarsal styloid fracture.

Treatment

Nondisplaced fractures are treated with foot placed in fracture boot or post-op shoes for 4 to 6 weeks. All displaced or angulated fractures should be referred to an orthopedic surgeon. Fracture of the fifth metatarsal styloid may be treated in a short leg walking cast for 3 to 6 weeks, until there is no tenderness over the base of the metatarsal, and radiographic healing is present.

Initial treatment of a Jones fracture is 6 weeks in a nonweight-bearing cast, then 4 to 6 weeks in a weight-bearing cast, orthosis or brace. Open reduction internal fixation and possibly bone grafting may be indicated in a highly competitive young athlete. These players should not return to their sport until the fracture is clinically and radiographically healed either with surgery or closed treatment.

SESAMOID FRACTURES

Definition and Epidemiology

Sesamoid bones are generally located in the first toe near the first metatarsal joint. Sesamoid fractures are rare in young athletes. Sprinting, basketball, and related sports which necessitate rapid velocity changes and repeated jumping place the young athlete at risk.

Mechanism

Repeated jumping can cause direct impact and fracture of the sesamoids. There may have been a hyperextension injury, such as catching the foot on artificial turf, and the area about the first metatarsophalangeal joint is usually swollen.

Clinical Presentation

Clinically the athlete will note several weeks of pain near the MTP joint of the first ray. There is usually local swelling and tenderness.

Box 28-1 When to Refer.
When to refer to orthopedics
■ Metatarsophalangeal fracture/dislocations
■ Acute ankle fractures
■ Osteochondritis dissecans of the talus
■ Chronic symptomatic ankle instability
■ Acute displaced fractures of the tibia and fibula
■ Severe tibiofibular syndesmotic disruptions
■ Acute Achilles rupture.

Diagnostic Imaging

X-rays show fracture through the sesamoid. Occasionally a bone scan or CT is useful to confirm or make the diagnosis.

Treatment

A short leg cast is placed for 4 to 6 weeks, but delayed union and nonunion are fairly common. In some cases surgical excision of the sesamoid is performed (Box 28-1).

REFERENCES

1. Menz MJ, Lucas GL. Magnetic resonance imaging of a rupture of the medial head of the gastrocnemius muscle. A case report. *JBJS*. 1991;73-A:1260-1262.
2. Sharma P, Maffulli N. Current concepts review tendon injury and tendinopathy: healing and repair. *JBJS*. 2005;87-A:187-202.
3. Schepsis A, Jones H, Haas A. Achilles tendon disorders in athletes. *Am J Sports Med.* 2002;30:287-305.
4. McGuigan F, Aierstok M. Disorders of the Achilles tendon and its insertion. *Curr Opin Orthop.* 2005;16:65-71.
5. Frank J, Jarit G, Bravman J, Rosen J. Lower extremity injuries in the skeletally immature athlete. *JAAOS.* 2007;15:356-366.
6. Setter K, Palomino K. Pediatric tibia fractures: current concepts. *Curr Opin Pediatr.* 2006;18(30):30-35.
7. Flynn J, Skaggs D, Sponseller P, Ganley T, Kay R, Leitch K. The operative management of pediatric fractures of the lower extremity. *JBJS.* 2002;84-A:2288-2300.
8. Zalavras C, Thordarson D. Ankle syndesmotic injury. *JAAOS.* 2007;15:330-339.
9. Amendola A, Williams G, Foster D. Evidence-based approach to treatment of acute traumatic syndesmosis (high ankle) sprains. *Sport Med Arthrosc Rev.* 2006;14(4): 232-236.
10. DiGiovanni BF, Partal G, Baumhauser JF. Acute ankle injury and chronic lateral instability in the athlete. *Clin Sport Med.* 2004;23:1-19.
11. Reid DC. *Sports Injury Assessment and Rehabilitation.* New York: Churchill Livingstone; 1992, Chapter 9:215-268.
12. Sullivan JA. Ligament injuries of the foot and ankle in the pediatric athlete. In: DeLee JC, Drez D, Miller MD, eds.

Orthopedic Sports Medicine, 2nd ed. Philadelphia: W.B. Saunders; 2003:2376-2390.
13. Cassillas MM. Ligament injuries of the foot and ankle in adult athletes. In: DeLee JC, Drez D, Miller MD, eds. *Orthopedic Sports Medicine,* 2nd ed. Philadelphia: W.B. Saunders; 2003:2323-2375.
14. Safran MR, Benedetti RS, Bartolozzi A, et al. Lateral ankle sprains: a comprehensive review part 1: etiology pathoanatomy histopathogenesis and diagnosis. *Med Sci Sport Exerc.* 1999;31(7 Suppl):S429-S437.
15. Safran MR, Zachazewski JE, Benedetti RS, et al. Lateral ankle sprains: a comprehensive review part 2: reatment and rehabilitation with emphasis on the athlete. *Med Sci Sport Exerc.* 1999;31(7 Suppl):S438-S447.
16. Harmon KG. The ankle examination. *Prim Care.* 2004;31: 1025-1037.
17. Magee DJ. *Orthopedic Physical Assessment,* 3rd ed. Philadelphia: Saunders; 1997, Chap 13:599-672.
18. Starkey C, Ryan JL. *Evaluation of Orthopedic and Athletic Injuries,* 2nd ed. Philadelphia: PA, FA Davis; 2002.
19. Smith AH, Bach BR. High ankle sprains: minimizing the frustration of a prolonged recovery. *Phys Sport Med.* 2004;32(12):9–14.
20. LeBlanc KE. Ankle problems masquerading as sprains. *Prim Care* 2004;31:1055-1067.
21. Lachmann LM, Kolb E, Koller MT, et al. Accuracy of Ottawa ankle rules to exclude fractures of the ankle and mid-foot: systematic review. BMJ. 2003;326-417. http://www.bmj.com/. Accessed February 23, 2005.
22. Stiell IG, Greenberg GH, McKnight D, et al. Decision rules for the use of radiography in acute ankle injuries: refinement and prospective validation. *JAMA.* 1993;269:1127-1132.
23. Stiell IG, Greenberg GH, McKnight RD, et al. A study to develop clinical decision rules for the use of radiography in acute ankle injuries. *Ann Emer Med.* 1992;21:384-390.
24. Glas AS, Pijnenburg Bas ACM, Lijmer JG, et al. Comparison of diagnostic decision rules and structured data collection in assessment of acute ankle injury. *CMAJ.* 2002;166(6):727-733.
25. Warren NP, Knottenbelt. The Ottawa ankle rules and missed fractures of the talus. Emj.bmjjournals.com accessed 23 February 2005.
26. Chande VT. Decision rules for current roentgenography of children with acute ankle injuries. *Arch Pediatr Adolesc Med.* 1995;149:255-258.
27. Plint AC, Bulloch B, Osmond MH, et al. Validation of the Ottawa ankle rules in children with ankle injuries. *Acad Emerg Med.* 1999;6:1005-1009.
28. Libetta C, Burke D, Brennan P, et al. Validation of the Ottawa ankle rules in children. *J Accid Emerg Med.* 1999;16:342-344.
29. Clark KD, Tanner S. Evaluation of the Ottawa ankle rules in children. *Pediatr Emerg Care.* 2003;19(2):73-78.
30. Boutis K, Komar L, Jaramillo D, et al. Sensitivity of a clinical examination to predict need for radiography in children with ankle injuries: a prospective study. *Lancet.* 2001;358(9299):2112-2121.
31. Bencardino J, Rosenberg ZS, Delfault E. MR imaging in sports injuries of the foot and ankle. *MRI Clin N Amer.* 1999;7(1):131-149.

32. Prentice WE. *Rehabilitation Techniques for Sports Medicine and Athletic Training*, 4th ed. New York, NY: McGraw-Hill; 2004.

33. Prentice WE. *Therapeutic Modalities for Sports Medicine and Athletic Training*, 5th ed. New York, NY: McGraw-Hill; 2003.

34. Omey M, Micheli L. Foot and ankle problems in the young athlete. *Med Sci Sport Exerc*. 1999;31(7):S470-S486.

35. Bazaz R, Ferkel R. Treatment of osteochondral lesions of the talus with autologous chondrocyte implantation. *Tech Foot Ankle Surg*. 2004;3(1):45-52.

Additional Readings

Copley L. Musculoskeletal infection in children. *Curr Opin Orthop*. 2005;16:445-450.

Denegar CR. *Therapeutic Modalities for Athletic Injuries*. Champaign, IL: Human Kinetics; 2000.

Edwards P, Wright M, Hartman J. A practical approach for the differential diagnosis of chronic leg pain in the athlete. *Am J Sports Med*. 2005;33:1241-1249.

Eiff MP, Smith AT, Smith GE. Early mobilization versus immobilization in the treatment of lateral ankle sprains. *Am J Sports Med*. 1994;22:83.

Frank J, Jarit G, Bravman J, Rosen J. Lower extremity injuries in the skeletally immature athlete. *JAAOS*. 2007;15: 356-366.

Horn D, Crisci K, Krug M, Pizzutillo P, MacEwen G. Dean. Radiologic evaluation of juvenile Tillaux fractures of the distal tibia. *JPO*. 2002;21:162-164.

Johnson E. Tennis leg. *Am J Phys Med Rehab*. 2000;79(3):221.

Loud K, Micheli L. Common athletic injuries in adolescent girls. *Curr Opin Pediatr*. 2001;13:317-327.

Marsh J, Daigneault J. Ankle injuries in the pediatric population. *Curr Opin Pediatr*. 2000;12:52-60.

Mattacola CG, Dwyer MK. Rehabilitation of the ankle after acute sprain or chronic instability. *J Athlet. Train*. 2002; 37:4.

Micheli L, Curtis C, Shervin N. Articular cartilage repair in the adolescent athlete: is autologous chondrocyte implantation the answer? *Clin. J. Sport. Med*. 2006;16(6):465-470.

Patel D, Janiski C. Ankle sprains in young athletes Part I: How to evaluate. *Contemp. Pediatr*. 2005;65-82.

Prentice WE. *Arnheim's Principles of Athletic Training: A Competency-Based Approach*, 11th ed. New York, NY: McGraw-Hill; 2003.

Shindle M, Foo L, Kelly R, et al. Magnetic resonance imaging or cartilage in the athlete: current techniques and spectrum of disease. *JBJS*. 2006;88-A supplement:27-46.

Tubin S, Brunet J. Traumatic dislocations of lesser toe joints. In: Orthopaedic Proceedings, Canadian Orthopaedic Association; May 31-June 4, 1997; Ontario, Canada.

Willems T, Witvrouw E, Verstuyft J, Vaes P, De Clercq D. Proprioception and muscle strength in subjects with a history of ankle sprains and chronic instability. *J. Athlet. Train*. 2002;37:4.

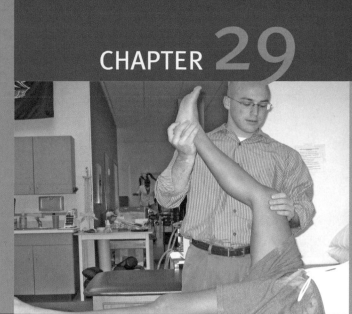

CHAPTER 29

Overuse Injuries of the Leg, Ankle, and Foot

Dilip R. Patel and E. Dennis Lyne

MEDIAL TIBIAL STRESS SYNDROME (SHIN SPLINTS)

Definition and Epidemiology

Shin splints (shin splint syndrome), preferably called medial tibial stress syndrome, is characterized by insidious onset activity-related leg pain caused by overuse and resultant musculotendinous and periosteal inflammation. It is the most common cause of chronic leg pain in runners but it has also been reported in basketball, tennis, and volleyball.

Pathogenesis

The underlying pathology is believed to be tibial periostitis secondary to chronic excessive stress at the bone–muscle junction. Repeated forceful dorsiflexion of the foot, repeated impact loading during foot strike, and excessive high-velocity foot pronation can lead to microtears at the soft tissue attachments, especially soleus muscle, to the periosteum of tibia.[1-3] This results in a musculotendinous inflammatory reaction. Poor shock absorption from shoes, hard running surface, rapid increase in the intensity of training, muscular weakness, and imbalances in strength of leg muscles, poor conditioning, and overweight are contributing factors.

Clinical Presentation

Athletes present with leg pain following a recent increase in running volume and intensity. Initially, the pain is felt during running and often relieved with continued running. With progressive severity, pain tends to recur at the end of the run and then felt throughout running with impairment of running. Pain and tenderness are localized along the middle third of the posteromedial border of the tibia (Figure 29-1). There may be relative weakness of the tibialis posterior and flexor hallucis longus muscles compared to the uninjured leg.

Differential Diagnosis

The differential diagnoses of exercise-related leg pain should include stress fracture of the tibia, exertional compartment syndrome, and other conditions (Tables 29-1 and 29-2).[1-3] Differentiating features of chronic leg pain are summarized in Table 29-3. An algorithm characterizing the clinical features of common conditions causing lower leg pain based on history and examination is presented in Figure 29-2.[1]

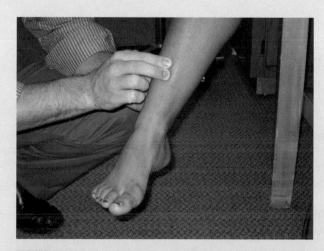

FIGURE 29-1 ■ Site of maximum pain and tenderness in medial tibial stress syndrome.

Table 29-1.

Causes of Chronic Leg Pain in Young Athletes

Relatively More Common
Medial tibial stress syndrome
Chronic exertional compartment syndrome
Stress fractures of tibia or fibula
Achilles tendonitis
Muscle strains

Relatively Less Common
Metabolic bone disease
Referred pain from spine, hip, or knee

Rare
Popliteal artery entrapment syndrome
Peripheral entrapment neuropathies (see Table 29-2)
Bone and muscle neoplasms
Osteomyelitis

Diagnosis

Diagnostic imaging

X-ray of the leg (tibia, fibula) in AP and lateral view is indicated in the evaluation of activity-related leg pain. In medial tibial stress syndrome, x-rays are usually normal. In some cases a thick tibial cortex and subperiosteal lucency on the anterior or medial aspect of the tibia may be seen. Characteristic longitudinal uptake pattern along the tibia is characteristically seen on a bone scan. MRI scan is highly specific and sensitive in the diagnosis of medial tibial stress syndrome as well as stress fracture. It is also useful to evaluate soft tissue pathology in the leg. A diagnostic studies algorithm in presented in Figure 29-3.[1]

Treatment

A period of relative rest from running (and jumping activity) is essential and the most effective treatment for medial tibial stress syndrome. During the period of healing and recovery, alternative activities such as swimming, water running, biking, and exercising on the elliptical machine are recommended. Modification of current level and type of activity is needed. Local application of ice is recommended. Shoes with good shock-absorbing capacity should be worn while excessive pronation should be corrected by using orthosis; a softer training surface is preferred. The athlete should follow a regular program of stretching and strengthening of leg muscles, especially the Achilles, tibialis anterior, and posterior tibialis muscles.

Preventive measures include a regimen of gradually increasing the level of activity, on-going stretching and strengthening exercises, and maintaining good running shoes. It may take from 6 to 8 weeks before returning to pre-injury level of activity. The most common cause of recurrence is too early return to running and is seen within the first 1 to 3 weeks of resumption of running. Athletes who fail conservative treatment should be referred to orthopedics for evaluation and consideration for surgical treatment.

CHRONIC EXERTIONAL COMPARTMENT SYNDROMES OF THE LEG

Definition and Epidemiology

Chronic exertional compartment syndromes of leg can affect one or more compartments of the leg (Figure 29-4) and are usually seen in long-distance runners.[1-3] Pain in the leg characteristically occurs at a certain point in running and is relieved with cessation of running. There may or may not be neurovascular symptoms and signs.

Mechanism

Vascular perfusion of the muscle is dependent on the normal arterial–venous pressure gradient and is most efficient when the muscle is in the relaxed state. Muscle contractions result in increase in the intramuscular

Table 29-2.

Peripheral Nerve Entrapment in Leg

Nerve	Site of Characteristic Pain	Site of Tingling Sensation on Tinel Test
Common peroneal nerve	Lateral leg and foot	From fibular neck with distal radiation
Superficial peroneal nerve	Lateral calf and dorsum of the foot	Few centimeters proximal to lateral malleolus
Saphenous nerve	Above the medial malleolus	From above medial malleolus with distal radiation to medial aspect of the foot

Table 29-3.

The Clinical Characteristics and Imaging Features of Common Causes of Shin Pain in Athletes

Site	Pain	Effect of Exercise	Associated Features	Tenderness	Investigations
Bone stress reaction or stress fracture	Localized, acute or sharp Subcutaneous medial tibial surface or fibula	Constant or increasing Worse with impact	Exacerbated by vibration (tuning fork) and ultrasound	Subcutaneous medial tibial surface or fibula	X-ray may be negative Use magnified views Look for callous or periosteal reaction MRI can stage severity and define prognosis but is nonspecific
Medial tibial periostitis	Diffuse pain on posterior medial border of tibia; variable intensity	Decreases as athlete warms up and stretches	Worse in the morning and after exercise. Pes planus	Posterior medial edge of tibia at muscular insertions	X-rays negative. Bone scan shows diffuse uptake. MRI shows diffuse edema and periosteal thickening.
Chronic exertional compartment syndrome	No pain at rest; ache, tightness, gradually building with exertion	Specific onset variable between athletes, usually 10–15 min into exercise Decreases with rest	Occasional muscle weakness or dysfunction with exercise. Paresthesia of nerve in affected compartment is possible	None at rest Antero and lateral more common with exertion Occasionally related to palpable muscle herniation (superficial peroneal nerve)	X-rays negative Bone scans negative Exertional compartment pressure testing is diagnostic Exertional MRI assessment may also be diagnostic
Popliteal artery entrapment	Pain in calf with exertion not anterolateral 'Atypical compartment syndrome'	Worse with exertion, especially active ankle plantarflexion	Pulses may be diminished with palpation or Doppler ultrasound with active plantarflexion	Rarely in proximal calf	X-rays negative MRI may reveal hypertrophic or abnormal insertion of medial gastrocnemius MRA (arteriography) with provocative maneuvers is diagnostic
Muscle–tendon injuries Strains Tendinopathy	Pain at pathological site with resisted stretch	Pre-exercise stretching usually helps	Good response to NSAIDs and ice	Pain can be at muscle belly, muscle–tendon junction, tendon, or tendon insertion	Rarely required X-rays usually negative MRI gives best view of soft tissue pathology

From Brukner P, Khan K, Bradshaw C, Hislop M, Hutchinson M. Shin pain. In: Brukner P, Khan K, eds. Clinical Sports Medicine, 3rd ed. New York: McGraw Hill Professional; 2007:557.

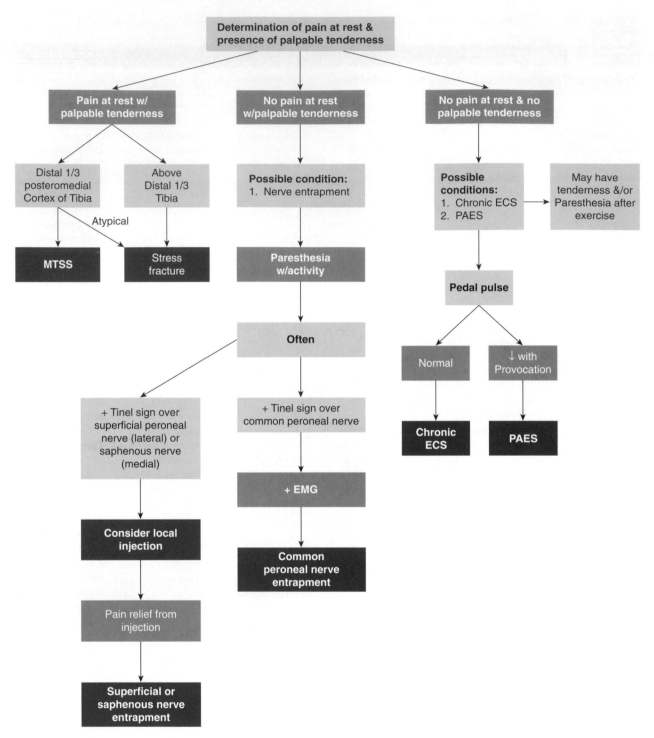

FIGURE 29-2 ■ History and examination algorithm for chronic leg pain. *(Adapted and redrawn from Edwards PH, Wright ML, Hartman JF. A practical approach to differential diagnosis of chronic leg pain in the athlete. Am J Sport Med 2005;33(8):1241–1249.)*

pressure, which is normally accommodated by an increase in the muscle volume. If the fascia that the muscle is contained in is unyielding, the intramuscular pressure will rise to a level that impairs the arterial-venous gradient and muscle perfusion. This will affect the muscle, vascular, and nerve function in that compartment. The pain in the compartment syndrome is believed to be caused by ischemia.

Clinical Presentation

Initially the runner feels aching or burning pain in the leg during running without any neurovascular symptoms or signs. The pain is characteristically predictable and tends to occur at a certain point in time during running and with certain intensity, with resolution after complete cessation of running for a certain period of

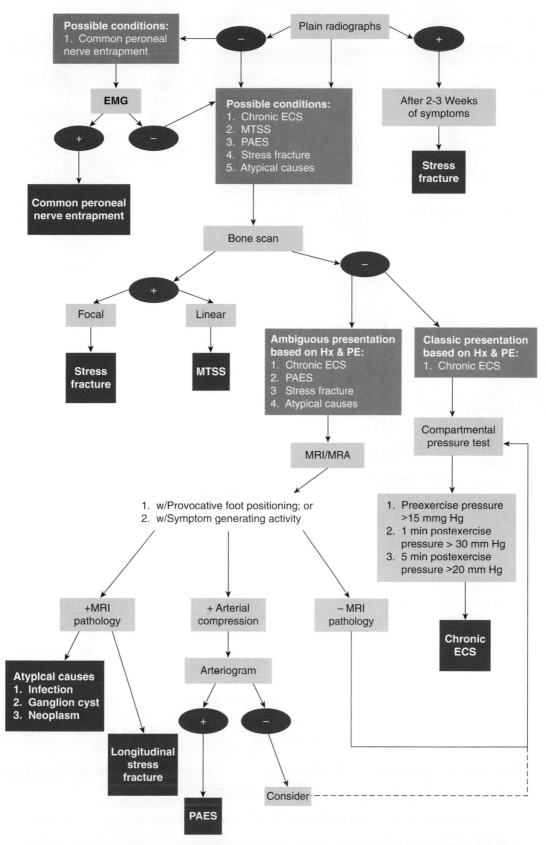

FIGURE 29-3 ■ Diagnostic studies algorithm for chronic leg pain. (*Adapted and redrawn from Edwards PH, Wright ML, Hartman JF. A practical approach to differential diagnosis of chronic leg pain in the athlete. Am J Sport Med 2005;33(8):1241–1249.*)

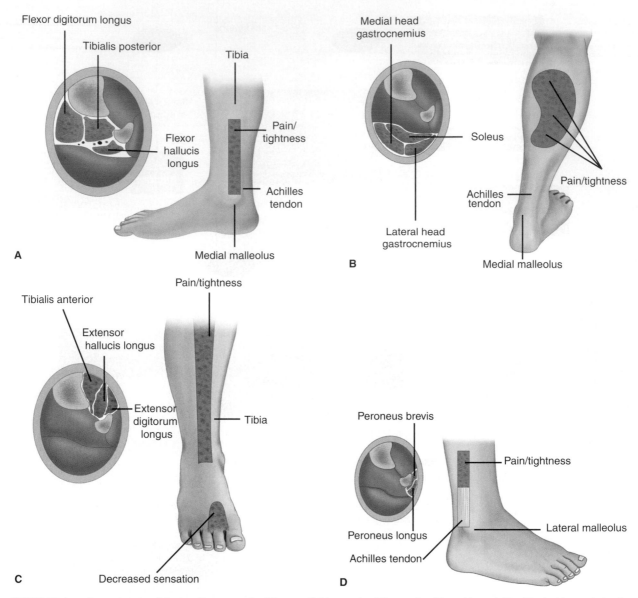

FIGURE 29-4 ■ Compartments of the leg. Deep posterior (**A**), superficial posterior (**B**), anterior (**C**), and lateral (**D**). (*Used with permission from Reid DC. Sports Injury Assessment and Rehabilitation. New York: Churchill Livingstone; 1992.*)

time. It may take from several minutes to hours for the pain to resolve. The symptoms and signs vary depending upon the particular compartment affected (Table 29-4).[3] In most cases, by the time the diagnosis of exertional compartment syndrome is made the symptoms have been present for almost 1 to 2 years. The anterior and lateral compartments are the most commonly affected accounting for 80% of all cases. The examination at rest during the time the athlete is pain-free is normal. When the athlete is having pain, there may be tenderness over the affected compartment. Once the diagnosis of leg compartment syndrome is entertained based on clinical evaluation, the athlete should be referred to orthopedic surgeon or other specialist with expertise in the condition for definitive diagnostic testing.

Diagnostic Studies

The diagnosis of the compartment syndrome is made by the measurement of intracompartmental pressure with the use of specific instrument. The diagnostic criteria are listed in Table 29-5.

Treatment

Running should be stopped. Leg massage, stretching, and use of NSAIDs may help relieve pain and discomfort. If the runner gives up running he or she may fully recover and remain asymptomatic without surgical intervention. However, most athletes will be reluctant to give up sports or running and the definitive treatment is fasciotomy and these athletes are

Table 29-4.

Symptoms and Signs of Specific Compartment Affected

Compartment	Lateral	Anterior	Superficial Posterior	Deep Posterior
Site of pain	Middle one-third of anterolateral leg	Anterior leg	Posterior middle third of leg	Distal one-third of posteromedial leg
Pain elicited by passive	Inversion and plantar flexion of ankle	Flexion of great toes. Inversion and plantar flexion of the ankle	Dorsiflexion of the ankle	Extension of the toes and dorsiflexion of ankle
Muscles affected	Peroneus longus and brevis	Tibialis anterior, extensor hallucis longus and extensor digitorum longus	Gastrocnemius and soleus	Flexor hallucis longus, flexor digitorum, and tibialis posterior
Motor weakness elicited with resisted	Eversion of the ankle	Extension of toes and dorsiflexion of ankle	Plantar flexion of ankle	Flexion of the toes and inversion of the ankle
Nerve affected	Superficial peroneal	Deep peroneal	Sural	Tibial
Site of paresthesia and cutaneous sensory loss	Web space between great and second toe	Dorsum of the foot	Lateral aspect of the foot	Plantar aspect of toes and foot
Arterial pulse that may be diminished		Dorsalis pedis		Posterior tibial

referred to orthopedics (Box 29-1). Generally, failure to improve pain after 3 months of nonoperative measures, fasciotomy is considered. Fasciotomy has been reported to relieve the pain in 90% of cases. Following fasciotomy, the athlete goes through rehabilitation over a period of 10 to 12 weeks. Regular running can be resumed gradually after the athlete is pain-free at rest and on initial trials at running, has no leg tenderness, and has gained previous level of leg muscle strength and flexibility. Most athletes can expect to return to unrestricted sport participation by 8 to 12 weeks following fasciotomy.

Table 29-5.

Criteria for Chronic Exertional Compartment Syndrome

Time of Pressure Measurement	Pressure Diagnostic of Compartment Syndrome
Resting or pre-exercise	Equal to or more than 15 mm Hg
1 minute postexercise	Equal to or more than 30 mm Hg
5 minute postexercise	Equal to or more than 20 mm Hg

FLAT FEET

Definition and Epidemiology

Flat feet or pes planus is characterized by loss of the medial arches of the feet. Pes planus is common in children up to the age of 6 years.[4–6] Flexible pes planus occurs in up to 15% of the overall population, and most of those affected have no symptoms. In a young athlete who competes in running or field sports, pes planus and overpronation of the foot may predispose him or her to knee, leg, or ankle pain, but less commonly than previously thought. Many great athletes have flexible flat feet, almost always bilateral.

Mechanism

Pes planus in most children is of flexible type. Because asymptomatic flat feet are common before age 6 years, a diagnosis of flexible flat feet is generally not made until after 6 years of age. The medial arch is lost while weight bearing and there is associated hyperpronation of the feet. Flexible flat feet in older children and adolescents are often associated with generalized ligamentous laxity and are an autosomal dominant condition. In flexible flatfoot the subtalar joint motion is preserved whereas rigid flat feet are characterized by loss of subtalar motion.[4–6] Causes of rigid flat feet include tarsal coalition, neuromuscular disease, tight Achilles, and familial trait.[6,7]

Clinical Presentation

Most children and adolescents with flexible flat feet are asymptomatic. Athletes may sometimes have activity-related pain. In flexible flat foot the longitudinal medial arch of the foot is lost while weight bearing, with foot going into hyperpronation. When the patient is asked to go up on his toes the arch is evident and the heel goes into inversion or varus (Figure 29-5).

Diagnostic Imaging

Weight-bearing lateral x-ray of the foot shows loss of the medial arch and the straight line relationship between the axis of the talus and the first metatarsal is lost. Heel valgus is evident on the weight-bearing AP x-ray.

Treatment

No treatment is indicated for asymptomatic flexible flat feet. Athletes can participate in all sports unrestricted. If the patient has activity-related pain in the foot, ankle, knee, or hip, biomechanics are assessed and orthotics may be considered. Overtreatment and unnecessary activity restrictions should be avoided.

POSTERIOR TIBIAL TENDON DYSFUNCTION

Definitions and Epidemiology

Tibialis posterior is the main dynamic stabilizer of the hind foot. It acts to resist the eversion of the foot. The function of the tendon can be affected by closed disruptions, stenosing tenosynovitis, or dislocations.[8] Dysfunction of the posterior tibialis is rarely reported in young athletes and is likely not recognized with a reported average time from symptom onset to diagnosis of more than a year.

Mechanism

Tibialis posterior muscle originates from the posterior surfaces of the tibia and fibula as well as the interosseous membrane (Figure 29-6). The tendon courses behind

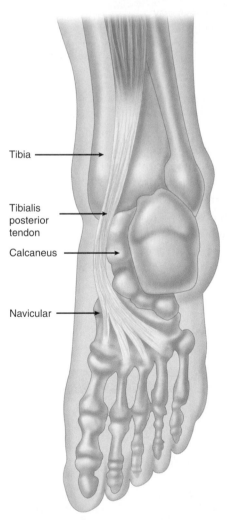

FIGURE 29-6 ■ Tibialis posterior anatomy. The tendon courses behind and below the medial malleolus at it enters the foot, to be inserted at multiple sites on the navicular, cuneiforms, and second, third, and fourth metatarsals.

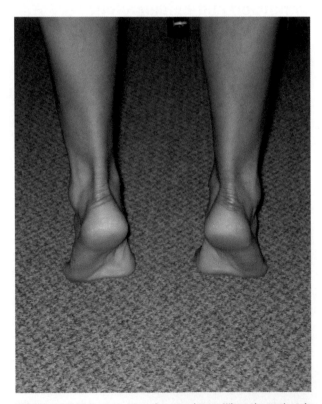

FIGURE 29-5 ■ Toe raise test for pes planus. When the patient is asked to go up on her toes the medial longitudinal arch is normally evident and the heel goes into inversion or varus as shown.

and below the medial malleolus as it enters the foot, to be inserted at multiple sites on the navicular, cuneiforms, and second, third, and fourth metatarsals. Chronic dysfunction of the tibialis posterior in the foot results in stretching of the ankle and foot ligaments, unopposed eversion of the foot, and eventually a flat foot.[8]

Clinical Presentation

Patient presents with a history of foot pain that is gradually progressive in nature. Pain is often worse with activities and especially ascending and descending stairs. There may or may not be an antecedent twisting ankle injury. Pain and tenderness are typically localized between the tip of the medial malleolus and the navicular bone. The foot is flat with loss of medial longitudinal arch and too many toes sign and single heel raise sign are positive (Figures 29-7 and 29-8).

Diagnostic Imaging

Weight-bearing AP and lateral x-rays of the foot and ankle will show increased talocalcaneal angle and inferior subluxation of the talus at the talonavicular articulation.

Treatment

In active athletes nonoperative measures (immobilization, casting, orthotics) have poor results and surgical reconstruction is generally indicated.

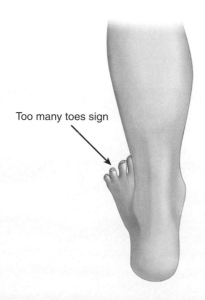

Too many toes sign

FIGURE 29-7 ■ Too many toes sign. In case of tibialis posterior dysfunction, with the patient standing full weight bearing the medial longitudinal arch is lost, the foot goes into valgus and hyperpronation, and looking from behind more than one toe are seen lateral to the foot.

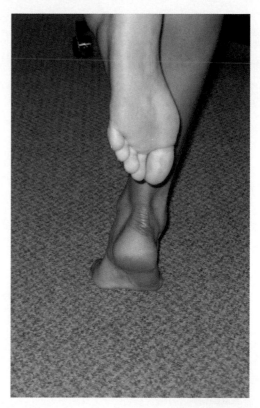

FIGURE 29-8 ■ Single heel raise test. Normally when the athlete is asked to raise the heel of one foot and bear all weight on that leg the heel goes into varus locking the hindfoot as shown. With weakness or dysfunction of the posterior tibialis tendon the athlete is not able to do the heel raise or the foot tends to roll on to the lateral border.

ACCESSORY NAVICULAR

Definition and Epidemiology

An accessory bone adjacent to the navicular has been reported in 15% to 25% of the general population. It is also known as prehallux, os tibiale externum, or navicular secundum.[6]

Mechanism

Three types of accessory navicular bones have been described: (i) a small accessory bone within the tibialis posterior tendon, (ii) an ossicle that is connected to the navicular bone by a cartilaginous bridge, and (iii) an accessory bone that is a remnant of navicular after the fusion of the accessory navicular with the navicular bone.[6] Chronic inflammation is the most common pathological change reported in accessory navicular. Other changes reported include areas of fracture and local hemorrhage.

Clinical Presentation

Accessory navicular is asymptomatic in many individuals. Patients present with medial foot pain that is

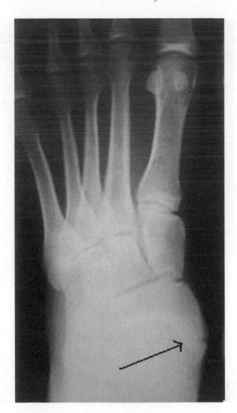

FIGURE 29-9 ■ X-ray of accessory navicular.

aggravated by running and jumping activities, and tight-fitting shoes. The swelling, pain, and tenderness are localized medially over the navicular bone just at the insertion of the posterior tibial tendon on the navicular. Pain is elicited on resisted inversion of the foot.

Diagnostic Imaging

An oblique x-ray directed from medial to lateral (external oblique) of the foot will show the accessory navicular (Figure 29-9), that is often visualized best on a CT scan.

Treatment

Most athletes will respond to a period of rest, local ice, NSAIDs, soft padding locally, avoiding tight-fitting shoes, and use of a shoe insert if the foot is hyperpronated. Often, short leg cast immobilization is needed if the pain is severe. Failure to respond to nonoperative measures and persistent severe pain are indications for simple excision of the accessory navicular.

TARSAL COALITION

Definition and Epidemiology

A tarsal coalition is a cartilaginous, fibrous, or bony bridge between two or more bones in the mid- or hind foot. Overall, coalitions occur in approximately 1% of the general population.[7] Calcaneonavicular and talocalcaneal coalitions are the most common, usually bilateral.[6]

Mechanism

Tarsal coalitions are because of failure of differentiation and segmentation of tarsal bones during early development. The coalitions usually become symptomatic during adolescence, at an average age of 13 years. At this time the coalition is attempting to ossify and will limit subtalar motion. Calcaneonavicular coalitions ossify at 8 to 12 years of age, and talocalcaneal coalitions later at 12 to 16 years of age. Pain is caused by fractures in the coalition. In adolescents with tarsal coalition, nonflexible flat and hyperpronated feet are common findings.

Clinical Presentation

The athlete with a symptomatic coalition presents with insidious onset of ankle or foot pain. These patients will give a history of frequent "ankle sprains," and pain in the midfoot or hindfoot because of added stress of joints around the coalition. Sports often precipitate or increase the pain and running on the uneven surface is especially painful. The examiner tests for a coalition by grasping the forefoot in one hand and attempting to invert and evert the heel with the other hand (Figure 29-10). This will give a sense of the mobility of the subtalar joint. In a coalition this motion is limited. Causes of foot pain are listed in Table 29-6 and 29-7.[5,6,9–11]

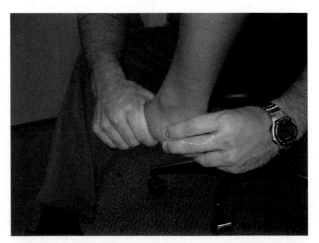

FIGURE 29-10 ■ Examination for tarsal coalition. Grasp the forefoot in one hand then invert and evert the heel with the other hand. This will assess the mobility of the subtalar joint. In tarsal coalition this motion is limited.

Table 29-6.

Causes of Foot Pain in Young Athletes

Relatively More Common
Poor fitting shoes
Tarsal coalition
Sever disease
Islelin disease
Achilles tendonitis
Ingrown toe nail
Friction blisters
Painful callus or corn
Bunion
Warts

Relatively Less Common
Peroneal tendonitis
Flexor hallucis longus tendonitis
Posterior tibial tendonitis
Stress fractures
Foreign body
Metatarsalgia
Plantar faciitis
Osteochondroses
Hypermobile flat feet
Accessory navicular
Cuboid syndrome
Spring ligament sprain
Sesamoiditis
Morton neuroma
Osteomyelitis
Neoplasms

Diagnostic Imaging

Plain films including an AP, lateral, and oblique foot views will often show the coalition (Figure 29-11). CT scan is useful to better demonstrate the extent of the coalition and is the study of choice. CT scan is indicated for surgical treatment planning.

Table 29-7.

Entrapment Neuropathies Causing Foot Pain

Nerve	Main Site of Paresthesias (Burning, Tingling)
Posterior tibial nerve	Plantar aspect of foot
Motor branch to abductor digiti quinti	Heel
Sural nerve	Lateral heel, lateral border of foot and fifth toe
Deep peroneal nerve	Dorsal and medial aspect of the foot
Superficial peroneal nerve	Dorsal aspect of the foot and ankle

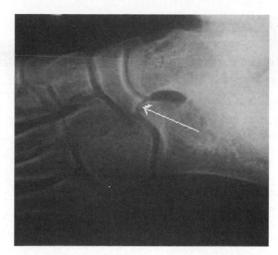

FIGURE 29-11 ■ X-ray of calcaneonavicular coalition.

Treatment

Initial treatment is often the use of orthotics to control foot motion, along with physical therapy for strengthening the foot and ankle muscles. In some cases with severe persistent pain, a short course of casting for 6 weeks or less is also effective. If the athlete is reasonably compliant and is not improving with conservative care, resection of the coalition should be done early, and not delayed until skeletal maturity. Resection of the coalition, especially in talocalcaneal bars, may restore motion, decrease pain, and improve foot and ankle function. The procedure usually consists of resection of the synchondrosis itself, with placement of an interposition graft of muscle or fat. Surgery is followed by a short period of rehabilitation before gradual return to sports.

SEVER DISEASE

Definition and Epidemiology

Sever disease is a traction apophysitis of the calcaneal apophysis, to which the Achilles tendon, the short muscles of the sole of the foot, and the plantar fascia attach.[5,6,9,12] It is most commonly seen in preteen to early teenage years in gymnasts, soccer players, and basketball players.

Mechanism

The secondary center of ossification of calcaneus appears at age 9 and fuses at approximately 16 years of age. The vertically oriented apophyseal plate of posterior calcaneus is subject to shearing and traction stresses from repetitive contractions of the gastroc-soleus complex.

Table 29-8.

Causes of Heel Pain

Achilles tendonitis
Calcaneus stress fracture
Calcaneus osteomyelitis
Entrapment neuropathies (see Table 29-6)
Haglund deformity
Os trigonum syndrome
Peroneal tendonitis
Plantar faciitis
Retrocalcaneal bursitis
Sever disease
Tibialis posterior tendinitis

Clinical Presentation

Onset of heel pain in Sever disease is usually associated with the beginning of a new sport or season, or an increase in running. It occurs more often in athletes with a tight gastroc-soleus complex, as well as in those with a pronated foot. The average age of onset is 8 to 13 years. Sever disease is a common cause of heel pain in the child athlete, and is bilateral in more than half of the children. On examination there will be tenderness medially and laterally to the heel. There is also sometimes associated Achilles tendonitis. Causes of heel pain in young athlete are listed in Table 29-8.[6,12]

Diagnostic Imaging

Diagnosis is apparent clinically and x-rays are normal (Figure 29-12). Imaging studies are usually not indicated unless to exclude other diagnostic considerations.

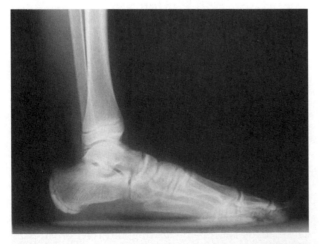

FIGURE 29-12 ■ X-ray in case of Sever disease typically shows the normal appearing posterior calcaneal apophysis.

Treatment

The primary treatment is stretching of the heel cord, avoidance of barefoot ambulation, and a heel cup or heel wedge until the athlete is asymptomatic. A period of rest from running or jumping activities usually is sufficient to resolve the pain. Athlete is generally ready to play sport within 6 to 8 weeks. This is a benign, self-limiting condition with no long-term complications and over treatment and unnecessary restriction of activities should be avoided.

ISELIN DISEASE

Definition and Epidemiology

Iselin disease is a traction apophysitis of the base of the fifth metatarsal, seen most commonly in young adolescents participating in sports that involve running and jumping.

Mechanism

The proximal apophysis of the tuberosity of the fifth metatarsal appears at 10 years of age in girls and 12 years of age in boys, and fuses after approximately 2 years. The tendon of the peroneus brevis is inserted at the base of the fifth metatarsal and is believed to contribute to inflammation of the apophysis because of repeated traction. A repeated inversion movement of the foot causes such traction on the peroneus brevis.

Clinical Presentation

The young adolescent athlete presents with activity-related localized pain over the lateral border of the foot. Pain is more intense while weight bearing, running, or jumping. There may be localized soft tissue edema and erythema and tenderness is elicited over the proximal fifth metatarsal. Pain can be exacerbated by eversion of the foot against manual resistance, as well as with extreme plantar flexion or dorsiflexion of the foot.

Diagnostic Imaging

Diagnosis is apparent clinically and x-ray is usually normal. In some cases an oblique view of the foot may show hypertrophy and fragmentation of the apophysis. Sometimes the apophysis fails to unite with the metatarsal and may be mistaken for a fracture (Figure 29-13).

Treatment

Most athletes will respond to a short period of rest, local ice, and NSAIDs if needed. Rarely, in case of severe

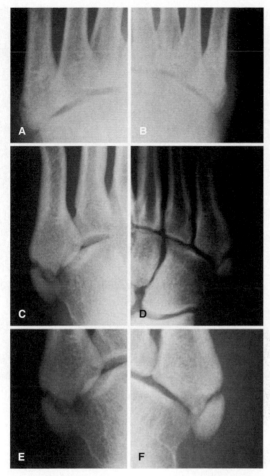

FIGURE 29-13 ■ X-ray of the foot in case of Iselin disease. (A, B) oblique radiographs of a 13-year-old basketball player with bilateral Iselin disease. (C, D) the same patient as a college freshman (18 years old) with nonunited secondary ossification centers that were symptomatic. (E, F) the patient as a college senior (21 years old); there is definite evidence of bilateral disease and nonunion, but only the left foot is symptomatic. (*Used with permission from Canale ST. Osteochondrosies and related problems of the foot and ankle. In: DeLee JC, Drez D Jr, Miller MD, eds. DeLee and Drez's Orthopaedic Sports Medicine, 2nd ed. Philadelphia: Saunders Elsevier; 2003, Figure 30K-50:2616.*)

persistent pain, immobilization of the foot and ankle in short leg walking cast may be needed. It is important to recognize the benign self-limited nature of this conditions and either overtreatment or overprotection or restriction from sports should be avoided.

JUVENILE OSTEOCHONDRITIS DISSECANS OF THE TALUS

Definition and Epidemiology

Osteochondritis dissecans (OCD) is an injury of the articular cartilage and underlying subchondral bone.

OCD of the talus occurs in association with ankle sprains and direct impact, either acute or repetitive, injuries to the foot and ankle. Based on the Berndt and Harty classification a type I OCD is a small area of compression of subchondral bone, type II injury is a partially detached osteochondral fragment, type III injury is a completely detached fragment without displacement from the fragment bed, and a type IV injury is a displaced osteochondral fragment.[13–15]

Inversion injuries of the ankle are more commonly associated with anterolateral cartilage injuries (44% of OCD lesions) whereas posteromedial lesions are associated more often with repetitive microtrauma (56% of OCD lesions).

Mechanisms

Osteochondritis dissecans of the talus can result from acute direct impact, ankle inversion dorsiflexion injuries, or from repetitive trauma with overloading of the cartilage of the ankle joint. Anterolateral talus lesion is usually traumatic, whereas posteromedial lesion can be genetic and benign.

Clinical Presentation

Most often the onset of pain is insidious, and there may be a history of preceding macrotrauma such as a severe inversion sprain. There may be a history of a recent increase in chronic ankle pain after a recent ankle sprain. Athletes will report recurrent ankle swelling, and often "weakness" of the ankle. The athlete will complain of chronic aching in the ankle, and occasionally catching or clicking. Pain on motion, tenderness over the anterolateral, or posteromedial talus, and often a small effusion are present.

Diagnostic Imaging

X-ray findings are shown in Figure 29-14. In some cases a bone scan or MRI may be needed to confirm the diagnosis and to aid in treatment planning.

Treatment

Initial treatment of types I and II OCD lesions in young athletes is casting and orthotics in young patients. Type III lesions on the medial side are initially treated the same way. All type IV lesions and the lateral type III lesions will require arthroscopic drilling, removal, or pinning to best enhance healing potential. In some cases larger OCD lesions may need cartilage transfer or grafting procedures.

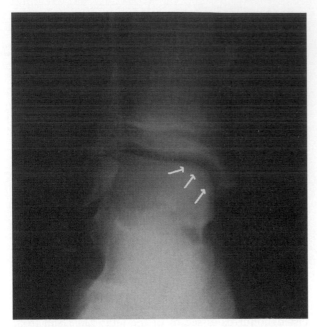

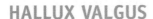

FIGURE 29-14 ■ X-ray of osteochondritis dissecans of talus.

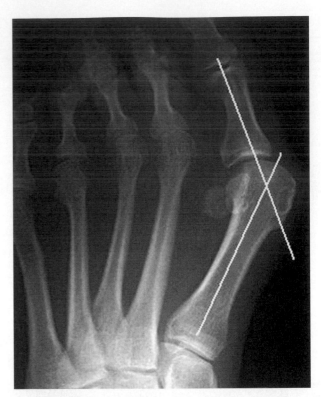

FIGURE 29-15 ■ X-ray hallux valgus.

HALLUX VALGUS

Definition and Epidemiology

Hallux valgus (bunion) is characterized by static subluxation of the first metatarsophalangeal (MTP) joint, accompanied by valgus deviation of the great toe and varus deviation of the first metatarsal.[16,17] Hallux valgus or adolescent bunion occurs in up to 22% to 40% of adolescents, more often in females, with a high prevalence in dancers.

Mechanism

In hallux valgus the first metatarsal deviates medially, is usually pronated, and the great toe deviates laterally with a prominent first MTP joint. There are a variety of factors associated with hallux valgus, including wearing of tight or pointed shoes, heredity, global ligamentous laxity, pes planus, and metatarsus primus varus.

Clinical Presentation

Patient presents with pain in great toe. The pain is particularly worse while in shoes and relieved when the foot is out of the shoe and is relaxed. Pressure over the local sensory nerve can cause paresthesia felt in the toe. With progressively increasing toe deformity, the patient tends to shift weight bearing laterally and develops forefoot pain. Patient should be examined standing to appreciate the deformity. Range of motion and pin prick sensation of the foot should be assessed.

Diagnostic Imaging

Weight-bearing AP and lateral views of the foot will best demonstrate the characteristic valgus deformity (Figure 29-15).

Treatment

Treatment begins with proper shoe wear, a firm-soled shoe with a high wide toe box, use of bunion pads, orthotics, and rehabilitation. However, if pain persists, the athlete may not be able to return to sports, and a realignment of the first metatarsal is often necessary. Recurrence in this age group is high however, ranging between 20% and 60% after surgical correction. Operative treatment should be delayed until skeletal maturity because recurrence is high in the skeletally immature.

SESAMOIDITIS

Sesamoid bones in the foot are most often present just under the head of the first metatarsal. Sesamoiditis is caused by overuse injuries in young athletes who push off the ball of their foot.[18] This injury occurs in ballet, tennis, basketball, and other jumping sports. The athlete may have an underlying pronated or cavus foot, and sometimes a hypermobile plantar flexed great toe. X-rays, AP lateral and oblique of the foot may not demonstrate any significant changes unless there is a bipartite sesamoid present or a true fracture exists, which is uncommon. Examination will demonstrate swelling and tenderness to palpation over the sesamoids, directly plantar to the first metatarsal head. These injuries are treated with orthotics with or without a relief cut out for the sesamoids, ice massage, rest, and NSAIDs as needed.

PLANTAR FACIITIS

Plantar fasciitis is relatively uncommon in young athletes but is seen often enough in adolescent athletes who run hills, are involved in jumping sports, or in speed work. A high arched or a rigid hindfoot which is in varus can predispose to this problem. In the adolescent with closed physes there will be heel or medial arch pain, and pain with weight bearing, worsened by climbing stairs or rising up on the toes. Pain and stiffness of the foot in the morning are common symptoms. Tenderness can be elicited along the medial edge of the fascia or at the anterior edge of the calcaneus. Imaging with x-rays may not be helpful, and heel spurs which are seen on plain films are not related to the pain of plantar fasciitis. Treatment includes Achilles stretches, rest, ice, NSAIDs, heel cups, orthotics, night splints, and rarely local soft tissue corticosteroid injections. Training errors and overtraining need to be corrected, and in rare severe cases which do not improve with these measures, a plantar fascial release can be done. Prognosis with conservative treatment in young athletes is excellent for complete resolution of the pain and full return to sports.

HAGLUND DEFORMITY

Haglund's deformity (pump bump) is a prominence which develops over the posterior superior calcaneus (Figure 29-16). It is because of shoe wear and occurs in male and female ice skaters, and in soccer players and runners. The bump is often palpable more laterally over the heel. There may be an associated retrocalcaneal bursitis or Achilles tendonitis, and often the hindfoot is in varus. Treatment includes wearing larger-size shoes, padding or a heel lift, and Achilles stretching and strengthening. Often the deformity will require excision in those with recurrent symptoms.

TENDONITIS

Flexor Hallucis Longus (FHL) Tendonitis

FHL tendonitis is more common in ballet dancers who repeatedly place their feet in extremes of plantar flexion, and in runners, field sports players, and gymnasts. The problem may be associated with a symptomatic os trigonum. Athlete with FHL tendonitis presents with pain in the foot that is exacerbated with resisted great toe flexion. The patient will also have discomfort posterior and inferior to the medial malleolus, which may extend along the tendon distal to the malleolus. Treatment is usually conservative, with icing, stretching, and then strengthening. Tenosynovectomy is needed in some cases that do not resolve with conservative care.

Achilles Tendonitis

Achilles tendonitis is more frequent in young athletes who have increased their training regimen significantly. The athlete will complain of pain along the Achilles tendon itself, and may have associated swelling. Hyperpronation of the foot, a recent rapid growth spurt, or inappropriate or inadequate shoe wear are also associated with Achilles tendonitis. Sports which involve running, jumping, cycling, or sudden stops such as vaulting and jumps in gymnastics are associated with this problem. Treatment begins with stretching, and then strengthening once motion is improved, orthotics, and possible heel lifts or cups, and some newer options have been reported.[19] The athlete's footwear must be looked at carefully, and running shoes should have a flexible forefoot with a firm heel, and be no more than 4 to 6 months old depending upon the athlete's training schedule.

Peroneal Tendonitis

Peroneal tendonitis is common in young dancers and ice skaters, but is seen in other running athletes as well.

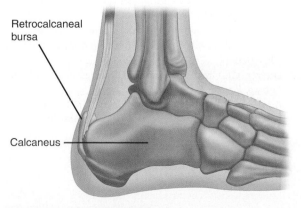

Retrocalcaneal bursa

Calcaneus

FIGURE 29-16 ■ Haglund deformity.

The athlete will complain of pain behind and distal to the lateral malleolus, and the area may be swollen. Resisted foot eversion will cause discomfort. X-ray may show fibula calcaneal impingement in eversion. These injuries are treated with stretches, ice, strengthening, and sometimes an ankle brace for use during sports. Debridement of the tendon may be needed in refractory cases.

Posterior Tibial Tendonitis

Posterior tibial tendonitis is uncommon in young athletes in general, but can be seen frequently in dancers and ice skaters, and in sports which involve running and rapid directional changes. The posterior tibial tendon inverts and plantar flexes the foot and supports the longitudinal arch. Examination will demonstrate pain on resisted ankle plantarflexion and inversion. The course of the tendon posterior to the medial malleolus and extending to the navicular may be tender to palpation. Those with pronated feet are more likely to have this problem, and there may be an associated accessory navicular present in some. Plain films may not be that helpful, and the MRI scan and bone scan will aid the physician in making the diagnosis. Treatment includes stretching, icing, and strengthening, and orthotics as well as occasional casting. In some cases a tenosynovectomy may be required.

Anterior Tibialis Tendonitis

Tibialis anterior tendonitis is usually seen in runners, and examination demonstrates point tenderness anteriorly where the tendon crosses the ankle joint. Treatment is stretching, icing, strengthening, orthotics, and occasional casting.

Conditions that should be referred to orthopedics are listed in Box 29-1.

Box 29-1 When to Refer.

Chronic exertional compartment syndromes of the leg
Popliteal artery entrapment syndrome
High-risk stress fractures of the tibia
High-risk stress fractures of the foot
Chronic symptomatic posterior tibial tendon dysfunction
Symptomatic tarsal coalition
Hallux valgus

REFERENCES

1. Edwards PH, Wright ML, Hartman JF. A practical approach to differential diagnosis of chronic leg pain in the athlete. *Am. J. Sport. Med.* 2005;33(8):1241-1249.
2. Reinking MF. Exercise-related leg pain in female collegiate athletes: the influence of intrinsic and extrinsic factors. *Am. J. Sport. Med.* 2006;34(9):1500-1507.
3. Reid DC. Exercise-induced leg pain. In: Reid DC. *Sports Injury Assessment and Rehabilitation.* New York: Churchill-Livingstone; 1992:269-300.
4. Sullivan JA. Pediatric flatfoot: evaluation and management. *J. Am. Acad. Orthop. Surg.* 1999;7:44-53.
5. Omey ML, Micheli LJ. Foot and ankle problems in the young athlete. *Med. Sci. Sport. Exerc.* 1999;31:S470.
6. Herring JA. Disorders of the foot. *Tachdjian's Pediatric Orthopaedics*, 3rd ed. New York: Saunders Elsevier; 2002:891-1038.
7. Bhone WH. Tarsal coalition. *Curr. Opin. Pediatr.* 2001;13:29-35.
8. Keene JS. Tendon injuries of the foot and ankle. In: DeLee JC, Drez D, Miller MD, eds. *Orthopaedic Sports Medicine*, 2nd ed. Philadelphia: Saunders Elsevier; 2002:2409-2445.
9. Pontell D, Hallivis R, Dullard MD. Sports injuries in pediatric and adolescent foot and ankle: common overuse and acute presentations. *Clin. Podiatr. Med. Sur.* 2006;23(1):209-231.
10. Kennedy JG, Knowles B, Dolan M, Bohne W. Foot and ankle injuries in adolescent runner. *Curr. Opin. Pediatr.* 2005;17(1):34-42.
11. Mann RA. Entrapment neuropathies of the foot. In: DeLee JC, Drez D, Miller MD, eds. *Orthopaedic Sports Medicine*, 2nd ed. Philadelphia: Saunders Elsevier; 2002:2474-2482.
12. Reid DC. Heel pain and problems of hindfoot. *Sports Injury Assessment and Rehabilitation.* New York: Churchill Livingstone; 1992:185.
13. Perumal V, Wall E, Babekir N. Juvenile osteochondritis dissecans of the talus. *J. Pediatr. Orthop.* 2007;27(7):821-825.
14. Canale S, Belding R. Ostochondral lesions of the talus. *J. Bone Joint Surg. Am.* 1980;62:97-102.
15. Chambers HG. Ankle and foot disorders in skeletally immature athletes. *Orthop. Clin. North Am.* 2003;34(3):445-459.
16. Easley ME, Trnka HJ. Current concepts review. Hallux valgus: pathomechanics, clinical assessment, and nonoperative management. *Foot Ankle Int.* 2007;28(5):654-659.
17. Robinson AH, Limbers JP. Modern concepts in the treatment of hallux valgus. *J. Bone Joint Surg. Br.* 2005;87(8):1038-1045.
18. Dietzen CJ. Great toe sesamoid injuries in the athlete. *Orthop. Rev.* 1990;19(11):966-972.
19. Alfredson H, Cook J. A treatment algorithm for managing Achilles tendinopathy: new treatment options. *Br. J. Sport. Med.* 2007;41(4):211-216.

CHAPTER 30

Thoracolumbar Spine Injuries

Dilip R. Patel and Dale Rowe

ANATOMY

Gross Anatomy

The gross anatomical features of the thoracolumbar spine are shown in Figures 30-1 to 30-6.

Developmental Anatomy[1–4]

The three ossification centers of each vertebra (one for the centrum and two for each neural arch) typically fuse between the age 2 and 6 years. Each vertebra

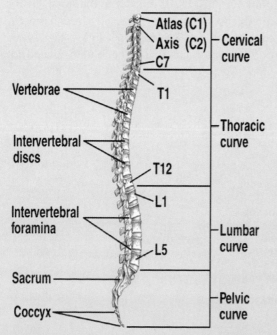

FIGURE 30-1 ■ Spine. (*Used with permission from Van De Graaff KM. Human Anatomy, 6th ed. New York: McGraw Hill; 2002, Figure 6-35, p. 161.*)

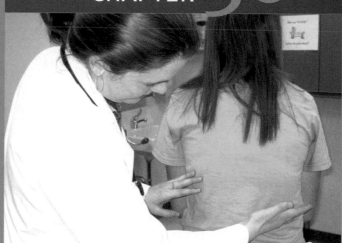

FIGURE 30-2 ■ Gross anatomy: thoracic spine. (*Used with permission from Van De Graaff KM. Human Anatomy, 6th ed. New York: McGraw Hill; 2002, Figure 6-35, p. 161.*)

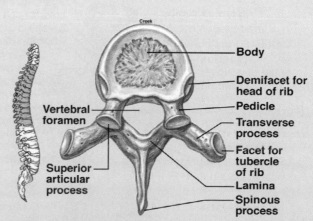

FIGURE 30-3 ■ Gross anatomy: lumbar spine. (*Used with permission from Van De Graaff KM. Human Anatomy, 6th ed. New York: McGraw Hill; 2002, Figure 6-36, p. 162.*)

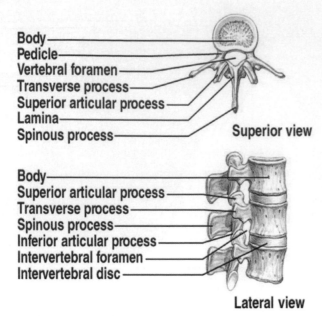

Body
Pedicle
Vertebral foramen
Transverse process
Superior articular process
Lamina
Spinous process **Superior view**

Body
Superior articular process
Transverse process
Spinous process
Inferior articular process
Intervertebral foramen
Intervertebral disc
Lateral view

FIGURE 30-4 ■ Gross anatomy: lumbar spine. (*Used with permission from Van De Graaff KM. Human Anatomy, 6th ed. New York: McGraw Hill; 2002, Figure 6-36, p. 162.*)

assumes adult characteristics by approximately age 8 years and oblique pattern is achieved by age 15 years. The vertebral body physes can be seen on x-ray by 8 years of age when they begin to ossify peripherally and are relatively thicker at the periphery (ring apophysis). Ossification is completed by 12 years of age. The physis begins to fuse with the vertebral body at approximately 14 years of age and the fusion is complete between the age 21 and 25 years. The physis contributes to the growth in height of the vertebral body whereas the ring apophysis contributes to the growth in breadth of the vertebral body.

The basic structure of the immature vertebral body and associated disk is depicted in Figure 30-7. The intervertebral disk is composed of a centrally located nucleus pulposus and peripheral annulus fibrosus, and the adjacent vertebral endplate. The nucleus pulposus in the immature spine is more resilient and elastic because of relatively higher water content compared to the mature spine.

The spinal canal achieves the adult volume by 6 years of age. There is an inherent difference between the spinal column and the spinal cord flexibility in the immature spine. The spinal column can be stretched up to 5 cm before it fails owing to disruption, whereas the spinal cord fails after 1 cm of stretch. This explains the phenomenon of spinal cord injury without radiological abnormality (SCIWORA) seen mostly in young children and predominantly affects the cervical spine. The spinal cord ascends to L1 by age 1 and therefore the neurological levels of spinal cord injury are the same as adult after age 1 year.

DEFINITIONS AND EPIDEMIOLOGY

Sport-related thoracolumbar injuries can involve soft tissue structures, the bony elements, or the spinal cord. Sport-related acute trauma is rare in young children and uncommon in adolescents. It is estimated that 80% of the injuries occur during practice, and acute injuries account for 60% of these.

Overuse injuries of the back are relatively more common in adolescent athletes. Sport-related injuries account for 10% to 15% of injuries to the spine. Overall, the prevalence of back pain from all causes has been reported to be between 20% and 30% in 11- to 17-year age group.[5–12] The incidence of back pain related to

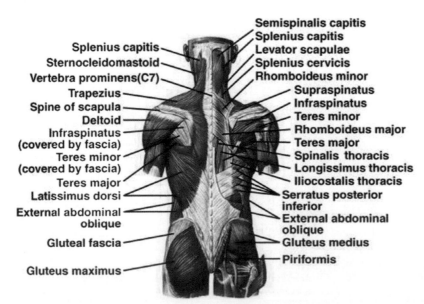

Splenius capitis
Sternocleidomastoid
Vertebra prominens(C7)
Trapezius
Spine of scapula
Deltoid
Infraspinatus
(covered by fascia)
Teres minor
(covered by fascia)
Teres major
Latissimus dorsi
External abdominal
oblique
Gluteal fascia
Gluteus maximus

Semispinalis capitis
Splenius capitis
Levator scapulae
Splenius cervicis
Rhomboideus minor
Supraspinatus
Infraspinatus
Teres minor
Rhomboideus major
Teres major
Spinalis thoracis
Longissimus thoracis
Iliocostalis thoracis
Serratus posterior
inferior
External abdominal
oblique
Gluteus medius
Piriformis

FIGURE 30-5 ■ Muscles of the back. (*Used with permission from Van De Graaff KM. Human Anatomy, 6th ed. New York: McGraw Hill, 2002.*)

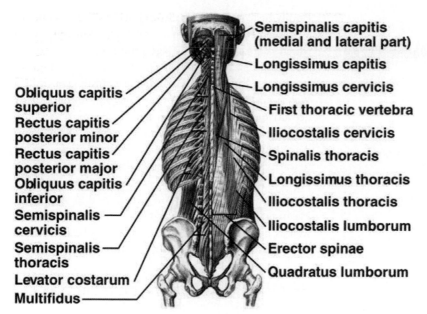

Semispinalis capitis
(medial and lateral part)
Longissimus capitis
Longissimus cervicis
First thoracic vertebra
Iliocostalis cervicis
Spinalis thoracis
Longissimus thoracis
Iliocostalis thoracis
Iliocostalis lumborum
Erector spinae
Quadratus lumborum

Obliquus capitis
superior
Rectus capitis
posterior minor
Rectus capitis
posterior major
Obliquus capitis
inferior
Semispinalis
cervicis
Semispinalis
thoracis
Levator costarum
Multifidus

FIGURE 30-6 ■ Muscles of the back. (*Used with permission from Van De Graaff KM. Human Anatomy, 6th ed. New York: McGraw Hill; 2002, Figure 9-25, p. 262, Figure 9-27, p. 265.*)

sports injuries vary widely depending upon the sport. The most common injuries are the acute soft tissue sprains, strains, and contusions.

Unlike in an acute injury, the cause and effect relationship between the chronic injury and symptoms or spine abnormalities cannot be always clearly established in young athletes. In adolescent athletes the most common underlying identified spine lesion is spondylolysis.

The severity of the lower back pain and abnormal findings of the spine are relatively increased during the adolescent growth spurt. Early age at onset and longer duration of sports participation may contribute to increased symptomatology.

MECHANISMS

The most common predisposing factor for thoracolumbar back pain in adolescent athletes has been reported to be a recent change in training regimen. Other reported predisposing factors include poor conditioning, relative core muscle weakness, decreased hamstring flexibility, increased lumbar lordosis, improper sport technique, and poor fit or use of equipment. Sports with relatively higher prevalence of back pain are listed in Table 30-1.[5–12]

Sport biomechanics play an important role in the type of stress and injury sustained in sports (Table 30-2). Flexion of the thoracolumbar spine has been shown to increase the pressure on the intervertebral disks, increase

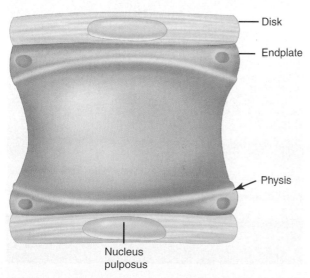

Disk

Endplate

Physis

Nucleus
pulposus

FIGURE 30-7 ■ Schematic diagram of immature vertebral body with disk.

Table 30-1.
Sports with a Relatively Higher Prevalence of Back Pain
Golf
Running
Weight lifting
Racquet sports
Gymnastics
Cheerleading
Dancing
Diving
Rowing
Basketball
Wrestling
Rugby
Ice hockey
American football
Fast bowling in cricket

Table 30-2.	

Biomechanics and Spine Injuries

Biomechanical Stress	Example of Sport
Compression of spine in vertical plane	American football, weight lifting
Rotational (torque) or shear force in horizontal plane	Throwing sports, golf, baseball
Tensile stress from excessive, repetitive motion	Gymnastics, ballet, cheerleading

the tension on the nerve root and dural sac, and increase the relative size of the intervertebral canal and the foramen. Extension of the spine will have the opposite effects.

Direct blows to the back can cause muscle contusions. Hyperextension of lumbar spine, as seen in football and gymnastics, is implicated in the development of spondylolysis. In gymnasts, a higher level of competition is correlated with a higher incidence of back problems. Studies suggest that floor exercises, the balance beam, uneven parallel bars, flips, and vaulting dismounts contribute to back injuries in gymnasts. In throwing sports, musculotendinous avulsions may occur from forceful sudden muscle contractions. In the adolescent athlete, the immature vertebral end plates may be injured from improper weight lifting. Lifting with spine in flexion, and moving from flexion to extension causes significant stress to the spine. Improper lifting techniques may cause injuries in ballet and figure skating. Twisting motions in tennis can cause musculotendinous strains and avulsions. Chronic poor posture may result in chronic ligamentous strain.

CLINICAL PRESENTATION

History should include the mechanism of injury and detailed history characterizing the pain. Pain should be characterized by onset, location, duration, progression, exacerbating factors and relieving factors. Is there night pain? Is there radiation of pain in legs? Ascertain past history of back pain or injury. Has the athlete sought any previous medical care?

Athlete will present with a history of back pain following acute trauma or activity-related chronic or recurrent pain. Back pain in a young child must be thoroughly investigated for specific etiology that may include infection, tumors, or developmental anomalies of the spine. Localization of pain may indicate possible etiology. Scheuermann disease is the most common identifiable cause of thoracic back pain. Spondylolysis most commonly affects the lower lumbar spine. Constitutional symptoms such a fever, rash, other joint pain, loss of appetite, and weight loss suggest systemic disease.

Family history and psychosocial history are essential in all adolescents to assess psychosomatic pain syndrome which is common in this age group. Although neurological injuries are rare, it is important to recognize symptoms and signs that indicate neurological injury that should prompt appropriate imaging and referral for definitive diagnosis and treatment.

General physical examination should focus on detecting signs that indicate systemic etiology. Sexual maturity rating or Tanner stage (see Figures 2-2, 2-3, and 2-4, Chapter 2) should be assessed and both lower extremities should be carefully examined. A systematic examination of the back and thoracolumbar spine as well as neurological examination should be conducted in all athletes with back injuries and pain.

Examination of Thoracolumbar Spine[13–16]

Athlete standing

- Gait: Observe for pain during full weight bearing or any protective posture. Also judge the degree of pain or discomfort.
- Observe the overall standing posture from behind and from side. Note any asymmetry. Note the normal thoracic (convex) and lumbar (lordotic) curves. Note listing. Note tendency to stand or walk with flexed hips and knees (crouching).
- Have the athlete bend over (flexion) and observe the spine from front, behind, and side of the athlete. Note scoliosis (Adam test) or kyphosis (Figure 30-8).

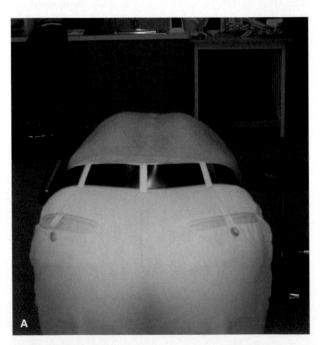

FIGURE 30-8 ■ Adam test. Have the athlete bend over and observe the spine from the front, behind (**A**) and side (**B**). Note asymmetry, scoliosis, or kyphosis. (*continued*)

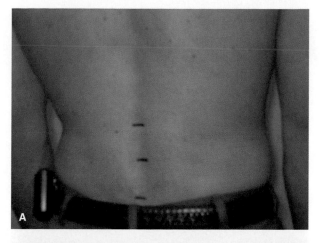

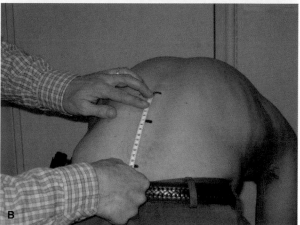

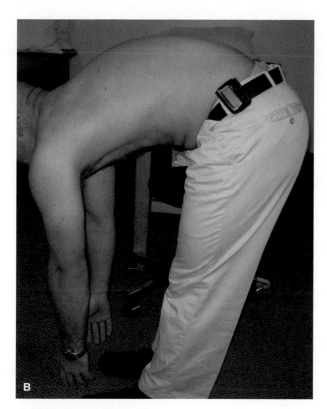

FIGURE 30-8 ■ (Continued)

- Observe from the front the symmetry of hips and alignment of iliac crests.
- Assess active range of motion of the spine (Table 30-3). Schober test (Figure 30-9) is helpful to measure the degree of flexion of the thoracolumbar spine. To measure the lateral flexion first mark the point on the lateral aspect of the thigh where the tip of middle finger reaches; followed by marking the point on lateral flexion. The distance between the two points is useful to assess the amount of lateral flexion.
- One-legged hyperextension test (Figure 30-10)
- Trendelenburg test (Figure 30-11)
- Assess the strength of the calf muscle by observing the ability of the athlete to do repeat unilateral heel raises (S1). Manual testing of plantar flexion is not reliable.

FIGURE 30-9 ■ Schober test. With the athlete standing, mark a point on the spine midway between the posterior superior iliac spines, second point 5 cm above and third point 10 cm below (**A**). Measure the distance between the most superior and the most inferior points. Ask the athlete to bend forward and measure the distance between the same points again (**B**). The degree of flexion of the lumbar spine is indicated by the difference between the measurements.

Assess the strength of the anterior tibialis muscle (ankle dorsiflexion) by having the athlete do heel walking (L5).
- Palpate and localize soft tissue and bony tenderness over the back, spine, and hips.

Athlete sitting

- Observe the athlete for any apparent discomfort as he or she moves from standing to sitting on the exam table. Observe the sitting posture from back, side, and front. Note asymmetry of shoulders or hips. Note the alignment of iliac crests.
- Tripod test (Figure 30-12)
- Slump test (Figure 30-13)

Athlete supine

- Note the level of anterior superior iliac spines
- Measure for both legs (a) the leg length from the anterior superior iliac spine to lateral malleolus; (b) girth at midthigh; and (c) girth at midcalf.

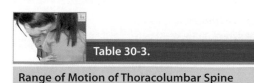

Table 30-3.

Range of Motion of Thoracolumbar Spine

Movement	Range (degrees)	
	Thoracic Spine	Lumbar Spine
Forward flexion	20–45	40–60
Extension	25–45	20–35
Lateral flexion (side bending)	20–40	15–20
Rotation	35–50	3–18

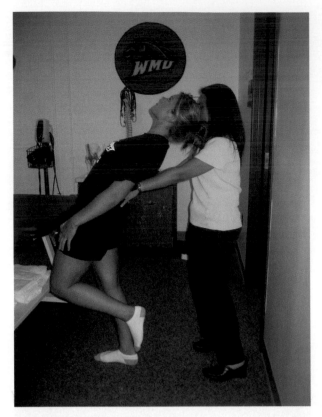

FIGURE 30-10 ■ One-legged hyperextension (Stork test). With the athlete standing on one leg have her extend the back. Repeat the same on the opposite leg. Pain is elicited on extension in case of pars interarticularis stress fracture of a lumbar vertebra. Pain is relatively more intense on the ipsilateral side.

- Assess quadriceps and hamstring flexibility (Figure 30-14)
- Assess strength (Table 30-4), sensation to pin prick (Table 30-5) and reflexes (Table 30-6) in both lower limbs
- Straight leg raise (Lasegue) test: Contralateral leg pain is characteristic of a disk herniation whereas, ipsilateral pain is characteristic of sciatica.
- Hoover sign (Figure 30-15)
- Patrick or FABER test (Figure 30-16)
- Gaenslin test (Figure 30-17)

Athlete prone

- Observe for thoracic kyphosis: Apparent kyphosis owing to postural round back disappears when the athlete extends the back while prone whereas a fixed deformity will persist.
- Femoral nerve stretch test (Figure 30-18)

DIAGNOSIS

Back pain in young children with certain "red flag" signs (Table 30-7) warrants a thorough evaluation. In addition to apparent acute or repetitive trauma, a number of other intrinsic (Table 30-8) and extrinsic (Table 30-9) conditions should be considered in the differential diagnosis of back pain in adolescents.[1,2,5–9,11,17,18]

AP, lateral, and oblique x-rays of the spine are the initial study of choice to assess back thoracolumbar spine injuries and pain. Other imaging studies such as bone scan, CT scan, or MRI scan may be indicated in the evaluation of specific conditions. The most useful screening laboratory studies are a complete blood count and erythrocyte sedimentation rate.

TREATMENT

Treatment of the athlete with thoracolumbar back injury and pain depends upon the specific condition. Conservative modalities include rest, pain management, therapeutic exercises, bracing, orthotics, improving biomechanics, improving sport techniques, and appropriate conditioning and training. Most athletes will respond to conservative treatment depending upon the nature of the specific condition causing the back pain; a few will need further orthopedic consultation (Box 30-1).

ACUTE SOFT TISSUE SPRAINS, STRAINS, AND MUSCLE CONTUSIONS

Acute soft tissue trauma is the most common back injury and cause of back pain in adolescent athletes. The athlete with *acute back strain/sprain*, who is otherwise in good health, should expect full recovery within few days. Absolute bed rest is no longer recommended. The athlete should be allowed to carry on daily activities as tolerated. Analgesics and muscle relaxants may help relieve pain during the acute phase. As the pain and general mobility improve, a back rehabilitation exercise program is started in consultation with a sports physical therapist. Basic exercises are shown in Appendix C. The goals of

Box 30-1 When to Refer.
Indications of orthopedic referral
Fractures of thoracolumbar spine
High-grade spondylolisthesis
Spondylolysis not responding to conservative treatment
Scheuermann kyphosis
Acute back pain with neurological symptoms and signs
Scoliosis of 20 degree or more in during peak growth
Significant scoliosis, progressive curve, atypical scoliosis
Diskitis and osteomyelitis
Acute disk herniation with neurological signs
Apophyseal fractures
Tumors of spine and cord

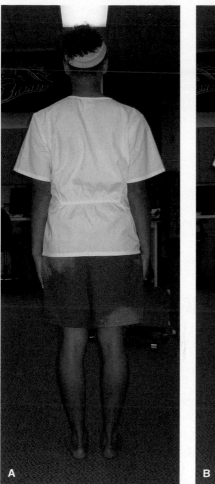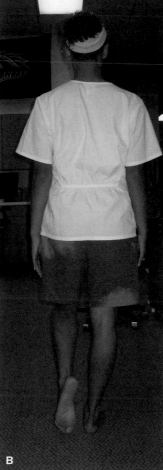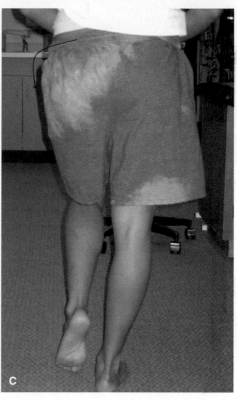

FIGURE 30-11 ■ Trendelenburg test. Have the athlete stand on one leg (**A**). Observe from behind. Normally the pelvis remains level or horizontal mainly because of the contraction of the gluteus medius of the leg that is weight bearing (**B**). Sagging of the hip of the leg lifted off the ground is suggestive of gluteus medius weakness of the weight-bearing leg (**C**).

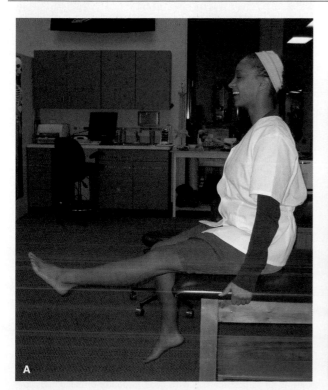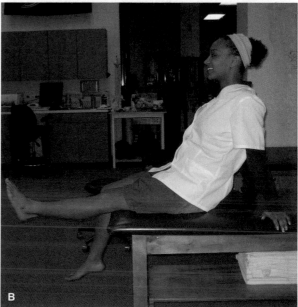

FIGURE 30-12 ■ Tripod test. The athlete is seated on the examination table with both hips and knees at approximately 90-degree flexion and straight back. The knee is then extended (**A**). If the hamstring on that side is tight or if the nerve roots are irritated, the athlete will extend her back to relieve the tension in hamstrings or on the sciatic nerve (**B**). Repeat on the other side.

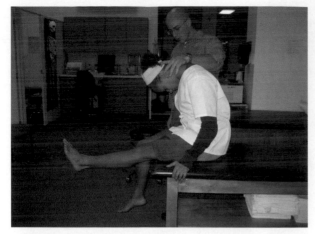

FIGURE 30-13 ■ Slump test. The athlete is seated on the examination table. She is asked to slump with flexion of spine and allowing the shoulders to sag forward. Sequentially, the examiner flexes the neck, followed by passive extension of the knee, and passive dorsiflexion of the foot. Sciatica type pain in the leg is considered positive test suggesting impingement of the dura or spinal cord or nerve root.

rehabilitation for acute back strains and sprains are to regain normal pain-free range of motion, improve core strength and stability, correct abnormal posture, improve biomechanics, and improve sport techniques.

Table 30-4.	
Strength Testing of Lower Extremity Muscles	
Muscle Group	**Neurological Level**
Abdominals	T7–T12
Hip flexors	L1–L2
Knee extensors	L3
Knee flexors	S2
Ankle dorsiflexors	L4
Ankle plantarflexors and evertors	S1
Hip extensors	
Great toe extensor	L5

THORACIC SCHEUERMANN DISEASE (JUVENILE DISK DISEASE)

Definition and Epidemiology

Scheuermann disease, seen in adolescents, is characterized by fixed kyphotic deformity of the spine. Sorenson's radiographic criteria are listed in Table 30-10. The diagnostic wedging is not seen before 10 years of age. The normal range of thoracic spine curve in sagittal plane is between 20 degrees and 40 degrees and a

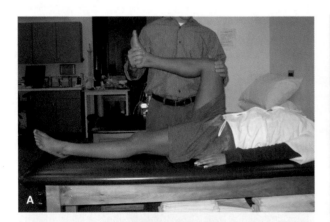

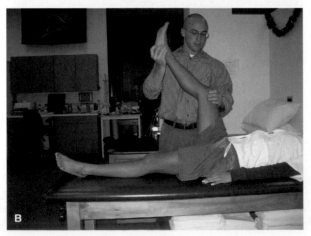

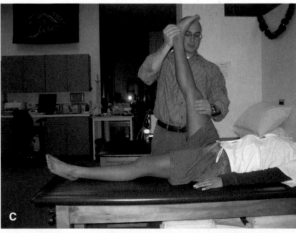

FIGURE 30-14 ■ Testing hamstring flexibility. With the athlete supine on the examination table, first fully flex the hip and knee (**A**), then bring the hip to 90 degree flexed position (**B**), and extend the knee as far as possible (**C**). With good flexibility of hamstrings, the knee can be extended to 180 degrees. The degree of lack of extension (popliteal angle) of the knee is a measure of hamstring tightness. Examine each leg separately.

Table 30-5.

Sensory Dermatomes of Lower Extremities

Area	Nerve Root Level
Medial midthigh	L2
Superior aspect of medial knee	L3
Medial arch of the foot	L4
Dorsum of the foot	L5
Lateral border of and plantar aspect of the foot	S1
Popliteal fossa	S2

Table 30-6.

Main Reflexes Tested in the Examination

Deep tendon reflex
Patellar (L4)
Achilles (S1)

Superficial reflexes
Abdominal: upper (T7–T9)
Abdominal: lower (T11–T12)
Cremasteric (T12–L1)

Pathologic reflex
Babinski (upper motor neuron lesion)

kyphotic deformity exceeding 45 degrees is considered abnormal. Males are affected more than females and most cases are seen between ages 10 and 15 years. Most have a positive family history of kyphosis. The reported incidence ranges between 0.4% and 10% during adolescence.[19] No studies have reported specific incidence or prevalence in athletes. Scheuermann disease is the most common identified cause of thoracic back pain in adolescents.

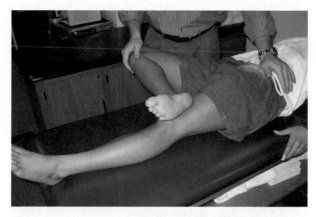

FIGURE 30-16 ■ Patrick or FABER test. With the athlete supine the leg is placed in a figure of 4 position (flexion, abduction, external rotation of the hip). Then it is lowered with gentle downward pressure over the knee while holding down the opposite hip. Positive test is indicated by pain or discomfort in the sacroiliac area iliopsoas or sacroiliac pathology.

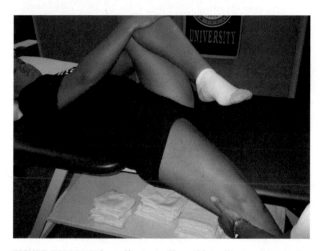

FIGURE 30-17 ■ Gaenslin test. The athlete lies supine on the examination table. Ask her to fully flex both legs, followed by having her move to the edge of the table and slowly extend the hip and lower the leg over the edge of the table. Repeat on the opposite leg. Pain in the sacroiliac joint area while extending the hip and lowering the leg is suggestive of sacroiliac pathology.

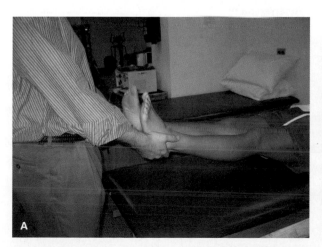

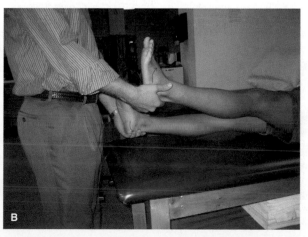

FIGURE 30-15 ■ Hoover test. With the athlete supine on the examination table ask her to raise her fully extended leg while cupping the heel of the opposite foot. Normally, a downward pressure is appreciated in the opposite leg, while the athlete attempts to raise the other leg. If no such downward pressure or bearing down is felt it is suggested that the athlete is not trying to raise the opposite leg, as in malingering.

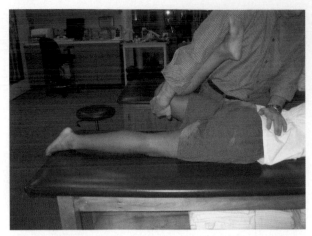

FIGURE 30-18 ■ Femoral nerve stretch test. Have the athlete lie prone. Extend the knee and hip of the affected leg followed by flexion of the knee and full extension of the hip. Radiating anterior thigh pain is a positive test indicating femoral nerve pathology.

Mechanism

The exact etiology is not known. Postulated contributing factors include genetic predisposition, hormonal abnormalities, collagen defects, juvenile osteoporosis, vitamin deficiencies, and repetitive microtrauma from sport participation or other physical stress to the spine.[5,6,8,19]

Clinical Presentation

Many adolescents initially remain asymptomatic and may first present with poor posture and kyphotic deformity. However, most present with dull aching thoracic back pain located between scapulae that is aggravated by physical activity, prolonged sitting, standing, and forward flexion. Pain tends to diminish as the adolescent approaches skeletal maturity. The severity of pain and progressive worsening of the kyphosis have poor correlation.

Kyphotic deformity is evident on Adam forward bending test in classic presentation. Many adolescents in the early stage may only have back pain for several weeks to months before progressive kyphosis develops, therefore

Table 30-7.

Red Flag Signs of Back Pain

Back pain in a child younger than 10 y
Pain that wakes the patient up from sleep
Pain lasting 2 or more months
Severe progressive pain
Continuous or constant pain
Pain at rest
Associated neurological signs
Associated systemic symptoms and signs

Table 30-8.

Intrinsic Causes of Back Pain in Adolescents

Acute pain
Acute fractures of the thoracolumbar spine
Acute musculotendinous strains and sprains
Acute spondylolysis
Muscle contusions
Disk herniation*

Chronic/insidious or recurrent pain
Lumbar spondylolysis and spondylolisthesis
Postural
Psychosomatic*
Hypermobility syndrome
Scheuermann disease
Diskitis and vertebral osteomyelitis*
Idiopathic juvenile osteoporosis
Lumbarization or sacralization
Spina bifida occulta
Facet joint syndrome*
Benign and malignant tumors of the spine or cord
Sacroiliac joint pain

Can be acute or chronic.

Scheuermann disease should be considered in any adolescent who presents with chronic or recurrent thoracic back pain. Occasionally, the pain is of sudden onset. The kyphosis should be differentiated from adolescent postural round back that disappears when the athlete hyperextends the back while prone. Patients also have decreased flexibility of hamstrings and exacerbated lumbar lordosis.

Table 30-9.

Extrinsic Causes of Back Pain in Adolescents

Referred pain
Abdominal or pelvic neoplasms
Acute appendicitis
Pancreatitis
Pyelonephritis
Renal stones
Urinary tract infection
Pelvic inflammatory disease
Pelvis osteomyelitis with or without abscess

Systemic disease
Leukemia
Inflammatory bowel disease
Spondyloarthopathy
Ankylosing spondylitis
Rheumatoid arthritis
Metabolic diseases
Neuromuscular disease
Myopathy

Diagnostic Imaging

X-ray findings include vertebral end plate irregularities, narrowing of the intervertebral disk space, anterior wedging and decreased height of the vertebrae, and Schmorl nodes (protrusion of nucleus pulposus into the vertebral body anteriorly) (Figure 30-19). In the classic presentation the apex of the kyphotic deformity is at T7-T8 level.

Treatment

Therapeutic exercises to improve flexibility (especially of hamstrings and lumbodorsal muscles and fascia) and core strength are recommended for all patients. Pain can be managed as needed by use of analgesics (Appendix D).

More definitive treatment is guided by the severity of the deformity and the remaining growth potential of the patient based on skeletal maturity. Patients with kyphosis less than 50 degrees can be managed conservatively with rehabilitation exercises and regular clinical and radiographic monitoring until they reach skeletal maturity. Orthopedic consultation should be obtained in all cases of Scheuermann disease. Adolescents who are skeletally immature and have kyhposis that exceeds 50 degrees, bracing is considered. Milwaukee brace is used initially full time for a period of 12 to 18 months followed by 12 hours per day until skeletal maturity.[8,9,17,19] Adequate improvement has also been reported with use of Boston brace for kyphosis with apex below T7. Curves that exceed 70 degrees, severe persistent pain, and progression of the curve are indications for considering surgical treatment.

Athletes with curves less than 50 degrees who have undergone rehabilitation and are asymptomatic may return to sports without restrictions. Athletes being treated with bracing may be allowed to participate in sports, with brace removed for the duration of game or practice, once they have started the rehabilitation and are pain-free.

Recurrent, activity-related back pain and restriction of some back extension are long-term problems

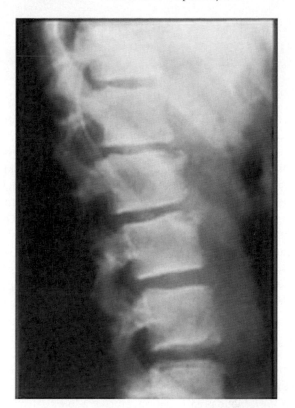

FIGURE 30-19 ■ X-ray of Scheuermann disease. Note vertebral end plate irregularities and Schmorl nodes.

seen in some patients; however, overall functional outcome has been reported to be very good.

THORACOLUMBAR (ATYPICAL) SCHEUERMANN DISEASE

Thoracolumbar Scheuermann disease is seen in adolescents who participate in sports that require repeated flexion and extension movements such as gymnastics. It has also been reported in adolescents who participate in wrestling, football, weight lifting, rowing, tennis, and bicycle racing. It is seen most commonly in male athletes with a peak incidence between 15 and 17 years of age.

Because of wedging of the vertebrae at the thoracolumbar spine there is a loss of lumbar lordosis and the back appears straight or mildly kyphotic. Other clinical features are similar to the thoracic type. Thoracolumbar Scheuermann disease generally is nonprogressive and treated with exercise and conditioning program and restriction of sport until the athlete is pain-free. Most athletes are able to return to sports after a period of approximately 6 months of conservative treatment. Bracing for a period anywhere from 3 to 12 months has also been used allowing athletes to return to sports within 2 to 3 months once pain-free.

Table 30-10.

Sorensen Radiographic Criteria for Scheuermann Disease

1 Anterior wedging exceeding 5 degrees of 3 consecutive vertebrae in the apex of the kyphosis
2 Irregular vertebral apophyseal lines with flattening and wedging of the apophysis
3 Disk space narrowing
4 Schmorl's nodes may be present

ADOLESCENT IDIOPATHIC SCOLIOSIS

Definitions and Epidemiology

Scoliosis is defined as a lateral curvature of the spine greater than 10 degrees as measured by using the Cobb method on a standing posteroanterior radiograph of the spine.[6,17,20] Vertebral rotation is associated with the lateral curvature. In Cobb method, a line is drawn through the superior surface of the uppermost vertebra of the curve. Another is drawn through the inferior surface of the lowermost vertebra of the curve. The angle at the intersection of lines drawn perpendicular to the above two lines is the Cobb angle or the curvature of the scoliosis (Figure 30-20). The reported prevalence of adolescent scoliosis is between 0.5% and 3%.

Mechanism

The exact mechanism or etiology of adolescent scoliosis is not known but believed to be multifactorial with strong genetic predisposition. During adolescent years, curve progression occurs in approximately 10% of cases of adolescent idiopathic scoliosis. Curve progression is a function of gender, remaining skeletal maturity at the time of diagnosis, and the magnitude of the curve at the time of diagnosis (Table 30-11).[17,20–28]

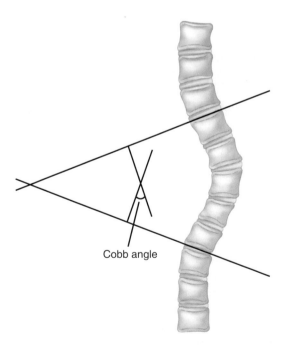

FIGURE 30-20 ■ Cobb angle measurement. In lateral radiograph of the spine in the Cobb method, a line is drawn through the superior surface of the uppermost vertebra of the curve. Another is drawn through the inferior surface of the lowermost vertebral of the curve. The angle at the intersection of lines drawn perpendicular to the above lines is the Cobb angle or the degree of curvature of the scoliosis.

Table 30-11.

Juvenile Scoliosis and Curve Progression[17,20–28]

- Thoracic curves are at a higher risk for progression compared with thoracolumbar or lumbar curves
- Females have 10 times higher risk for curve progression
- The risk for curve progression is highest during first 2 y of peak height velocity, that is 11–13 y in girls and 13–15 y in boys
- The risk for curve progression is highest during Sexual Maturity Rating 2
- Curve of 30 degrees or more at the onset of puberty progresses rapidly and presents a 100% prognosis of surgery
- Curves between 21 degrees and 30 degrees at the onset of puberty have a 75% prognosis for surgery
- Curve progression velocity of 1 degree per month during pubertal growth represents 100% prognosis for surgery
- Surgery is indicated for curves of 40 degrees or more during peak height velocity
- Curve progression is difficult to predict before onset of puberty
- Fusion of all elbow epiphyses marks the end of pubertal growth, typically at bone age of 13 y in girls and 15 y in boys

Clinical Presentation

Adolescent idiopathic scoliosis can be asymptomatic. Pain and deformity may become apparent with larger curves and with progression of the curve. Spine should be examined at all preventive visits during adolescent years, typically once a year. Measure leg length (from anterior superior iliac spine to medial malleolus) to rule out leg length inequality. Have the standing patient bend forward as far as he or she can, with both upper extremities extended and palms held together hanging down. Observe from the front of the patient for a thoracic hump on one side indicating scoliosis. This is called Adam's test. Also observe the spine from side to note any kyphosis. Determine the sexual maturity rating of the patient.

Diagnostic Imaging

A scoliosis series is indicated to assess the degree of scoliosis as measured by Cobb angle. Periodic radiographic evaluation is indicated based on the initial degree and risk of progression of the scoliosis.

Treatment

Adolescents with idiopathic scoliosis at sexual maturity rating of 2 with curves more than 20 degrees should be referred to pediatric orthopedic or spine specialist. Those whose curves are less than 20 degrees, and are less likely to progress as determined by gender and remaining skeletal maturity can be followed by the pediatrician every 6 months with clinical and radiologic evaluation to assess the curve. In a meta analysis of nonoperative interventions for scoliosis treatment, bracing 23 hours daily was been shown to be effective in preventing curve progression.[22] Exercise programs are not effective. Surgery is considered in rapidly progressive curves, and curves more than 45 degrees.

Asymptomatic athletes are allowed unrestricted sport participation. Participation decision should be individualized in consultation with orthopedic surgeon for those with painful high-degree curves, those being treated with bracing, and those who had surgical correction.

LUMBAR SPONDYLOLYSIS

Definition and Epidemiology

Spondylolysis refers to stress fracture of the pars interarticularis (isthmic type); most lesions are bilateral (80%) and affect L 5 (95%) (Figure 30-21).[29] It is one of the most common and significant conditions that causes back pain in adolescent athletes, reported in almost 50% of cases of sport-related low back pain in adolescents.[29,30] The incidence of spondylolysis is 6% in the general population compared with 50% in gymnasts, 40% in Alaskans, and 13% in Eskimos. A higher incidence is seen in ballet, gymnastics, competitive cheerleaders, football linemen, weight lifting, wrestling, diving, volleyball, and fast bowlers in cricket. The mean age at diagnosis in athletes is around 15 to 16 years, but can occur at earlier ages.

Mechanism

Repetitive axial loading and rotation, especially in an extended lumbar spine, is the most important contributing mechanism leading to fatigue fracture of the pars interarticularis.[30,31]

Clinical Presentation

Many athletes with spondylolysis are asymptomatic and may or may not progress to symptomatic lesions. Athletes with symptomatic spondylolysis generally present with insidious onset, recurrent, activity-associated, low back pain. Athlete may also present with a history of sudden onset on pain with acute spondylolysis as reported in competitive cheerleading and gymnastics. The pain is localized to low back, nonradiating, and dull aching to sharp. Pain is also reported in buttocks and back of the thigh. Patients do not have any neurological symptoms or signs.

Decreased flexibility of the hamstrings and lumbodorsal muscles and fascia is seen in almost all symptomatic athletes and may be the only and/or initial presenting sign. Increased lumbar lordosis and a relative weakness of abdominal muscles are also common findings. Lower back pain can be reproduced or exacerbated by one-leg hyperextension movement of the lumbosacral spine (Figure 30-10).

Diagnostic Imaging

There is no universally accepted consensus for imaging protocol, and the decision to proceed with any particular imaging study and its timing should be

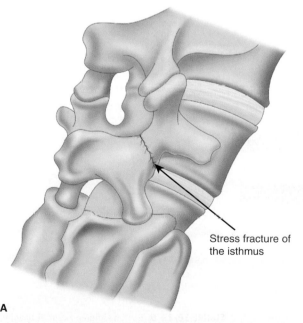

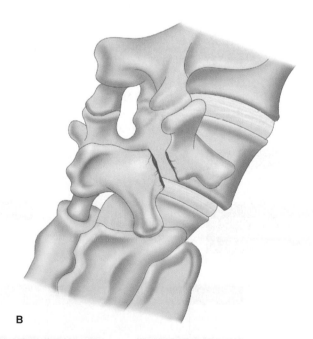

Stress fracture of the isthmus

A

B

FIGURE 30-21 ■ Schematic drawings of spondylolysis (**A**), and spondylolisthesis (**B**).

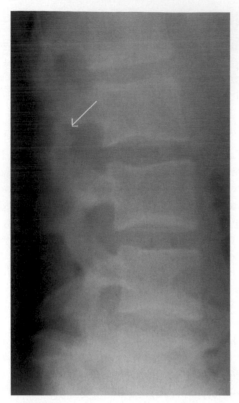

FIGURE 30-22 ■ X-ray of spondylolysis. Note the pars defect at L2 on this lateral radiograph.

determined on an individual basis based on the findings on clinical evaluation and particular circumstances of the athlete.

Plain films are initial study of choice and should include anteroposterior, lateral, (Figure 30-22) and oblique views of the lumbosacral spine, although some have questioned the value of routinely obtaining oblique

views. One study has reported that 85% of the lesions can be detected on coned-down lateral x-ray of the lumbosacral junction.[6,7] In a classic lesion the characteristic pars defect is most evident on the oblique view, and described as the scotty dog with a collar appearance. Like other stress fractures, x-rays may not be positive until after 1 to 2 weeks. Plain films are useful to detect any associated anomalies such as spina bifida occulta and other congenital vertebral anomalies, as well as spondylolisthesis.

The need for and appropriateness of additional imaging studies should be ideally considered in consultation with the radiologist locally. A bone scan or a single photon emission computed tomography scan are highly sensitive in the diagnosis if the plain films are normal, and to determine the acuity of the fracture; and a computed tomography scan is useful to delineate the defect. The bone scan and SPECT scan require injection of radiographic dye, and radiation exposure which is also a consideration for CT scan.

Increasingly, magnetic imaging resonance scan is being used as a next step in cases where initial x-rays are negative. MRI scan is useful in detecting early or acute lesions, delineating the anatomic nature of the pars defect, and detect any spinal or soft tissue pathology. An imaging protocol used at the Boston Children Hospital is depicted in Figure 30-23.[6,7]

Treatment

Most athletes with spondylolysis can be managed conservatively. Symptomatic athletes should refrain from sports and hyperextension activities until pain-free, which may take a few days to several weeks.[29,31–34]

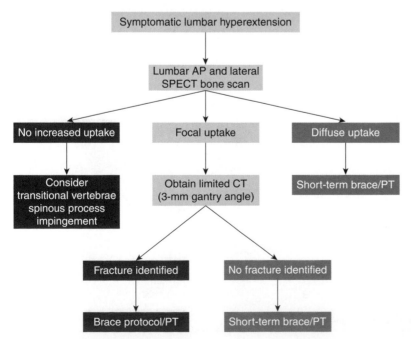

FIGURE 30-23 ■ Boston Children Hospital Imaging Protocol for Spondylolysis.

Athletes should work with knowledgeable sports physical therapist or athletic trainer for rehabilitation program focused on core stabilization, strengthening, and flexibility exercises. Return to sport is allowed once the athlete is pain-free, has normal examination, and has undergone rehabilitation. Failure of conservative treatment and recurrent or persistent pain is an indication for orthopedic consultation.

For acute symptomatic lesions, a treatment protocol is used at the Children's Hospital Boston, is summarized below.[6,7]

(a) Diagnosis of symptomatic spondylolysis is confirmed at the initial visit after clinical and radiographic evaluation (Figure 30-23). The athlete is restricted from sports, physical therapy is started, and modified Boston brace is prescribed (Boston overlap brace fitted at 0 degree of extension). Athlete is allowed stationary bike exercise, and swimming (except butterfly and breast stroke). Brace is worn for 23 of 24 hours daily.

(b) Athlete is seen 4 to 6 weeks later. If the pain has resolved and examination is normal he or she is allowed to return to sports with continued bracing, and progressive physical therapy. Persistent pain at this point indicates an evaluation to identify any additional contributing conditions.

(c) After 4 months of treatment, a CT scan is obtained. If there is a bony union or pain-free nonunion, the athlete is weaned off the brace and allowed full sports participation. If there is persistent pain and no evidence of bony union a trial of electrical stimulation is considered with continued bracing.

Failure of conservative treatment as indicated by persistent pain after 9 to 12 months of treatment is an indication for operative intervention.

Table 30-12.

Wiltse-Newman Classification of Spondylolisthesis

I Dysplastic
II Isthmic
  (a) Disruption of the pars interarticularis due to stress fracture
  (b) Elongation of the pars without disruption due to repetitive healed microfractures
  (c) Acute fracture of the pars interarticularis
III Degenerative
IV Traumatic
V Pathologic

SPONDYLOLISTHESIS

Definition and Epidemiology

Spondylolisthesis is characterized by forward slippage of a vertebra over the one just below it, most commonly of L5 over S1.[17,29] Spondylolisthesis is a common complication of bilateral spondylolytic lesions. Wiltse–Newman classification of types of spondylolisthesis is described in Table 30-12. Isthmic type is the most common type seen in adolescent athletes. The overall incidence and epidemiologic characteristics are similar to those of spondylolysis.

Mechanism

The basic mechanism is similar to that of spondylolysis, and generally occurs as a complication of bilateral spondylolytic defects at the same vertebral level.

Clinical Presentation

Athlete presents with gradual onset, aching pain in the lower back, buttocks, or the posterior thigh. The pain is aggravated with physical activities, especially those involving repeated flexion, extension, and rotation. In some cases spondylolisthesis is asymptomatic. Patient often assumes characteristic posture while standing or walking with increased hip and knee flexion or crouched posture (known as the Phalen-Dickson sign).[29] On examination there is hamstring tightness (80% of patients), and exacerbated lumbar lordosis and a step-off over the lumbar spine may be palpated. Lumbar radicular symptoms are rare, and may be present in high-grade spondylolisthesis. Lower limb strength, sensation, and reflexes should be tested.

Diagnostic Imaging

Lateral x-ray of the lumbosacral spine is sufficient in most cases to diagnose and assess the degree of slippage. Meyerding classification of the degree of slippage is described in Figure 30-24.[29,30] MRI scan is indicated if the patient has neurological symptoms or signs to evaluate for other causes such as disk herniation in conjunction with spondylolisthesis.

Treatment

The risk for progression is higher for younger athletes and they should be followed regularly until skeletal maturity. Initial treatment of patients with low-grade (grade I and II) spondylolisthesis without neurological signs is similar to that of patients with symptomatic

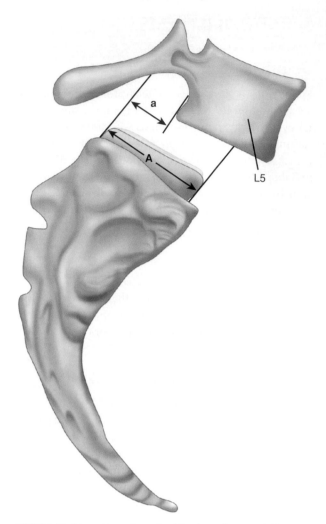

FIGURE 30-24 ■ Meyerding classification of spondylolisthesis. Grade 1 is less than 25% slip, grade 2 is 26% to 50% slip, grade 3 is a 51% to 75% slip and grade 4 is 76% to 99% slip. The percentage of the slip is determined based on the radiographic measurements (lateral view of the spine) using the formula $a/A \times 100$, where a is the distance between the posterior edge of the inferior endplate of the proximal vertebra and the posterior edge of the superior endplate of the vertebral below it and A is the distance between the anterior and posterior edge of the superior endplate of the distal vertebra.

acute spondylolysis that includes restriction of sports until asymptomatic, physical therapy, and bracing. All patients with high-grade lesions and those with neurological signs should be referred to orthopedic surgeon for definitive further evaluation and treatment that includes different surgical options.

DISK HERNIATION

Definition and Epidemiology

Herniation of the intervertebral disk into the spinal canal is rare in children and adolescents with a reported incidence of between 0.8% and 3.2%.[5,7,17] The incidence is generally equal between males and females. Most commonly affected levels are L4-L5 and L5-S1. Weight lifting, gymnastics, wrestling, and collision sports are high-risk sports for disk herniation.[2–11]

Mechanism

Disk herniation can result either from acute or repetitive trauma. In skeletally immature adolescents compression force during forward flexion can result in disk herniation and may involve herniation of the disk vertically through the end plate. In many adolescents with disk herniation, other congenital spine anomalies are found such as spina bifida occulta, transitional vertebra, or congenital spinal stenosis.

Clinical Presentation

Athlete may present with a history of sudden onset pain related to a particular activity or insidious onset, intermittent activity-related pain of several weeks or months duration. A clear history of acute trauma is elicited in only 40% to 50% of the patients. The most common presenting symptoms are back and leg pain and stiffness that are exacerbated with activity. The pain may or may not radiate to legs and generally neurological signs are absent in most children and adolescents (Table 30-13).[14,17] Pain is also exacerbated by coughing, sneezing, or sitting. In some athletes lumbar radicular signs may be elicited. Most have limitation of lumbosacral spine movement and mild scoliosis may be detected in some patients. Positive straight leg raise sign is the most common finding present in almost all patients. Listing toward the side of herniation may also be present. Hamstring tightness is common and early sign of disk herniation.

Diagnostic Imaging

MRI is the study of choice to detect disk herniation and any neurological compromise. Positive MRI scan findings must be correlated with clinical findings because many individuals have abnormalities on MRI scan that are of no clinical significance.

Treatment

In the absence of neurological signs the initial treatment is conservative with relative rest, restriction from sports and initiating physical therapy. Most adolescents respond well to conservative treatment over a period of several weeks, typically 6 to 12 weeks. Failure of clinical improvement with conservative treatment

Table 30-13.

Common Radicular Syndromes of the Lumbar Spine				
Disk Level	Nerve Root	Motor Deficit	Sensory Deficit	Reflex Compromise
L3–L4	L4	Quadriceps (knee extension)	Anterolateral thigh Anterior knee Medial leg and foot	Patellar
L4–L5	L5	Extensor hallucis longus (great toe extension)	Lateral thigh Anterolateral leg Middorsal foot	Medial hamstrings
L5–S1	S1	Gastrocnemius Soleus Flexor digitorum longus Tibialis posterior (ankle plantar flexion)	Posterior leg Lateral foot	Achilles

and presence of any neurological signs (initially or later) are indications for surgical consultation for definitive treatment. Some advocate more aggressive surgical treatment for young athletes with disk herniation. Prognosis in young athletes is excellent for return to full sport participation following appropriate treatment.

SLIPPED VERTEBRAL APOPHYSIS (FRACTURE OF RING APOPHYSIS)

Definition and Epidemiology

A fracture through the weak osteocartilagenous junction between the vertebral body and its apophysis results in displacement and protrusion into the spinal canal of the fractured segment along with the associated intervertebral disk.[8,17] This injury is unique to adolescents, more common in males, and most commonly involves the inferior apophysis of L4. Most cases are reported in wrestling and gymnastics.

Mechanism

Apophyseal fractures and displacement can result from either acute or repetitive trauma from compressive loads applied to the spine during flexion.

Clinical Presentation

In general, symptoms and signs are similar to that of acute central disk herniation. The athlete typically presents with acute lumbar pain with onset during activity usually weight lifting or other sports that require

hyperflexion of lumbar spine. Pain may be described as burning and radiate into the leg. The pain is exacerbated by sitting, coughing, and sneezing. Pain is also elicited by contralateral straight leg raise. Because of posterior central protrusion lumbar, radicular signs may be elicited on examination; however, neurological findings are uncommon in most adolescents which may delay diagnosis.

Diagnostic Imaging

AP and lateral x-rays of the lumbar spine may or may not show the bony avulsion. A CT scan and/or MRI scan may be indicated to further delineate the injury.

Treatment

Patient should be restricted from sports and referred to orthopedics for definitive treatment. Most consider surgical excision of the fractured fragment as the treatment of choice.

FRACTURES OF THE THORACOLUMBAR SPINE

Definitions and Epidemiology

Acute fractures of the thoracolumbar spine are uncommon in youth sports; most are owing to motor vehicle accidents, falls or abuse in the very young child and approximately 25% may be associated with neurological injury.[1,8,10] Fractures of the thoracolumbar spine have been reported in adolescents participating in collision sports such as American football, ice hockey, and rugby.

Most are seen in adolescents more than 16 years of age in whom the fracture characteristics are similar to those seen in adults. The most frequently injured area is from T4 to T12.[1,2,8,17] Spinal cord injury without a bony fracture (spinal cord injury without radiographic abnormality), most affecting the cervical spine, is a unique injury seen mostly in very young children whereas vertebral apophyseal and endplate injuries are unique to adolescents.

Mechanisms

The key mechanisms for spine fractures include (a) sudden hyperflexion of the spine with or without vertebral body compression; (b) distraction of the spine; and (c) shearing force.[1,2,8,17] Axial loading or compression of the flexed or straight spine can cause a vertebral body compression or a burst fracture seen in sports. Fracture of the apophysis of the spinous process, mostly of the thoracic spine, can result from sudden distraction force.

Clinical Presentation

The athlete typically is injured in a collision sport and present with a history of acute onset back pain with or without neurological findings. Most will present on the field or in the emergency department following the injury and should be further evaluated and treated by physicians with expertise in the management of spinal trauma.

Diagnostic Imaging

According to the Denis theory the spinal column is divided into three segments (Figure 30-25).[1,2,17] Based on findings on imaging studies the fractures are classified as either stable or unstable. Fractures that involve either 1 column or have intact middle column are considered stable whereas fractures that involve 2 columns are considered unstable. Initial x-rays are done with the athlete still immobilized appropriately following the spine injury protocol, followed by CT scan and MRI scan in case of neurological findings to better delineate the injury.

Treatment

Pediatric athletes with acute traumatic spine fractures should be referred to orthopedic surgeon for further evaluation and definitive management with long-term follow-up.

SI Joint Pain

SIJ is a diarthrodial joint with minimal movements in transverse or longitudinal planes not exceeding 2 to 3 degrees.[35] The prevalence of low back pain directly related to SIJ in young athletes is not known. SIJ pain has been reported most commonly in rowing and cross-

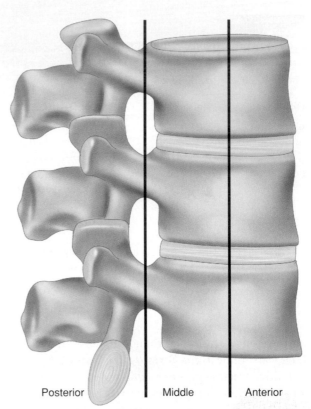

FIGURE 30-25 ■ Denis 3-column of spine. The spine is divided into three columns: anterior (anterior longitudinal ligament, anterior half of the annulus fibrosus, and anterior half vertebral body), middle (posterior longitudinal ligament, posterior half of the annulus fibrosus, and posterior half vertebral body), and posterior (osseous and ligamentous structures posterior to the posterior longitudinal ligament or interspinous ligaments).

country skiing. Pain may be in the lower back, buttocks, back of thighs or pelvis. Tenderness may be localized over the SIJ and pain may be elicited or exacerbated with some provocative tests such as FABER and Gaenslen. The diagnosis is mainly based on history and examination findings. Imaging studies may be indicated to exclude other causes of pain. Chronic SIJ pain may be difficult to treat. In addition to relative rest, modification of activities, and use of NSAIDs various other treatment modalities have been reported with variable success in individual cases. These include manual or manipulative treatment, prolotherapy, intra-articular injections of local anesthetics and corticosteroids, and radiofrequency neurotomy.[35–38] Athletes with significant chronic pain should be referred to experts with experience in treating SIJ pain and dysfunction.

REFERENCES

1. Clark P, Letts M. Trauma to the thoracic and lumbar spine in the adolescent. *Can J Surg.* 2001;44(5):337-345.
2. Ferguson RL. Thoracic and lumbar spine trauma of the immature spine. In: Herkowitz HN, Garfin SR, Eismont

FJ, Bell GR, Balderston RA, eds. *Rothman-Simeone The Spine*, 5th ed. Philadelphia: Saunders; 2005:603-612.

3. Lamon RD. Growth and maturation of the spine from birth to adolescence. *J Bone Joint Surg.* 2007;89-A:3-7.

4. Dimeglio A. Growth in pediatric orthopaedics. *J Pediatr Orthop.* 2001;21:549-555.

5. Waicus KM, Smith BW. Back injuries in the pediatric athlete. *Curr Sport Med Rep.* 2002;1:52-58.

6. Curtis C, d'Hemecourt P. Diagnosis and management of back pain in adolescents. *Adoles Med.* 2007;18(1):140-164.

7. d'Hemecourt PA, Gerbino PG, Micheli LJ. Back injuries in the young athlete. *Clin Sport Med.* 2000;19(4):663-679.

8. Richards BS, McCarthy RE, Akbarnia BA. Back pain in childhood and adolescence. *AAOS Instruct Course Lectures.* 1999;48:525-542.

9. Karol LA. Back pain in children and adolescents, Chap 31. In: Herkowitz HN, Garfin SR, Eismont FJ, Bell GR, Balderston RA, eds. *Rothman-Simeone The Spine*, 5th ed. Philadelphia: Saunders;2005:493-506.

10. Jones GT, Macfarlane GJ. Epidemiology of low back pain in children and adolescents. *Arch Dis Childhood.* 2005;90:312-316.

11. Bono CM. Low-back pain in athletes. *J Bone Joint Surg Am.* 2004;86-A(2):382-396.

12. Trainor TJ, Wiesel SW. Epidemiology of back pain in the athlete. *Clin Sport Med.* 2002;21(1):93-103.

13. Hoppenfeld S. *Examination of Spine and Extremities: Physical Examination of the Lumbar Spine.* Philadelphia: Appleton-Lange; 1976:237-263.

14. Hoppenfeld S. *Orhtopedic Neurology: A Diagnostic Guide to Neurologic Levels.* Baltimore: Lippincott Williams Wilkins; 1997.

15. Magee DJ. *Orthopedic Physical Assessment*, 3rd ed. Philadelphia: WB Saunders; 1997:331-433.

16. Dutton M. *Orthopedic Examination, Evaluation, and Intervention.* New York: McGraw Hill Medical; 2004:1152-1336.

17. Herring JA. Back pain. *Tachdjian's Pediatric Orthopaedics*, 3rd ed. Philadelphia: Saunders Elsevier; 2002:95-108.

18. Dormans JP, Moroz L. Infection and tumors of the spine in children. *J Bone Joint Surg Am.* 2007;89:79-97.

19. Sorensen KH. Scheuermann's Juvenile Kyphosis: Clinical Appearance, Radiography, Aetiology and Prognosis. Copenhagen: Munksgaad; 1964.

20. Parent S, Newton PO, Wenger DR. Adolescent idiopathic scoliosis: etiology, anatomy, natural history, and bracing. *AAOS Instructional Course Lectures.* 2005;54:529-536.

21. Dolan LA, Weinstein SL. Surgical rates after observation and bracing for adolescent idiopathic scoliosis: an evidence based review. *Spine.* 2007;32(19 supp):S91-100.

22. Rowe DE, Bernstein SM, Riddick MF, Adler F, Emans JB, Gardner-Bonneau D. A meta analysis of the efficacy of non-operative treatments for idiopathic scoliosis. *J Bone Joint Surg Am.* 1997;79(5):664-674.

23. Charles YP, Daures JP, de Rosa V, Dimegglio A. Progression risk of idiopathic juvenile scoliosis during pubertal growth. *Spine.* 2006;31(17):1933-1942.

24. Sanders JO, Browne RH, McConnell SJ, Margraf SA, Coney TF, Finegold DN. Maturity assessment and curve progression in girls with idiopathic scoliosis. *J Bone Joint Surg Am.* 2007;89(1):64-73.

25. Tanner JM, Whitehouse RH. Clinical longitudinal standards for height, weight, height velocity and the stages of puberty. *Arch Dis Chil.* 1976;51:170-179.

26. Greulich WW, Pyle SI. *Radiographic Atlas of Skeletal Development of Hand and Wrist*, 2nd ed. Stanford, CA: Stanford University Press; 1959.

27. Dimeglio A, Charles YP, Daures JP, et al. Accuracy of the Sauvergrain method in determining skeletal age during puberty. *J Bone Joint Surg.* 2005;87-A:1689-1696.

28. Perdriolle R, Vidal J. Thoracic idiopathic scoliosis curve progression and prognosis. *Spine.* 1985;10:785-791.

29. Mooney JF. Spondylolysis and spondylolisthesis, Chap 36. In: Herkowitz HN, Garfin SR, Eismont FJ, Bell GR, Balderston RA, eds. *Rothman-Simeone The Spine*, 5th ed. Philadelphia: Saunders; 2005:586-602.

30. Cavalier R, Herman MJ, Cheung EV, Pizzutillo PD. Spondylolysis and spondylolisthesis in children and adolescents: diagnosis, natural history, and nonsurgical management. *J Am Acad Orthop Surg.* 2006;14: 417-424.

31. McCleary MD, Congeni JA. Current concepts in the diagnosis and treatment of spondylolysis in young athletes. *Curr Sport Med Rep.* 2007;6(1):62-66.

32. Congeni J, McCulloch J, Swanson K. Lumbar spondylolysis. A study of natural progression in athletes. *Am J Sport Med.* 1997;25(2):248-253.

33. Miller SF, Congeni J, Swanson K. Long-term functional and anatomical follow-up of early detected spondylolysis in young athletes. *Am J Sport Med.* 2004;32(4):928-933.

34. Stasinopoulos D. Treatment of spondylolysis with external electrical stimulation in young athletes: a critical literature review. *Br J Sport Med.* 2004;38:352-354.

35. Brolinson PG, Kozar AJ, Cibor G. Sacroiliac joint dysfunction in athletes. *Curr Sport Med Rep.* 2003;2:47-56.

36. Foley BS, Buschbacher RM. Sacroiliac joint pain. *Am J Phys Med Rehab.* 2006;85(12):997-1006.

37. Hansen HC, McKenzie-Brown AM, Cohen SP, et al. Sacroiliac joint interventions: a systematic review. *Pain Phys.* 2007;10:165-184.

38. Rabago D, Best TM, Beamsley M, Patterson J. A systematic review of prolotherapy for chronic musculoskeletal pain. *Clin J Sport Med.* 2005;15:376.

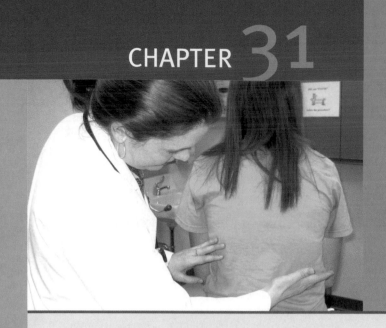

CHAPTER 31

Stress Fractures

Steven Cline and Dilip R. Patel

DEFINITIONS AND EPIDEMIOLOGY

A stress fracture is a fatigue fracture resulting from repetitive, excessive load applied to a normal bone.[1-4] On the other hand a "normal" amount of load applied to a weak or structurally abnormal bone results in an insufficiency fracture.

The reported incidence and the site of stress fracture vary by sport (Table 31-1).[1-3] Stress fractures are more frequent in track and field athletes than in other sports. The incidence can range from 3% in soccer players to 15% in runners, and stress fractures account for between 7% and 20% of all injuries seen in sport medicine clinic.[5] Overall, stress fracture of the tibia is the most common. Stress fractures are more common in females, some studies reporting a rate 10 times higher than males.

MECHANISM

Stress fractures are caused by overuse. Bone is constantly remodeling, and under the repetitive stress of athletics resorption of the bone in a particular area (e.g., the lateral femoral neck or the tibial shaft in runners) may outpace bone formation (Figure 31-1). This follows an increase in training intensity, often within 6 to 8 weeks of the change. High-performance athletes often have a protein calorie imbalance and train so intensely that it is difficult for them to take in adequate protein, calcium, and other nutrients without eating a high-calorie, high-protein diet.[6,7] It is theorized that multiple factors contribute to eventual fatigue fracture of the bone, and in addition to the excessive physical activity, other factors include bone density at the site, the geometry of the bone, the direction of the load, the vascular supply at the site, the muscle attachments, and the specific sport.[1-4,8]

Female athletes participating in sports that require maintaining a thin body habitus may engage in weight control by restricting caloric intake at the same time expending significant calories. This is often complicated by menstrual irregularities, amenorrhea, and a hypoestrogenic state. In addition to caloric deficit, these athletes also have dietary intake deficient in calcium, vitamins, and other essential nutrients. A higher incidence of stress fractures is reported in these female athletes.

Table 31-1.

Stress Fracture by Sport

Sport	Fracture
Aerobics	Fibula, tibia
Ballet dancing	Tibia
Baseball	Humerus, scapula, rib, patella
Basketball	Patella, tibia, calcaneus
Cricket	Humerus
Curling	Ulna
Fencing	Pubic ramus
Gymnastics	Pars interarticularis
Handball	Metacarpal
Javelin	Ulna
Jumping	Pelvis, femur
Running	Tibia, fibula, metatarsal, tarsal
Soccer	Tibia, metatarsal
Skating	Fibula
Swimming	Tibia, metatarsal
Tennis	Ulna, metacarpal

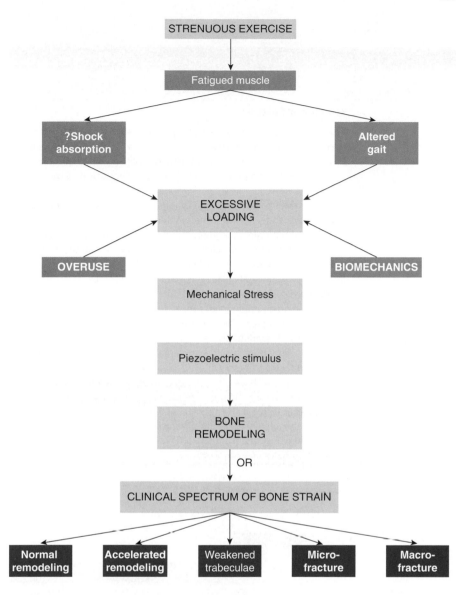

FIGURE 31-1 ■ Possible evolution of stress reaction and stress fracture of bone. *(Used with permission from Reid DC. Sports Injury Assessment and Rehabilitation, NY: Churchill Livingstone, 1992, Fig 6-14, p 123.)*

CLINICAL PRESENTATION

The cardinal symptom of stress fracture is activity-related insidious onset pain generally with a history of preceding increase in the volume and intensity of the physical activity. Initially the pain may be mild and only during activity. The athlete typically continues to play until the intensity of the pain increases and the pain may occur even at rest. By then athlete is not able to effectively continue to play. Key elements to be ascertained in the history are listed in Table 31-2.

The physical examination may reveal localized tenderness if the involved bone is superficial. In case of lower extremity stress fractures the athlete may have pain on weight bearing. Depending upon the site of the stress fracture there may be pain on movement of the joint. The differential diagnosis of bone pain and tenderness must always include benign or malignant neoplasm of the bone and osteomyelitis.

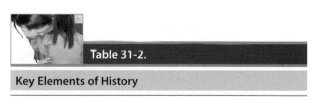

Table 31-2.

Key Elements of History

Characteristics of the pain
Type, intensity, volume, duration, and change in the level of activity
Known medical condition that may affect bone
Therapeutic medication that may cause osteopenia
Caloric intake, dietary habits, nutrient intake
Attempt to lose weight, methods to lose weight
Past history of stress fractures
Menstrual history in female athletes
Use of anabolic androgenic steroids
Systemic symptoms such as fever, joint pain, undue fatigue, unintended weight loss, loss of appetite
Symptoms associated with pain such as tingling, numbness

Table 31-3.

High-Risk Stress Fractures

Fracture	Key Clinical Features
Femoral neck (Figure 31-2)	Insidious onset groin or anterior thigh pain. Pain may be referred to the knee. Often night time pain in the groin. Pain on weight bearing, limping, and antalgic gait. Pain with internal and external rotation of the hip at the end of the range of motion. Diagnosis may be delayed up to 14 weeks.
Patella	Insidious onset pain on the patella aggravated with knee extension. Localized tenderness over the patella.
Anterior cortex of the tibia (Figure 31-3)	Leg pain with running and jumping that progresses to pain at rest. Pain and tenderness localizes over the middle third of the anterior tibia. May have palpable thickening over the area.
Medial malleolus	Insidious onset medial ankle pain. Localized tenderness.
Talus	Gradual onset of lateral ankle or subtalar pain. Pain on ankle movements. Ankle pain on jumping and running. Foot may be hyperpronated.
Tarsal navicular (Figure 31-4)	Nonspecific foot pain often radiates to medial arch. Pain on weight bearing and standing on toes with the foot in equinus or on hopping on toes. Tenderness over the proximal navicular. Diagnosis may be delayed for up to 4 months.
Fifth metatarsal at the junction of proximal diaphysis and tuberosity	Pain in the foot with weight bearing. Pain aggravated after prolonged walking or running. Localized tenderness over the proximal fifth metatarsal. Pain may be aggravated with inversion of the ankle.
Sesamoids of great toe	Often disabling pain under the great toe. Localized tenderness. Pain is of gradual onset. Pain aggravated with hyperextension of great toe and athlete trying to push off.

Clinically stress fractures can be grouped into high risk (Table 31-3) and low risk (Table 31-4).[9–15] High-risk stress fractures are important to recognize early to prevent complications that include delayed or nonunion, local avascular necrosis, and progression to a complete fracture.

DIAGNOSTIC IMAGING

Plain x-rays are usually the initial study indicated when a stress fracture is suspected. X-rays show periosteal reaction, cortical lucency, or a fracture line in the cortex of the bone, whereas focal necrosis without periosteal reaction is typically seen in cancellous bone.[3] X-rays have a high rate of false negative results and remain normal for 2 to 3 weeks of onset of symptoms.

Technetium-99 diphosphonate bone scan is highly sensitive and positive within 3 days of onset of symptoms. Localized area of increased uptake in all three phases (phase I or blood flow or angiographic phase, phase II or the blood pool or soft tissue phase, and phase III or delayed images phase) is the characteristic finding. Radionuclide scan is nonspecific and is also positive in other conditions such as osteomyelitis and

Table 31-4.

Low-Risk Stress Fractures

Upper extremity
- Clavicle
- Scapula
- Humerus
- Olecranon
- Ulna
- Radius
- Scaphoid
- Metacarpals

Thorax, spine, pelvis
- Ribs
- Pars interarticularis
- Sacrum
- Pubic rami

Lower extremity
- Femoral shaft
- Tibial shaft
- Fibula
- Calcaneus
- Metatarsal shaft

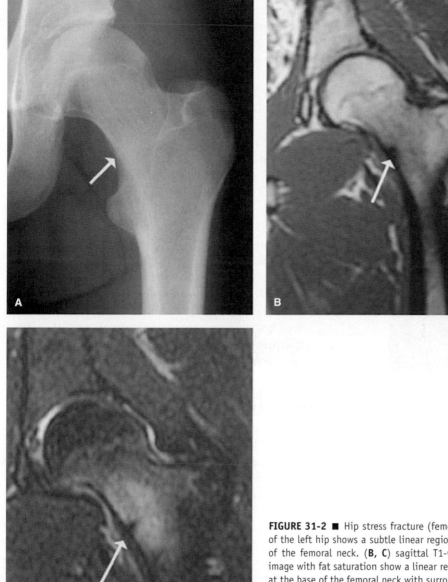

FIGURE 31-2 ■ Hip stress fracture (femoral neck). (**A**) Anteroposterior radiograph of the left hip shows a subtle linear region of sclerosis (arrow) in the medial aspect of the femoral neck. (**B, C**) sagittal T1-weighted image and sagittal T2-weighted image with fat saturation show a linear region of decreased signal intensity (arrows) at the base of the femoral neck with surrounding edema. (*Used with permission from, Sanders TG, Fults-ganey C. Imaging of sports-related injuries. In: DeLee JC, Drez D Jr, Miller MD, eds. DeLee and Drez's Orthopaedic Sports Medicine, 2nd ed. Philadelphia: Saunders Elsevier; 2003, Figure 16A-21, p. 577.*)

osteoid osteoma. The resolution of the radionuclide scan images can be enhanced by single-photon emission computed tomography (SPECT).

Magnetic resonance imaging (MRI) scan is the diagnostic study of choice in the evaluation of stress fractures. A band-like fracture line is the characteristic finding in case of a stress fracture. The MRI may also show an amorphous alteration of the bone marrow signal or periosteal reaction, a finding consistent with stress reaction or prefracture stage. A classification system for grading stress fractures based on

findings of radionuclide and MRI studies is presented in Table 31-5.[3]

TREATMENT

Injury rehabilitation for stress fractures is divided into three stages: (1) the acute stage, (2) recovery, and (3) enhancement stage. During the acute stage the focus is on allowing the injury to heal and decreasing symptoms. Activity is usually quite limited and the athlete

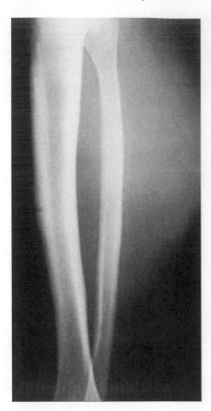

FIGURE 31-3 ■ Stress fracture of the anterior cortex of the tibia. Note the linear black line in the anterior cortex.

may be placed in a nonweight-bearing cast or orthosis. The recovery stage begins when the athlete is pain-free and imaging studies show healing of the injury. The athlete is then gradually advanced in strength and flexibility training, and when pain-free with 75% to 80% of normal strength, the enhancement stage is begun. During this stage further strengthening, core fitness, and sport-specific techniques are added. The core and strength and conditioning facets of this phase should be continued after return to play has occurred to prevent further injury.

Under treating a high-risk stress fracture such as a tension sided femoral neck fracture can lead to catastrophic failure of the bone, prolonged loss of playing time, and can lead to severe long-term sequelae for the young athlete. Athletes with low-risk stress fractures may be allowed to return to play with specific limitations in many cases, and high-risk stress fracture patients should be kept from play and treated aggressively.[9] The management and return to play strategies for high-risk stress fractures are summarized in Table 31-6 and for low-risk stress fractures in Table 31-7.

Another tenet which must be adhered to is to optimize the nutritional status of the athlete. Beyond the female athletic triad, many athletes overtrain, and in relative terms do not consume enough protein and calories to sustain the large catabolic demands they place on their bodies. This leaves them more susceptible to stress fractures and other injuries.

The overall differential of leg pain as well as stress fractures must always include compartment syndrome, medial tibial stress syndrome, infections, and tumor. Any child with pain in a long bone or joint deserves a careful and meticulous workup and appropriate imaging and laboratory studies. Laboratory studies should include serum calcium, phosphorus, alkaline phosphatase and nutritional parameters, as well as a complete blood count and erythrocyte sedimentation rate. Early referral to the appropriate specialist, in particular with an apparent tumor to the orthopedic oncologist is the best course of treatment (Box 31-1).[16]

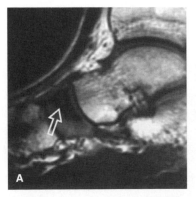
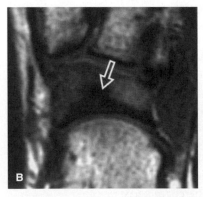
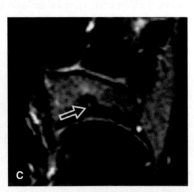

FIGURE 31-4 ■ Tarsal navicular stress fracture. (**A**) sagittal T1-weighted image shows gray signal marrow edema in the dorsal aspect of the navicular adjacent to the site of a sagittal plane stress fracture (arrow). (**B**) Coronal T1-weighted image shows a linear black stress fracture line extending from the talonavicular articular surface in the dorsal aspect of the central navicular (arrow). (**C**) Coronal T2-weighted image shows bright signal marrow edema surrounding the fracture line (arrow), involving the proximal articular surface of the navicular. (*Used with permission from Smith DK, Gilley JS. Imaging of sports injuries of the foot and ankle. In: DeLee JC, Drez D Jr, Miller MD, eds. DeLee and Drez's Orthopaedic Sports Medicine, 2nd ed. Philadelphia: Saunders Elsevier; 2003, Figure 30B-25, p. 2214.*).

Table 31-5.

Radiologic Grading System of Stress Fractures

Grade	Radiograph	Bone Scan	MRI	Treatment (weeks of rest)
1	Normal	Mild uptake confined to one cortex	Positive STIR* image	3
2	Normal	Moderate activity, larger lesion (confined to unicortical area)	Positive STIR and T2-weighted images	3–6
3	Discrete line (+/–) Periosteal reaction (+/–)	Increased activity	No definite cortical (>50% width of bone) Positive T1- and T2-weighted images	12–16
4	Fracture or periosteal reaction	More intense bicortical uptake	Fracture line Positive T1- and T2-weighted images	16+

*Short T1 inversion recovery.
Used with permission from Boden BP, Osbahr DC, Jimenez C. Low-risk risk factors. Am. J. Sport. Med. 2001;29(1):100-111.

Table 31-6.

Management of and Return-to-Play Strategies for High-Risk Stress Fractures

Anatomic Site	Complications	Suggested Treatment	Level of Data
Femoral neck	Displacement Nonunion Avascular necrosis	Tension: Strict NWB or bed rest Surgical fixation RTP when healed Compression: NWB until pain-free with radiographic evidence of healing, then slow activity progression RTP after no pain on examination or with any activities Surgical fixation (optional)	Level C (expert opinion) Level D (case series)
Anterior tibia	Nonunion	Nonoperative: NWB until pain-free with ADL; pneumatic leg splints	Level A (RCT)
	Delayed union	RTP with slow progression after nontender and pain-free with ADL (9 mo)	Level B (nonrandomized)
	Fracture progression	Operative: Intramedullary nailing RTP is usually faster (2–4 mo)	Levels C and D
Medial malleolus	Fracture progression Nonunion	Nonoperative: (no fracture line) 4–6 wk pneumatic casting Avoid impact; rehabilitation RTP when nontender, no pain with ADL Operative: (fracture line, nonunion, or progression) ORIF with bone graft	Levels C and D
Tarsal navicular	Nonunion	Nonoperative: NWB cast 6–8 wk, then WB cast 6–8 wk	Levels C and D
	Delayed union Displacement	RTP is gradual after pain-free with ADL Orthotics and rehabilitation suggested Operative: (Complete, nonunion) RTP only when healed	

(continued)

Table 31-6. (Continued)

Management of and Return-to-Play Strategies for High-Risk Stress Fractures

Anatomic Site	Complications	Suggested Treatment	Level of Data
Talus	Nonunion Delayed union	Nonoperative: NWB cast 6–8 wk RTP is gradual after pain-free with ADL Orthotics and rehabilitation suggested Operative: Reserved for nonunion	Level C
Patella	Displacement Fracture completion	Nonoperative: (Nondisplaced) Long-leg NWB cast 4–6 wk Rehabilitation following RTP is gradual after pain-free with ADL Operative: Horizontal – ORIF Vertical – lateral fragment excision RTP when healed	Level C
Seasmoids	Nonunion Delayed union Refracture	Nonoperative: NWB 6–8 wk RTP is gradual after pain-free with ADL Operative: Excision if fail nonoperative	Level C

Fifth metatarsal	Nonunion
	Delayed union
	
	Refracture
		Nonoperative: (No fracture line)
		NWB cast 4–6 wk followed by WB cast
		    until healed
		RTP after nontender and pain-free
		Operative: (Fracture line, nonunion, or
		    individual at high risk for refracture)
		Intramedullary screw fixation
		RTP 6-8 week, early ROM/rehabilitation
			Levels C and D

ADL, activities of daily living; NWB, non-weight bearing; ORIF, open reduction with internal fixation; RCT, randomized controlled trial; ROM, range of motion; RTP, return to play; WB, weight bearing.
Used with permission from Diehl JJ, Best TM, Kaeding CC. Classification and return-to-play considerations for stress fractures. Clin. Sport. Med. 2006;17-28. Philadelphia: Saunders Elsevier.

Table 31-7.

Low-Risk Stress Fracture Treatment Guide

Symptoms	Goal	Treatment Suggestions
Any level of pain	Heal injury	Titrate activity to a pain-free level for 4–8 wk depending on the grade of injury Braces/crutches Modify risk factors
Pain with no functional limitations	Continue participation	Titrate activity to a stable or decreasing level of pain Closely follow Modify risk factors
Pain with functional limitation	Continue participation	Decrease activity level to point at which pain level is decreasing and until a functional level of pain has been achieved, then titrate activity to stable or continued decrease level of pain. Modify risk factors
Limiting pain intensifies despite functional activity modification (i.e., unable to continue to perform at any reasonable functional level despite activity modification)	Heal injury	Complete rest Immobilization Surgery Modify risk factors

Used with permission from Diehl JJ, Best TM, Kaeding CC. Classification and return-to-play considerations for stress fractures. Clin. Sport. Med. 2006;17-28. Philadelphia: Saunders Elsevier.

> **Box 31-1 When to Refer.**
>
> ■ Orthopedic consultation is generally indicated in high-risk stress fractures because of high risk for delayed union, nonunion, and avascular necrosis, and progression to complete fracture. Some of these fractures may require operative intervention.
> ■ Osteomyelitis indicates consultation with orthopedics and infectious disease specialist
> ■ Bone tumors indicate consultation with orthopedic oncologist

REFERENCES

1. Matheson GO, Clement DB, McKenzie DC, et al. Stress fracture in athletes. *Am J Sport Med.* 1987;15:46-58.

2. McBryde AM. Stress fractures in athletes. *J Sport Med.* 1975;3:212-217.

3. Boden BP, Osbahr DC, Jimenez C. Low-risk stress fractures. *Am J Sport Med.* 2001;29(1):100-111.

4. Carpenter D, Matheson G, Carter D. Stress fractures and stress injuries in bone. In: Garrick J, ed. *Orthopedic Knowledge Update: Sports Medicine III.* Chicago, IL: American Academy of Orthopedic Surgeions; 2004:273-283.

5. Fredericson M, Jennings F, Beaulieu C, Matheson G. Stress fractures in athletes. *Top Magn Reson Imaging.* 2006; 17(5):309-325.

6. Harmon K. Lower extremity stress fractures. *Clin J Sport Med.* 2003;13(6):358-364.

7. Salminen S, Bostman O, Kiuru M, Pihlajamaki H. Bilateral femoral fatigue fractures an unusual fracture in a military recruit. *CORR.* 2006;456:259-263.

8. Bolin D, Kemper A, Brolinson G. Current concepts in the evaluation and management of stress fractures. *Curr Rep Sport Med.* 2005;4:295-300.

9. Johansson C, Ekenman I, Tornkvist H, et al. Stress fracture of the femoral neck in athletes: the consequences of a delay in diagnosis. *Am J Sport Med.* 1990;18:524-528.

10. Torg JS, Pavlov H, Cooley LH, et al. Stress fractures of the tarsal navicular: a retrospective review of twenty-one cases. *JBJS-A.* 1982;64:700-712.

11. Chen R, Shia D, Ganesh V Kamath, Thomas A, Wright R. Troublesome stress fractures of the foot and ankle. *Sport Med Arthrosc Rev.* 2006;14(4):246-251.

12. Shelbourne KD, Fisher DA, Rettig AC, et al. Stress fractures of the medial malleolus. *Am J Sport Med.* 1988;16:60-63.

13 Smith A. The skeletally immature knee: what's new in overuse injuries? Instructional Course Lectures. *AAOS.* 2003;52:691–697.

14. Hutchinson M, Ireland ML. Overuse and throwing injuries in the skeletally immature athlete. *Instructional Course Lectures, AAOS.* 2003;52:25–36.

15. Diehl JJ, Best TM, Kaeding CC. Classification and return-to-play considerations for stress fractures. *Clin Sport Med.* 2006;25:17-28.

16. Kaeding C, Yu J, Wright R, Amendola A, Spindler K. Management and return to play of stress fractures. *Clin J Sport Med.* 2005;15(6):442-447.

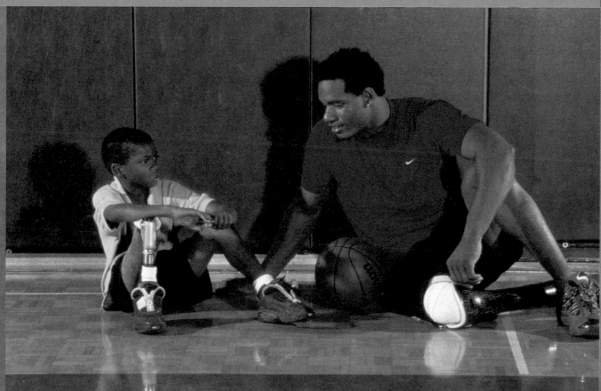

Team Physician, Emergencies, and Other Topics

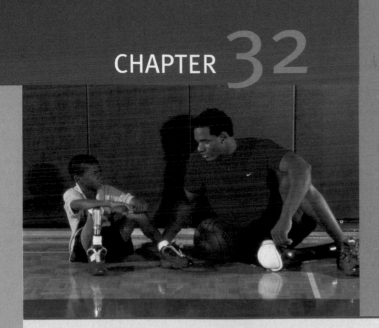

CHAPTER 32

Team Physician

*Daniel G. Constance and
Robert J. Baker*

TEAM PHYSICIAN ROLE AND RESPONSIBILITIES

The team physician is the medical team leader who is ultimately responsible for the safety and care of the athlete. The day-to-day role of the team physician varies dependent on the situation and the members of the sports medicine team that may include an athletic trainer, school nurse, dentist, nutritionist, psychologist, and other physician specialists. The team physician's role should be a formal relationship with the team, even if volunteer. This agreement, among other things, should include complete autonomy in medical decisions and guarantees against acts of coercion. It is important to specifically avoid conflicts of interest, so that the safety and health of the athlete are the first priority of the physician.

The Team Physician Consensus Statements (Appendixes 32-1 and 32-2) outline the qualifications and responsibilities of the team physician and provide guidance for sideline preparedness for the team physician.[1,2]

The consensus statement further defines the duties of the team physician.[1] A full range of Consensus and Position Statements relevant to team physician are easily accessible at the websites for the American College of Sports Medicine (www.acsm.org) and the American Academy of Family Physicians (www.aafp.org), and all physicians assuming responsibilities of a team physician should be familiar with these guidelines.[1–5]

Medicolegal Aspects

The responsibilities of the team physician present a few unique medicolegal situations. One major difference that may exist is that athletes are typically highly motivated and may aggressively push to return to play. In addition, there may be third parties such as parents or coaches that challenge physician decisions regarding delay of return-to-play. In the case of the a young athlete, the physician should be cognizant of the parent–child relationship that may interfere with treatment or return-to-play. Additionally, there is a potential conflict-or-interest when the physician is employed by the sports team. The team physician must specifically be aware of and avoid or mitigate conflicts of interest and be mindful that their primary responsibility is to the safety and health of the athlete.

When acting as a treating physician, the physician–athlete relationship remains fiduciary in nature. Therefore, the same principles apply in sports medicine as in the general practice of medicine. The team physician must use the knowledge, skills, and care that are ordinarily possessed by prudent members of their specialty, given the state of medical science at the time care was rendered.[6] Evaluations and medical decision making must be documented whether in-office, athletic training room, gym, or on the field. The same principles of informed consent apply to the team physician. In general, the athlete, and if a minor, his or her parents, must have all material information regarding the diagnoses, treatment options, as well as risks and benefits of those options explained in lay terms, so that they may make a truly informed decision. The team physician must also be mindful of issues related to disclosure of information. Generally, there should be explicit written consent for information to be provided to parties other than the athlete. However, in the case of the physician employed by the team, where records are the property of the team, the physician must be mindful of the implications of what records may contain.

Issues regarding exclusion of athletic participation are another area of potential legal action. If a physician is performing a preparticipation medical screening for the purpose of athletic participation, and there is not a treatment relationship present, the courts have set the precedent that the traditional patient–physician relationship is not present and torts for medical malpractice have been dismissed. However, a contractual relationship exists and the physician is still responsible to inform the athlete of findings made during the examination, and need for further investigations and care. Additionally, athletes should be informed of the limits of the screening examination. As long as exclusions from participation are based on the best medical information available, the courts have upheld these medical exclusions. The Rehabilitation Act and the Americans with Disabilities Act require balancing the physical disabilities a person may have with the personal risks and safety of the sport. Ultimately any decision for exclusion should include evaluation of the condition, risks to the athlete and others, and safety equipment that may mitigate risks. The legal atmosphere in sports medicine continues to evolve and the team physician should continue to monitor those changes, through participation in national and local medical societies.

Table 32-1.

Secondary Survey

A → Airway
　　Need for advanced/definitive airway
　　Trachea midline
　　Subcutaneous emphysema

B → Breathing
　　Supplemental oxygen
　　Pneumothorax
　　Wheezing
　　Need for beta agonist

C → Circulation
　　Pulse volumes
　　Blood pressure
　　Intravenous access
　　Severe bleeding
　　Jugular venous distension (tension pneumothorax, tamponade)

D → Deformity/disability
　　Altered level of consciousness
　　Cervical spine
　　Major joint dislocation
　　Fractures

E → Exposure/environment
　　Checking occult injuries
　　Hyperthermia/hypothermia

General Approach to Emergencies on the Field

As with all aspects of medical care, the on-field emergency starts with the basic life support (BLS) principles of the primary survey. The primary survey includes initial evaluation of the ABCDs: (1) airway, (2) breathing, (3) circulation, and (4) defibrillation. Fortunately, in most athletic settings, this is easily accomplished when seeing the athlete with a major injury calling out in pain. However, the physician should always remember to return to the primary survey should the situation fail to improve, or worse yet, deteriorate. Once the primary survey is complete, the physician can continue to the secondary survey following the principles of advance cardiac life support (ACLS), pediatric advanced life support (PALS), and advanced trauma life support (ATLS). The secondary survey includes a head-to-toe evaluation of the ABCDEs as listed in Table 32-1. Any injury that is serious or of potential seriousness should prompt the physician to activate the medical protocol for emergent or urgent transport to an appropriate facility for continued evaluation and treatment.

REFERENCES

1. Herring SA, Bergfeld JA, Boyd J, et al. Team physician consensus statement. *Med Sci Sport Exerc.* 2000;32(4):877.
2. Herring SA, et al. The team physician and conditioning of athletes for sports: a consensus statement. *Med Sci Sport Exerc.* 2001;33(10):1789-1793.
3. Herring SA, Bergfeld J, Boyd J, et al. Sideline preparedness for the team physician: a consensus statement. *Med Sci Sport Exerc.* 2001;35(5):846-849.
4. Herring SA, Bergfeld J, Boyd J, et al. Mass participation event management for the team physician: a consensus statement. *Med Sci Sport Exerc.* 2003;36(11):2004-2008.
5. Herring SA, Bergfeld JA, Boyd J, et al. The team physician and return-to-play issues consensus statement. *Med Sci Sport Exerc.* 2002;34(7):1212-1214, 849.
6. Sanders AK, Boggess BR, Koenig SJ, et al. Medicolegal issues in sports medicine. *Clin Orthop Relat Res.* 2005;433:38-49.

Additional Readings

American College of Surgeons. *Advanced Trauma Life Support Course Student Manual.* 7th ed. American College of Surgeons; 2007.

American Heart Association. *Advanced Cardiac Life Support Course Provider Manual.* Dallas, TX: American Heart Association; 2005.

Kleiner DM, Almquist JL, Bailes J, et al. *Prehospital Care of the Spine-Injured Athlete.* Inter-Association Task Force for Appropriate Care of the Spine-Injured Athlete. Dallas, TX: National Athletic Trainers' Association; 2001.

Team Physician Consensus Statement

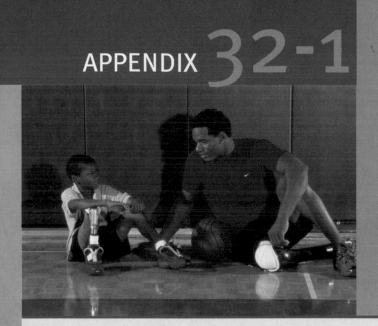

Summary

The objective of the Team Physician Consensus Statement is to provide physicians, school administrators, team owners, the general public, and individuals who are responsible for making decisions regarding the medical care of athletes and teams with guidelines for choosing a qualified team physician and an outline of the duties expected of a team physician. Ultimately, by educating decision makers about the need for a qualified team physician, the goal is to ensure athletes and teams are provided the very best medical care.

The Consensus Statement was developed by the collaboration of six major professional associations concerned about clinical sports medicine issues: American Academy of Family Physicians, American Academy of Orthopaedic Surgeons, American College of Sports Medicine, American Medical Society for Sports Medicine, and the American Osteopathic Academy of Sports Medicine. These organizations have committed to forming an ongoing project-based alliance to "bring together sports medicine organizations to best serve active people and athletes."

Expert Panel

Stanley A. Herring, M.D., Chair, Seattle, Washington
John A. Bergfeld, M.D., Cleveland, Ohio
Joel Boyd, M.D., Edina, Minnesota
William G. Clancy, Jr., M.D., Birmingham, Alabama
H. Royer Collins, M.D., Phoenix, Arizona
Brian C. Halpern, M.D., Marlboro, New Jersey
Rebecca Jaffe, M.D., Chadds Ford, Pennsylvania
W. Ben Kibler, M.D., Lexington, Kentucky
E. Lee Rice, D.O., San Diego, California
David C. Thorson, M.D., White Bear Lake, Minnesota

Team Physician Definition

The team physician must have an unrestricted medical license and be an M.D. or D.O. who is responsible for treating and coordinating the medical care of athletic team members. The principal responsibility of the team physician is to provide for the well-being of individual athletes—enabling each to realize his/her full potential. The team physician should possess special proficiency in the care of musculoskeletal injuries and medical conditions encountered in sports. The team physician also must actively integrate medical expertise with other healthcare providers, including medical specialists, athletic trainers, and allied health professionals. The team physician must ultimately assume responsibility within the team structure for making medical decisions that affect the athlete's safe participation.

Qualifications of a Team Physician

The primary concern of the team physician is to provide the best medical care for athletes at all levels of participation. To this end, the following qualifications are necessary for all team physicians:

- Have an MD or DO in good standing, with an unrestricted license to practice medicine
- Possess a fundamental knowledge of emergency care regarding sporting events
- Be trained in CPR
- Have a working knowledge of trauma, musculoskeletal injuries, and medical conditions affecting the athlete

In addition, it is desirable for team physicians to have clinical training/experience and administrative skills in some or all of the following:

- Specialty Board certification
- Continuing medical education in sports medicine
- Formal training in sports medicine (fellowship training, board recognized subspecialty in sports medicine [formerly known as a certificate of added qualification in sports medicine])
- Additional training in sports medicine
- Fifty percent or more of practice involving sports medicine
- Membership and participation in a sports medicine society
- Involvement in teaching, research and publications relating to sports medicine
- Training in advanced cardiac life support
- Knowledge of medical/legal, disability, and workers' compensation issues
- Media skills training

Duties of a Team Physician

The team physician must be willing to commit the necessary time and effort to provide care to the athlete and team. In addition, the team physician must develop and maintain a current, appropriate knowledge base of the sport(s) for which he/she is accepting responsibility.

The duties for which the team physician has ultimate responsibility include the following:

Medical management of the athlete

- Coordinate preparticipation screening, examination, and evaluation
- Manage injuries on the field
- Provide for medical management of injury and illness
- Coordinate rehabilitation and return to participation
- Provide for proper preparation for safe return to participation after an illness or injury
- Integrate medical expertise with other health care providers, including medical specialists, athletic trainers and allied health professionals
- Provide for appropriate education and counseling regarding nutrition, strength and conditioning, ergogenic aids, substance abuse, another medical problems that could affect the athlete
- Provide for proper documentation and medical record keeping

Administrative and logistical duties

- Establish and define the relationships of all involved parties
- Educate athletes, parents, administrators, coaches, and other necessary parties of concern regarding the athletes
- Develop a chain of command

- Plan and train for emergencies during competition and practice
- Address equipment and supply issues
- Provide for proper event coverage
- Assess environmental concerns and playing conditions

Education of a Team Physician

Ongoing education pertinent to the team physician is essential. Currently, there are several state, regional and national stand-alone courses for team physician education. There are also many other resources available. Information regarding team physician specific educational opportunities can be obtained from the organizations listed to the right.

Team physician education is also available from other sources such as: sport-specific (e.g., National Football League Team Physician's Society) or level-specific (e.g., United States Olympic Committee) meetings; National Governing Bodies' (NGB) meetings; state and/or county medical societies' meetings; professional journals; and other relevant electronic media (Websites, CD-ROMs).

Conclusion

This Consensus Statement establishes a definition of the team physician, and outlines a team physician's qualifications, duties, and responsibilities. It also contains strategies for the continuing education of team physicians. Ultimately, this statement provides guidelines that best serve the health care needs of athletes and teams.

Source: Permission to reprint this statement is granted by the project-based alliance for the advancement of clinical sports medicine contingent upon the statement being reprinted in full, without alteration and on proper credit given to the alliance as shown, "Reprinted with permission of the project-based alliance for the advancement of clinical sports medicine, comprised of the American Academy of Family Physicians, the American Academy of Orthopaedic Surgeons, the American College of Sports Medicine, the American Medical Society for Sports Medicine, the American Orthopaedic Society for Sports Medicine, and the American Osteopathic Academy of Sports Medicine© 2000.")

- American Academy of Family Physicians (AAFP) 11400 Tomahawk Creek Pkwy. Leawood, KS 66211-2672 1-800-274-2237
- American Academy of Orthopaedic Surgeons (AAOS) 6300 N. River Road Rosemont, IL 60018 1-800-346-AAOS

- American College of Sports Medicine (ACSM)
  401 W. Michigan Street
  Indianapolis, IN 46202-3233
  (317) 637-9200
- American Medical Society for Sports
  Medicine (AMSSM)
  11639 Earnshaw
  Overland Park, KS 66210
  (913) 327-1415

- American Orthopaedic Society for Sports Medicine
  6300 N. River Rd., Suite 200
  Rosemont, IL 60018
  (847) 292-4900
- American Osteopathic Academy of Sports Medicine
  (AOASM)
  7611 Elmwood Ave., Suite 201
  Middleton, WI 53562
  (608) 831-4400

Sideline Preparedness for the Team Physician: A Consensus Statement

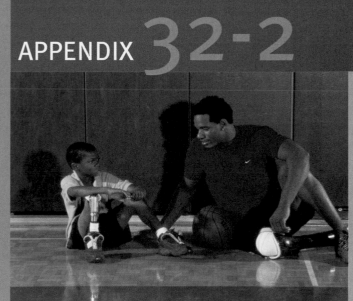

Summary

The objective of the Sideline Preparedness Statement to provide physicians who are responsible for making decisions regarding the medical care of athletes with guidelines for identifying and planning for medical care and services at the site of practice or competition. It is not intended as a standard of care, and should not be interpreted as such. The Sideline Preparedness Statement is only a guide, and as such, is of a general nature, consistent with the reasonable, objective practice of the health care professional.

Individual treatment will turn on the specific facts and circumstances presented to the physician at the event. Adequate insurance should be in place to help protect the physician, the athlete, and the sponsoring organization.

The Sideline Preparedness Statement was developed by a collaboration of six major professional associations concerned about clinical sports medicine issues; they have committed to forming an ongoing project-based alliance to "bring together sports medicine organizations to best serve active people and athletes." The organizations are American Academy of Family Physicians, American Academy of Orthopaedic surgeons, American College of Sports Medicine, American Medical Society for Sports Medicine, American Orthopaedic Society for Sports Medicine, and the American Osteopathic Academy of Sports Medicine.

Expert Panel

Stanley A. Herring, MD, Chair, Seattle, Washington
John Bergfeld, MD, Cleveland, Ohio
Joel Boyd, MD, Edina, Minnesota
Per Gunnar Brolinson, DO, Toledo, Ohio
Timothy Duffy, DO, Columbus, Ohio
David Glover, MD, Warrensburg, Missouri
William A. Grana, MD, Oklahoma City, Oklahoma
Brian C. Halpern, MD, Marlboro, New Jersey
Peter Indelicato, MD, Gainesville, Florida
W. Ben Kibler, MD, Lexington, Kentucky
E. Lee Rice, DO, San Diego, California
William O. Roberts, MD, White Bear Lake, Minnesota

Sideline Preparedness Statement Definition

Sideline preparedness if the identification of and planning for medical services to promote the safety of the athlete, to limit injury, and to provide medical care at the site of practice or competition.

Goal

The safety and on-site medical care of the athlete is the goal of the sideline preparedness. To accomplish this goal, the team physician should be actively involved in developing an integrated medical system that includes:

- Preseason planning
- Game-day planning
- Postseason evaluation

Preseason Planning

Preseason planning promotes safety and minimizes problems associated with athletic participation at the site of practice or competition.
The team physician should coordinate:

- Development of policy to address preseason planning and the preparticipation evaluation of athletes

- Participation of the administration and other key personnel in medical issues
- Implementation strategies

Medical Protocol Development

It is essential that

- Prospective athletes complete a preparticipation evaluation

    In addition, it is desirable that:

- The preparticipation evaluation be performed by an MD or DO in good standing with an unrestricted license to practice medicine
- A comprehensive preparticipation evaluation form be used (e.g., the form found in the current edition of Preparticipation Physical Evaluation ©)*
- The team physician has access to all preparticipation evaluation forms
- The team physician review all preparticipation evaluation forms and determine eligibility of the athlete to participate
- Timely preparticipation evaluations be performed to permit the identification and treatment of injuries and medical conditions

Administrative Protocol Development

It is essential for the team physician to coordinate:

- Development of a chain of command that establishes and defines the responsibilities of all parties involved
- Establishment of an emergency response plan for practice and competition
- Compliance with Occupational Safety and Health Administration (OSHA) standards relevant to the medical care of the athlete
- Establishment of a policy to assess environmental concerns and playing conditions for modification or suspension of practice or competition
- Compliance with all local, state, and Federal regulations regarding storing and dispensing pharmaceuticals
- Establishment of a plan to provide for proper documentation and medical record keeping

    In addition, it is desirable for the team physician to coordinate:

- Regular rehearsal of the emergency response plan
- Establishment of a network with other health care providers, including medical specialists, athletic trainers and allied health professionals
- Establishment of a policy that includes the team physician in the dissemination of any information regarding the athlete's health
- Preparation of a letter of understanding between the team physician and the administration that defines the obligations and responsibilities of the team physician

Game-Day Planning

Game-day planning optimizes medical care for injured or ill athletes. The team physician should coordinate:

- Game-day medical operations
- Game-day administrative medical policies
- Preparation of the sideline "medical bag" and sideline medical supplies

Medical Protocol

It is essential for the team physician to coordinate:

- Determination of final clearance status of injured or ill athletes on game-day prior to competition
- Assessment and management of game-day injuries and medical problems
- Determination of athletes' same-day game return to participation after injury or illness
- Follow-up care and instructions for athletes who required treatment during or after competition
- Notifying the appropriate parties about an athlete's injury or illness
- Close observation of the game by the medical team from an appropriate location
- Provision for proper documentation and medical record keeping

    In addition, it is desirable for the team physician to coordinate:

- Monitoring of equipment safety and fit
- Monitoring of postgame referral care of injured or ill athletes

Administrative Protocol

It is essential for the team physician to coordinate:

- Assessment of environmental concerns and playing conditions
- Presence of medical personnel at the competition site with sufficient time for all pregame preparations
- And plan with the medical staff of the opposing team for medical care of the athletes
- Introductions of the medical team to game officials
- Review of the emergency medical response plan
- Checking and confirmation of communication equipment
- Identification of examination and treatment sites

    In addition, it is desirable for the team physician to coordinate:

- Arrangements for the medical staff to have convenient access to the competition site
- A postgame review and make necessary modifications of medical and administrative protocols.

On-Site Medical Supplies

The team physician should have a game-day sideline "medical bag" and sideline medical supplies. The following is a list of "medical bag" items and medical supplies for contact/collision and high-risk sports.

It is highly desirable for the "medical bag" to include:

General

- Alcohol swabs and povidone iodine swabs
- Bandage scissors
- Bandages, sterile/nonsterile, band-aids
- D-50%-W
- Disinfectant
- Gloves, sterile/nonsterile
- Large bore angiocath for tension
- Pneumothorax (14–16 gauge)
- Local anesthetic/syringes/needles
- Paper
- Pen
- Sharps box and red bag
- Suture set/steri-strips
- Wound irrigation materials (e.g., sterile normal saline, 10–50 cm³ syringe)

Cardiopulmonary

- Airway
- Blood pressure cuff
- Cricothyrotomy kit
- Epinephrine 1:1000 in a prepackaged unit
- Mouth-to-mouth mask
- Short-acting beta agonist inhaler
- Stethoscope

Head and neck/neurologic

- Dental kit (e.g., cyanoacrylate, Hank's solution)
- Eye kit (e.g., blue light, fluorescein stain strips, eye patch pads, cotton tip applicators, ocular anesthetic and antibiotics, contact remover, mirror)
- Flashlight
- Pin or other sharp object for sensory testing
- Reflex hammer

It is highly desirable for sideline medical supplies to include:

General

- Access to a telephone
- Extremity splints
- Ice
- Oral fluid replacement
- Plastic bags
- Sling

Head and neck/neurologic

- Face mask removal tool (for sports with helmets)

- Semirigid cervical collar
- Spine board and attachments

In addition, it is desirable for the "medical bag" to include:

General

- Benzoin
- Blister care materials
- Contact lens case and solution
- 30% Ferric subsulfate solution (e.g., Monsel's—for cauterizing abrasions and cuts)
- Injury and illness care instruction sheets for the patient
- List of emergency phone numbers
- Nail clippers
- Nasal packing material
- Oto-ophthalmoscope
- Paper bags for treatment of hyperventilation
- Prescription pad
- Razor and shaving cream
- Rectal thermometer
- Scalpel
- Skin lubricant
- Skin staple applicator
- Small mirror
- Supplemental oral and parental medications
- Tongue depressors
- Topical antibiotics

Cardiopulmonary

- Advanced Cardiac Life Support (ACLS) drugs and equipment
- IV fluids and administration set
- Tourniquet

In addition, it is desirable for sideline medical supplies to include:

General

- Blanket
- Crutches
- Mouth guards
- Sling psychrometer and temperature/humidity activity risk chart
- Tape cutter

Cardiopulmonary

- Automated external defibrillator

Head and neck/neurologic

- A sideline concussion assessment protocol

There are many different sports, levels of competition, and available medical resources that must all be considered when determining the on-site medical bag and sideline medical supplies.

Postseason Evaluation

Postseason evaluation of sideline coverage optimizes the medical care of injured or ill athletes and promotes continued improvement of medical services for future seasons.

The team physician should coordinate:

■ Summarization of injuries and illnesses that occurred during the season
■ The improvement of the medical and administrative protocols
■ Implementation strategies to improve sideline preparedness

Medical Protocol

It is essential for the team physician to coordinate:

■ A postseason meeting with appropriate team personnel and administration to review the previous season
■ Identification of athletes who require postseason care of injury or illness and encourage follow-up

In addition, it is desirable for the team physician to coordinate:

■ Monitoring of the health status of the injured or ill athlete
■ Postseason physicals
■ An off-season conditioning program

Administrative Protocol

It is essential for the team physician to coordinate:

■ Review and modification of current medical and administrative protocols

In addition, it is desirable for the team physician to coordinate:

■ Compilation of injury and illness data

Ongoing education pertinent to the team physician is essential. Information regarding team physician-specific educational opportunities can be obtained from the six participating organizations:

■ American Academy of Family Physicians
  11400 Tomahawk Creek Pkwy
  Leawood, KS 66211-2672
  Tel.: 1-800-274-2237
  Website: www.aafp.org
■ American Academy of Orthopaedic Surgeons
  6300 N. River Road
  Rosemont, IL 60018
  1-800-346-AAOS
  Website: www.aaos.org

■ American College of Sports Medicine
  401 W. Michigan Street
  Indianapolis, IN 46202
  Tel.: (317) 637-9200
  Website: www.acsm.org
■ American Medical Society for Sports Medicine
  11639 Earnshaw
  Overland Park, KS 66210
  Tel.: (913) 327-1415
  Website: www.amssm.org
■ American Orthopaedic Society for Sports Medicine
  6300 N. River Rd., Suite 200
  Rosemont, IL 60018
  Tel.: (847) 292-4900
  Website: www.sportsmed.org
■ American Osteopathic Academy of Sports Medicine
  7611 Elmwood Ave., Suite 201
  Middleton, WI 53562
  Tel.: (608) 831-4400
  Website: www.aoasm.org

*Preparticipation Physical Evaluation, 2nd ed. McGraw Hill Publishing, 1997.

Conclusion

This Consensus Statement outlines the essential and desirable components of sideline preparedness for the team physician to promote the safety of the athlete, to limit injury, and to provide medical care at the site of practice or competition. This statement was developed by the collaboration of six major professional associations concerned about clinical sports medicine issues: American Academy of Family Physicians, American Academy of Orthopaedic Surgeons, American College of Sports Medicine, American Medical Society for Sports Medicine, American Orthopaedic Society for Sports Medicine, and the American Osteopathic Academy of Sports Medicine.

Source: Permission to reprint this statement is granted by the project-based alliance for the advancement of clinical sports medicine contingent upon the statement being reprinted in full, without alteration and on proper credit given to the alliance as shown, "Reprinted with permission of the project-based alliance for the advancement of clinical sports medicine, comprised of the American Academy of Family Physicians, the American Academy of Orthopaedic Surgeons, the American College of Sports Medicine, the American Medical Society for Sports Medicine, the American Orthopaedic Society for Sports Medicine, and the American Osteopathic Academy of Sports Medicine© 2000."

CHAPTER 33

Maxillofacial and Dental Injuries

Joseph D'Ambrosio

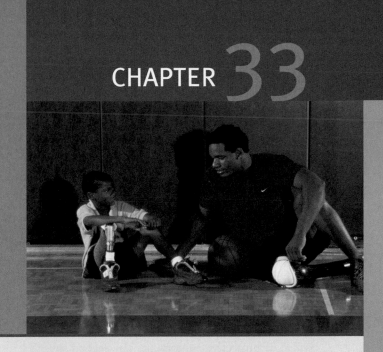

DEFINITIONS AND EPIDEMIOLOGY

Oral injuries account for 30% of sports injuries and each athlete participating in a contact/collision sport has a 10% chance of such an injury.[1] Intrusive displacement of the anterior teeth as a result of falls is the most common injury in children with primary dentition, whereas fractures of the crown are the most common injuries in adolescents and adults.[1–10] More than half of dental injuries involve maxillary incisors. The highest incidence of oral injuries has been reported in baseball and biking.[1–10] The American Academy of Pediatric Dentistry definitions of dento-alveolar injuries are summarized Table 33-1.

Studies over several decades have looked at the factors involved in facial and dental injuries and their epidemiology.[1–11] It must be remembered that over the past 20 years many amateur and professional sports organizations have encouraged and/or mandated the use of protective equipment which has resulted in significant reductions in such injuries. Many experts have been quick to point out, however, that as there is no mandatory reporting of such injuries, the true incidence is almost certainly much higher than what is reported in the literature.

MECHANISMS

Trauma to the face during sports participation may result in several common outcomes. The first of these involves fractures of the facial bones; i.e., the maxilla, the mandible, and/or the dental alveolar ridge. Whenever injuries to the face and dental structures occur there is a possibility for life-threatening injury and the examiner should always follow the ABCs of basic life support.[4,12,13] The extent of such an examination depends on the

Table 33-1.

American Academy of Pediatric Dentistry Definitions of Dental Injuries

Injury	Definition
Infraction	Incomplete fracture (crack) of the enamel without loss of tooth structure
Crown fracture— uncomplicated	An enamel fracture or an enamel–dentin fracture that does not involve the pulp
Crown fracture— complicated	An enamel–dentin fracture with pulp exposure
Crown/root fracture	An enamel, dentin, and cementum fracture with or without pulp exposure
Root fracture	A dentin and cementum fracture involving the pulp
Concussion	Injury to the tooth-supporting structures without abnormal loosening or displacement of the tooth
Subluxation	Injury to tooth-supporting structures with abnormal loosening but without tooth displacement
Lateral luxation	Displacement of the tooth in a direction other than axially. The periodontal ligament is torn and contusion or fracture of the supporting alveolar bone occurs
Intrusion	Apical displacement of tooth into the alveolar bone. The tooth is driven into the socket, compressing the periodontal ligament and commonly causes a crushing fracture of the alveolar socket
Extrusion	Partial displacement of the tooth axially from the socket. The periodontal ligament usually is torn
Avulsion	Complete displacement of tooth out of socket. The periodontal ligament is severed and fracture of the alveolus may occur

nature of the injury and the clinical presentation of the athlete. One should remember that any injury to the face and dental structures is an injury to the head with potential concussion and/or neurological compromise. Once the ABCs have been appropriately evaluated a brief neurological examination is often indicated.[4,12,13]

The most frequently encountered physiologic mechanism is "deceleration injury" caused by contact of a moving player with the ground, with another player, with protective equipment, or with obstacles adjacent to the field of play (i.e., the outfield fence in baseball, the goal post in football, or a tree in downhill skiing).[12,14–18] The likelihood and severity of injury is determined by many factors including the age and development of the player, the competitive level, and the presence or absence of protective equipment. The second mechanism of injury is "acceleration" type injury caused by contact of the facial structures with a moving object such as a baseball, baseball bat, or hockey stick. Many injuries combine the aspects of acceleration and deceleration as when two outfielders collide when chasing down a fly ball. Given the kinetic energy which is released in such collisions there is greater potential for serious injury to facial structures.

DIAGNOSES AND TREATMENT

Fractures of the Facial Bones

Fractures of the maxilla

Fractures of the maxilla occur along suture lines and for that reason are fairly easy to understand.[17] Such injuries are exceedingly rare and require a great deal of kinetic energy applied to cause such disruption. In fact, maxillary fractures are much more common in motor vehicle accidents than they are in sports. The classification of maxillary fractures was described decades ago by Renee LeFort and is presented in Figure 33-1.[17] It should be noted that because of the relative lack of development of the lower and mid-face in the preschooler, maxillary fractures are an uncommon occurrence.

Subsequent to any injury resulting in severe blunt trauma to the face, especially in the presence of abrasions, lacerations, or ecchymoses the examiner should consider the possibility of a LeFort type of fracture.[3,12,16,19] Facial asymmetry is the first clue to maxillary fractures. Palpation of the zygomatic arches and the maxilla may reveal "step off" of the bones or mobility of bony segments suggestive of fractures.

It is important to palpate the nasal cartilage and nasal bones: excessive mobility of the entire maxilla or of the nasal bridge may be indicative of a LeFort II or

III fracture. Any suggestion of maxillary fracture requires emergent imaging and evaluation by a facial trauma specialist. LeFort I fractures require intermaxillary (maxilla to mandible) fixation with orthodontic brackets and wires. LeFort II or III fractures may also require further fixation of the maxillary segment to the base of the skull. Depending on the findings and the necessary intervention, the athlete will usually be unavailable for 6 to 12 weeks, and the return to play decision is best left up to the trauma specialist involved. Early return to play has been associated with displacement of the maxillary segments and later significant malocclusion.

Fractures of the mandible

Because of its relative prominence in older children and adults, fractures of mandible occur at a relatively higher frequency than those of the maxilla. The mid and lower face (mandible) is relatively underdeveloped in the preschooler and fractures of the mandible are uncommon.[5,7,17] The first part of the examination after trauma to the mandible is, as before, visual inspection to assess asymmetry. The examiner should then palpate along the body, angle, and ramus bilaterally to look for any evidence of bony discontinuity ("step-off") or mobility. Ask the athlete to open the mouth and assess the degree of opening, since decreased opening of the mouth may indicate damage to the TMJ or mandibular fracture. The athlete should then be asked to close the mouth completely into a "normal bite." It may be possible to assess the occlusion to see if the maxillary and mandibular teeth articulate correctly.

It is important to note that many athletes may have malocclusion prior to the traumatic injury (Figure 33-2). A simple and reliable way to evaluate for occlusion is to ask the athlete to open and close the mouth several times and to clench the teeth together. If the athlete has a sense that the teeth are not coming together properly or if there is significant pain with clenching, it is a good indicator of fracture or TMJ disruption. If there is any doubt about the diagnosis, continued play is contraindicated and a panoramic x-ray is required.

As with long bone fractures, fracture points of the mandible are located at maximum stress points and "weak areas" related to anatomy. Figure 33-3 shows these stress points which are the angle, the neck, and the anterior symphysis.

Fractures of the zygomatic bones

Fractures of the zygomatic bones are uncommon before 12 years of age, because they have not yet fully developed. The fracture results from a direct impact to face. The athlete may complain of diplopia and feeling of numbness on the cheek. On examination, there is localized ecchymosis, swelling, and tenderness over the zygomatic bone.

Tenderness can be elicited on palpation of the roof of the mouth. In athletes with zygomatic fracture, eye injury should be ruled out and the athlete should be referred to ophthalmology and maxillofacial surgery for further evaluation and management.

TEMPEROMANDIBULAR JOINT TRAUMA

The temperomandibular joint is quite unique in structure and function. A glance at Figure 33-4 serves to

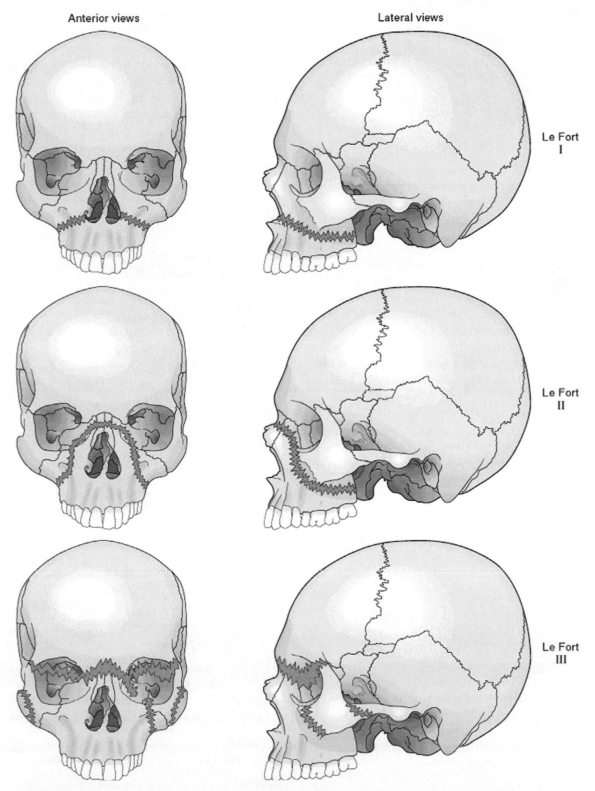

Anterior views   Lateral views

Le Fort I

Le Fort II

Le Fort III

FIGURE 33-1 ■ Le Fort classification of fractures of the maxilla. (*Used with permission from Current Diagnosis and Treatment in Emergency Medicine. New York: McGraw Hill Medical, 2007, Figure 23-5.*)

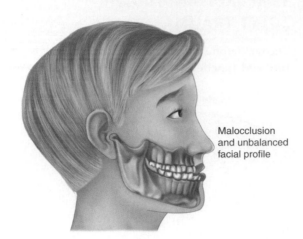

FIGURE 33-2 ■ Malocclusion of the jaw. (*Source: Medline Plus, United States National Library of Medicine and National Institutes of Health.*)

remind us that the structure is actually a U-shaped long bone with a "ball and socket" joint on each end. The unique feature of the TMJ is the articular disk composed of fibrocartilagenous tissue positioned between the two bones that form the joint. The TMJs are the only synovial joints in the human body with such an articular disk. The disk divides each joint into two compartments. The lower joint compartment formed by the condyle of the mandible and the articular disk is involved in rotational (hinge) movement which accounts for approximately the first 20 mm of mandibular opening. The upper joint compartment formed by the articular disk and the glenoid fossa of the temporal bone is involved in translational movements (sliding the

lower jaw forward or side to side). The TMJ is thus a ginglymoarthroidial joint, referring to its dual functions of "hinge" (ginglymo-) and "gliding"(arthroidial-) movement. When mild to moderate direct force is applied to the mandible, damage to the TMJ is much more often the case than is fracture of the facial bones.

The articular disk is comprised of a fibrous and avascular central area which is ideally placed between the condyle and the fossa particularly during mastication. Anteriorly and posteriorly to this area the disk is less fibrous and much more vascular. Trauma to the mandible may result in displacement of the articular disk anteriorly such that load-bearing forces are applied to the posterior disk area. Pain and TMJ dysfunction occur as a result of the sensory nerve inervation of this portion of the articular disk. The displaced disk may reposition during opening or closing of the mouth with a loud "pop" or "click" and usually brief but considerable pain. Anterior dislocation may also result in a situation

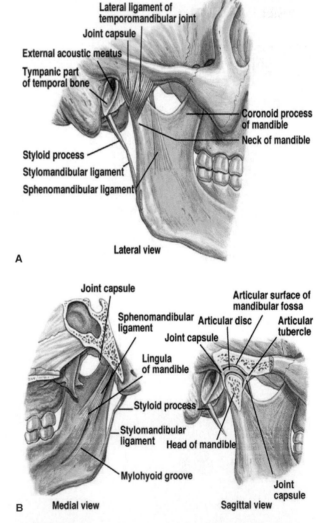

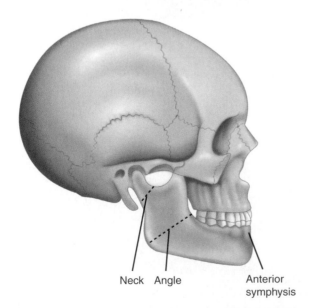

FIGURE 33-3 ■ Stress points of mandible are located at the angle, the neck, and the anterior symphysis.

FIGURE 33-4 ■ Temperomandibular joint anatomy. (*Used with permission from Van de Graaff. Human Anatomy, 6th ed. New York: McGraw Hill, 2002.*)

in which the disk is "locked" in position anterior to the condyle. In such cases there will be no "popping" or "clicking" of the joint with opening or closing of the mouth. The most notable feature will be limited opening of the mouth, usually accompanied by significant pain with mandibular movement. Careful observation of the mandible during opening of the mouth will reveal that it deviates to the side of the dislocated TM joint as there is no gliding function on that side.

Acute TMJ injury is rarely an emergency and is not usually a contraindication to continued play. The athlete should be encouraged to obtain a dental evaluation as soon as possible to ensure that the articular disk is not locked anterior to the condyle. Chronic TMJ dysfunction if left untreated can lead to permanent derangement of the joint components with chronic pain and decreased function. The exception to this rule is the mandible, which is locked in an open or closed position. This requires manipulation of the mandible by a trained professional usually a dentist, oral surgeon, or ER physician, most often with sedation.

A properly fitting mouthguard is essential in protecting the teeth and TMJ from direct trauma. The exact mechanism of how mouthguard prevents the trauma is not fully understood, but may involve either the "cushioning" or the energy dissipating effect or both. There is evidence that by disarticulating the teeth and opening the mouth slightly as well as positioning the mandible slightly forward the mouthguard increases the space between the condyle and the fossa and helps retain the disk in position between these bony structures.

DENTO-ALVEOLAR INJURIES

Anatomy of the Tooth

The tooth is basically composed of three main structural layers: enamel, dentin, and pulp tissue (Figure 33-5). The visible portion of the tooth in the oral cavity is referred to as the crown and is composed of an inorganic enamel matrix. This material is one of the hardest and most durable in nature and allows the tooth to function over a lifetime of many decades. The portion of the tooth below the gingival margin and encased in bone is referred to as the root. The root is not covered with enamel but with a material called cementum. Underneath the enamel layer (and also under the cementum of the root) is a layer of dentin which, although quite hard, is significantly softer and more porous than enamel. In the center of the tooth beneath this layer of dentin there is a "cavity" referred to as the pulp chamber. The pulp chamber contains the nerves, blood vessels, and supporting connective tissues which make up the living portion of the tooth. These vital tissues may be compromised where they enter the pulp chamber through a small opening at the apex of the root, if the tooth is displaced or avulsed from trauma.

Fractures of the Tooth

Fractures of the crown

Enamel fractures. Fractures of the crown may involve the enamel only, enamel and dentin, or enamel dentin and pulp.[3,11,12,14,18] Fractures of enamel are in general cosmetic in nature and often may be completely asymptomatic (Figure 33-6). They require no urgent attention and a dentist will either smooth off the fracture or, if larger, may bond a tooth-colored resin to restore the lost tooth structure. The most commonly fractured teeth are the maxillary incisors an honor which stems largely from their prominence in the dental arch.

Enamel and dentin fractures. Fractures which involve the dentin result in mild to severe thermal sensitivity to liquids and even to cold air. These injuries require more rapid repair, although generally are not urgent or emergent. The athlete is usually able to avoid pain by limiting foods and beverages to those which are at room temperature.

Enamel, dentin, and pulp fractures. Tooth fractures that expose vital pulp tissues are the most problematic and need urgent dental attention. If the exposed pulp area is small, the dentist may be able to cover it with a protective material and subsequently restore the crown. If the exposure is large and/or dental intervention is not urgently obtained, the prognosis is less favorable and may result in eventual root canal therapy to remove the dead or infected pulp tissues and to seal up the pulp chamber. With any of the above tooth fractures

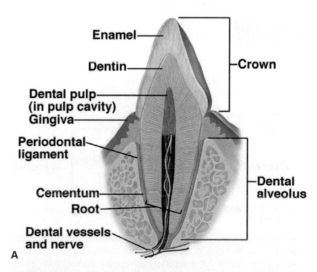

FIGURE 33-5 ■ **(A)** Anatomy of tooth. (*Used with permission from Van de Graaff. Human Anatomy, 6th ed. New York: McGraw Hill, 2002.*) (*continued*)

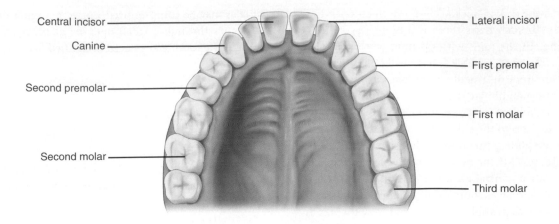

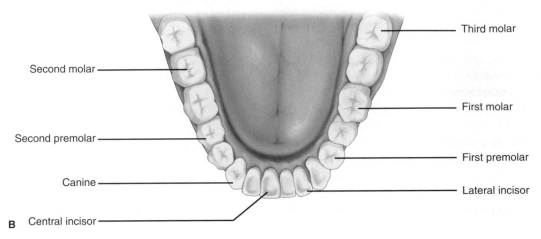

FIGURE 33-5 ■ *(Continued)* **(B)** *(Source: Medline Plus, United States National Library of Medicine and National Institutes of Health.)*

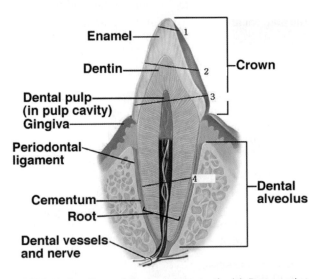

FIGURE 33-6 ■ Types of fracture of the tooth. (1) Fractures that involve enamel only. (2) Fractures that involve enamel and dentin. (3) Fractures that involve enamel, dentin, and the pulp. (4) Fractures that involve the root. (*Adapted with permission from Van de Graaff. Human Anatomy, 6th ed. New York: McGraw Hill, 2002.*)

there is really no contraindication to continued sports participation. Clearly, if the injury occurred while the athlete was not using an appropriate mouthguard it should serve as a wake up call to do so in the future!

Fractures of the root

Vertical fractures. Complications of tooth fracture occur when the fracture is more vertical and involves the root structure. Fortunately these types of fractures are uncommon, but when they occur they may result in severe pain as the tooth fragment often remains attached to gingiva and to bone. Dental intervention should be sought urgently as the fragment of tooth will need to be detached from the gingiva and tooth socket (bone) using local anesthetic. These teeth are also much more complicated to repair and depending on the extent of the damage the dentist will need to make a decision as to the possibility of successful repair versus extraction and replacement with an implant or prosthesis. Once again such a fracture does not indicate an absolute need to refrain from sports participation, but the athlete will likely be unable to insert a well-fitting mouthguard as this will result in displacement of the tooth fragment and considerable pain.

Horizontal or oblique fractures.

One further type of fracture seen almost exclusively with the anterior dentition is the oblique or horizontal root fracture. This fracture remains entirely below the crest of the tooth and presents a whole host of challenges to the dentist. Such a fracture should always be suspected if the tooth or teeth in question are mobile and the only definitive modality to diagnose is a dental x-ray. Panoramic films are useful and often available to the physician, but a periapical x-ray done in the dental office is much more sensitive and also better at documenting the degree of separation of the root fragments. As with all mobile teeth after trauma, the athlete should be advised to assume a soft diet and to see a dentist as soon as possible.

Definitive treatment of root fractures.

The definitive treatment for root fractures involves splinting of the crown to adjacent teeth using wire and acrylic bonding materials. This stabilization allows for the regeneration of periodontal ligament and the repair of damaged bone in the tooth socket. If successful the cementum layer of the root will develop a "callus" just as happens with cortical bone in the axial skeleton. The prognosis for retention of the crown depends on many factors, but overall the greater the distance between the crown and the fracture line (i.e. the longer the portion of root remaining attached to the crown above the fracture) the more likely the tooth will be successfully stabilized and retained. If a root fracture is suspected or confirmed the athlete will be unable to insert a mouthguard and contact sports are contraindicated. Once the crowns are splinted or other dental intervention is completed the dentist should provide recommendations for an appropriate return to play.

Displacement (Luxation) of Tooth

If sufficient force is applied to the incisal edge of an anterior tooth, the tooth may be intruded into the socket. Physiologically this involves disruption of the periodontal ligament fibers and compression (fracture) of the alveolar bone of the tooth socket. Although rare, it is possible for a tooth to be intruded up into the nasal cavity or into the maxillary sinus. It is not uncommon for maxillary primary teeth to be fully intruded to the extent that they are not apparent on clinical examination and are thought to be avulsed. Whenever an "avulsed" tooth cannot be located, it is important to obtain appropriate dental x-rays to confirm that the tooth is indeed gone!

If lateral forces are applied to the incisor teeth they may be "luxated" or displaced anteriorly (through the buccal plate) or posteriorly (into the palate). As with intrusion, this results in disruption of the periodontal ligament and sectional fracture of the alveolar bone.

In any case of tooth displacement there are several immediate actions which are required and urgent dental intervention is advised. If the tooth is tipped buccally or palatally one should place the forefinger over the palatal root and the thumb over the buccal root area and gently compress the bony alveolar plates while simultaneously "torquing" the tooth into more ideal position. This is especially important for teeth which are moved palatally and may prevent full closure of the mouth because of contact of the lower incisors against the luxated maxillary tooth. This occurs most commonly with pre-school athletes who still have primary upper incisors in place.

Avulsion of the Tooth

Complete avulsion of primary and permanent incisors is not an uncommon occurrence. If the avulsed tooth cannot be located and verified to be intact then an immediate x-ray is indicated to locate the missing tooth and/or tooth fragments. Complete intrusion into the socket is a possibility, as is swallowing or aspiration of the tooth. A chest x-ray should be obtained.

An avulsed permanent tooth should be retrieved and handled by the crown only. If the athlete or bystander is willing, the tooth should be gently cleaned of all debris and immediately replaced in the socket and held in place with gentle finger pressure. The buccal and palatal alveolar plates are then compressed between thumb and forefinger and the tooth is torqued (if necessary) into alignment with adjacent teeth. Emergent dental intervention is indicated to temporarily splint the tooth in place and allow healing of the bone and periodontal ligament. During transport to the dental office the tooth may be held in position by biting down on a gauze pad, handkerchief, or clean rag. The patient also needs to be placed on antibiotic coverage as bacteria will obviously be present on the root surface.

There is very little data to indicate the optimal antibiotic regimen, but most practitioners have experienced good results with amoxicillin-trimethoprim, clindamycin, or first-generation cephalosporins. Updating tetanus immunization is also important, given that most avulsed teeth are found in contact with soil. Return to play should be determined by the dental specialist who performs the splinting procedure, and usually requires a 4- to 8-week period. The splint may remain in place from 10 days up to several weeks. Once the splint is in place for an appropriate period of time, it is required for further repair of the bone and for fabrication of a new custom mouthguard. A decision tree for an avulsed tooth is presented in Figure 33-7.

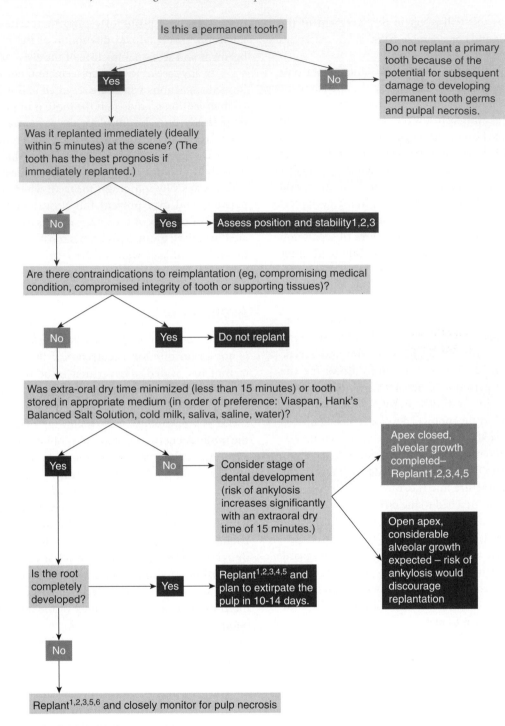

FIGURE 33-7 ■ American Academy of Pediatric Dentistry decision tree for the initial management of avulsed tooth.

1. Obtain a radiograph to verify position.
2. Flexible splinting for 7 days is indicated. Additional splinting may be required with concomitant bone fracture
3. Consideration should be given to antibiotic therapy and tetanus immunization.
4. Use of a root surface preconditioning protocol may help delay/prevent the expected replacement resorption process.
5. Holding the tooth by the crown, irrigate with sterile saline and gently replant with digital pressure.
6. Use of a preconditioning protocol may enhance pulp revascularization.

PREVENTION OF TOOTH INJURIES

The development of organized sports at all levels and the subsequent evolution of the appropriate regulatory and governing bodies has dramatically reduced the incidence of sports-related injuries to the face and dental structures. The use of protective equipment began in youth and amateur sports and later expanded into high

Table 33-2.

American Society for Testing and Materials Classification of Mouthguards

Type I Stock mouthguards
Purchased over-the-counter
Used without modification
Held in place by clenching the teeth
Least efficacious

Type II Mouth formed mouthguards
Also called boil and bite mouthguards
Commercially available
Made from thermoplastic material
Used after immersing in hot water
Adapted in mouth by pressure from biting
Most widely used type
Efficacy variable

Type III Custom fabricated mouthguards
Specifically made for the individual athlete
Made on a dental model of athlete's mouth
Made using either vaccum-forming or heat-pressure lamination technique
Most effective

school and college athletics. Currently, the use of such protective devices has expanded into professional sports and will undoubtedly continue to do so in the future. Science and technology of the late 20th and now the 21st century have produced incredibly strong and lightweight plastics and metal alloys which have allowed protective sports equipment to function without adversely affecting the performance of the athlete. The helmet and protective pads now used in American football at all levels have reduced the number of facial and dental injuries in that sport. Mouthguards are mandatory in football, ice hockey, lacrosse, and field hockey.

The dental mouthpiece or mouthguard (Table 33-2) remains arguably the most important device in terms of reduction of dental injuries, in particular those injuries to teeth and the dentoalveolar ridge (Box 33-1).[1,5,11,14,16,20-22]

Box 33-1 When to Refer.

Appropriate referral should be made to dentist, dental surgeon, maxillofacial surgeon, plastic surgeon, otolaryngologist or other specialists depending upon the nature of the trauma
Conditions to be referred include:
■ Tooth fractures
■ Tooth avulsions
■ Tooth luxations
■ Significant orofacial soft tissue trauma
■ Facial bone fractures
■ Fractures and dislocations of the temperomandibular joint

REFERENCES

1. Choy MMH. Children, sports injuries and mouthguards. *Hawaii Dent J.* 2006;11-13.
2. Kumamoto D, Maeda Y. Global trends and epidemiology of sports injuries. *J Pediatr Den Care.* 2005;11(2):15-25.
3. American Academy of Pediatric Dentistry. Guideline on Management of Acute Dental Trauma. www.aapd.org. 7/20/2008
4. Ranalli DN, Demas PM. Orofacial injuries from sport: preventive measures for sports medicine. *Sport Med.* 2002;32(7):409-418.
5. Ranalli DN. Dental injuries in sports. *Curr Sport Med Rep.* 2005;4:12-17.
6. Hill CM, Burford K, Martin A, et al. A one year review of maxillofacial sports injuries treated in an accident and emergency department. *Br J Oral Maxillofac Surg.* 1998; 36:44-47.
7. Cornwell H. Dental trauma due to sport in the pediatric patient. *CDA J.* 2005;33(6):457-461.
8. Beachy G. Dental injuries in intermediate and high school athletes: a 15-year study at Punahou School. *J. Athlet Train.* 2004;39(4):310-315.
9. Kvittem B, Hardie N, Roettger M, et al. Incidence of orofacial injuries in high school sports. *J Pub Health Dentist.* 1998;58(4):288-293.
10. Tesini DA, Soporowski NJ. Epidemiology of orofacial sports-related injuries. *Dent Clin North Am.* 2000;44(1):1-18.
11. American Academy of Pediatric Dentistry. Policy on Prevention of Sports-Related Orofacial Injuries. www.aapd.org. 7/20/2008
12. Lephart SM, Fu FH. Emergency treatment of athletic injuries. *Dent Clin North Am.* 1991;35(4):707-717.
13. Crow RW. Diagnosis and management of sports related injuries to the face. *Dent Clin North Am.* 1991;35(4): 719-732.
14. Honsik KA. Emergency treatment of dentoalveolar trauma. *Phys Sport Med.* 2004;32(9):10-14.
15. Romeo SJ, Hawley CJ, Romeo MW, et al. Facial injuries in sports. *Phys Sport Med.* 2005;33(4):19-23.
16. Hildebrandt JR. Dental and maxillofacial injuries. *Clin Sport Med.* 1982;1:449-468.
17. Tanaka N, Hayashi S, Amagasa T, et al. Maxillofacial fractures sustained during sports. *J Oral Maxillofac Surg.* 1996;54:715-719.
18. Ranalli DN. Sports dentistry and dental traumatology. *Dent Traumatol.* 2002;18:231-236.
19. Romeo SJ, Hawley CJ, Romeo MW, et al. Sideline management of facial injuries. *Curr Sport Med Rep.* 2007;6:155-161.
20. Newsome P, Tran D, Crooke M. The role of the mouthguard in the prevention of sports-related dental injuries: a review. *Int J Pediatr Dent.* 2001;11:396-404.
21. Gooch BF, Truman BI, Griffin SO, et al. A comparison of selected evidence reviews and recommendations on interventions to prevent dental caries, oral and pharyngeal cancers, and sports-related craniofacial injuries. *Am J Prev Med.* 2002;23(1S):55-80.
22. ADA Council on Access, Prevention and Interprofessional Relations; ADA Council on Scientific Affairs. Using mouthguards to reduce the incidence and severity of sports-related oral injuries. *JADA.* 2007;137:1712-1720.

CHAPTER 34

Acute Head and Neck Trauma

Robert J. Baker

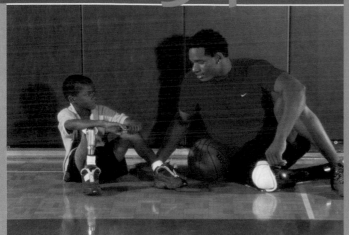

HEAD TRAUMA

Epidemiology

Participation in sports carries an inherent risk of head and neck injury. A relatively larger ratio of head to body places children at further risk for injury. This ratio decreases as children approach adolescence. Injuries to the head include scalp lacerations, skull fractures, brain injuries, and intracranial bleeding.

Of the 6000 neck injuries that occur annually among children a quarter of these are related to sports. High-risk sports are football, rugby, ice and field hockey, soccer, diving, gymnastics, cheerleading, and wrestling. Sports-related catastrophic neck injuries resulting in paralysis are rare with a prevalence of 2 per 100,000.[1–7] Head and neck injury risk has long been a concern and cause for injury surveillance in contact sports such as football and hockey. As a result, changes in rules and techniques have helped to decrease injury rates. The National Collegiate Athletic Association (NCAA) injury surveillance system recently reported an injury rate of 2.34 and 0.61 per 1000 athlete-exposures (AE) for head and neck respectively in football.[3] These rates were the highest of all sports. Other sports with significant risk were wrestling (1.27 AE head, 0.39 AE neck), lacrosse (1.08 AE head, 0.12 AE neck), and gymnastics (0.4 AE head, 0.28 AE neck). Hockey had an injury rate of 1.47 AE for the head and no significant neck injuries, owing to rule changes regarding checking from behind. While most head injuries were concussions, most neck injuries were strains.

SKULL FRACTURES

Definition

Most sports-related skull fractures occur in the frontal and parietal bones. These fractures can be classified as either linear or depressed.[6–9]

Mechanism

Low-energy blunt trauma over a wide area of the skull can result in a linear fracture. Most of the fractures seen in children are a result of falls and bicycle accidents. These fractures involve the entire thickness of bone and can continue through the vasculature, resulting in the epidural hematoma. Contact of the skull with a projectile, such as a baseball, to the temple can result in a depressed fracture of the frontal or parietal bones. These fractures result from high-energy direct blow to a relatively small surface. The fracture may be comminuted and either open or closed. Since open fractures may need surgical evaluation and management, it is important to evaluate the athlete for associated laceration.

Clinical Presentation

While loss of consciousness can occur, these athletes are often lucid. Concussion symptoms can present later. Other complications such as seizures can also occur. Epidural bleeding can be subtle and result quickly in worsening neurological function and even death. For this reason, any athlete who sustains this type of injury should be observed closely.

Diagnostic Imaging

The imaging study of choice for severe head injury is a CT scan. Skull CT scan will confirm the fracture and also show evidence of bleeding or brain injury. The scan should be thin sliced bone windows. If bloody fluid is present in the nose or ear, a paper tissue maybe used to identify presence of cerebrospinal fluid. The "ring" sign is indicated when a halo of fluid is present on the tissue beyond the blood. A positive "ring" sign should raise suspicion for a basilar skull fracture.

Treatment

Generally, outcome of skull fracture is good in the absence of neurological symptoms. In most cases without neurological signs, observation for 24 hours is all that is necessary. Patients with open fractures, evolving symptoms, and persistent symptoms should be referred to neurosurgery. Return to play should be delayed until the skull fracture has fully healed and patient is asymptomatic.[7–9]

EPIDURAL HEMATOMA

Definition

Trauma of the head can lead to bleeding between the dura and the skull in the epidural space resulting in an epidural hematoma.[7–9]

Mechanism

As the bleeding expands, intracranial pressure is increased resulting in death in up to 20% of patients. The acceleration–deceleration mechanism is thought to cause shearing which results in tearing of blood vessels in the epidural space. Fractures from a blunt trauma can directly tear superficial arteries.

Clinical Presentation

Because it is often bleeding from arteries, hemorrhage can occur quickly. Athletes with epidural bleeding can potentially progress to death within 6 to 8 hours.[8] They can be quite lucid and symptom-free during this period. A subtle progressive headache may be the initial sign. As the brain stem becomes compressed, the athlete will demonstrate decreased pupil response, decreased consciousness, and abnormal posturing.

Diagnostic Imaging

CT scan is the study of choice although the hematoma may be seen on MRI as well (Figure 34-1). There is often

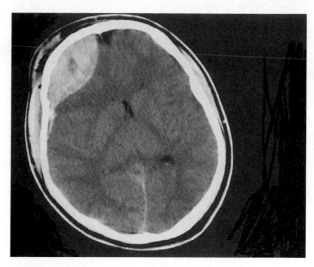

FIGURE 34-1 ■ CT scan showing epidural bleeding.

association of epidural hematoma and subdural hematoma and both may be seen on scans.

Treatment

Once the epidural hematoma is identified, surgical referral is necessary. With a timely neurosurgical intervention full recovery is possible. Return to play is individualized and based on risk factors related to possible bleeding disorder or anatomical abnormality.

SUBDURAL HEMATOMA

Definition

Blood collecting between the dura and the arachnoid space is known as subdural hematoma, and can be acute or chronic. Acute subdural hemorrhage accounts for most deaths caused by sport-related head trauma.

Mechanism

Following head trauma the bridging veins in the subdural space can tear and result in bleeding. Compared to the epidural bleeding which results from arterial injury and forms quickly, subdural bleeding forms more slowly. Thus, the course and progression are slower.

Clinical Presentation

Like the epidural hematoma there is a high mortality rate associated with the subdural hematoma. Mortality related to subdural hematoma can approach 60% to 80%.[7–9] Symptoms may have a more gradual onset

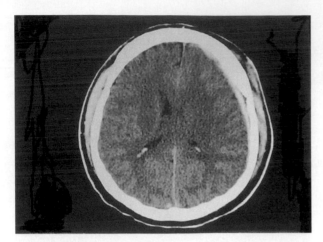

FIGURE 34-2 ■ CT scan showing subdural bleeding.

over days rather than hours as is seen with epidural hematomas. Often neurological symptoms such as numbness, headache, disorientation, amnesia, inability to concentrate, ataxia, lethargy, nausea, vomiting, and slurred speech are present. Occasionally, seizures may occur. Sometimes only subtle personality changes are present. Many of these symptoms are similar to those seen with concussion and athlete with persistent post-concussion symptoms should be evaluated for sub-dural bleed.

Diagnostic Imaging

Subdural hematoma should be visible on CT scan. MRI will show changes as well, though the imaging study of choice is the CT scan (Figure 34-2). Bleeding disorders should be considered in the differential diagnosis. Athletes may be at greater risk if taking aspirin or NSAIDs which can interfere with blood clotting.

Treatment

Athletes with subdural hematoma should be referred expeditiously for neurosurgical evaluation and further management. Full recovery is possible and return to play is individualized based on the presence of risk factors.

SUBARACHNOID HEMORRHAGE

Definition

In subarachnoid hemorrhage the blood collects in the subarachnoid space, between the arachnoid and pia mater as a result of blood vessel or brain parenchyma injury. This is a very rare occurrence in sport-related head trauma.

Mechanism

Trauma to the blood vessels in the pia mater or in the brain can lead to leakage of blood in the subarachnoid space.

Clinical Presentation

Headache is usually associated with subarachnoid hematoma. The same neurological symptoms of nausea, vomiting, confusion, loss of consciousness, or even seizure are associated with this bleeding. Intraocular hemorrhage may occur. Progression can be rapid with a 50% overall survival, with 10% to 15% mortality before arriving to the hospital.[7–9]

Diagnostic Imaging

CT scan or MRI may show subarachnoid bleeding. Occasionally, lumbar puncture is required to identify the bleeding. Vascular anatomy should be evaluated by either CT scan or MR angiogram. A cerebral aneurysm may be present as an underlying cause.

Treatment

Neurosurgery consultation is indicated in patients with subarachnoid hemorrhage. Recovery can be varied and the mortality rate is high even in the best of hands. Recurring headaches are a common complication. Some will have persistent neurological deficits.

INTRACEREBRAL HEMORRHAGE

Head trauma can cause bleeding within the brain tissue itself. Coagulation abnormalities should be considered as well as possible aneurysms or arteriovenous malformation. Rapidly progressive neurological symptoms such as headache, ataxia, slurred speech, weakness, inability to concentrate, and confusion will be present. CT scan can often identify the bleeding within brain tissue. Treatment is supportive, with referral to neurosurgery.

SCALP LACERATIONS

The scalp can be lacerated by contact typically encountered with sports, even in noncontact sports. If there is a significant blunt trauma to the head, more serious underlying injuries such as a skull fracture or serious neurological compromise because of bleeding should be ruled out. The laceration may be associated with an underlying open skull fracture.

Blood flow to the scalp is very good and even small lacerations can bleed extensively. The presence of scalp hair can interfere with visualization. Anesthesia with lidocaine with epinephrine can relieve pain and decrease bleeding to allow adequate evaluation. In children, this may be difficult. Most scalp lacerations are superficial and are closed easily. Rarely, deeper sutures are required to allow for closure. Staples are a widely used option for closure of the scalp laceration. If the edges are smooth and regular, adhesive could be used, otherwise, nonabsorbable suture works well. Since these lacerations are usually dirty, irrigation with 200 cm³ normal saline will adequately cleanse the site. Healing is usually rapid and sutures or staples may be removed as early as 1 week.

CERVICAL SPINE INJURIES

Definition and Epidemiology

It is estimated that there are 1.4 million high-school and college-age players.[1-3] Cervical spine injuries affect 15% of these players.[1-3] Between 1977 and 1989, 128 players suffered a permanent spinal cord injury.[1-3,7] This translates to about 10 spinal cord injuries per year. Half of college football players with neck injury showed x-ray changes. Worldwide, the sport of rugby has the highest risk of neck injury. A retrospective descriptive case series study of cervical spinal injury (CSI) in school-aged children injured in community-based rugby football reported 125 children with CSI, most (97%) were boys.

Mechanism

Serious cervical spine fractures are most likely to occur with the head flexed to 30 degrees while axially loaded from the top of the head.[7] This position tends to place the cervical spine in a straight column (Figure 34-3). An axial load to the column will result in failure or the burst fracture at mid-column (C3-C5). This results in not only an unstable spinal column, but fracture fragments can transect the spinal cord resulting in permanent quadriplegia. Rule changes making the use of the head as an initial point of contact in football illegal, has decreased spinal injuries. Instructing athletes in football and hockey to keep their head up during contact has also decreased catastrophic neck injuries.

Clinical Presentation

The most common presenting complaint was neck pain with 43% having neurological symptoms, and half had associated concussion. The examination should include a quick mental status examination looking for disorientation from concussion or possible hematoma of the brain. The neurological examination should assess both motor and sensory functions. Next, the neck should gently be palpated for tenderness. This should be done with care not to move the athlete. If there is no tenderness on palpation and isometric testing does not cause pain, active range of motion of the neck can be checked. If active range of motion of the neck is full and there is no suspicion of back or abdominal injury, the athlete may be brought to a sitting position or standing position to recheck range of motion. Finally, Spurling test is performed to check for nerve root irritation (Figure 34-4).

A   B   C   D

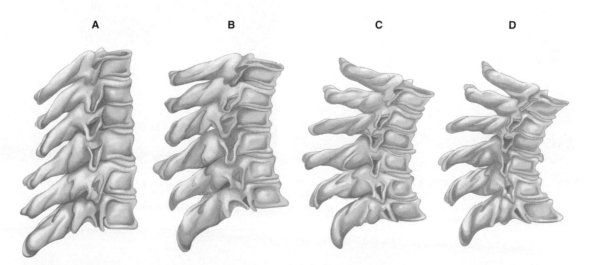

FIGURE 34-3 ■ Mechanism of cervical spine failure and fracture. Cervical spine normally maintains a slight lordosis. In this alignment and in neutral alignment **(A)** a compressive axial force is more effectively dissipated by the muscles and ligaments of cervical spine and neck. When the cervical spine sustains an axial load in a flexed position **(B)**, it tends to buckle and deform resulting in fracture and dislocation **(C, D)**.

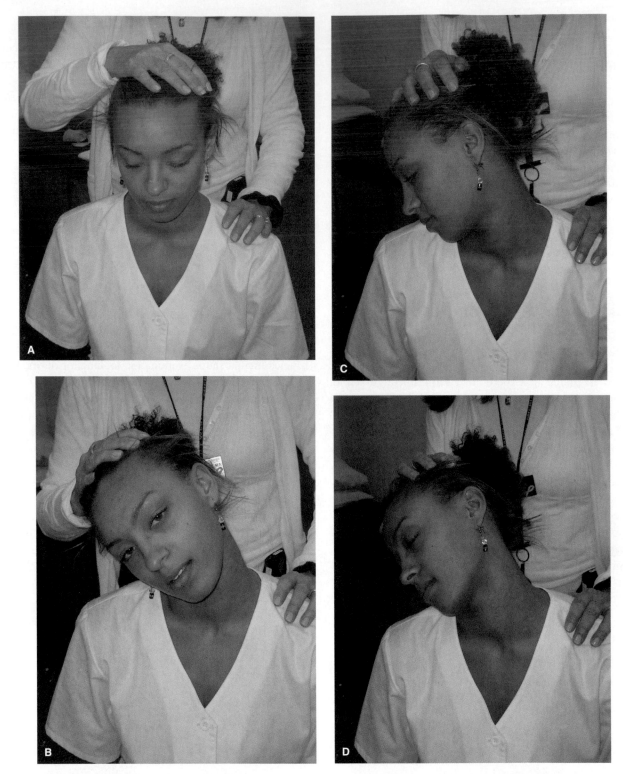

FIGURE 34-4 ■ Spurling test. The athlete bends the neck laterally and the examiner, from behind the athlete, applies axial pressure on the head. Radiation of pain down the arm toward the arm on the side the neck is flexed constitutes a positive test and indicates pressure on the cervical nerve root. If no pain is experienced with this initial position the examiner may apply axial pressure to the head with athlete's neck in extension and lateral rotation.

Athletes who experience numbness, tingling, dysthesias, weakness, or pain in extremities should not be allowed to return to play.[10–21] They should be worked up further. The athlete with normal neurological examina-tion, pain-free cervical range of motion, normal strength, sensation, and reflexes, and normal axial load testing (Spurling test) may perform provocative sport-specific testing. If these tests are pain-free the athlete is safe to return to sports. Following any neurological injury, the athlete must have 90% of his full range of motion and 90% of his full strength to return to sports.[10–21]

Diagnostic Imaging

Initial x-rays should include AP, lateral, odontoid, and oblique views. The oblique views allow better visualization of the facets, foramen, and posterior elements. The flexion and extension views allow evaluation of segmental movement and possible instabilities. Subsequent testing may include CT scan, or MRI. In young athletes, less then 8 years, fractures can be difficult to identify on plain films. CT scan can help identify specific fractures. MRI can be helpful in identifying acute fractures as well as soft tissue injuries involving the disk, spinal cord, and nerve roots.

Associated with the fracture, there may be ligamentous involvement and instability. While ligaments are not visible on x-rays, instabilities may be evident on plain films by appreciating cervical alignment. On the lateral cervical view, three columns should align (Figure 34-5). The anterior margin of the vertebral bodies should align in a smooth, continuous lordotic curve. The posterior margins of the vertebral bodies should align in a smooth continuous lordotic curve. The third and final column is formed by anterior margin of the spinous processes. Disruption of any two columns should raise suspicion for an unstable cervical spine. CT scan of the neck can help identify cervical fractures with greater accuracy. Any athlete with an abnormal cervical spine x-ray should receive a CT scan with thin cuts through the level of abnormality to clearly characterize the cervical fracture.

Treatment

Athlete with neck and cervical spine injuries should be managed by trained personnel following the standard principles of advanced life support and trauma life support.[6,7,21] The unconscious downed athlete should not be moved, EMS should be immediately activated and athlete should be appropriately boarded, immobilized, and transported to the emergency department.[10–21]

An algorithm for on-field evaluation of the conscious athlete with cervical spine injury is presented in Figure 34-6.[20] The EMS should be activated to assist with immobilization and removal of the athlete. If a neck collar is available this could be applied. However, hard cervical collars should not be used in athletes with helmet, neck roll or shoulder pads, because these devices will interfere with fit and function of the hard collar. Studies have shown an increased neck motion and manipulation during application of the collar in these

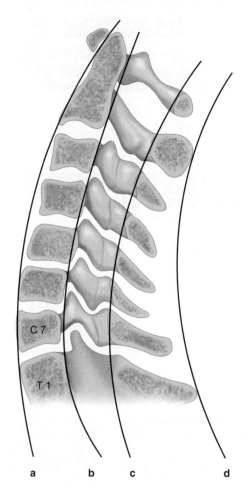

FIGURE 34-5 ■ Schematic illustration of lateral radiograph of the cervical spine. Normally the anterior vertebral body line **(A)**, posterior vertebral body line **(B)**, the spinolaminar line **(C)**, and the line along the spinous processes **(D)**, should be aligned in a smooth continuous curve.

athletes. The neck of the helmeted athlete can be immobilized by taping the helmet to the spine board. Sand bags or pillows along each side of the neck can help to further immobilize the head and neck. Appropriately trained personnel should log roll and immobilize the athlete on the spine board. Football helmets should not be removed. The face mask can be removed from the helmet to allow airway management or CPR if necessary. If it becomes necessary to remove the helmet, the shoulder pads should also be removed. The athlete's head will fall into hyperextension as the shoulders are elevated by the shoulder pads. If available, the National Institute of Neurological Disorders and Stroke recommends intravenous methyl prednisolone within 8 hours at an initial dose 30 mg/kg bolus over 15 minutes, followed by 5.4 mg/kg/h over next 23 hours. Inter-Association Task Force Guidelines for appropriate care of the spine-injured athlete are presented in Table 34-1.

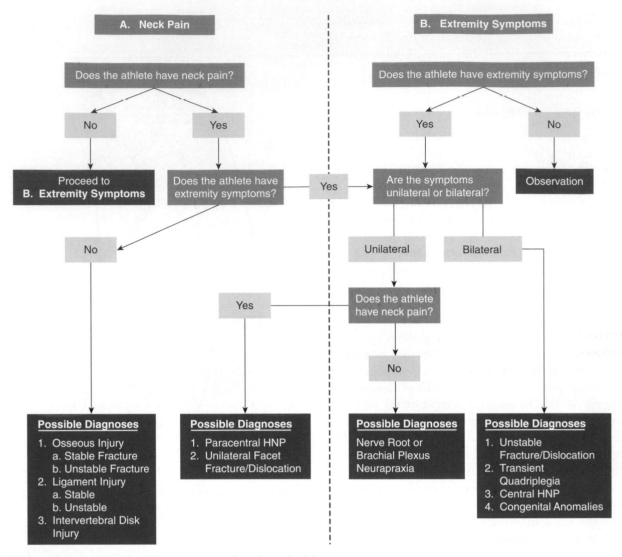

FIGURE 34-6 ■ Algorithm for on-field evaluation of cervical spine injury.

Table 34-1.

Inter-Association Task Force Guidelines for Appropriate Care of the Spine-Injured Athlete

General guidelines

■ Any athlete suspected of having a spinal injury should not be moved and should be managed as though a spinal injury exists.

■ The athlete's airway, breathing, circulation, neurological status, and level of consciousness should be assessed.

■ The athlete should not be moved unless absolutely essential to maintain airway, breathing, and circulation.

■ If the athlete must be moved to maintain airway, breathing, and circulation, the athlete should be placed in a supine position while maintaining spinal immobilization.

■ When moving a suspected spine-injured athlete, the head and trunk should be moved as a unit. One accepted technique is to manually splint the head to the trunk.

■ The Emergency Medical Services system should be activated.

Face mask removal

■ The face mask should be removed prior to transportation, regardless of current respiratory status.

■ Those involved in the prehospital care of injured football players should have the tools for face mask removal readily available.

Football helmet removal

The athletic helmet and chin strap should only be removed:

■ if the helmet and chin strap do not hold the head securely, such that immobilization of the helmet does not also immobilize the head;

(continued)

Table 34-1. *(Continued)*

Inter-Association Task Force Guidelines for Appropriate Care of the Spine-Injured Athlete

- if the design of the helmet and chin strap is such that, even after removal of the face mask, the airway cannot be controlled nor ventilation provided;
- if the face mask cannot be removed after a reasonable period of time;
- if the helmet prevents immobilization for transportation in an appropriate position.

Helmet removal

Spinal immobilization must be maintained while removing the helmet.

- Helmet removal should be frequently practiced under proper supervision.
- Specific guidelines for helmet removal need to be developed.
- In most circumstances, it may be helpful to remove cheek padding and/or deflate air padding prior to helmet removal.

Equipment

Appropriate spinal alignment must be maintained.

- There needs to be a realization that the helmet and shoulder pads elevate an athlete's trunk when in the supine position.
- Should either the helmet or shoulder pads be removed—or if only one of these is present—appropriate spinal alignment must be maintained.
- The front of the shoulder pads can be opened to allow access for CPR and defibrillation.

Additional guidelines

- This task force encourages the development of a local emergency care plan regarding the prehospital care of an athlete with a suspected spinal injury. This plan should include communication with the institution's administration and those directly involved with the assessment and transportation of the injured athlete.
- All providers of prehospital care should practice and be competent in all of the skills identified in these guidelines before they are needed in an emergency situation.

SPECIFIC INJURIES

Cervical Spine Fractures

Cervical fractures can occur at any cervical level. In sports, the most common mechanism is axial loading with the neck slightly flexed.[7] In football, this can occur if the tackler or running back drops his head and looks down, while making initial contact with the head. In hockey, this mechanism can occur as the athlete drops his head prior to contacting the boards with his head. Gymnasts and divers are exposed to these mechanisms as they fall from a height on the head. Axial loading of the cervical spine often results in burst fracture of the vertebral body. Fatigue of the bony column commonly occurs in the middle resulting in burst fracture. Axial loading in diving can result in burst fracture of C_1, which is known as a Jefferson Fracture. Hyperflexion, hyperextension, lateral bending, and rotation can contribute to extensive neck injury resulting in cervical fractures.

Once a cervical fracture is suspected or identified, referral to orthopedic or neurosurgeon should be initiated. The surgeon will guide and direct the management and return to play based on experience. In the case of well-healed fractures and single level fusion with no neurological sequelae, athletes may be allowed to return to sports, possibly even contact sports. Athletes with multiple level cervical fusion may be allowed to return to noncollision, noncontact, and low-risk sports.

Cervical Sprain

Cervical ligaments stabilize the cervical spine. The anterior longitudinal, posterior longitudinal, and ligamenta flavum may be injured by forced flexion or extension of the neck.[17] Collision sports such as wrestling, football, and rugby put the neck at risk. Athletes present with pain and spasm of the neck. Neck range of motion will be limited. Also, there is commonly midline cervical tenderness. Plain films should be taken if there is midline tenderness or if there is a limited range of motion. Often these x-rays appear normal. Lateral films with the neck in flexion and extension can identify instabilities. MRI can help identify cervical instabilities as well as neurological compromise.

Stable cervical sprains can be managed conservatively with relative rest and pain control. When the athlete is pain-free, he should begin a rehabilitation program to return neck range of motion and strength. Only when full pain-free range of motion and strength has returned can the athlete begin to return to sport. Unstable cervical sprains should be referred to orthopedic or neurosurgeon for management. Initially, the neck should be immobilized in a cervical collar. Return to play will be determined based on surgical procedure.

Cervical Strain

The most common neck injuries in young athletes are cervical strains. Resisted extension, flexion, or lateral flexion can result in tearing of the cervical musculature.

Direct trauma to the cervical muscles can result in muscle injury as well. Pain will be localized to the isolated muscle group injured. Pain is increased with resisted force. Range of motion in the isolated direction may be limited by pain. If pain is midline, over the spinous processes, x-rays are indicated. Occasionally, avulsion fractures of the spinous process are associated with cervical strains.

Treatment includes pain control and relative rest from sports. Rehabilitation may be necessary to retain range of motion and strength. No athlete should return to sports until full pain-free range of motion and strength has returned.

Spear Tackler Spine

Poor tackling technique in football can lead to the loss of lordotic curve of the spine. Athletes who repeatedly make initial contact with the head are at risk for developing spear tackler spine. These athletes may present with neck pain or may have no symptoms at all. In the later case, loss of cervical lordosis should prompt further investigation. Lateral x-rays will show a straightening of the cervical spine (Figure 34-7).

The combination of abnormal alignment of the cervical spine and poor technique places the athlete with spear tackler spine at risk for fracture and permanent spinal cord injury.[7,17,22–24] When this condition is identified, the athlete should be disqualified from contact/collision sport participation. Prolonged rest may sometimes reverse the loss of normal alignment.

Stingers and Burners

Injuries involving the brachial plexus are commonly referred to as "burners or stingers." Fifty percent of high school football players experience these injuries during their sport participation.[25,26] Symptoms are often transient and resolve spontaneously. Thus, athletes may experience a "burner or stinger" without reporting the incident. Three common mechanisms for burner and stingers are described (Figure 34-8).[7,25,26] Injuries can predominantly affect either the nerve root or the brachial plexus (Table 34-2), however mixed injury can also occur. Effects of brachial plexus lesions are summarized in Table 34-3.

Often repeat examination will show full return of strength, sensation, and range of motion within 48 hours. Although symptoms usually resolve in most athletes, persistent neurological symptoms, bilateral symptoms and signs, and recurrent episodes of burners, justify further workup including neurosurgical consultation and advance imaging.

No athlete should return to participation with symptoms or weakness. However, prognosis is good for full recovery after the initial episode. Athletes can return without further risk. For football players, a neck roll or cowboy collar can be attached to the shoulder pads to allow proper neck positioning and protect against brachial plexus compression.

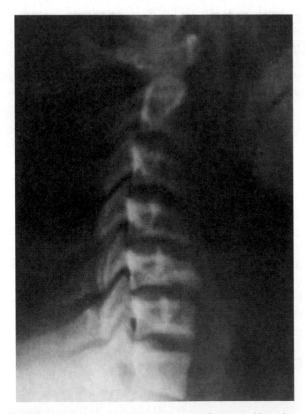

FIGURE 34-7 ■ Lateral cervical spine x-ray of spear tackler spine.

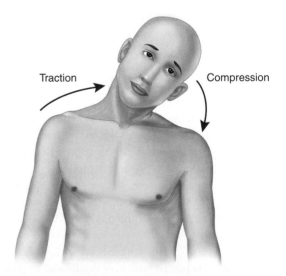

FIGURE 34-8 ■ Mechanisms of burner or stinger. Brachial plexus or cervical nerve roots can be injured with either traction or compression as a result of sudden forceful lateral flexion of the neck.

Table 34-2.

Differentiation Between Brachial Plexus and Nerve Root Lesions

Brachial Plexus Lesions	Nerve Root Lesions
1. Numbness and burning of entire arm, hand, and fingers	1. Numbness and burning confined to one or more definable dermatomes
2. Sensation loss over two to four dermatomes	2. Sensation loss confined to a definable dermatome
3. Complete transient paralysis of arm	3. Partial transient paralysis of arm
4. Tenderness over brachial plexus	4. No tenderness over brachial plexus
5. No tenderness over neck posteriorly	5. Tenderness over neck posteriorly
6. Increase in symptoms with passive movement of neck to *opposite side*	6. Hyperflexion, extension, or lateral flexion of neck to *same side* as the symptoms may cause symptoms
7. Symptoms do not occur with downward pressure on head with chin in supraclavicular fossa on same side as lesion	7. Symptoms occur with downward pressure on head with chin in supraclavicular fossa on same side as lesion

Note: It may not be possible to differentiate these two because the symptoms and signs may be mixed.
From Roy S, Irvin R. Sports Medicine. Englewood Cliffs, NJ: Prentice-Hall, Inc; 1983:259.)

Cervical Cord Neuropraxia and Transient Quadriplegia

Cervical cord neuropraxia can result in temporary symptoms of burning, loss of sensation, and tingling with or without extremity weakness. This is referred to as transient quadriplegia.[27–30] Full recovery is usually within minutes, though it can possibly take up to 2 days or more to resolve. In football, the incidence of transient quadriplegia has been reported to be seven cases in 10,000 athletes. Hyperflexion and hyperextension of the neck are described as the inciting mechanisms. Under the extreme of these motions, the central cervical canal can become relatively stenosed (functional stenosis) resulting in injury to the spinal cord.

Athletes with cervical spinal stenosis would be at an increased risk for transient quadriplegia as well as permanent spinal cord injury. The initial management

Table 34-3.

Effects of a Brachial Plexus Lesion

Nerve Root	Symptoms: Pain, Numbness, Tingling	Signs: Sensation Impairment	Weakness	Reflexes Absent
C4	Supraclavicular and shoulder area	Supraclavicular and shoulder area	On attempting to resist forced lateral flexion of the neck to the opposite side	
C5	Outer border of upper arm	Outer border of upper arm	Shoulder abduction Elbow flexion	Biceps Supinator
C6	Down radial side of arm to include radial side of hand	Radial side of forearm, thumb, and index fingers	Shoulder abduction Elbow flexion Pronation and supination Wrist flexion and extension	Biceps Supinator
C7	Down arm to hand including middle finger	Middle finger and corresponding area on palmar aspect of hand	Shoulder adduction Elbow extension Wrist flexion and extension Finger flexion and extension	Triceps Flexor finger jerk
C8	Down ulnar side of forearm to include ulnar side of hand	Ulnar side of forearm, ring, and little finger	Elbow extension Finger flexion and extension	Flexor finger jerk
T1	Inner border of mid- and upper arm	Inner border upper arm	Finger abduction and adduction	

From Roy S, Irvin R. Sports Medicine. Englewood Cliffs, NJ: Prentice-Hall, Inc; 1983:260.

Box 34-1 When to Refer.

■ All athletes with significant head and neck trauma must be managed in the appropriate acute care medical setting by a team of expert clinicians that may include orthopedics, neurosurgery, spine surgery, otolaryngology, and others as appropriate.

■ Appropriate specialist consultation should be obtained for other conditions such as spear tackler spine, bilateral neurological symptoms and signs, cervical cord neuropraxia, and transient quadriplegia.

should be the same as for any spinal cord injured athlete and all athletes with episodes of cervical cord neuropraxia and transient quadriplegia should be referred to neurosurgery for further evaluation, management, and to guide the return to play decisions[7,11,15,22,25,27–31] (Box 34-1).

REFERENCES

1. Pizzutillo PD. Injury of the cervical spine in young children. *Instr Course Lect.* 2006;55:633-639.

2. Powell J D. High School Football Injury Surveillance Study Highlights, National Athletic Trainers Association. 1995. www.nata.org/prevention/95highlights. Accessed April 12, 1998.

3. Clarke KS. Epidemiology of athletic neck injury. *Clin Sport Med.* 1998;17(1):83-97.

4. National Collegiate Athletic Association. *Sports Medicine Handbook 2005-2006.* 18th ed. Indianapolis, IN; National Collegiate Athletic Association; 2005.

5. Thomas B, McCullen G. Cervical spine injuries in football players. *J Am Acad Orthop Surg.* 1999;7:338.

6. Dimberg EL, Burns TM. Management of common neurologic conditions in sports. *Clin Sports Med.* 2005;24(3): 637-662, ix.

7. Banerjee R, Palumbo MA, Fadale PD. Catastrophic cervical spine injuries in the collision sport athlete, part 1: epidemiology, functional anatomy, and diagnosis. *Am J Sports Med.* 2004;32(4):1077-1087.

8. Torg JS. *Athletic Injuries of the Head, Neck, and Face,* 2nd ed. Philadelphia, PA: Lea and Febiger 1992.

9. Cantu RC. Head injuries in adults. In: DeLee JC, Drez D, Miller MD, eds. *Orthopedic Sports Medicine.* 2nd ed. Philadelphia, PA: Saunders; 2003:769-774.

10. Stevenson KL, Adelson D. Pediatric sport-related head injuries. In: DeLee JC, Drez D, Miller MD, eds. *Orthopedic Sports Medicine.* 2nd ed. Philadelphia, PA: Saunders; 2003:775-790.

11. Cooper L. Acute disposition of neck injuries. *Curr Sports Med Rep.* 2005;4:24-26.

12. Hutchinson M, Tansey J. Sideline management of fractures. *Curr Sports Med Rep.* 2003;2:125-135.

13. Dec KL, Cole SL, Metivier S. Screening for catastrophic neck injuries in sports. *Curr Sports Med Rep.* 2007;6:16-19.

14. Ellis JL, Gottlieb JE. Return to play decisions after cervical spine injuries. *Curr Sports Med Rep.* 2007;6:56-61.

15. Herman MJ. Cervical spine injuries in the pediatric and adolescent athlete. *Instr Course Lect.* 2006;55:641-646.

16. Lebrun CM. Care of the high school athlete: prevention and treatment of medical emergencies. *Instr Course Lect.* 2006;55:687-702.

17. Sanchez AR 2nd, Sugalski MT, LaPrade RF. Field-side and prehospital management of the spine-injured athlete. *Curr Sports Med Rep.* 2005;4(1):50-55.

18. Cooper L. Acute disposition of neck injuries. *Curr Sports Med Rep.* 2005;4(1):24-26.

19. Boden BP, Prior C. Catastrophic spine injuries in sports. *Curr Sports Med Rep.* 2005;4(1):45-49.

20. Banerjee R, Palumbo MA, Fadale PD. Catastrophic cervical spine injuries in the collision sport athlete, part 2: principles of emergency care. *Am J Sports Med.* 2004;32(7):1760-1764.

21. Waninger KN. Management of the helmeted athlete with suspected cervical spine injury. *Am J Sports Med.* 2004; 32(5):1331-1350.

22. Zmurko MG, Tannoury TY, Tannoury CA, et al. Cervical sprains, disc herniations, minor fractures, and other cervical injuries in the athlete. *Clin Sports Med.* 2003;22(3):513-521.

23. Morganti C. Recommendations for return to sports following cervical spine injuries. *Sports Med.* 2003;33(8):563-573.

24. Vaccaro AR, Klein GR, Ciccoti M, et al. Return to play criteria for the athlete with cervical spine injuries resulting in stinger and transient quadriplegia/paresis. *Spine J.* 2002;2(5):351-356.

25. Eddy D, Congeni J, Loud K. A review of spine injuries and return to play. *Clin J Sports Med.* 2005;15(6):453-458.

26. Cantu RC. Stingers, transient quadriplegia, and cervical spinal stenosis: return-to-play criteria. *Med Sci Sports Exerc.* 1997;29(Suppl):S233-S235.

27. Kasow DB, Curl WW. "Stingers" in adolescent athletes. *Instr Course Lect.* 2006;55:711-716.

28. Torg JS. Cervical spinal stenosis with cord neuropraxia: evaluations and decisions regarding participation in athletics. *Curr Sports Med Rep.* 2002;1:43-46.

29. Castro FP Jr. Stingers, cervical cord neurapraxia, and stenosis. *Clin Sports Med.* 2003;22(3):483-492.

30. Allen CR, Kang JD. Transient quadriparesis in the athlete. *Clin Sports Med.* 2002;21(1):15-27.

31. Cantu RV, Cantu RC. Current thinking: return to play and transient quadriplegia. *Curr Sports Med Rep.* 2005;4(1): 27-32.

Additional Readings

American College of Surgeons. *Advanced Trauma Life Support Course Student Manual.* 7th ed. American College of Surgeons, 2007.

American Heart Association. *Advanced Cardiac Life Support Course Provider Manual.* Dallas: American Heart Association; 2005.

Kleiner DM, Almquist JL, Bailes J, et al. *Prehospital Care of the Spine-Injured Athlete.* Inter-Association Task Force for Appropriate Care of the Spine-Injured Athlete, National Athletic Trainers' Association, Dallas, 2001.

CHAPTER 35

Physically Challenged Athletes

Dilip R. Patel and
Donald E. Greydanus

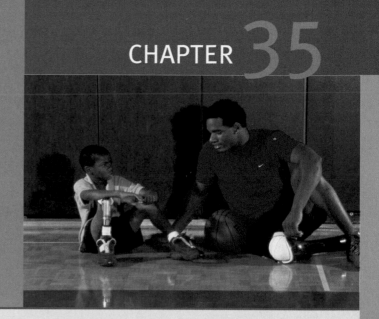

DEFINITIONS

Athletes with neuromotor and sensory disorders (Table 35-1) have a wide range of abilities.[1–7] The World Health Organization International Classification of Functioning, Disability, and Health (ICF) terminology is summarized in Table 35-2.[8–10]

The older terminology defined a *handicap* as a disadvantage for a given individual, resulting from impairment or a disability that limits or prevents the fulfillment of a role that is normal (depending on age, sex, and social as well as cultural factors) for that individual. Americans with Disabilities Act defines a disability as an impairment that limits a major life activity; either a record of such an impairment in the preparticipation or physician's notes, or a perception by the public that an impairment limits major activity of life, are also considered as evidence of disability.[11]

The term, *adapted sport*, refers to a sport that is modified or especially designed for an athlete with disability.[4,5] The athlete may either participate with others who have no disabilities (integrated settings) or only with other athletes with disabilities (segregated settings). *Paralympic Games* (Table 35-3) include athletes who have physical disabilities or visual impairment, whereas *Special Olympics* is a sports training and competition program for persons with intellectual disability (mental retardation) age 8 years and older, irrespective

Table 35-1.

Neuromotor and Sensory Disabilities

Amputations
Cerebral palsy
Traumatic brain injury
Spinal cord injuries
Spina bifida
Neuromuscular disorders
Neurocognitive disabilities
Visual impairment
Hearing impairment
Disabilities associated with chronic medical diseases

Table 35-2.

WHO International Classification of Functioning, Disability, and Health

Normal Function	Lack of Normal Function
Body functions	*Impairments*
The physiological functions of the body	Problems in the body function as a significant deviation or loss
Body structures	*Impairments*
Anatomical parts of the body	Problems in structure as a significant deviation or loss
Activity	*Activity limitations*
The execution of a task or action by an individual	Difficulties an individual may have in executing activities
Participation	*Participation restrictions*
Involvement in a life situation	Problems an individual may have in involvement in life situation
Functioning	*Disability*
A global term used to encompass body functions, body structures, activities, and participation	A global term used to encompass problems with body functions, body structures, activity limitations, and participation restrictions

http://www.who.int/classifications/icf/en/.

Table 35-3.

Paralympic Games

Alpine skiing
Archery
Athletics (track & field)
Basketball
Bocce
Curling
Cycling
Equestrian
Fencing
Goalball
Ice hockey
Ice sledge hockey
Judo
Lawn bowls
Nordic skiing
Powerlifting
Rowing
Sailing
Shooting
Soccer (football)
Swimming (aquatics)
Table tennis
Tennis
Volleyball
Wheelchair dance
Wheelchair rugby

of their abilities.[4,5,12] Athletes with other disabilities such as those with muscular dystrophy, multiple sclerosis, chronic juvenile arthritis, osteogenesis imperfecta, ataxia, are all categorized as *les austres* (meaning "others").

Persons with disability should be referred to appropriately so as to maintain respect and dignity. A preferred way to address these individuals is the "person first" approach, e.g. a person with cerebral palsy instead of a cerebral palsy victim; in this manner, one refers to a person with a disability rather than to a disabled person.

EPIDEMIOLOGY

An estimated 12% of the school-aged children in the United States are physically challenged; there are

Table 35-4.

Paralympic Athletes

Spinal cord injuries
Limb amputations
Cerebral palsy
Blindness and other visual impairments

Table 35-5.

Epidemiological Characteristics of Musculoskeletal Injuries in Physically Challenged Athletes

The incidence and pattern of musculoskeletal injuries in physically challenged athletes are similar to those in able-bodied athletes
Overuse injuries are the most common injuries
For acute injuries, soft-tissue injuries (skin abrasions, strains, sprains, contusions) are the most common injuries
Acute fractures and dislocations are uncommon
The site and type of injury vary depending upon particular sport and specific disability
Prosthesis, orthoses, and other adaptive equipment influence the type and pattern of injuries
Most injuries are considered minor (7 or less days of time loss from sports)

approximately 40 million physically challenged persons in the United States.[1,13,14] It is estimated that there are more than three million individuals with physical and mental disabilities involved in organized athletic competition in the US; and many more in recreational sports. Participation opportunities for the physically and mentally challenged athletes have increased over the past several decades with between 3000 and 6000 Paralympic athletes (Table 35-4) participating at various levels of competition. Several investigators have analyzed the epidemiology of musculoskeletal injuries in athletes with physical and sensory disabilities and key findings are summarized in Table 35-5.[15–30]

PATHOGENESIS AND CLINICAL PRESENTATION

Pathophysiology and clinical presentations differ depending upon specific disorder or physical disability. For ease of discussion, key elements of pathophysiology, clinical presentations, and major medical concerns (Table 35-6) for specific disorders are reviewed together below with comments on relevant and any unique aspects of management.[31–36]

Spinal Cord Injury (SCI)

Fortunately, spinal cord injuries in children and adolescents are not common; however, they have significant lifelong consequences for independent living as well as sport participation. These athletes are predisposed to injuries related to use of wheelchairs, prostheses, and other adaptive devices, not unlike other athletes who are

Table 35-6.

Major Medical Concerns in Physically Challenged Athletes

Hyperthermia
Hypothermia
Autonomic dysreflexia
Neurogenic bowel
Neurogenic bladder
Latex allergy
High risk for pressure sores
Heterotrophic calcification
Osteopenia

wheelchair bound.[28,37–39] Individuals with SCI are at risk for specific medical problems related to loss of motor and sensory function as well as lack of control of autonomic function (dysautonomia) below the level of the lesion, including impaired thermoregulation and autonomic dysreflexia.[40–56]

Thermoregulation

Temperature regulation is impaired in athletes with spinal cord injury, especially with lesions above T8. Both, hyperthermia and hypothermia have been reported to be serious problems in these athletes. Impaired sweating below the lesion level reduces the effective body surface area available for evaporative cooling. There is also venous pooling in lower limbs, and decreased venous return, which also reduces heat loss by convection and radiation. This can lead to increased body temperature and hyperthermia. Certain medications (e.g., anticholinergics) taken by these athletes can also increase the risk of hyperthermia.

On the other hand in cooler conditions, such as swimming, there is an increased risk for hypothermia. Impaired vasomotor and sudomotor neural control, decreased muscle mass below the lesion, and possible impaired central temperature-regulating mechanisms, all contribute to the development of hypothermia. There is a lack of shiver response below the level of the lesion. These athletes also lack sensation below this level and thus may not be aware of wet clothes. Problems with appropriate temperature regulation can occur even within milder ambient temperature ranges. Adequate hydration must be maintained, and the athlete should be removed from sports activity at the first sign of any problem. Awareness of these issues and education of athletes and coaches are key to prevention.

Autonomic dysreflexia

Autonomic dysreflexia has been known to occur in athletes with spinal cord injuries above T6. There is a loss of inhibition of the sympathetic nervous system, which leads to an acute uncontrolled sympathetic response manifested by sweating above the lesion, chest tightness, headache, apprehension, acute paroxysmal hypertension, hyperthermia, cardiac arrhythmias, and gastrointestinal disturbances. A number of stimuli below the level of the lesion can trigger such a response; these include urinary tract infection, bladder distension, bowel distention, pressure sores, tight clothing, and acute fractures. Awareness of the potential for autonomic dysreflexia is the key to prevention. At the first signs of this syndrome the athlete should be removed from the sports activity, any recognized offending stimulus should be eliminated, and the athlete should preferably be transported to an emergency facility for further management. In most cases this is a self-limited response; however, persistent hypertension and cardiac arrhythmias can occur.

A phenomenon of self-induced autonomic dysreflexia, known as 'boosting,' has been recognized over the past several years, especially in wheelchair athletes seeking to improve their race times. These athletes will knowingly trigger such a response, by inducing a trigger such as distending the bladder. They may drink large amount of fluids, strap legs very tightly, or clamp their catheters to induce bladder distention. Self-induced lower leg fractures have also been reported. The exact mechanism of performance enhancement effects is not known; however, it is hypothesized that it is in part caused by increased blood flow to working muscles, and glycogen sparing caused by increased utilization of adipose tissue which is induced by increased catecholamines. This has been shown to enhance performance and reduce race time and give the athlete an advantage. It is important to recognize that self-induced dysreflexia poses serious health risks for the athlete and this practice is considered an ergogenic aid which is not sanctioned by sport governing bodies.

Meningomyelocele

Children with meningomyelocele are at an increased risk for obesity (prevalence of up to 75%) for whom participation in sports and other physical activities is especially therapeutic.[1] Approximately 75% of these lesions occur at the lower lumbar and sacral levels with loss of motor and sensory function below the lesion level. The presence of hydrocephalus can adversely affect cerebral function; increased intraventricular pressure and dilatation can damage the motor cortex and lead to development of spasticity above the level of the lesion.[1–3,32] Children with meningomyelocele also have deficits in both hand to eye and foot to eye coordination. They have decreased aerobic power, decreased endurance, decreased peak anaerobic power, and mechanical inefficiency similar to others with neuromuscular disorders.[4,51–53] The level of the lesion and severity of hydrocephalus are important factors influencing the ability to participate in sports.[2,10] Children with meningomyelocele are categorized according to the functional level of the spinal cord lesion.

Because of poor soft tissue support, increased local pressure and lack of sensation below the lesion level, these children are prone to develop localized skin breakdown, with resultant pressure sores and ulcers. They are also at an increased risk for ligament sprains because of lack of strong musculotendinous units around the involved joints. Decreased muscle strength and strength imbalance increase the risk for muscle strains in these athletes. Children with meningomyelocele lack the appropriate loading of their bones because of the lack of weight-bearing activities; this, often combined with nutritional inadequacy, may lead to osteopenia and increased risk for fractures. Fractures may occur following minimal trauma and may initially be mistaken for localized infection because of erythema and swelling. Because of lack of sensation, these athletes do not feel pain, further delaying the diagnosis of a fracture.

Bowel and bladder control

Children with meningomyelocele, spinal cord injuries, and other neuromuscular disabilities have difficulty with bladder control (neurogenic bladder) and bowel control (neurogenic bowel). Different bowel and bladder routines, accidents, and odor may cause embarrassment for the child. In the context of sports participation, the athlete may be too preoccupied with the sport to adhere to a prescribed bladder or bowel regimen. Some athletes may be on a scheduled voiding regimen, requiring clean intermittent catheterization, or may have an indwelling catheter. There is also the problem of access to appropriate facilities in a timely fashion. These factors and others (as inadequate hydration) lead to an increased risk for urinary tract infections in these athletes. A regular regimen of voiding, ensuring adequate hydration (before, during, and after the sports activity), and using appropriate sterile voiding techniques will prevent urinary retention and associated complications. In addition to a neurogenic bladder, these athletes also have problems with constipation and stool retention that require following a regular bowel regimen.

Latex allergy

The prevalence of latex allergy in children with myelomeningocele is between 60% and 70%.[35,36,57] Thus, latex allergy is an important consideration while working with athletes who have spina bifida. This information should be ascertained from the athlete or the family, so that during medical emergency one can avoid using latex gloves with these athletes. Other articles containing natural rubber latex should also be avoided.

Sources of latex in the medical setting include gloves, stethoscope tubing, blood pressure cuffs, catheters, wound drains, bandages, bulb syringes and others; household sources include balloons, condoms, shoe soles, erasers, some toys, sport equipment, and others.

Hydrocephalus and shunt

The presence and severity of hydrocephalus and a ventriculoperitoneal (VP) shunt in children with meningomyelocele are major factors affecting the functional level and ability of these athletes to participate in sports. The VP shunt system is generally protected under the skin; however, it is at risk of injury if the overlying skin sustains sufficient impact to cause a laceration. Such an injury requires immediate evaluation by a neurosurgeon. Athletes with cerebrospinal fluid shunts are not necessarily restricted from sport participation simply because of the presence of this shunt. They should wear appropriate helmet/headgear for protection.

Associated conditions

Children with the associated Arnold-Chiari type 2 malformation should be restricted from activities that have significant risk of injury to the cervical spine; these include sports such as diving and football. Children with progressively worsening extremity strength, scoliosis, and bowel and bladder function should be evaluated for possible hydromyelia and tethered cord. These athletes should be restricted from further sports participation until after appropriate orthopedic and neurosurgical intervention and reassessment of their functional abilities. Examples of high-risk sports for children with spina bifida include football, cheerleading, scuba diving, water skiing, polo, and bobsledding.

Cerebral Palsy

Cerebral palsy is characterized by spasticity, athetosis, and ataxia. Fifty percent of athletes with cerebral palsy participate in wheelchair sports and the other 50% are ambulatory. Multiple factors affect the ability of athletes with cerebral palsy to optimally perform in sports, influence the risk for injury, and can have implications for developing training programs for athletes with cerebral palsy (Table 35-7).[58–73]

Athletes with cerebral palsy are at increased risk for overuse syndromes, muscle strains, chronic knee pain, patellofemoral problems, and chondromalacia patellae. Progressively decreased flexibility of hamstrings and quadriceps contributes to proximal patellar migration. Normal hip development is affected because of decreased flexibility and increased spasticity around the hips. This eventually contributes to the development of coxa valga, acetabular dysplasia, and hip subluxation. Hip flexion contractures and tight hamstrings can lead

Table 35-7.

Factors that Increase the Risk of Injury and Adversely Affect Ability to Participate in Sports in Athletes with Cerebral Palsy

Decreased musculoskeletal flexibility
Decreased muscle strength and endurance
Muscle strength and flexibility imbalance (i.e., relatively stronger flexors compared to extensors)
Progressively worsening spasticity
Progressively increasing joint contractures
High energy cost of movement (decreased mechanical efficiency)
Decreased anaerobic power and capacity
Decreased aerobic capacity
Increased cost of breathing (decreased lung volume and stiff thoracic cage)
Perceptual motor deficiencies
Visual impairment
Hearing impairment
Impaired hand eye coordination
Cognitive delay and retardation

to increased lumbar lordosis, chronic back pain, and spondylolysis. Some athletes find it difficult to control rackets and bats because of impaired hand–eye coordination; athletes with perceptual problems may also have difficulties in throwing and catching. Many will develop ankle and foot deformities affecting sport participation and requiring orthopedic management. The presence of tonic neck reflexes can adversely affect effective development of certain sport skills, such as use of bats, hockey sticks, or rackets.

Athletes with cerebral palsy benefit from carefully designed conditioning programs which should include appropriately supervised strength training and flexibility exercises. Strength training should take into account the differential tone and spasticity in different muscle groups so that the training is directed to appropriate muscle groups to optimize muscle balance. Stretching, started after a period of warm-up, should be slow and sustained to prevent activation of stretch reflex. Specific training can also help improve ataxia and coordination.

Wheelchair Athletes

Wheelchair athletes include those with cerebral palsy, spina bifida, and spinal cord injuries. Sports with descending order of injury risk for wheelchair athletes are track, basketball, road racing, tennis, and field events. In wheelchair athletes, overuse injuries are the most common injuries, shoulders and wrists are the most frequently injured regions and[74–76] shoulder pain is a common complaint; specific shoulder injuries include

rotator cuff impingement, rotator cuff tendonitis, biceps tendonitis, and tear of the long head of biceps tendon. Soft tissue injuries (most commonly seen in track, road racing, and basketball) include lacerations, abrasions, and blistering affecting arms and hands. Peripheral entrapment neuropathies is common in wheelchair athletes, the most common of which is the carpal tunnel syndrome, reported in 50% to 75% of the athletes.[74–76] In athletes with spinal cord injuries and meningomyelocele, painless hip dislocations can occur. Some athletes may develop progressive neuromuscular scoliosis limiting their cardiorespiratory capacity.

Pressure sores

Wheelchair athletes with spinal cord injuries and myelomeningocele are especially at risk for developing pressure sores. The wheelchair athlete's knees are at a higher level than the buttocks, a position that leads to increased pressure over the sacrum and ischial tuberosities for prolonged periods of time. Because of lack of pain and touch sensation, skin lesions remain asymptomatic. With delay in recognition, pressure sores can become infected. Thus, frequent, meticulous skin examinations are necessary for early detection of problem pressure areas. Any sores must be promptly treated to prevent complications. There must be adequate local padding to relieve pressure. The athlete should have appropriate chair size and fit, and should be educated to frequently change position.

Athletes with Limb Amputations

Use of assistive/adaptive devices, prostheses, and orthoses is common in athletes with limb amputations; these devises should be of proper fit and checked and adjusted regularly as the physical growth of the child or adolescent progresses.[37–39] Sports governing bodies have rules allowing or disallowing participation of athletes with prosthetic devices; currently, high school interscholastic athletics allow athletes to wear these devices in many sports including football, wrestling, soccer, and baseball. The factors considered include the type of amputation and prosthesis as well as the potential for harm to others or unfair advantage for the athlete because of the prosthetic device. Prostheses can increase local skin pressure and contribute to abrasions, blisters, and skin rash. Prepatellar, infrapatellar and pretibial bursitis in the below-knee amputee can result from socket irritation.

Athletes with lower limb amputation compensate by increasing lateral flexion and extension of the lumbar spine, potentially leading to back pain. Amputees are also prone to hyperextension injuries of the knee. Skills requiring balance are adversely affected in persons with amputation of a limb because of alteration of the center of gravity, especially in lower limb amputees.

In the skeletally immature athlete, overgrowth of the stump is a common problem. The overlying skin and soft tissue may breakdown because of friction and pressure during sports. Awareness of this problem is key to early detection because often these athletes lack pain sensation in extremities and may not be aware of the presence of these skin lesions. Increased bony prominence and local erythema indicate consideration of stump overgrowth and further evaluation. A skeletally immature child and adolescent may need periodic stump revisions until skeletal growth is complete.

Athletes with Visual Impairment

Visual impairment is a general term that refers to both partial sight as well as total blindness. A person with partial sight is only able to read using large print and/or proper magnification. A person who is not able to read large print even with magnification is considered blind; a person with total blindness is unable to perceive a strong light shone directly into his or her eyes. Legal blindness refers to visual acuity of 20/200 or less in the better eye even with correction, or a field of vision so narrowed that the widest diameter of the visual field subtends an angular distance no greater than 20 degrees (20/200).

Visual impairment does not necessarily cause motor disabilities per se; rather, it is the *lack* of experience in physical activities that may limit or delay the development or acquisition of specific motor skills.[4,77] Thus, sports participation is an important experience for the visually impaired to learn and improve movements as well as motor skills.

The United States Association for Blind Athletes promotes various sport activities for visually impaired athletes 14 years of age and older. The USABA classification for sports, based on residual vision, has these three categories: **B1** (from no light perception at all in either eye up to light perception and inability to recognize objects or contours in any direction and at any distance); **B2** (from ability to recognize objects or contours up to a visual acuity of 20/60 and/or limited visual field of 5 degrees); and **B3**: 2/60 to 6/60 (20/200) vision and/or field of vision between 5 and 20 degrees.[4,10,77]

Visually impaired athletes compete in a variety of sports including skiing, track and field events, wrestling, swimming, tandem cycling, power lifting, goal ball, judo, gymnastics, running, bicycling, baseball, bowling, and golf. Sport participation is facilitated by use of guides, such as sighted guide, a tether or guide wire, or a sound source, depending upon the degree of visual impairment.

Deaf Athletes

In the United States, deaf individuals consider themselves to belong to a subculture of the American society, and many do not consider themselves disabled. Many prefer the term *Deaf* with an uppercase D, rather than the person first terminology used to describe persons with other impairments.[4,5,10] Hearing loss can range from *mild* (hearing threshold of 27 to 40 decibels) to *profound* (hearing threshold of greater than 90 decibels). The age at which deafness occurs is an important factor in developing communication strategies for the Deaf. A child may be deaf since birth and thus before the development of speech (*prelingual deafness*) or may develop deafness later in childhood after the phase of speech development (*post lingual deafness*, usually after first 3 years of life). Some deaf persons may have associated damage to the vestibular apparatus affecting balance, otherwise most Deaf persons do not have any motor or physical deficits, in the absence of genetic or other disorders.[4,10,78]

Deaf athletes can potentially participate in all sports with athletes who do not have deafness. Sometimes, as is true for those with *unilateral* deafness, some minimal additional visual cues may be helpful; athletes with unilateral and bilateral deafness may be at some disadvantage in team sports, because of not being able to perceive voice directions from teammates and visual cues should be used instead of auditory cues for communication. Coaches should be made aware of this issue as well. In the United States, USA deaf Sport Federation promotes and organizes sports events for deaf athletes.

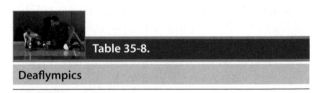

Table 35-8.

Deaflympics

Alpine skiing
Athletics (track & field)
Badminton
Basketball
Bowling
Cycling
Ice hockey
Ice sledge hockey
Nordic skiing
Orienteering
Shooting
Snowboarding
Soccer (football)
Swimming (aquatics)
Table tennis
Team handball
Tennis
Volleyball
Water polo
Wrestling

Deaf athletes do not generally qualify to participate in either the Paralympics or Special Olympics and at elite level have special summer and winter Deaflympics (Table 35-8) in which both the athletes and officials are deaf. The athlete must have a hearing loss of 55 decibels or greater in the better ear to qualify for participation in Deaflympics and hearing aids are not allowed during the competition.

MANAGEMENT

The value of sport participation for the athlete with disability is well recognized. Sport participation provides a positive social experience for these athletes. It is an opportunity for athletes and families to share their experiences with others. Sports participation can positively affect psychological, social, and moral developmental domains for the child and the adolescent, regardless of the presence of disability. Participation can enhance personal motivation, foster independence, improve coping abilities, allow athletes opportunity for social comparison, foster competitiveness and teamwork, and build self-confidence. In this section general principles of management of physically challenged athletes are presented.

Classification of Athletes

Classification of physically challenged athletes based on their functional abilities is the most important essential first step in determining the individual athlete's level of participation in sports or physical activities in general.[2,4–6,9,10,32,36] Classifying athletes with disabilities helps level the playing field, so that athletes with similar functional abilities compete against each other and will help ensure fairness in competition. The classification must also take into account the nature of the specific sport as well as any adaptive equipment used by the athlete. In addition to medical physicians, athletic trainers as well as specially trained and certified classification specialists are responsible for classification. Such a process involves a medical and a technical classification. Medical classification delineates the basic disability present, and does not necessarily provide information on the *functional* ability of the athlete for a given activity.

Functional or technical classification is based on observation of the athlete while playing his or her sport. FCS has been used for shooting, swimming, table tennis, and track and field events; it also includes athletes with spinal cord injuries, cerebral palsy, amputation, and visual impairment. Each disability sport organization (Table 35-9) may also use its own disability-specific classification system for sponsored events.

 Table 35-9.

Disability Sport and Other Related Organizations

Organization	Website
United States Paralympics	http://www.usparalympics.org
Disabled Sports USA	http://www.dsusa.org
Dwarf Athletic Association of America	http://www.daaa.org
National Disability Sports Alliance	http://www.ndsaonline.org
Special Olympics International	http://www.specialolympics.org
USA Deaf Sports Federation	http://www.usadsf.org
U.S. Association of Blind Athletes	http://www.usaba.org
Wheelchair Sports USA	http://www.wsusa.org
American Association of Adapted Sports Programs	http://www.aaasp.org
America's Athletes with Disabilities	http://americasathletes.org
Challenged Athletes Foundation	http://www.challengedathletes.org
Paralyzed Veterans of America	http://www.pva.org
United States Disabled Athletes Fund	http://www.blazesports.com
We Media Sports	http://www.wemedia.com
Women's Sports Foundation	http://www.womenssportsfoundation.org
World T.E.A.M. Sports	http://www.worldteamsports.org
International Paralympic Committee	http://www.paralympic.org
Cerebral Palsy—International Sports and Recreation Association	http://www.cpisra.org
Comité Internationale des Sports des Sourds	http://www.ciss.org
International Sports Federation—Intellectual Disability	http://www.inas-fid.org
International Blind Sports Association	http://www.ibsa.es
International Sports Organization for the Disabled	No web site
International Stroke Mandeville Wheelchair Sports Federation	http://www.wsw.org.uk

Source: *Disability Sports at the Disability Sports Website, Department of Kinesiology, Michigan State University,* http://edweb6.educ.msu.edu/kin866.

Pre-participation Evaluation

Whereas functional classification of physically challenged athletes provides the basis to match the athlete with appropriate level of physical activity with similarly challenged athletes, preparticipation evaluation as the next step forms the basis for assessing the individual athlete's general health and any specific medical conditions and treatment needs.

Preparticipaton evaluation (PPE) is an essential component of injury and illness prevention strategy in all athletes. Pediatricians and other physicians working with athletes should be familiar with the *Preparticipation Physical Evaluation Monograph*, which provides detailed guidelines for conducting PPE.[79–83] There are no specific guidelines especially designed for PPE of the physically challenged athlete. The general approach to the PPE of disabled athletes should be similar to those without disability. Often the focus is so much on the primary condition causing the disability, that the examiner may overlook common medical issues apart from the primary disability (or *diagnostic overshadowing*).

A detailed history is the mainstay of any PPE. It has been suggested that PPE for the athletes with disabilities should be preferably done by a team of medical professionals who are involved in the longitudinal care of these athletes and who know their baseline functioning. These athletes should be examined in an office setting, and the mass or station method should be avoided. The examiner(s) should be cognizant of disability-specific medical issues for the athlete. In addition to the history and physical examination, careful evaluation of the prosthetics, orthotics, and assistive/adaptive devices being used should be accomplished by a knowledgeable health care professional to ensure adequacy and proper fit.

Sport Participation Guidelines

Athletes with physical disabilities participate in a number of sports depending upon the specific disability and the demands of the sport. Use of adaptive equipment and modification of rules further enhance the sport participation experience for these athletes.

A number of factors should be considered in matching the athlete to the right sport, not unlike those for the athlete without disabilities. Among the many factors to be considered in determining the eligibility of a given athlete to participate in a particular sport include current health status of the athlete, level of competition and position played, psychological maturity of the athlete, adaptive and protective equipment, modification of the sport, and parents' and athlete's understanding of the inherent risks of injury. Thus, considering the disability and functional level of the athlete (based on appropriate classification) in conjunction with all other factors, the athlete should be matched to an appropriate sport on an individual basis.

Use of Therapeutic Medications

Many athletes with disabilities are likely to be on various therapeutic medications for associated medical disorders. The potential side effects of these medications and effects on performance should be considered while working with these athletes. The coaches, athletes, parents, and other staff should be familiar with the athlete's treatment regimen and potential medication side effects. One should also inquire about over-the-counter drugs and nutritional supplements the athlete may be taking to assess potential for drug interaction or other inadvertent effects. Thermoregulation can be adversely affected by sympathomimetics and anticholinergics. Volume depletion and dehydration are potential problems with diuretics and excessive caffeinated beverage usage. Other considerations include cardiovascular side effects of beta blockers as well as sedating effects of narcotic analgesics, muscle relaxants, and some antiepileptic drugs.

Use of Performance-Enhancing Aids

Just like athletes with no disability, the athletes with disabilities are not immune from pressure to succeed and enhance their performance by various means. No specific data are available on the prevalence of drug or supplement use for performance enhancement by athletes with disabilities. However, one should be cognizant about such a possibility while working with these athletes; thus, they should also be screened for using ergogenic drugs and supplements.

ATLANTOAXIAL INSTABILITY AND DOWN SYNDROME

Athletes with Down syndrome generally do not fall under the category of physically challenged athletes and they participate in Special Olympics. Because the question of atlantoaxial instability often arises while taking care for athletes with Down syndrome, it is briefly reviewed here.[79–83] Atlantoaxial instability has been reported in 15% of persons with Down syndrome. Children with Down syndrome have abnormal collagen resulting in increased ligamentous laxity and decreased muscle tone. Laxity of the annular ligament of C1 and hypotonia contribute to the AAI; approximately 2% of children with AAI may be symptomatic because of subluxation. Symptoms suggestive of atlantoaxial subluxation (AAS) include easy fatigueability, abnormal gait, neck pain, limited range of motion of the cervical spine, torticollis, incoordination, spasticity, hyperreflexia, clonus, extensor

Box 35-1 When to Refer

Patients with conditions that predispose them to significant physical and cognitive challenges are ideally managed by multidisciplinary teams in the setting of Medical Home.

plantar reflex, sensory deficits and other upper motor neuron and posterior column signs. Asymptomatic AAI is a concern for athletes because of increased risk for spinal cord injury during sport participation.

It has been a common practice to obtain lateral cervical spine radiographs in flexion, extension, and neutral positions, to screen for asymptomatic AAI. A 4.5 mm or more space between the posterior aspect of the anterior arch of the atlas and the odontoid process (*atlanto-dens interval*) is considered evidence of instability. Magnetic resonance imaging (observed MRI of cervical spine in flexion, extension, and neutral) is most sensitive in identifying neural canal compromise related to AAI and AAS. Radiologic studies in asymptomatic AAI may not identify all at-risk athletes, and it is difficult to predict those at-risk for future spinal cord injury. Past and current history of symptoms is the most important part of the assessment of AAI.

Athletes with Down syndrome participate in sports under the umbrella of Special Olympics. Because of increased risk for spinal cord injury from atlantoaxial subluxation during excessive flexion-extension movements, certain sports are contraindicated for persons with AAI: contact/collision sports, gymnastics, diving, pentathlon, butterfly stroke, high jump, soccer, diving starts in swimming, and certain warm-up exercises involving neck flexion–extension. Special Olympics guidelines require all athletes with Down syndrome be screened by lateral neck radiographs, initially before participating in sport programs. Some recommend periodic reassessment every 3 to 5 years, although some experts doubt the value of periodic screening if the initial screening was normal. The highest risk for AAS has been reported to be between 5 and 10 years of age (Box 35-1).

ACKNOWLEDGMENT

This chapter was adapted with permission from Patel DR, Greydanus DE. The pediatric athlete with disabilities. *Pediatr Clin North Am.* 2002;49:803-827. Copyright Elsevier 2002.

REFERENCES

1. Batshaw ML, ed. *Children with Disabilities.* 5th ed. Baltimore: Paul Brookes Publishing Co; 2007.

2. Chang FM. The disabled athlete. In: Stanitiski CL, Delee JL, Drez D, eds. *Pediatric and Adolescent Sports Medicine.* Philadelphia, PA: WB Saunders; 1994:48-75.

3. Clark MW. The physically challenged athlete. *Adolesc. Med.* 1998;9:491-499.

4. Winnick JP, ed. *Adapted Physical Education and Sport.* Champaign, IL: Human Kinetics; 2000.

5. Paciorek MJ, Jones JA. *Sports and Recreation for the Disabled.* 2nd ed. Carmel, IN: Cooper Publishing Group; 1994.

6. DePauw KP, Gavron SJ. *Disability and Sport.* Champaign, IL: Human Kinetics; 1995.

7. Adams RC, McCubbin JA. *Games, Sports, and Exercises for the Physically Disabled.* 4th ed. Philadelphia, PA: Lea and Febiger; 1991.

8. WHO International Classification of Functioning, Disability and Health. Geneva: World Health Organization; 2001.

9. Ploeg HP, Beek AJ, Woude LHV, et al. Physical activity for people with a disability: a conceptual model. *Sports Med.* 2004;34(10):639-649.

10. Goldberg B. *Sports and Exercise for Children with Chronic Health Conditions.* Champaign, IL: Human Kinetics; 1995.

11. Nichols AW. Sports medicine and the Americans with Disabilities Act. *Clin J Sports Med.* 1996;6:190-195.

12. Reynolds J, Stirk A, Thomas A, et al. Paralympics: Barcelona 1992. *Br J Sports Med.* 1994;28:14-17.

13. Halpern BC, Bochm R, Cardone DA. The disabled athlete. In: Garrett WE, Kirkendall DT, Squire DL, eds, *Principles and Practice of Primary Care Sports Medicine.* Philadelphia, PA: Lippincott Williams & Wilkins; 2001:115-132.

14. Bergeron JW. Athletes with disabilities. *Phys Med Rehabil Clin N Am.* 1999;10:213-228.

15. Ferrara MS, Buckley WE, McCann BC, et al. The injury experience of the competitive athlete with a disability: prevention implications. *Med Sci Sports Exerc.* 1991;24:184-188.

16. Ferrara MS, Buckley WE, Messner DG, et al. The injury experience and training history of the competitive skier with a disability. *Am J Sports Med.* 1992;20:55-60.

17. Steadward RD, Wheeler GD. The young athlete with a motor disability. In: Bar Or, ed. *The Child and Adolescent Athlete.* London: Blackwell Science;1996:493–522.

18. Wilson PE, Washington RL. Pediatric wheelchair athletics: sports injuries and prevention. *Paraplegia* 1993;31:330-337.

19. Ferrara MS, Peterson CL. Injuries to athletes with disabilities: identifying injury patterns. *Sports Med.* 2000;30:137-143.

20. Ferrara MS, Buckley WE. Athletes with disabilities injury registry. *Adapt Phys Activ Q* 1996;13:50-60.

21. Ferrara MS, Davis RW. Injuries to elite wheelchair athletes. *Paraplegia* 1990;28:335-341.

22. Ferrara MS, Richter KJ, Kaschalk SM. Sport for the athlete with a physical disability. In: Scuderi GR, McCann PD, Bruno PJ, eds. *Sports Medicine: Principles of Primary Care.* St. Louis: Mosby-Year Book, Inc; 1997:598-608.

23. Ferrara MS, Palutsis GR, Snouse S, et al. A longitudinal study of injuries to athletes with disabilities. *Int J Sports Med.* 2000;21:221-224.

24. Groah SL, Lanig IS. Neuromusculoskeletal syndromes in wheelchair athletes. *Semin Neurol.* 2000;20:201-208.

25. Kegel B, Malchow D. Incidence of injury in amputees playing soccer. *Palaestra* 1994;10:50-54.

26. Laskowski ER, Murtaugh PA. Snow skiing injuries in physically disabled skiers. *Am J Sports Med.* 1992;20:553-557.

27. McCormack DAR, Reid DC, Steadward R, et al. Injury profiles in wheelchair athletes: results of a retrospective survey. *Clin J Sports Med.* 1991;1:35-40.

28. Richter KJ, Hyman SC, Mushett CA, et al. Injuries in world class cerebral palsy athletes of the 1988 South Korea Paralympics. *J Osteopath Sports Med.* 1991;7:15-18.

29. Taylor D, Williams T. Sports injuries in athletes with disabilities: wheelchair racing. *Paraplegia* 1995;33:296-299.

30. Nyland J, Snouse SL, Anderson M, et al. Soft tissue injuries to USA paralympians at the 1996 summer games. *Arch Phys Med Rehabil.* 2000;81:368-373.

31. Dec KL, Sparrow KJ, McKeag DB. The physically-challenged athlete: medical issues and assessment. *Sports Med.* 2000;29:245-258.

32. Booth DW. Athletes with disabilities. In: Harries M, Williams C, Stanish W, et al., eds. *Oxford Textbook of Sports Medicine.* 2nd ed. New York: Oxford University Press; 1998:634-645.

33. American College of Sport Medicine (ACSM). *ACSM's Exercise Management for Persons with Chronic Diseases and Disabilities.* Champaign, IL: Human Kinetics; 1997.

34. Batts KB, Glorioso JE Jr, Williams MS. The medical demands of the special athlete. *Clin J Sports Med.* 1998;8:22-25.

35. Lai AM, Stanish WD, Stanish HI. The young athlete with physical challenges. *Clin Sports Med.* 2000;19:793-819.

36. Wind WM, Shwend RM, Larson J. Sports for the physically challenged child. *J Am Acad Orthop Surgeons.* 2004;12:126-137.

37. Goldberg B, Hsu J, eds. *Atlas of Orthoses and Assistive Devices. American Academy of Orthopedic Surgeons.* 3rd ed. St Louis, MO: Mosby; 1997.

38. Herring JA, Birch JG, eds. *The Child with a Limb Deficiency.* Rosemont, IL: American Academy of Orthopedic Surgeons; 1998.

39. Shephard RJ. Sports medicine and the wheelchair athlete. *Sports Med.* 1988;5:226-247.

40. Maki KC, Langbein WE, Reid-Lokos C. Energy cost and locomotive economy of handbike and rowcycle propulsion by persons with spinal cord injury. *J Rehabil Res Dev.* 1995;32:170-178.

41. Armstrong LE, Maresh CM, Riebe D, et al. Local cooling in wheelchair athletes during exercise-heat stress. *Med Sci Sports Exerc.* 1995;27:211-216.

42. Bhambhani YN, Holland LJ, Eriksson P, et al. Physiological responses during wheelchair racing in quadriplegics and paraplegics. *Paraplegia* 1994;32:253-260.

43. Braddom RL, Rocco JF. Autonomic dysreflexia: a survey of current treatment. *Am J Phys Med Rehabil.* 1991;70:234-241.

44. Burnham R, Wheeler GD, Bhambhani Y, et al. Autonomic dysreflexia in wheelchair athletes. *Clin J Sports Med.* 1994;4:1-10.

45. Erickson RP. Autonomic hyperreflexia: pathophysiology and medical management. *Arch Phys Med Rehabil.* 1980;61:431-440.

46. McCann BC. Thermoregulation in spinal cord injury: the challenge of the Atlanta Paralympics. *Spinal Cord* 1996;34:433-436.

47. Sawka MN, Latzka WA, Pandolf KB. Temperature regulation during upper body exercise: able-bodied and spinal cord injured. *Med Sci Sports Exerc.* 1989;21:S132-S140.

48. van der Woude LHV, Bakker WH, Elkhuizen JW, et al. Anaerobic work capacity in elite wheelchair athletes. *Am J Phys Med Rehabil.* 1997;76:355-365.

49. Burnham R, Wheeler G, Bhambhani Y, et al. Intentional induction of autonomic dysreflexia among quadriplegic athletes for performance enhancement: efficacy, safety, and mechanism of action. *Clin J Sports Med.* 1994;4:1-10.

50. Harris P. Self-induced autonomic dysreflexia ("boosting") practiced by some tetraplegic athletes to enhance their athletic performance. *Paraplegia* 1994;32:289-291.

51. Cooper RA, Horvarth SM, Bedi JF, et al. Maximal exercise response of paraplegic wheelchair road racers. *Paraplegia* 1992;30:573-581.

52. Dallmeijer AJ, Kappe YJ, Veeger D, et al. Anaerobic power output and propulsion technique in spinal cord injured subjects during wheelchair ergometry. *J Rehabil Res Dev.* 1994;31:120-128.

53. Davis GM. Exercise capacity of individuals with paraplegia. *Med Sci Sports Exerc.* 1993;25:423-432.

54. Jacobs PL, Nash MS. Exercise recommendations for individuals with spinal cord injury. *Sports Med.* 2004;34(11):727-751.

55. Bhambhani Y. Physiology of wheelchair racing in athletes with spinal cord injury. *Sports Med.* 2002;32(1):23-51.

56. Randolph C. Latex allergy in pediatrics. *Curr Prob Pediatr.* 2001;31:135-153.

57. Taft LT, Matthews WS, Molnar GE. Pediatric management of the physically handicapped child. *Adv Pediatr.* 1983;30:13-60.

58. Lockette K, Keyes AM. Conditioning with physical disabilities. Champaign, IL: Human Kinetics; 1994.

59. Miller P, ed. Fitness programming and physical disability. Champaign, IL: Human Kinetics; 1995.

60. Sheppard RJ. *Physical Activity for the Disabled.* Champaign, IL: Human Kinetics; 1988.

61. McCann C. Sports for the disabled: the evolution from rehabilitation to competitive sport. *Br J Sports Med.* 1996;30:279-280.

62. Shephard RJ. Benefits of sport and physical activity for the disabled: implications for the individual and for society. *Scand J Rehabil Med.* 1991;23:51-59.

63. Bhambhani YN, Holland LJ, Steadward RD. Maximal aerobic power in cerebral palsied wheelchair athletes: validity and reliability. *Arch Phys Med Rehabil.* 1992;73:246-252.

64. Damiano DL, Abel MF. Functional outcomes of strength training in spastic cerebral palsy. *Arch Phys Med Rehabil.* 1998;79:119-125.

65. Figoni SF. Exercise responses and quadriplegia. *Med Sci Sports Exerc.* 1993;25:433-441.

66. MacPhail HEA, Kramer JF. Effect of isokinetic strength training on functional ability and walking efficiency in adolescents with cerebral palsy. *Dev Med Child Neuro.* 1995;37:763-775.

67. Parker DF, Carriere L, Hebestreit H, et al. Muscle performance and gross motor function of children with spastic cerebral palsy. *Dev Med Child Neurol.* 1993;35:17-23.

68. Parker DF, Carriere L, Hebestreit H, et al. Anaerobic endurance and peak muscle power in children with spastic cerebral palsy. *Am J Dis Child.* 1992;146:169-173.

69. Pitetti KH. Exercise capacities and adaptations of people with chronic disabilities: current research, future directions, and widespread applicability. *Med Sci Sports Exerc.* 1993;24:421-422.

70. Richter KJ, Gaebler-Spira DG, Mushett CA. Sport and the person with spasticity of cerebral origin. *Dev Med Child Neurol.* 1996;38:867-870.

71. Unnithan VB, Clifford C, Bar-Or O. Evaluation by exercise testing of the child with cerebral palsy. *Sports Med.* 1998;26:239-251.

72. Carroll KL, Leiser J, Paisley TS. Cerebral palsy: physical activity and sport. *Curr Sports Med Rep* 2006;5:319-322.

73. Klenck C, Gebke K. Practical management: common medical problems in disabled athletes. *Clin J Sports Med.* 2007;17:55-60.

74. Boninger ML, Robertson RN, Wolff M, et al. Upper limb nerve entrapment in elite wheelchair racers. *Am J Phys Med Rehabil.* 1996;75:170-176.

75. Burnham R, May L, Nelson E, et al. Shoulder pain in wheelchair athletes: the role of muscle imbalance. *Am J Sports Med.* 1993;21:238-242.

76. Burnham RS, Steadward RD. Upper extremity peripheral nerve entrapments among wheelchair athletes: prevalence, location, and risk factors. *Arch Phys Med Rehabil.* 1994;75:519-524.

77. Makris VI. Visual loss and performance in blind athletes. *Med Sci Sports Exerc.* 1993;25:265-269.

78. Palmer T, Weber KM. The deaf athlete. *Curr Sports Med Rep* 2006;5:323-326.

79. Sanyer ON. Down syndrome and sport participation. *Curr Sports Med Rep* 2006;5:315-318.

80. Caird MS, Wills BPD, Dormans JP. Down syndrome in children: the role of the orthopaedic surgeon. *J Am Acad Orthop Surg.* 2006;14:610-619.

81. American Academy of Pediatrics: Atlantoaxial instability in Down syndrome: subject review. *Pediatrics.* 1995;96: 151-154.

82. Torg JS, Ramsey-Emrhein JA. Management guidelines for participation in collision activities with congenital, developmental, or postinjury lesions involving the cervical spine. *Clin J Sports Med.* 1997;7:273-291.

83. American Academy of Pediatrics, American Academy of Family Physicians, American Orthopedic Society for Sports Medicine, American Medical Society for Sports Medicine, American Osteopathic Society for Sports Medicine. *Preparticipation Physical Evaluation Monograph.* 3rd ed. New York: McGraw Hill; 2005.

Additional Readings

Disability Sports at the Disability Sports Website, Department of Kinesiology, Michigan State University, http://edweb6. educ.msu.edu/kin866.

CHAPTER 36

Conditions and Injuries of the Eyes, Nose, and Ears

Robert J. Baker

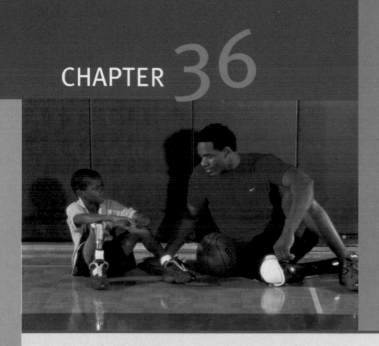

EYE INJURIES

Of the 100,000 eye injuries that occur annually, 40% occur during sports or recreational activities.[1] Foreign bodies and lacerations are the most common and generally can be treated by the pediatrician. Globe lacerations, retinal hemorrhage, and retinal detachments can lead to permanent vision loss and should be referred to an ophthalmologist (Box 36-1). Orbital hemorrhage and hyphema can look dramatic but usually resolve with minimal treatment.

Use of appropriate protective eyewear will decrease the risk of corneal abrasion. Good supervision, equipment of good repair, and rules enforcement can further decrease the risk of these eye injuries. For outdoor sports, the area should be inspected for potential obstacles such as tree branches. Appropriate eye protection should be used in high-risk sports such as hockey, football, baseball, softball, basketball, tennis, racquet sports, lacrosse, and swimming. Regular glasses and contacts are not adequate protection. The eye wear should include lenses of polycarbonate 3 mm thick. Frames should be of polycarbonate and molded to the temples, not hinged. Lens treatment with fog resistance will improve vision under environmental conditions (Table 36-1). Proper fitting by an experienced ophthalmologist may improve compliance. Full face protectors either of polycarbonate shield or wire cage should be

Box 36-1 When to Refer.

Recommended Referral for Eye Injuries in Sports

Symptoms	Physical Findings	Diagnosis	Comment
"Gravel sensation"	Visible foreign object not easilyremoved with cotton or tissue	Embedded foreign object	Slit-lamp examination may be required with small spud for removal
Loss of vision	Irregularity of the globe Herniation of viteous of eye Full thickness laceration of the eyelid	Laceration of the globe Ruptured globe	Surgical repair of the globe
Proptosis interfering with vision Pain	Hemorrhage and swelling	Orbital hemorrhage with increased intraocular pressure	Intraocular pressure measurement
"Eight-ball" eye Loss of visual field	Totally black anterior chamber Persistent blood in the anterior chamber	Hyphema large or not resolving in 3 days	Hemorrhage aspiration may be necessary
"Flash" sensation Loss of part of visual field	Irregularity of retina on ophthalmoscopic exam	Detached retina Retinal hemorrhage	May need surgical/laser repair
Loss of vision in one eye	Irregularity of the pupil	Dislocated lens	Surgical reduction and repair
Blurred vision with upward gaze only	Inability to gaze upward with involved eye	Fracture of the floor of the orbit	Surgical reduction and repair of sinus

Table 36-1.

Recommended Eye Protectors for Selected Sports*

Sport	Minimal Eye Protector	Comment
Baseball/softball, youth batter or base runner	ASTM F910	Face guard attached to helmet
Baseball/softball, fielder	ASTM F803 for baseball	ASTM specifies age ranges
Basketball	ASTM F803 for basketball	ASTM specifies age ranges
Bicycling	Helmet plus streetwear ANSI Z80, industrial ANSI Z87.1, or sports ASTM F803 eyewear	Use only polycarbonate lenses; excellent plano industrial spectacles are available that are inexpensive and give good protection from wind and particles
Boxing	None available; not permitted in sport	Sport contraindicated for functionally one-eyed
Fencing	Protector with neck bib	Test requirements of the International Federation of Fencing
Field hockey (both sexes)	Goalie: full face mask; others: ASTM F803 for women's lacrosse	Protectors that pass ASTM F803 for women's lacrosse also pass for field hockey; should have option to wear helmet with attached face mask
Football	Polycarbonate eye shield attached to helmet-mounted wire face mask	
Full-contact martial arts functionally	None available; not permitted in sport	Contraindicated for one-eyed
Ice hockey	ASTM F513 face mask on helmet; goaltenders ASTM F1587	HECC or CSA certified full face shield
Lacrosse, men's	NOCSAE face mask attached to lacrosse helmet	
Lacrosse, women's	ASTM F803 for women's Lacrosse	Should have option to wear helmet with attached face mask
Paintball	ASTM F1776 for paintball	
Racket sports (badminton, tennis, paddle tennis, handball, squash, and racquetball)	ASTM F803 for specific sport	
Soccer	ASTM F803 for any selected sport	No specific standard for soccer; currently, eye protectors that comply with ASTM F803 for any specified sport are recommended
Street hockey	ASTM F513 face mask on helmet	Must be HECC or CSA certified
Track and field	Streetwear/fashion eyewear	Use only polycarbonate lenses
Water polo/swimming	Swim goggles with polycarbonate lenses	
Wrestling	No standard is available	Custom protective eyewear can be fabricated

*For sports in which a face mask or helmet with eye protector is worn, functionally one-eyed athletes, and those who have had previous eye trauma or surgery, and for whom their ophthalmologists recommend eye protection, must also wear sports protective eyewear that conforms to ASTM F803 requirements.

used in hockey. Wire cage face protectors are most commonly used in lacrosse and football.

SPECIFIC EYE INJURIES

Foreign Body

Definitions and epidemiology

Dust and debris may become trapped in the eye of the athlete. Especially of high risk are outdoor sports,

contact sports, and team sports. Foreign body in the eye is the most common sports-related eye injury.

Mechanism

With exposure to environmental elements as well as sports equipment, foreign bodies can lodge in the eye.

Clinical presentation

The athlete with a foreign body in the eye will complain of pain, irritation, possibly a "gravelly feeling" in the eye. The irritation is made worse with blinking and rubbing.

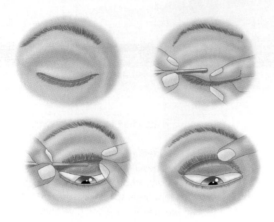

FIGURE 36-1 ■ Examination under the eyelid is done by gently everting the upper lid over a cotton tip applicator as shown.

Irritation can result in conjunctival injection. Excessive tearing is a common associated symptom.

Diagnosis

The entire eye should be evaluated to locate the foreign body which often lodges under the upper or lower eyelid. The upper eye lid should be everted by gently inverting the closed lid over a cotton tip applicator (Figure 36-1). The foreign body lodged under the lid can lead to corneal abrasions with movement of the eye.

Treatment

Instilling a topical anesthetic in the eye will help relieve pain and keep the athlete more comfortable during the examination. When the foreign body is located, the corner of a tissue or a wisp of cotton can be used to remove the foreign body. Symptoms usually resolve when the foreign body is removed. The anesthetic should not be administered on a regular basis, as this can lead to damage to the eye.[2] If the foreign body cannot be removed or is embedded, the ophthalmologist will need to remove it with a spade and slit lamp. Rarely, a CT scan may be necessary to localize the foreign body. Protective eyewear may be required for a short period of time, but athlete can usually return to activity immediately after removal of the foreign body. Ice may be applied for pain relief.

Lacerations

Definitions and epidemiology

Blunt trauma, sharp objects, even inferior or improperly worn eyewear can result in lacerations of the eye lid or globe. Superficial lacerations are the most common eye injuries related to sports. Most sports-related trauma does not result in globe laceration.

Mechanism

Blunt trauma from a small sharp object most commonly results in superficial eyelid lacerations. The natural reflex is closure of the eyelids as potential danger to the eye is sensed. With lower-energy trauma the damage may be limited to superficial tissue. High-energy trauma could result in globe lacerations.

Clinical presentation

The athlete will often recall a specific trauma, usually of a smaller object size. Often there will be pain swelling and hemorrhage present. Anatomic disruption may be subtle on initial inspection. Visual acuity is often decreased with globe lacerations. Obvious anatomic deformity may be readily apparent.

Diagnosis

Lacerations of the eyelid can be subtle and may have normal appearing eye. Lacerations of the external surface of the eye lid should be inspected to determine if there is a full-thickness laceration or the lid margin is involved.[3] The eye lid which is swollen shut should not be forcibly opened to avoid possible herniation of globe contents. Globe lacerations are associated with decreased acuity and if deep put vision at risk. Referral to the ophthalmologist is recommended.

Corneal abrasions and foreign bodies may be associated with lacerations. Full eye examination including visual acuity, ocular motion, lid motion, and under surface of the lid should be performed. If the trauma is related to a larger object, an orbital fracture should also be considered.

Treatment

Superficial lid lacerations may be repaired by delicate suturing well-approximated edges while avoiding injury to the globe. Eyelid lacerations usually heal quite well with very little scar. The athlete should be referred to ophthalmology if the laceration involves the full thickness of the lid or the lid margin. The athlete should be referred if a globe laceration is suspected (Box 36-1).

Corneal abrasion

Definitions and epidemiology

The cornea is the clear covering of the anterior aspect of the eye lens. Defects in the cornea can result in inference of light penetration through the lens and focus on to the retina. A nontransparent cornea will result in decreased vision. The eyes are shielded from large object by the hard bony orbit. The eyes are also protected from smaller particles by eye lashes and eye lids. Racquet sports and baseball, for example, place the eyes at risk from contact with a fast moving ball. In any team sport even limited contact places the eye at risk of corneal abrasions.

Mechanisms

In team sports, the most common mechanism of abrasion is the "finger in the eye," usually from another athlete. Outdoor sports can have added risk of debris blown into the eye. Finally other objects such as balls, bats, sticks, and pucks, can pose a similar risk.

Clinical presentation

The most common symptom of corneal abrasion is a very painful eye. This may be described as a gritty feeling which is increased with eye movements. These symptoms can be an indication of a foreign body as well. Other associated complaints include headache, blurred vision, photophobia, and watery eyes. Often the athlete will relate a specific ocular trauma; however, there may be no other trauma than rubbing of the eyes.

Diagnosis

On inspection, the conjunctiva may appear injected. Instillation of topical anesthetic (e.g., tetracaine) will help to relieve the athlete's pain and allow full examination of the eye. Full examination of the eye with specific attention to check under the eyelids is important to identify any foreign body. Foreign bodies resting on the eyelid or the cornea may be elevated and removed with a tissue or gauze. Embedded objects are best removed by the ophthalmologist in an appropriate setting. Instillation of flourescein and examination under blue light will identify the extent of the abrasion as dye uptake lights up brightly.

Treatment

Full healing without complication is the usual prognosis; however, the athlete should be re-examined daily until the abrasion is healed. These usually heal within 3 days. The involved eye should be protected from light exposure during the healing process. Sunglasses to protect the eyes from sunlight exposure are helpful, but patching has not been shown to be effective. Athletes with contact lenses should remove contacts while symptomatic. The athlete diagnosed with a corneal abrasion should be kept out of contact sports or high-risk sports until healed.[4] Natural tears or other wetting solution can offer some symptomatic relief. Topical nonsteroidal anti-inflammatories could be used as well. Antibiotic eye drops are generally not required unless there are signs of infection.

Orbital Hemorrhage

Definitions and epidemiology

Depending on the velocity and size of object involved, trauma to the orbit can result in orbital hemorrhage and edema. More significant trauma may result in orbital fractures. These injuries may occur in any sport because of equipment or other athletes. Contact sports raise the most risk.

Mechanisms

Direct trauma to the eye and orbit will result in hemorrhage and swelling. The classic "black eye" appears when hemorrhage occurs around the orbit.

Clinical presentation

Vision is usually not directly affected after orbital hemorrhage, though swelling around the eye can interfere with the visual field. Swelling in the orbit can increase pressure behind the globe and lead to proptosis. In this case, the upper lid may not close completely.

Diagnosis

Orbital hemorrhage is associated with significant trauma and severe injuries such as facial fractures and globe injuries. These should be ruled out in the athlete that presents with hemorrhage. Vision is usually preserved; however, proptosis can be significant and interfere with the athlete's vision. Increased intraocular pressure can complicate the picture and should be evaluated immediately.[5] This will be marked by increase in pain and proptosis. In severe cases, the eye may be difficult to fully evaluate to rule out complications. Athletes in which case athletes should be referred to an ophthalmologist.

Treatment

Prognosis is good for a complete resolution of the hemorrhage without long-term complications. Symptomatic treatment with ice and NSAIDs for pain control is all that is needed. The athlete should not return to sport until a complete field of vision has returned.

Hyphema

Definitions and epidemiology

Hyphema is the term for blood that collects in the anterior chamber of the eye. This injury often occurs as a result of trauma in contact sports.

Mechanisms

Blunt trauma to the eye can cause tearing and bleeding in any location. Hemorrhage in the anterior chamber does require a significant amount force. Therefore, when hyphema does occur, there are likely other associated injuries to the eye.

Clinical presentation

Bleeding in this area can be subtle and overlooked. Rebleeding can be massive and fill the entire chamber. Because of the appearance of the eyes, this has been referred to as "eight-ball" hemorrhage.[3] The small initial amounts of blood may not obscure the lens and go unnoticed by the athlete.

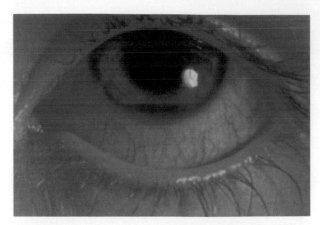

FIGURE 36-2 ■ Hyphema. Small hyphema layering out in the inferior portion of the anterior chamber. (*Used with permission from Brunette DD, Chapter 70, Figure 70-9. In: Marx JA, (Ed in chief). Rosen's Emergency Medicine, 6th ed. Philadelphia: Mosby Elsevier; 2006.*)

Diagnosis

Blood will collect beneath the cornea and a meniscus of blood can be appreciated inferiorly as the athlete's eye is examined in the upright position (Figure 36-2). The eye and vision should be carefully checked, as there may be associated more serious eye injuries.

Treatment

Commonly hyphema resorbs without squealae. Rarely the blood can permanently stain the cornea. If the blood does not resorb within 3 days, ophthalmology should be consulted (Box 36-1). Rebleeding can occur, so the athlete should be restricted from activity for 4 days.[3] During this time regular re-evaluation of the eye should be performed to monitor resolution.

Retinal Hemorrhage

Definitions and epidemiology

Following blunt trauma to the eye, face, or head, bleeding can occur from the retina. Valsalva maneuvers associated with heavy effort (e.g., weightlifting) can increase interocular pressure and produce bleeding from the retina.

Mechanisms

Retinal hemorrhages occur as the result of direct trauma to the head or eye. Occasionally effort, usually with valsalva, or decreased oxygen saturation can lead to retinal hemorrhage as well.

Clinical presentation

While hemorrhage can occur from multiple areas of the retina, these may be located in the periphery of the visual field. Subtle loss of vision at the edges may not be readily identified by the athlete. Should bleeding occur in the macula or center of vision, visual acuity will be affected.

Diagnosis

Findings can be subtle, even asymptomatic especially if small or involve only the periphery. Central hemorrhage can result in vision loss and should be referred for examination and treatment by an ophthalmologist. Full examination of the retina under pupil dilation should be performed to identify peripheral hemorrhages.

Treatment

Depending on necessary treatment, the athlete may need to be restricted from sports for 6 weeks or longer.

Retinal Detachment

Definitions and epidemiology

As a result of direct trauma to the head, face, or eye, the retina can be injured. Structural abnormalities of the eye such as high myopia, Marfan's syndrome, degeneration of the pigmented epithelium, sensory retina, or vitreous body, may predispose the athlete to these injuries.

Mechanisms

Trauma can cause separation of the superficial and deep layers of the retina. Retinal tissue tears and holes can develop as well. Three classifications of detachments are described.[6] Rhegmatogenous retinal detachment is the most common and traumatic in nature. These occur when there is a break in the sensory retina allowing fluid from the vitreous to separate the rods and cones from the villi of the pigment epithelium.[6] Tractional detachment occurs following contraction of fibrous vitreous bands pulling the sensory retina off the pigment epithelium. This is chronic, progressive, and asymptomatic. Exudative retinal detachment results from an abnormal collection of fluid which separates the retinal layer. This detachment often affects the macula and central vision.

Clinical presentation

Small retinal injuries can progress over time without appropriate treatment. Total vision loss can occur. The athlete may complain of free-floating objects, and scotoma. Flashes with or without pain can mark the onset of retinal injury. If central or macula retina is involved, visual acuity will be affected.

Diagnosis

As the retina separates, the characteristic vascular pattern seen through the superficial retina tissue will not be visualized on ophthalmoscope examination. Dilation of the pupil will be necessary to appreciate peripheral detachments. Visual field defects will be present in area of detachment as well.

Treatment

As surgery is often necessary for any athlete with suspected retinal injury, the athlete should be referred to an ophthalmologist (Box 36-1). Return to activity will be dependent on the extent of damage and should be determined in consultation with the ophthalmologist. In general, 2 weeks off of contact sports at a minimum is necessary.

Rupture of the Globe

Definitions and epidemiology

Increased pressure on the globe can lead to failure of the supporting tissue. Increased intraocular pressure can occur as a direct result of trauma to the eye. Indirectly, swelling and hemorrhage can lead to increased eye pressure.

Mechanisms

Direct trauma to the eye or even the head can result in significant trauma to the eye. Swelling of the eye, as a result of trauma, can lead to increased pressure and further injury to the globe. Contact of the globe with a sharp object like a broken stick, bat, fishing hook, even a finger can also lead to rupture or serious injury to the globe. Contact sports, team sports, and sport with sticks or bats can place the young athlete at risk for globe injuries.

Clinical presentation

Significant eye pain and deformity may be obvious. Vision is compromised as well. Examination of the eye should be gentle as to not cause further damage to the eye.[3] Forceful opening of the lid could lead to herniation of globe contents.

Diagnosis

Diagnosis is usually based on pain and obvious deformity. If suspicion is high regarding globe rupture, referral to an ophthalmologist on an emergent basis will be necessary (Box 36-1). If there is an obvious embedded foreign object in the globe, it should not be removed prior to transfer.

Treatment

Generally the globe injuries should be transferred for emergent care by an ophthalmologist. Removing foreign objects from the eye may only result in further injury and should be avoided. Rather the eye and the object should be covered to protect and avoid further trauma. Covering the eye with a paper cup will accommodate most objects.

Return to play would be based on whether full vision returns. If full vision does not return the recommendation would be the same as for a single-eyed athlete.

Dislocation of Lens

Definitions and epidemiology

Tearing of the lens supporting structures can lead to dislocation of the lens. A partial tear can result in subluxation of the lens. The lens may remain in a relative normal position, but slightly off center. Complete dislocation can result in complete displacement of the lens into the anterior chamber or posterior chamber. Young athletes with Marfan's syndrome will be at increased risk for lens dislocation.

Mechanisms

A significant trauma to the eye or head is required to dislocate the lens for most normal athletes. Motor sports, extreme sports, football, or hockey could possibly result in such significant trauma.

Clinical presentation

Visual acuity is decreased and on examination, irregular astigmatism is appreciated. Visual correction will be changed. Iris stability is lost and tremulous ocular movement may be present.

Diagnosis

On examination visual acuity will be decreased. Irregularity of the pupil may be readily identified. The above-mentioned motion irregularities may be identified as extraocular motions and are tested.

Treatment

If a lens dislocation is suspected, referral to ophthalmology is appropriate (Box 36-1). Treatment may require surgical removal of the lens. Because treatment is varied based on the extent of injury, prognosis is likewise variable.[3]

Fracture of the Floor of the Orbit

Definitions and epidemiology

Orbital floor fractures are rare prior to the age of 7. Younger children may sustain fracture of the paranasal sinus or orbital roof. There may be pneumatization of the paranasal sinuses or CNS injury with these other locations.[7]

Mechanisms

Direct trauma to the anterior aspect of the eye can result in fracture of the floor of the orbit. The mechanism is because that of increased pressure within the orbit as the result of a projectile, often softball, and baseball or tennis ball. As the ball contacts the anterior rim of the orbit, intraorbital pressure increases. The floor of the orbit is often the thinnest of bone and thus fractures into the maxillary sinus below. The inferior muscles and soft

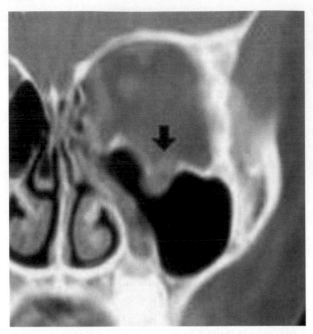

FIGURE 36-3 ■ CT scan showing fracture of the floor of the orbit.

tissue of the eye can then herniate through the defect. Impingement of the soft tissue leads to the common finding of decreased upward gaze in the involved eye.

Clinical presentation

As the eyes become disconjugate with upward gaze, the athlete may note diplopia or double vision. This diplopia is usually limited to upward gaze only. Other findings are periorbital edema, enophthalmos and subconjunctival ecchymosis.[8]

Diagnosis

Plain films including Water's view can be helpful, but CT scan of the orbits is the definitive test (Figure 36-3). Late complications include sinusitis, orbital infection permanent restriction of eye movement, and enophthalmos.

Treatment

The athlete should be referred to an ophthalmologist for further evaluation especially if upward gaze is limited (Box 36-1).

EAR INJURIES

Cauliflower Ear

Definitions and epidemiology

In spite of the availability of protective head gear, injuries to the ear in contact sports such as wrestling still occur. The presentation of the cauliflower ear is classic after direct external ear trauma or traction.

Mechanism

Trauma or traction on the pinna of the ear leads to the collection of blood and swelling between the perichondrium and cartilage of the ear. Once formed the hematoma is not fully reabsorbed. The hematoma organizes and leaves the ear with permenant ear deformity.

Clinical presentation

The athlete will complain of pain and deformity of the external ear. Redness and obvious swelling of the pinna of the ear is present.

Treatment

To prevent permanent deformity, the fluid should be aspirated under sterile technique. The aspiration should be performed within 48 to 72 hours after formation. Delay will result in the formation of scar tissue and may not be possible to drain (Box 36-2). In order to prevent re-collection, pressure packing should be provided.[9] This can be achieved with colloidian. Some will sew in buttons on the front and back of the ear. It may take 2 weeks for the ear to heal. During this time the ears should be protected by head gear.

Tympanic Membrane Rupture

Definitions and epidemiology

Direct blow to the opening of the external ear canal can result in high pressure change across the tympanic membrane. The high pressure change will result in failure or rupture of the tympanic membrane. Contact sports, in which direct blows can occur, place the young

Box 36-2 When to Refer.			
Recommended Referral for Ear Injuries in Sports			
Symptoms	**Physical Findings**	**Diagnosis**	**Comment**
Irregularity of the pinna of the ear	Persistent swelling despite drainage and packing	Cauliflower ear	Surgical drainage and reconstruction of the ear
Erythema and pain of the external ear		Possible organization of swelling	Antibiotics for infection
Hearing loss		Possible infection	
Pain	Defect in the tympanic membrane	Tympanic membrane rupture	Repair of the tympanic defect

athlete at risk. High divers are also at risk as similar pressure changes can occur at the time of water entry.

Mechanism

Trauma to the external ear can increase external canal pressure resulting in significant pressure change across the membrane resulting in a tear.[10] This rapid pressure change is common in divers at the time the ears enter the water. Blunt trauma, penetrating objects, and extreme noise can also result in tympanic membrane tears.

Clinical presentation

Athletes will complain of mild ear pain and partial hearing loss. Purulent or bloody discharge may be present in ear canal. The athlete may also complain of tinnitus, vertigo, or otorrhea. The tear is visible on internal ear inspection with otoscope. Weber and Rinne test may indicate conductive hearing loss.

Treatment

Most tears resolve with conservative management. Systemic antibiotics (i.e., amoxicillin, azithromycin, or cephalexin) may be necessary if signs of infection are present (Box 36-2). Analgesics for pain control may be prescribed. Topical antibiotics, analgesics, and steroids should not be used. The ears will need to be protected during healing time by covering. Ear plugs can both protect and prevent this injury.

INJURIES OF THE NOSE

Nasal Fractures

Definitions and epidemiology

The nasal fracture is the most common type of facial fracture. The nasal fracture accounts for more than 50% of facial fractures.[11] Injuries to the nose are common in contact sports and most sports with balls, pucks, bats, sticks, or clubs.

Mechanism

The common mechanism for fracture of the nasal bone is direct trauma to the bridge of the nose. Anatomically, the anterior two-thirds of the nose is cartilage, while the nasal bones form the proximal one-third of the nose. Direct trauma to the anterior aspect of the nose often results in injury to the cartilage of the nose. This can result in cartilage fracture, dislocation, or nasal septum fractures. Lateral trauma often results in fractures to the nasal bones.

Clinical presentation

Oftentimes the displacement is obvious. However, the physician may have a difficult time identifying this deformity because of swelling. Also, if the athlete has sustained prior injury to the nose, it may be difficult to distinguish old injury from new. A recent photo or driver's license photo may help in this regard. Complications such as swelling and bleeding following any traumatic facial injury can lead to airway obstruction and cause apprehension in the athlete. Generally, this is not life threatening. High-energy trauma to the anterior nose can potentially result in fracture of the cribiform plate and leakage of cerebrospinal fluid.[12] If this is suspected, the young athlete should be referred immediately to otolaryngology.

Diagnosis

The diagnosis of the nasal fracture is often on inspection and palpation of the nose. The nasal bones and cartilage should be palpated for deformity and crepitous. The internal nares should be inspected using the speculum to identify hematoma and/or source of bleeding. Anterior bleeding is often easily seen and treated to control bleeding. If a hematoma is identified, it should be drained immediately. Posterior bleeding should be controlled and raise suspicions of possible sinus fracture.

Because the nasal fracture is primarily a clinical diagnosis, imaging is not always necessary. If the trauma was high energy, a fracture is suspected but not visible, a septal fracture, or a sinus injury is suspected, further imaging may be helpful. Plain films with lateral and water's view can be helpful first step (Figure 36-4). To fully evaluate the sinus, a CT scan may be necessary.

Treatment

Face protectors in contacts sports such as hockey, football, and lacrosse, can prevent these types of injuries. Nasal fracture with obvious deformity should be referred to ENT surgeon for definitive evaluation and treatment within 2 weeks (Box 36-3). Usually the athlete may return early to conditioning and in 4 to 6 weeks to contact sports with adequate protection. Several nasal protection devices are available, but are usually expensive.

Epistaxis

Bleeding or epistaxis can occur anteriorly or posteriorly. Direct pressure to the base of the nose of the upper lip may initially help control bleeding. Anterior bleeding can often be identified and cauterized using silver nitrate or other cautery as available. Topical applications of vasoconstrictor medication or petroleum gel can help control bleeding and allow the athlete to return to play.

Posterior bleeding can be difficult to control. The athlete will be irritated by the feel of posterior drainage and the foul taste in the throat. Packing may be necessary to tamponade the bleeding.[13] Referral to ENT

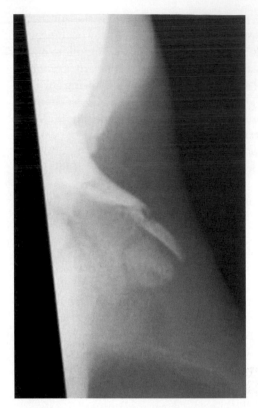

FIGURE 36-4 ■ Lateral x-ray of the nose showing nasal fracture.

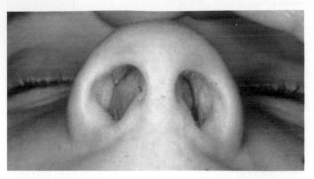

FIGURE 36-5 ■ Septal hematoma in a 6-year-old child. (*Used with permission from Krakovitz PR, Koltai PJ. Pediatric fractures. In: Cummings CW, et al., eds. Cumming's Otolaryngology: Head and Neck Surgery, 4th ed. Philadelphia: Mosby Elsevier, Fig 202-21, 2005.*).

specialist is often necessary (Box 36-3). The physician should be suspicious of possible sinus fracture where posterior bleeding is present.

Septal Hematoma

Septal hematoma of the nose can occur with any nose trauma. This is bleeding along the cartilage septum of the nose which forms a hematoma. This can occur bilaterally or unilaterally. Left untreated, there can be resorption of the cartilage resulting in the saddle, or flat nose deformity. This can lead to long-term breathing problems of the nose and upper airway. This deformity is identified on speculum examination of the anterior nose (Figure 36-5). There will be an obvious asymmetry of the septum. The septum may appear blue tinged and bulging on the involved side.[14] The athlete may complain of breathing problems because of slight obstruction. The hematoma should be drained early (Box 36-3).

REFERENCES

1. American Academy of Pediatrics. Policy statement: Protective eyewear for young athletes. *Pediatrics.* 2004;113(3):619-622.
2. Weber TS. Training room management of eye conditions. *Clin Sports Med.* 2005;24:681-693.
3. Petrigliano FA, Williams RJ. Orbital fractures in sport. *Sports Med.* 2003;33(4):317-322.
4. Wilson SA, Last A. Management of corneal abrasions. *Am Family Phys.* 2004;70(1):123-128.
5. Rodriguez JO, Lavina AM, Agarwal A. Prevention and treatment of common eye injuries in sports. *Am Family Phys.* 2003;67(7):1481-1488.
6. Lui E. Retinal detachments and tears. In: Bracker M, ed. *The 5 Minute Sports Medicine Consult.* Philadelphia: Lippincott Williams & Wilkins; 2001:520-521.
7. Romeo SJ, Hawley CJ, Romeo MW, et al. Sideline management of facial injuries. *Curr Sports Med Rep.* 2007; 6:155-161.
8. Schabowski S. Fracture, blow out. In: Bracker M, ed. *The 5 Minute Sports Medicine Consult.* Philadelphia: Lippincott Williams & Wilkins; 2001:80-79.

Box 36-3. When to Refer.

Recommended Referral for Nasal Injuries in Sports

Symptoms	Physical Findings	Diagnosis	Comment
Pain and swelling in nose following trauma	Deformity of nose	Nasal fracture Deviated septum	Reduction may be necessary
Bleeding with iron taste in mouth	Bleeding not responding to anterior pressure or cautery	Epistaxis with posterior bleeding	Packing necessary
Trauma with pain and difficulty breathing through nose	Swelling of nasal septum on involved nares	Septal hematoma	Immediate drainage of the hematoma

Rib films should be requested if multiple fractures are suspected. Because the ribs are often difficult to fully evaluate on plain films, a CT scan may show rib fractures more clearly than plain x-ray. The CT scan will be even more beneficial in evaluating underlying organ injury in case of multiple rib fractures or when associated complications are suspected.

Treatment

Most rib fractures generally heal well without any need for specific treatment. Pain control is important to allow the athlete to take full breaths and prevent atelectasis. A binder may give some relief of pain. Nonunion of these fractures are rare. Multiple rib fractures with associated flail chest may require open reduction internal fixation (ORIF) to stabilize the chest. The athlete can return to conditioning as soon as the pain is tolerable. Contact sports should be limited for 3 weeks. Some have recommended contact sports be limited up to 3 months.

Pneumothorax

Definition and epidemiology

Pneumothorax occurs as air collects between the plural membrane and chest wall. Pneumothorax is a rare occurrence in sports. Most cases reported in the literature are the result of trauma related to participation in football with a peak age of onset at 16 to 24 years, and young children rarely experience these injuries.[2]

Pathogenesis

In athletes, pneumothorax can result from direct chest trauma or spontaneously from rupture of the apical blebs. Activities such as weightlifting can result in increased pressure in the chest which can lead to rupture of a bleb.[3] Rib fractures can be associated with this injury.

Clinical presentation

The athlete experiences chest pain on deep inspiration, shortness of breath, and tachycardia. Breath sounds are diminished over the affected area. The pneumothorax may be stable or may be expanding or "tension" pneumothorax (Figure 37-2). The tension pneumothorax is a medical emergency and should be identified clinically when there is rapidly deteriorating shortness of breath (Figure 37-3). Trachea may be deviated to the uninvolved side. A rattling sound or sensation in the anterior chest is known as Hagemen's sign and indicates pneumomediastinum.

Diagnosis

If clinical signs suggest tension pneumothorax in an unstable patient, treatment should be started rather

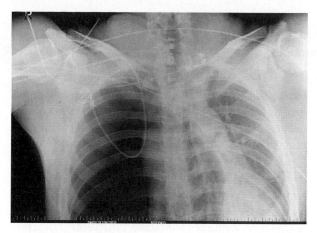

FIGURE 37-2 ■ Tension pneumothorax with collapse of right lung field and deviation of heart and trachea.

than delayed while awaiting an x-ray. For the stable patient with pneumothorax, the x-ray should be obtained to confirm the diagnosis and treatment based on percent of lung collapse.

Treatment

The tension pneumothorax can be aspirated immediately with 14 gauge needle inserted in the second intercostal space. Placement of a chest tube or catheter will allow the lung to re-expand. Percentage of lung collapse is estimated on the chest film. Stable pneumothorax less than 20% can be observed and managed conservatively. Pneumothorax greater than 20% should be re-expanded with placement of chest tube. Oxygen administration is indicated and will help with dyspnea. In cases of recurrent pneumothorax, surgical pleurodesis will be required. Return to sports should not be attempted prior to 2 weeks following complete resolution with gradual return to unrestricted sports participation over the subsequent 8 to 12 weeks.

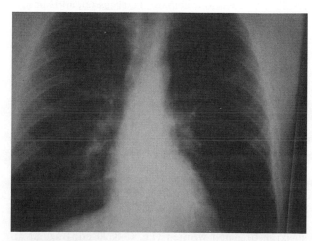

FIGURE 37-3 ■ Pneumothorax involving 40% of lung field.

Cardiac Contusion

Direct trauma to the anterior chest wall can result in concussion of the heart. Should this concussion occur during the repolarizing cycle of the heart, arrythmias can occur.[4] This leads to ventricular fibrillation and sudden cardiac death. Commotio cordis, as this is sometimes called, has resulted in deaths in young children.

Pericardial Tamponade

Direct trauma to the anterior chest can lead to the accumulation of fluid in the pericardial sac or pericardial tamponade. As fluid accumulates, the cardiac function is compromised. The ventricles cannot fill, cardiac output decreases, and cardiogenic shock results. The classic findings on examination are jugular vein distention, hypotension, and muffled heart sounds. The ECG may show sinus tachycardia with electrical alternans and PR segment depression.[4] Immediate decompression under ultrasound guidance is the treatment. Full recovery is expected with early intervention and the athlete can return to sports following recovery.

Prevention of Chest Trauma

Any young athlete participating in contact sports should use the appropriate protective equipment. In football and hockey, shoulder pads that are appropriately fitted and in good repair will protect the upper ribs. Protective rib pads, which cover the lower ribs, are available for contact sports as well. For baseball players, catchers should use appropriate chest protectors.

Breast Contusions and Lacerations

Definitions and epidemiology

Direct trauma following a collision with opposing player, projectile, or stick to the chest or breast area may result in a contusion, hematoma, abrasion, and/ or laceration of the breast. With the exception of horse bite in equestrian sports, chest and breast injuries are rarely reported in the literature. This may because of less severity of injury, rare occurrence, and or gender differences in the incidence of such injuries. Accident-prone sports such as biking, road racing, mountain biking, skiing, and rodeo may have a higher risk for these injuries. Though most collision sports such as hockey, football, baseball, and field hockey provide some chest protection for at-risk players, trauma can occur.[5]

Pathogenesis

Velocity of the unsupported breast can be significant, so large breasted women (i.e. C & D cup) are at an increased risk. Poor fitting of protective equipment will put the athlete at risk especially in collision sports. Hard or metal bra parts such as straps, metal hooks, clips, and underwire can cause breast injury in athletes.

Clinical presentation

Athletes presenting with local pain following trauma may be associated with bruising, swelling, or laceration of the breast tissue. Nipples can become irritated and painful because of chaffing. Males with gynecomastia are at an increased risk by virtue of added breast tissue. On examination swelling, mass, bruising, and hematoma can be identified. Masses should be localized and characterized in terms of density, consistency, movement, and pulsation. Axillary lymphadenopathy should be also noted.

Rarely, hematomas may become secondarily infected. Trauma of the chest and breast may lead to Mondor's disease or thrombophlebitis of superficial breast veins. Occasionally, breast trauma and pain will uncover tumors and masses. Complications following trauma include fat necrosis, induration, mastitis, scarring, and calcification.

Diagnosis

Imaging such as x-ray or bone scan may be indicated if an underlying fracture (i.e. stress fracture or pathological fracture) is suspected. While malignant masses are rare in children, concerning abnormalities may be evaluated by ultrasound. A mammogram would be reserved for males or older females with abnormalities.

Treatment

Contusion and hematoma should be treated with local ice application and oral pain medications as needed. The laceration should be repaired within 6 hours. These may be closed either with suture or steri-strips. Suture may be the best option to close subcutaneous dead space. While most hematomas resolve spontaneously, surgical aspiration may be indicated if the mass is enlarging, the mass appears infected, or calcifications are present. Masses thought to be cysts or hematomas may be aspirated under local anesthesia.[5] Suspicious masses should be referred for biopsy and excision.

Following a contusion or hematoma of the breast, females, especially large breasted women, should wear a supportive bra. Added pressure for the lacerated breast may be achieved by firm dressing and support worn at night. In most cases, the athlete may return to sports following healing of the contusion or laceration.

Prevention of Nipple Injury

The nipple of the breast can become irritated in even young athletes. If nipples are irritated by clothing, a bandage may be applied to the nipple. Tape should not be directly applied to the nipple; however, gauze or Telfa pads with Vaseline may be secured with tape over the irritated nipple. Females who experience recurrent problems with chaffing, should consider proper fitting of the sports bra. Temperature extremes can make the nipples more susceptible to injury.[5] Cooling across the sweat-soaked cotton shirt can cause pain, abrasions, and lacerations of the nipples. Appropriate clothing with newer synthetic materials which wick moist and "breath" will often alleviate this problem.

BLUNT ABDOMINAL TRAUMA

Definitions and Epidemiology

High-velocity sports such as skiing, biking, skate boarding, snow boarding, and motor sports can result in abdominal trauma. Contact sports also place the young athlete at risk. Abdominal trauma accounts for approximately 10% of trauma in the pediatric population and the most commonly injured organs are the spleen and the kidney.[2]

Pathogenesis

Because of proportionally larger abdominal organs in relation to adults, children are at a higher risk for abdominal organ injury. Younger children anatomically have a relatively smaller abdominal space. However, they also have less soft tissue protection and abdominal organs have more elastic attachments which could result in greater energy distributed to the abdominal organs.

Relatively larger kidneys along with a relatively smaller rib cage leave the pediatric kidneys more exposed to trauma, especially from the posterior. Often underlying kidney anomalies are identified at the time of evaluation following trauma.

Clinical Presentation

Any time the athlete sustains significant trauma to any part of the body, the physician should consider the possibility of internal organ injuries. A head to toe evaluation should include auscultation of the lungs for decreased breath sounds, and localization of abdominal or chest pain to light and deep palpation. Guarding and rebound on the abdominal examination should raise suspicion of internal organ injury. Flank pain, hematuria, and inability to void can indicate a severe kidney or collecting system injury. A significant amount of internal bleeding can occur in the abdomen or pelvis with relatively little outward signs. With rapid blood loss, shock, hypotension, and tachycardia can present early (Table 37-1).

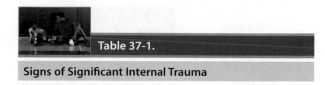

Table 37-1.
Signs of Significant Internal Trauma
Decreased breath sounds
Hypotension
Tachycardia
Tachypnea
Resound abdominal tenderness
Rigid abdomen
Flank pain and tenderness
Abdominal guarding
Post-traumatic hematuria
Inability to void

Splenic rupture

It is thought that splenomegaly puts the athlete at increased risk for rupture. Spleen size is often difficult to assess on physical examination. Some have considered CT or ultrasound studies to evaluate size. Because of significant variation in spleen size in the population, a single study does not necessarily correlate with spleen enlargement. Studies have shown that comparing spleen size in the acute case to a baseline may help identify spleen enlargement for the individual athlete. In most cases, this is not possible. Left upper quadrant pain that radiate to the left shoulder or neck, Kehr's sign, is associated with spleen injury. Findings of a left lower rib fracture should raise concern for a spleen rupture. In the case of spleen rupture, the blood loss is not always rapid. Athletes may present several days after the injury in significant distress.

Liver injuries

Right upper quadrant abdominal pain can indicate a liver injury including hematoma and laceration. Pain may radiate to the right shoulder and neck because of diaphragmatic irritation. Left lower rib fractures should raise suspicion of liver injury.

Hollow viscus injuries

The hollow viscus can rupture at any location as a result of trauma. Because the duodenum is attached in the second and fourth part, the most common location is the third part of the duodenum.[6] The athlete may experience severe abdominal pain, nausea, and vomiting with perforation. The abdomen may be tender, distended, and rigid. Rebound and guarding may be present. Fever and diffuse pain indicate possible peritonitis.

Abdominal wall contusion

The abdominal wall injury is often difficult to differentiate from deeper injuries just on the basis of physical examination alone. The athlete may have significant

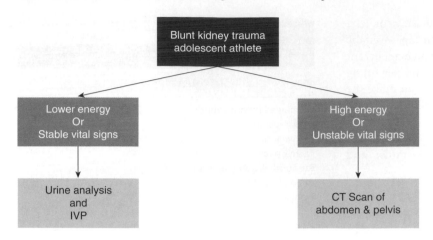

FIGURE 37-4 ■ Schematic of management of kidney and collecting system injury following trauma.

abdominal pain, even nausea and vomiting. Auscultation for bowel sounds can identify deeper injury. While the presence of bowel sounds is reassuring, absence can be associated with internal organ injury. Palpation should begin with light touch to evaluate deformity, hematoma, and muscle tearing that has occurred in the abdominal wall. Guarding and rebound tenderness on deep palpation indicate internal organ injury. Rigidity and distension are likewise findings on examination that should raise concern for internal injury. Finally, signs and symptoms of shock indicates significant blood loss and deserve further work up.

Abdominal wall hematoma

Muscle tears in the abdominal wall can lead to significant bleeding and hematoma. Because there is relatively larger room for expansion within the fascia, hematomas can be quite large. Though rare, there have been cases of abdominal wall compartment syndrome. Risk fractures that predispose to bleeding are associated with worse outcomes. Aspirin should probably be avoided in these athletes. Athletes may experience nausea and vomiting. Guarding and tenderness may be present and straight leg raise may increase the abdominal pain. A localized mass may be palpable later in the course as the hematoma organizes.

Kidney injury

Trauma to the back or flank can result in injury to the kidney. Injury to the kidney and collecting system in young children suggests the possibility of abnormal anatomy or function. For this reason most would recommend a more aggressive workup of the young athlete with this type of injury. Inability to void, flank pain, and shock following trauma should raise concern for a kidney or collecting system injury. The athlete with inability to void should be catheterized. Hematuria may be present with kidney hematoma, collecting system rupture, or kidney fracture.

Diagnosis

Diagnosis of abdominal injuries can be difficult owing to often subtle signs and symptoms. Signs of shock can present quickly. Therefore, an athlete with significant trauma should be suspected of having a serious abdominal injury. Laboratory studies such as blood counts, enzyme levels, urine analysis, ultrasound, and plain x-rays can often assist in rapid diagnosis. Advanced studies such as CT scan and MRI can assist with more difficult diagnoses (Figure 37-4). To fully evaluate the kidney and collecting system, IVP, ultrasound, and CT scan may be necessary.[7] Cystouerthrogram will help with identifying problems of the lower collecting system. Arteriogram can help in evaluation of the kidney (Figure 37-5).

Treatment

When there is a possibility of internal organ injury, the athlete should be limited in oral intake. This will reduce the risk of aspiration should urgent surgery be required. Until a firm diagnosis is established, pain should not be

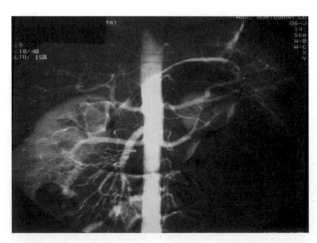

FIGURE 37-5 ■ Aortogram of left kidney showing laceration with no flow to inferior pole of left kidney.

treated aggressively with narcotics. The athlete with abdominal trauma and suspected internal organ injury should be immediately transported to the hospital for fluid resuscitation.

Not all *splenic ruptures* require surgery. If the bleeding is contained and has tamponade, then careful inpatient observation may be all that is necessary. The athlete will require bed rest and repeat studies. Serial physical examinations should be performed carefully, as to not cause rebleeding. Liver lacerations can lead to a significant amount of bleeding and will often require surgery. A hematoma that is stable may only require careful observation.

Treatment of *hollow viscus rupture* will include nothing by mouth, fluid, antibiotics, and surgical repair. Full return to activity will usually take 6 weeks.[6] If internal injuries can be ruled out abdominal wall contusions can be managed conservatively. Gradual return to activity will limit further abdominal wall irritation. Depending on the severity of the abdominal injury many athletes will be able to return to activity within 2 weeks. More severe injuries may take 8 to 12 weeks for the athlete to return to unrestricted sport participation. Management of abdominal wall hematoma is generally conservative, provided there are no bleeding complications, as is the usual case. Depending on activity, return to sports may take 4 to 12 weeks.

Hematomas of the kidney usually resolve with observation, whereas kidney fractures often are associated with significant bleeding and require repair. Extensive damage may necessitate nephrectomy. Fortunately, this is rare in sports-related trauma. Because of functional reserve, one kidney may be adequate.[7] Sport participation by athletes with solitary functioning kidney is reviewed in Chapter 13.

GENITOURINARY INJURIES

Injuries of the Ureters, Bladder, and Urethra

The pelvic organs of children are relatively smaller than their adult counterparts, making pelvic injuries less common. Trauma to the trunk or perineum can result in injury to the lower collecting system. Pelvic fractures may have associated injuries to the bladder or urethra. Ureteral injuries occur in isolation only rarely. Blunt lower abdominal trauma can lead to contusion or rupture of the bladder. Ureteral avulsion has been reported in children following blunt trauma. The abdominal position of the bladder in children can place it at greater risk for traumatic injury. Children may injure the urethra by the "straddle" mechanism.[8] Contact of the perineum with the cross bar of the bicycle can cause

injury to the urethra. In females, there may be labial hematoma causing urinary retention. Signs and symptoms of ureter injury include flank pain, possible mass, hematoma, hematuria, fever chills, and even shock. Bladder and urethral injury can result in hematuria, urethrorrhagia and inability to void. The perineum should be examined to evaluate bruising. Blood at the meatus may be found with urethral injury. The upper collecting system should be evaluated with IVP first.[8] Then the voiding cystourethrogram can be performed. Tear in the bladder, ureter, or urethra will need to be surgically repaired to prevent fistula.

Testicular Trauma

Testicular trauma causes significant pain and swelling. Torsion of the testicle can occur following trauma. This should be considered if the cremasteric reflex is diminished. Early referral to surgery/urology is recommended. Transillumination can differentiate a cyst from solid mass. Ultrasound with Doppler can identify masses and torsion of the testicle. After serious injury is ruled out, the main treatment is pain control. Exercise and stretching may relieve spasms. Ice and oral analgesics may be necessary.

Box 37-1 Indications for Referral of Abdomen, Genitourinary, and Chest Complaints.

Abdomen
1. Severe abdominal pain
2. Lower rib fractures with abdominal pain
3. Abdominal distention
4. Rebound or guarding on physical examination
5. Enlarged liver
6. Enlarged spleen
7. Fever
8. Signs of shock

Genitourinary
1. Hematuria
2. Flank pain
3. Urinary retention
4. Testicular swelling or deformity
5. Fever
6. Signs of shock

Chest
1. Multiple rib fractures
2. Upper rib fractures
3. Open rib fractures
4. Increasing shortness of breath
5. Hageman's sign
6. Deviation of the trachea
7. Jugular venous distention
8. Open chest wound
9. Arrhythmias
10. Cardiac arrest
11. Fever
12. Signs of shock

The "jock strap," or athletic supporter is an under garment which can prevent testicular trauma from excessive movement from running and jumping. In contact sports as well as sports where missiles or sticks may contact the body, male athletes should use a protective cup in the athletic supporter to cover the genitals (Box 37-1).

REFERENCES

1. Baker R. Fracture, rib. In: Bracker M, ed. *5 Minute Sports Medicine Consult.* Philadelphia: Lippincott, Williams & Wilkins; 2001:150-151.

2. Putukian M. Pneumothorax and pneumomediastinum. *Clin Sports Med.* 2004;23:443-454.

3. Ciocca M. Pneumothorax in a weight lifter: The importance of vigilance. *Phys Sports Med.* 2000;28(4):97-103.

4. Vincent GM, McPeak H. Commotio cordis: a deadly consequence of chest trauma. *Phys Sports Med.* 2000;28(11):31-39.

5. Greydanus DE, Patel DR, Baxter TL. The breast and sports: issues for the clinician. *Adolesc Med.* 1998:9(3):533–550.

6. Hunt A, Dorshimer G, Kissick J, et al. Isolated jejunal rupture after blunt trauma. *Phys Sports Med.* 2001; 29(11):39-46.

7. Homes FC, Hunt JJ, Sevier TL. Renal injury in sport. *Curr Sport Med Rep.* 2003;2:103-109.

8. Baker R. Ureteral, bladder and urethral injuries. In: Bracker M, ed. *5 Minute Sports Medicine Consult.* Philadelphia: Lippincott, Williams & Wilkins; 2001:564-565.

Additional Readings

Baker R. Chest and breast lacerations and contusions. In: Bracker M, ed. *5- Minute Sports Medicine Consult.* Philadelphia: Lippincott, Williams & Wilkins; 2001: 388-389.

Gregory PL, Biswas AC, Batt ME. Musculoskeletal problems of the chest wall in athletes. *Sports Med.* 2002;32(4):235-250.

Morton DP, Callister R. Characteristics and etiology of exercise-related transient abdominal pain. *Med Sci Sports Exerc.* 2000;32(2):432-438.

Porter AM. Marathon running and the caecal slap syndrome. *Br J Sports Med.* 1982;16(3):178.

Putukian M, Potera C. Don't miss gastrointestinal disorders in athletes. *Phys Sports Med.* 1997;25(11):80.

Rifat S, Gilvydis RP. Blunt abdominal trauma in sports. *Curr Sport Med Rep.* 2003;2:93-97.

Steinbrunn BS, Zera RT, Rodriguez JL. Mastalgia: tailoring treatment to type of breast pain. *Postgrad Med.* 1997;102(5):183-194.

CHAPTER 38

Environment-Related Conditions

Daniel G. Constance and Robert J. Baker

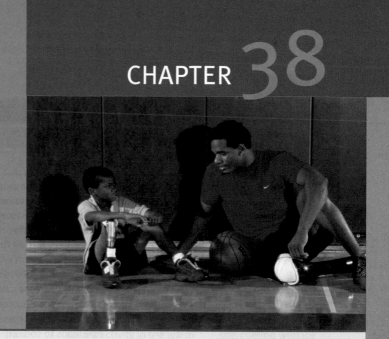

HEAT-REALTED ILLNESS

Definitions and Epidemiology

Heat illnesses exist on a spectrum of seriousness. An athlete need not experience symptoms of mild then moderate then severe heat illness to have heat stroke. The exact epidemiology is poorly defined and varies widely dependent on the study population and environmental conditions.

Definitions, pathogenesis, clinical presentations, and key principles of treatment of heat-related illnesses are summarized in Table 38-1.[1-8]

Pathogenesis

Pathogenesis is summarized in Table 38-1.[1-8] Risk factors are summarized in Table 38-2. Core body temperature is determined by the balance of heat generation and dissipation. A major contribution to the total thermal load is the generation of heat from exercising muscle. At maximal effort, skeletal muscle generates as much as 20 times the energy at rest. However, muscle energy generation is inefficient and as much as 75% is converted to heat, providing a major thermal load to the body systems. Additional thermal load is provided by the environment itself through radiant heat and convection in the environment. Dissipation of heat from the body to the environment is a combination of convection, radiation, and evaporative loss. But as the ambient temperature and humidity increase, the body becomes dependent on evaporative loss. At 23°C (74°F), 71% of heat dissipation is dependent on evaporative loss versus 100% dependence on evaporative loss at 35°C (95°F).[9] Logic dictates that ambient temperatures approaching 35°C, and high relative humidity, will decrease the efficacy of evaporative heat loss. It is noted that although core temperature above 40°C (104°F) is the definition for exertional heat stroke, higher core temperatures have been recorded in asymptomatic elite athletes. Therefore, the elevation of core temperature alone does not indicate heat illness.

The body's response to increasing core temperature is vasodilatation of the skin capillaries to dissipate heat. At the same time, there is vasodilatation of the skeletal muscle to provide oxygen and nutrients to the working muscle. As the skin temperature increases, neural regulation increases sweat loss. This sweat loss is hypotonic or isotonic. Thus, initially there may be no significant electrolyte loss. However, as exercise and sweating continues over longer endurance activities, continued loss of sweat can influence the loss of electrolytes.

Clinical presentation, diagnosis, and treatment are summarized in Table 38-1.

Prevention

Prevention of heat-related illnesses includes providing for a period of acclimatization, modification of activities based on the heat index, and access to electrolyte sports beverages. The process of acclimatization includes physiological adaptations that allow for increased peripheral blood flow, earlier onset of sweating, and greater volume of sweat. Acclimatization occurs over a period of 7 to 14 days where the athlete is gradually introduced to increasing levels and duration of physical activity.

Although weather forecasts may provide some information regarding the ambient temperature, relative

Patients with HAPE present with dyspnea, chest tightness, cough, fatigue, and "gurgling" in the lungs. Onset is usually 24 to 72 hours after arrival at altitude. Symptoms may present insidiously or as acute exertional dyspnea with progressive worsening at night. Tachypnea, tachycardia, orthopnea, rales on auscultation, cyanosis, pink-frothy sputum, and coma may be present.

Patients with HACE present initially with symptoms of AMS to include headache, nausea, vomiting, insomnia, but continue to develop progressive mental status changes. Onset can be within hours of arriving at altitude and usually presents within 5 days. Signs include ataxia, mental status changes, focal neurologic deficits, stupor, and coma. HACE can occur with HAPE. Fundoscopic exam may show retinal hemorrhages and papilledema.

Diagnosis

Diagnosis of the altitude illnesses is based on the history of recent ascent, symptoms, and signs. HAPE would show as pulmonary edema on chest x-ray. Pulse oximetry, and blood gas analysis would show hypoxia if not on current oxygen therapy. On MN imaging of the brain, HACE would show appear as white matter edema.

Treatment

Mild AMS may be treated with aspirin for headaches, antiemetics for nausea, restrictions on ascending further until symptoms resolve, and monitoring for signs of HAPE or HACE. The patient should be discouraged from physical activity and to remain rested and well hydrated. Acetazolamide or dexamethasone have been used; however, the definitive treatment for failure of symptoms to resolve or for more severe symptoms is supplementary oxygen and descent 500 to 1000 m.[8,12,15]

The most important treatment for HAPE and HACE is immediate descent. Supplemental high-flow oxygen at 4 to 6 LPM should be used as descent proceeds. The use of portable hyperbaric chambers while awaiting evacuation and during descent is useful. Dexamethasone and acetazolamide should be started. In isolated cases of HAPE, nifidepine sublingually reduces pulmonary resistance, but should not be used if there are symptoms of HACE.

Prevention

Most altitude illness can be prevented with appropriate acclimatization strategies. Gradual ascent is the rule of thumb. Once at altitude, avoid heavy exertion for 2 to 3 days. Above 2000 m, daily ascent should be limited to 300 to 600 m, with an extra day of rest every 1200 m ascended. Continue with regular meals and hydration. Alcohol, sedatives, and daytime sleeping should be avoided as the decreased respiratory drive may worsen hypoxia.

Medications that have been used during acclimatization and extreme high altitude, above 4000 m, include acetazolamide and dexamethasone, and have shown to be efficacious at reducing the incidence of AMS. Because of the risk for rebound illness, dexamethasone is recommended to be used for treatment only.

DIVING ILLNESS

Definitions and Epidemiology

Scuba diving has gained in popularity over the years, and although rare in most areas, a basic knowledge of diving illnesses is appropriate for the physician. Although a number of injuries can occur with diving including contact with marine life and physical hazards, these are variable dependent on the location.

More then 1000 diving-related injuries per year have been reported and 10% of these are fatal.[16] Barotrauma occurs when an air-filled body space fails to equilibrate to the prevailing pressures of the environment and causes tissue injury.[12,16] Decompression sickness is the liberation of gas bubbles within organ tissues because of the changes in gas tension between the dive state and returning to surface atmospheric pressure. Nitrogen narcosis is the change in mental status associated with increased nitrogen in the central nervous system that occurs at depth.[16]

Pathogenesis

The pathogenesis of barotrauma is explained by Boyle's Law that states, at a constant temperature, the volume of a gas is inversely proportional to the pressure. Therefore during descent to depth and increasing pressure, a gas that is within an air-filled space and not allowed to equilibrate will compress and the volume will decrease causing "under-pressure" and damage to tissues. The same holds true for ascent from depth; if the gas has been allowed to equilibrate at depth but on ascent cannot equilibrate, as the outside pressures decrease with ascent, the volume of the gas will expand and cause "over-pressure" injuries. These injuries can occur in any of the air-filled spaces of the body, most commonly the middle ear, inner ear, sinuses, lungs (pleural and mediastinal spaces), dental, and can even develop air emboli.

Decompression sickness and nitrogen narcosis are explained by Henry's Law. This law states that when the temperature is constant, the concentration of a gas dissolved in a fluid is directly proportional to the partial pressure of the gas. As the diver descends while breathing and the pressure from the depth increases, the partial pressures of the gasses inhaled increase in the blood stream, and therefore in the tissues. At depths deeper then 30 m (100 feet) the concentration of nitrogen in the central nervous system appears to cause mental status changes, explaining nitrogen narcosis. If ascent proceeds too quickly without the time needed for equilibration of the pressures between tissues, blood stream, and lungs, gas bubbles may form in the tissues or blood stream involving multiple organs, causing decompression illness.

Clinical Presentation

Symptoms of barotrauma are dependent on the structures involved. Pulmonary barotrauma presents with the typical symptoms of pneumothorax or pneumomediastinum. Arterial gas embolism may affect any end organ secondary to arterial occlusion for the emboli and may include heart (arrhythmia, myocardial infarction), brain (cerebrovascular accidents), kidneys (hematuria, renal failure), and other organs. Middle ear barotrauma presents with pain, hearing loss, and vertigo. Rupture of the tympanic membrane can occur. Sinus barotrauma presents with pain, epistaxis, and headache. Dental barotrauma can occur if infection or fillings are in place that allow for air space compression and expansion.

Decompression illness can affect multiple organs and the presentation depends on the organs affected. Musculoskeletal involvement usually presents in 30 to 60 minutes and is associated with "the bends" or joint pain, more commonly in the shoulder and elbow then knee or hip, that intensifies over the subsequent 2 days. Cutaneous manifestations include pruritis of the trunk that usually resolves within 30 minutes. Lymphatic involvement typically causes localized edema and pain. Neurologic involvement commonly involves the spinal cord and innervation of the upper lumbar and lower thoracic areas, leading to paresthesias and possible paraplegia. Other neurologic manifestations may include memory impairment and ataxia or "the staggers." Pulmonary manifestations include "the chokes" or chest pain, wheezing, and pharyngeal irritation. Emboli within the right heart can lead to right heart failure and cardiac collapse.

Nitrogen narcosis presents at depth as changes in mental status, personality, and neuromuscular coordination occurs. A major danger with nitrogen narcosis is the irrational behavior that may result, leading to poor judgment and drowning or decompression illness. Nitrogen narcosis typically resolves rapidly with ascent.

Diagnosis

Diagnosis of diving injuries is based on the pattern of the various illnesses and presenting symptoms. Treatment should proceed based on the history and presentation. There is no specific laboratory or imaging modality that provides a definitive diagnosis.

Treatment

Treatment of diving injuries is dependent on the organs involved. Pneumothorax and pneumomediastinum require emergent decompression of the potential spaces. The use of 100% O_2 is indicated in most situations while awaiting transportation to a hyperbaric unit for definitive treatment. Patients with right heart failure should be placed in the left lateral decubitus and slight Trendelenburg position to encourage forward flow.

Definitive treatment of air emboli from barotrauma and decompression sickness includes hyperbaric oxygen therapy. Although the best outcomes with hyperbaric therapy are noticed in the 4 to 6 hour time frame, treatment days later has shown improvement. Although delayed treatment is associated with risk of long-term poor prognosis. The National Diver's Alert Network at Duke University can provide assistance with locating the nearest hyperbaric treatment facility.

Prevention

Prevention of diving injuries relies on appropriate medical clearance for diving activities and following proper dive techniques to include decompression stops. Medical conditions that increase the risk for diving illness include pregnancy, asthma, chronic obstructive pulmonary disease, previous pneumothorax, cystic fibrosis, bronchiectasis, interstitial lung disease, history of thoracic surgery, patent foramen ovale, right-to-left shunts, ventricular arrhythmias, and congenital prolonged QT syndrome.

EXERCISE-RELATED URTICARIA AND ANAPHYLAXIS

Definitions and Epidemiology

Exercise-related allergic reactions include cholinergic urticaria, exercise-induced anaphylaxis, variant exercise-induced anaphylaxis, and food-dependent exercise-induced anaphylaxis. Approximately half of the cases of exercise-induced anaphylaxis are food dependent. Exercise-induced urticaria is a cholinergic urticaria associated with the development of 2 to 4 mm hives on the body that are pruritic but not associated with pulmonary or systemic symptoms. Urticatia or angioedema can be potentially life threatening because of upper airway sensitivity, hypotension, and syncope. The epidemiology of exercise-related allergic reactions is not well defined.[12,13,17]

Pathogenesis

Cholinergic urticaria presents with exercise, but also with warmer environments and emotional stress. There is an exaggerated cholinergic response that leads to mast cell degranulation and release of histamine. The histamine release leads to the development of pruritic hives.

Anaphylaxis is similarly a histamine response; however, the release of histamine is not well understood. Classic anaphylaxis is generally caused by antigen activation and a hypersensitivity reaction. The activation of the immune system with exercise is less well understood. In many cases there is an interaction of specific food or medication and exercise. Exposure to either the food or exercise by itself does not cause a reaction; however, when the specific food or medication is taken in close proximity to exercise, anaphylaxis develops. Numerous foods and medications have been implicated including celery, wheat, shellfish, chicken, aspirin, NSAIDs, antibiotics, and alcohol.

Clinical Presentation

Cholinergic urticaria presents as the body begins to warm during exercise, and typically starts early in exercise as pruritic hives that are 2 to 4 mm in size on the trunk and neck, later involving the extremities. Cholinergic urticaria may present with other body warming activities including a warm shower.

Exercise-induced anaphylaxis generally presents with fatigue, pruritis, warmth, erythema, and large urticarial lesion approximately 10 to 15 mm in diameter. This may progress to choking, stridor, and collapse. Variant type exercise-induced anaphylaxis differs from the classic exercise-induced anaphylaxis in that the urticarial lesions are small, 2 to 4 mm, and resemble cholinergic urticaria.

Diagnosis

Diagnosis of exercise-induced urticaria and exercise-induced anaphylaxis is based on the clinical evaluation, and in most cases, testing is not needed.

Cholinergic urticaria can be reproduced with raising the body temperature 0.5°C to 1.5°C passively or by immersing an extremity in warm water at 40°C to 42°C. Intradermal testing with methacholine chloride can be used for testing of cholinergic urticaria. These tests will cause the development of the typical small urticaria. However, the sensitivity of these tests is low and provides little information. Testing for food allergies may be helpful in exercise-induced anaphylaxis to help identify possible food/exercise interactions. However, as stated previously, many of these cases do not show sensitivity to the food in isolation from exercise, while other athletes actually show sensitivity to multiple foods.

Treatment

Cholinergic urticaria is usually self-limiting and treatment is symptom based. Use of antihistamines helps with the pruritis. H1 and H2 blockers can be used; however, there is little data available on efficacy. Athletes should be observed for any deterioration as the overlap of symptoms with variant type exercise-induced anaphylaxis.

Treatment of anaphylaxis requires recognition and emergent treatment with epinephrine. General supportive care is required until the athlete recovers and may require fluid resuscitation, H1 and H2 blockers, and supplemental oxygen. Although some athletes with known exercise-induced anaphylaxis report improvement with simply stopping activities, all athletes with

---

Box 38-1 When to Refer: Environment-Related Conditions.

- Exertional heat stroke (core body temperature above 40°C)—emergency department treatment and critical care management
- Gangrene secondary to frost bite or trench foot require surgical evaluation
- Cold urticaria associated with anaphylaxis requires evaluation in the emergency department. Immunology consultation is recommended
- Moderate to severe hypothermia (core body temperature below 32°C) requires emergency department treatment and critical care management
- Lightening strike victims—emergency department evaluation for cardiopulmonary arrest, blast injuries, burns, and fractures. Cardiology evaluation for all victims
- All cases of high-altitude pulmonary edema (HAPE), and high-altitude cerebral edema (HACE) require emergency department treatment and critical care management
- Diving injuries associated with barotrauma air emboli and decompression sickness, to include pneumothorax, pneumomediastinum, heart failure, and neurological manifestations require emergent transport and treatment at a hyperbaric treatment facility. (contact The National Diver's Alert Network at Duke University for closest facility)
- Exercise-induced anaphylaxis should be initially treated in the field and evaluated in the emergency department. Consultation with an immunologist is recommended.

known exercise-induced anaphlaxis should have an Epi-Pen available at all times when they are exercising.

Prevention

Symptoms of cholinergic urticaria can be minimized with the use of H1 and H2 blockers. Avoidance of exercising on hot and humid days may be prudent if this is a known trigger. There may be a level of acclimatization that allows for increased participation in warmer environments.

It is strongly advised athletes notify others they exercise with of their condition, wear medical alert identification, never exercise alone, and always have an Epi-Pen available. Identification of possible food triggers is important as it is reported that half of the cases are food dependent. Use of food/exercise logs may be helpful in defining the interaction. Once a food is identified, exercise should be avoided for 4 to 6 hours after ingestion of that food[17] (Box 38-1).

REFERENCES

1. Armstrong LE, Casa DJ, Millard-Stafford M, et al. American College of Sports Medicine position stand: exertional heat illness during training and competition. *Med Sci Sports Exerc.* 2007;39:556-572.
2. Binkley HM, Becket J, Casa DJ, et al. National Athletic Trainers' Association position statement: exertional heat illness. *J Athl Training.* 2002;37(3):329-343.
3. American Academy of Pediatrics Committee on Sports Medicine and Fitness: Climatic heat stress and the exercising child. *Pediatrics.* 2000;106:158-159.
4. Sawka M, Burke L, Eichner ER, et al. American College of Sports Medicine position stand: exercise and fluid replacement. *Med Sci Sport Exerc.* 2007;39:377-390.
5. Casa DJ. National Athletic Trainers' Association position statement: fluid replacement for athletes. *J Athl Training.* 2000;35(2):212-224.
6. Noakes T. Fluid replacement during marathon running: position statement of International Marathaon Medical Directors Association. *Clin J Sports Med.* 2003;13(5): 309-318.
7. Lebrun CM. Care of the high school athlete: prevention and treatment of medical emergencies. *AAOS Instructional Course Lectures* 2006;55:687-702.
8. Griffin LY. Emergency preparedness: things to consider before game starts. *AAOS Instructional Course Lectures.* 2006;55:677-686.
9. Walsh KM, et al. National Athletic Trainers' Association position statement: lightening safety for athletics and recreation. *J Athl Training.* 2000;5(4):471-477.
10. Castellani JW, Young AJ, Ducharme MB, et al. American College of Sports Medicine position stand: prevention of cold injuries during exercise. *Med Sci Sports Exerc.* 2006;38(11):2012-2029.
11. Roberts WO. Cold-related injury. In: Garrett WE, Kirkendall DT, Squire DL, eds. *Principles and Practice of Primary Care Sports Medicine.* Philadelphia: Lippincott, Williams & Wilkins; 2001.
12. Seto CK, Way D, O'Connor N. Environmental illness in athletes. *Clin Sports Med* 2005;24(3):695-718.
13. Butcher JD. Exercise-induced asthma in the competitive cold weather athlete. *Curr Sports Med Rep.* 2006;5(6): 284-288.
14. Sallis R, Chassay CM. Recognizing and treating common cold-induced injury in outdoor sports. *Med Sci Sports Exerc.* 1999;31(10):1367-1373.
15. Gallagher SA, Hackett PH. High-altitude illness. *Emerg Med Clin North Am.* 2004;22(2):329-355.
16. Benton PJ, Glover MA. Diving medicine. *Travel Med Inf Dis.* 2006;4(3):238-254.
17. Hosey RG, Carek PJ, Goo A. Exercise-induced analphylaxis and urticaria. *Am Family Physician.* 2001;64(8):1367-1374.

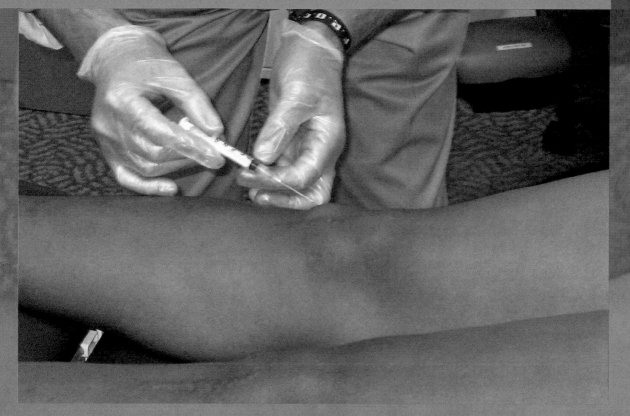

Appendices

A. Introduction to Bracing, Splinting, and Casting

B. Soft Tissue Injections, Joint Injections, and Aspiration

C. An Illustrated Guide to Some Common Exercises

D. Analgesic and Nonsteroidal Anti-Inflammatory Drugs

E. Resources for Further Education and Involvement

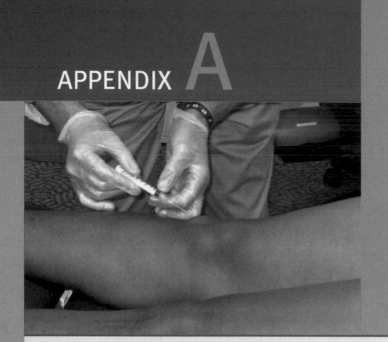

APPENDIX A

Introduction to Bracing, Splinting, and Casting

Eugene Diokno

BRACES

In the active pediatric population, the two most commonly injured areas for which braces have been used are the knee and ankle. One might have seen those football offensive linemen with large mid-thigh-to-calf hinged knee brace. Basketball players may be lacing up ankle braces on top of taped ankles and underneath those high-cut shoes. These are used for both acute and chronic conditions. For some athletes, they may gear them up for purely "cosmetic" reasons. The role and effectiveness of bracing for prevention and treatment of musculoskeletal injuries remain controversial; however, because of positive responses from the users, and minimal side effects, they are still widely used.[1]

Braces have generally been categorized into the following types: (1) prophylactic, to prevent or reduce severity of injury, (2) functional, to provide stability, and (3) rehabilitative, to augment postoperative care and recovery. A prophylactic knee brace is used to prevent injury; for example, the medial collateral ligament (MCL) injury during a valgus stress, or cruciate ligament sprains during a rotational stress (Figure A-1). Some find it cumbersome, but for athletes who are at high risk for such injuries (i.e., football offensive linemen, defensive linemen, linebackers, tight ends), might feel that this gives them a sense of protection.

A functional knee brace is used to provide stability to the joint; for example, control of knee joint rotation and anteroposterior translation for an anterior cruciate ligament (ACL) deficient knee.[2] This brace can come in the hinge-postshell or the hinge-poststrap types. It has an extension stop to guard against hyperextension. It has been recommended for select patients, including those who have poor motor control and pro-

prioception with the intention that the brace will increase their spatial awareness and better anticipate an impending event.[3]

A rehabilitative or postoperative brace is most commonly used for post-ACL reconstructive surgery and the nonoperated ACL-deficient knee. It is also used after repair of PCL, MCL, LCL, meniscus, or in managing nondisplaced epiphyseal fractures.[4] This type of brace has bilateral bars that span the thigh and leg with adjustable hinges at the knee that have extension and flexion stops to control the range of motion. This allows for different postoperative rehabilitation protocols. The use of this brace might not change the outcome of ACL reconstruction but it is still commonly used during the vulnerable postoperative period as it offers some protection from external forces and helps remind the patient of the risk of graft failure.[3] In 2001, the American Academy of Pediatrics released a technical report stating it does not recommend prescribing prophylactic knee braces because of the lack of solid evidence but has accepted the use of knee sleeves, functional braces, and postoperative braces on account of their subjective performance in the clinical setting.[4]

The knee sleeves are sometimes referred to as patellofemoral braces. The simplest one is a knee support, with or without a patellar cutout or donut, and may or may not come padded on the patellar area. This is usually made of neoprene which provides warmth. Aside from relieving discomfort, it provides compression and maybe even increases proprioception. Knee sleeves also come with a lateral buttress, which can be a "lateral J" or "hinged H"[5] or even C-shaped (Figure A-2). Indications for this include patellar subluxation or dislocation and patellofemoral syndrome.

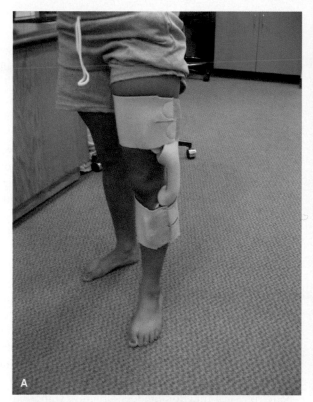

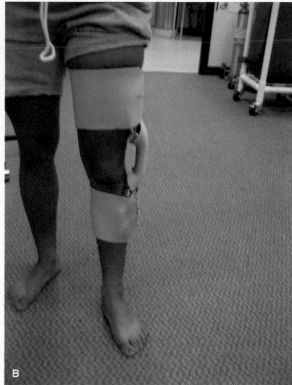

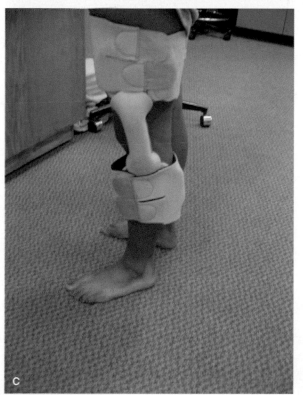

FIGURE A-1 ■ Unilateral hinged brace used for knee collateral ligament injuries.

The knee immobilizer (Figure A-3) is a light weight wide elastic strapping used for the purpose of complete knee immobilization in the face of an acute injury or for immediate postsurgical care. The length of its use depends on the specific condition but as a rule of thumb, it is preferred that the knee should resume its range of motion as soon as it is indicated to prevent stiffness and muscle atrophy with misuse. For patellar tendinitis or Osgood-Schlatter disease, a knee strap (i.e., Chopat®) has also been used as an adjunct to treatment (Figure A-4).

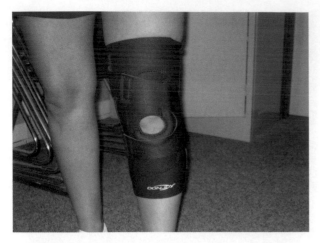

FIGURE A-2 ■ Knee or patellofemoral sleeve with buttress.

Ankle injuries commonly occur not only during participation with recreational or competitive sports but also with normal everyday activities. For the acute management of lateral ankle sprain, the use of Aircast® brace (Figure A-5) showed better improvement of function compared to the elastic bandage.[6] This type of semirigid support has preinflated air cells with adjustable Velcro® straps.[7] In children with isolated distal fibular fractures, which are considered low-risk, this removable brace has been demonstrated to be more effective than the below-the-knee walking cast.[8]

While considering the use of a prophylactic brace in prevention of ankle injuries, it is important to consider the presence of risk factors like sports that involve vigorous jumping, landing, and cutting maneuvers (i.e., basketball, volleyball, soccer) and prior history of ankle injuries.[9] In these situations, the use of taping and bracing could be of some benefits.[10,11] It has been argued that bracing is more cost-effective after taking into account not just the relatively lower expense with ankle brace but the manpower and time resource demanded by placing athletic tape on two ankles per athlete. The lace-up (Swede-O®) ankle support mimics a figure-of-eight construction to provide medial and lateral stability[7] (Figure A-6).

SPLINTS

Splints are another class of immobilization devices that are widely used for different indications. Wrist splints (Figure A-7) are an acceptable mode of immobilization for buckle fractures in children (i.e., removable volar splint).[12] In a randomized-controlled study comparing the splint with a short arm cast, the splinted group had better physical functioning, less difficulty with a number of daily activities and returned to play earlier.[13]

Finger splints come in foam-lined aluminum splints in different shapes and forms: straight, curved, baseball, or frog. Stax finger splints, useful in mallet

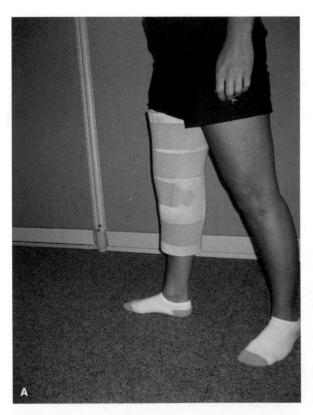

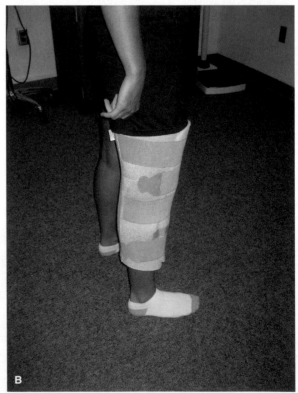

FIGURE A-3 ■ Knee immobilizer.

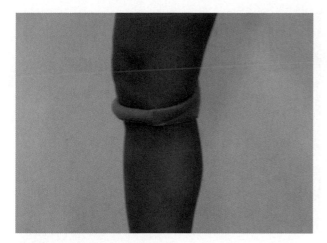

FIGURE A-4 ■ Chopat knee strap.

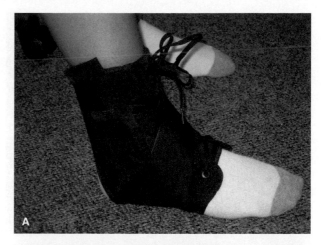

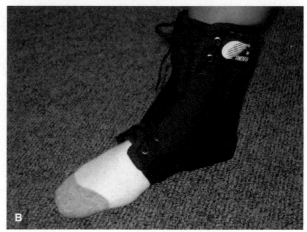

FIGURE A-6 ■ Lace up ankle brace.

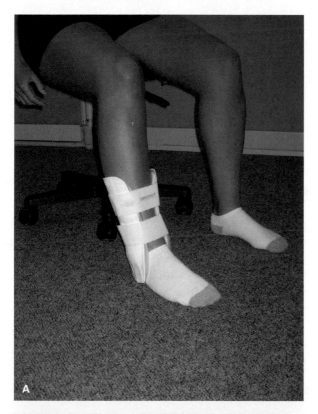

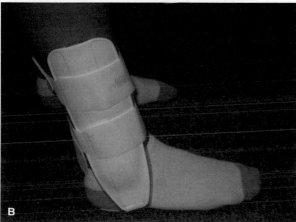

FIGURE A-5 ■ Airstirrup ankle brace.

fingers (Figure A-8), come in different sizes which come in handy as the swelling improves and one would need to change to a smaller size. In lieu of the half-inch cloth tape, one might opt for a buddy loop or strap for managing certain phalangeal fractures (Figure A-9).

Shoulder sling support can be used for easing discomfort after an acromioclavicular (AC) sprain, but is not recommended for extended use. It is best to resume range of motion as soon as it is tolerated. The figure-of-eight bandage is commonly used for clavicular fractures but a lot of younger children do not tolerate keeping this on for prolonged periods of time. For the older child, it serves as a reminder to hold back from high-risk activities as the fracture heals.

CASTS

Frequently, a splint is applied first in an urgent care or emergency room setting anticipating loosening of a cast as the initial swelling subsides to be replaced with a cast a few days later. The one-joint-above-and-one-joint-below-the-fracture rule generally applies to achieve maximal immobilization which is crucial in unstable or

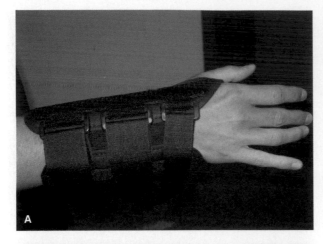

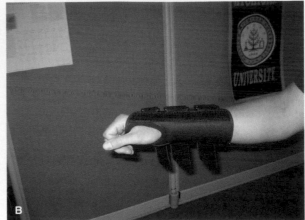

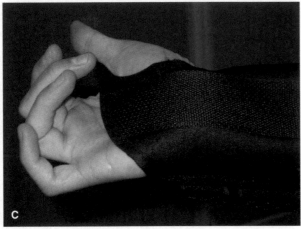

FIGURE A-7 ■ Views of a wrist splint.

potentially unstable fractures.[14] Instructions for cast care should be a routine part of discussion of fracture management as well as timely monitoring and continued re-evaluation as deemed appropriate for the specific fracture.

Cast materials are usually of the plaster and fiberglass type, the latter coming in a myriad of colors which has become a cosmetic plus for children and young teens. The traditional padding consisting of the stockinette and web roll prevents patients from getting the cast wet. There is also a waterproof liner available made up of Gore-tex® which is the same material used in waterproof outdoor apparel. This offers some convenience in an already difficult situation especially when caring for fractures in the preschool age children. Application of a fiberglass short arm cast is shown in Figure A-10A to A-10N. Different casts

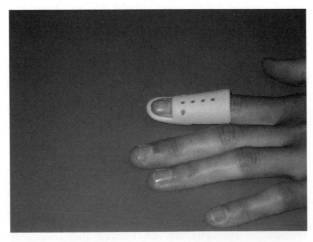

FIGURE A-8 ■ Finger splint to immobilize distal interphalangeal joint (for mallet finger).

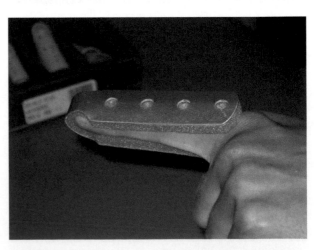

FIGURE A-9 ■ Finger splint used for simple phalangeal fractures.

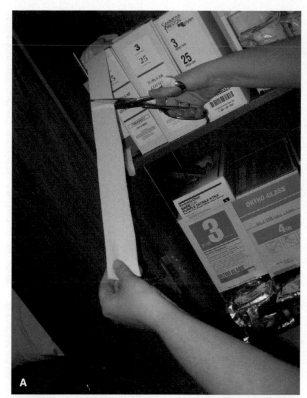

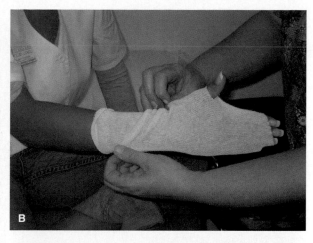

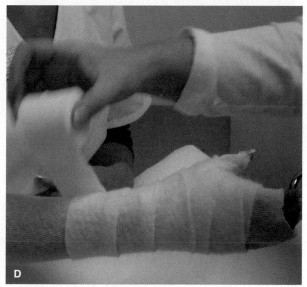

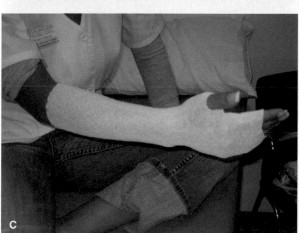

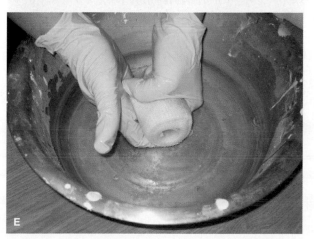

FIGURE A-10 ■ Application of a short arm thumb spica cast. Before applying the cast the skin must be cleaned and dried. A stockinette is first applied over the extremity followed by a roll of cotton padding over it (A–D). The stockinette ends are kept clear so they can be later rolled over the edges of the cast. A cotton padding is applied over it, with each turn overlapping the preceding turn by one-half its width (E–H). The fiberglass roll (or plaster roll) is soaked in water (cold for fiberglass) and gently squeezed (I). It is then applied from distal to proximal rolling it in the same direction as the cotton wadding (K,L). Each turn should overlap the preceding turn of plaster roll by half. The roll should be smoothened at each turn. Before the last roll is applied the stockinette is rolled over its proximal and distal ends to smoothen them out and then the final roll is applied (M). The desired position of the extremity should be maintained throughout the process and until the cast is set (hardened) (N). The hand should be generally held in the position of function (as if holding a can). *(continued)*

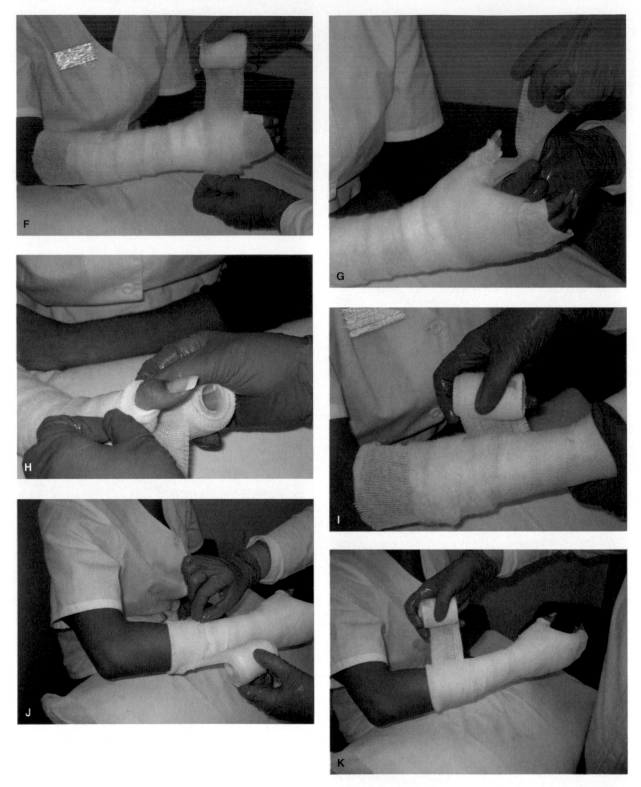

FIGURE A-10 ■ *(Continued).*

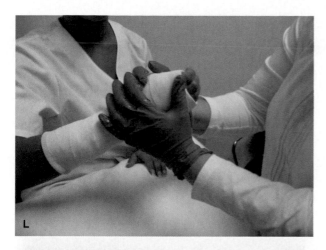

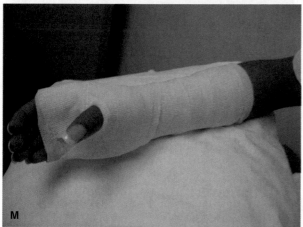

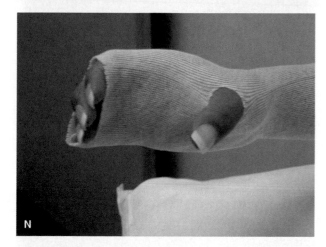

FIGURE A-10 ■ *(Continued).*

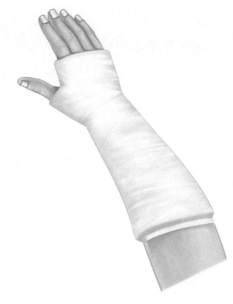

FIGURE A-11 ■ Short arm cast used in simple fractures of the wrist and hand.

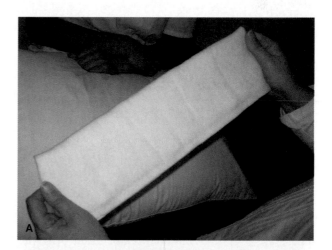

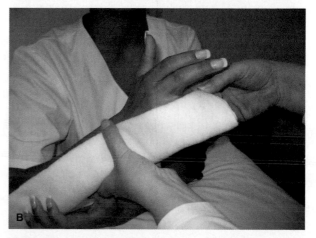

FIGURE A-12 ■ Ulnar gutter splint used for fractures of the metacarpals of the ring and little fingers. *(continued)*

are basically descriptive of the area and length they cover (Figures A-11 to A-14).

ORTHOTICS AND SHOE WEAR

Aside from injuries, feet and ankle problems are said to be the second most common musculoskeletal

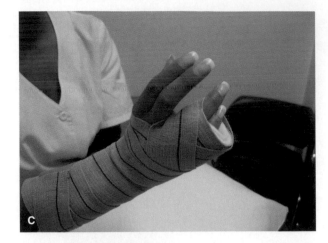

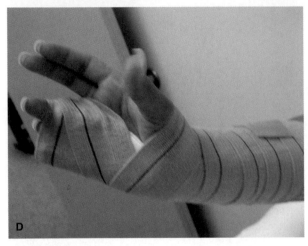

FIGURE A-12 ■ *(Continued).*

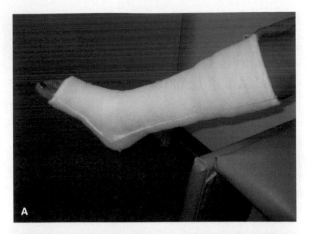

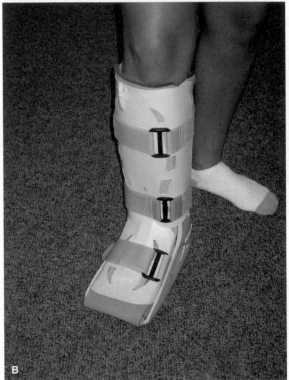

FIGURE A-13 ■ Short leg cast and cast brace used for simple fractures of the foot and ankle.

problem especially in children younger than 10 years of age.[15] Use of orthotics has a role in managing these problems and frequently also alleviates symptoms getting referred proximally to the knees and hips. There are over-the-counter prefabricated orthotics which includes heel cushions, arch supports, and full insoles. The second type is the customized orthosis which is a prefabricated one on top of which is added features like a pad or cushion. The third type is the custom molded and as the name implies, this is custom-made for a specific individual (Figure A-15A to A-15F).[16]

Children with pes planus or flat feet when symptomatic may need arch support to correct the pronated feet. Heel cups can be prescribed for Sever disease or calcaneal apophysitis (Figure A-16A and A-16B). Heel lifts may augment leg-length discrepancies. Other conditions that include orthotics as part of their nonsurgical management are tarsal coalition and sinus tarsi syndrome while turf toe and metatarsal stress fracture may require the use of hard-sole shoes.[15]

In the realm of prevention, choosing the right foot wear especially for the runner athlete is essential

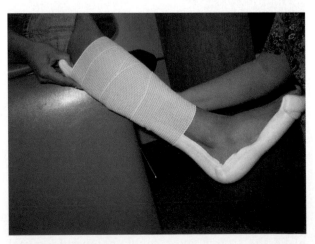

FIGURE A-14 ■ Posterior leg splint used for initial immobilization of the foot and ankle.

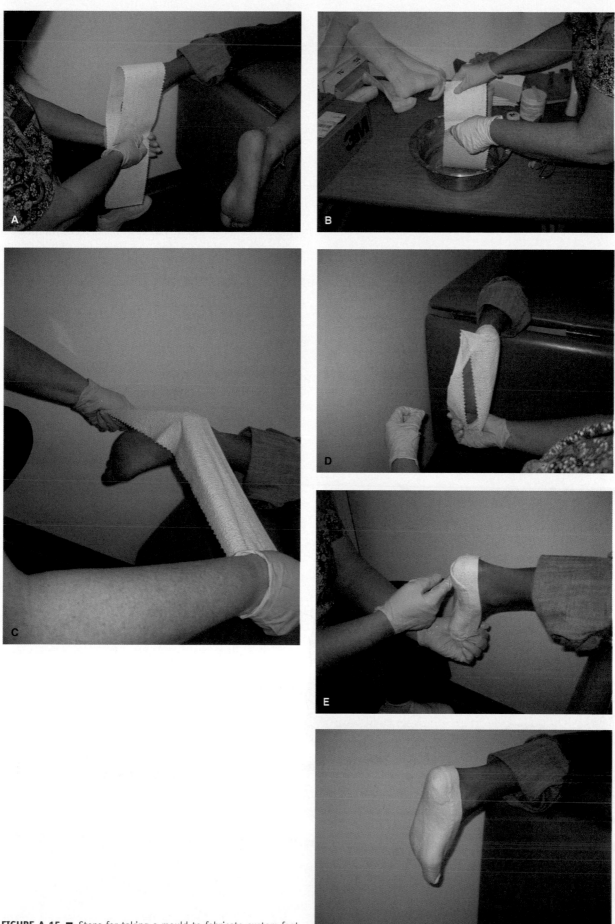

FIGURE A-15 ■ Steps for taking a mould to fabricate custom foot orthotics is shown.

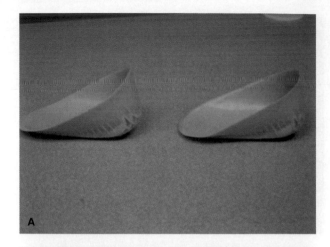

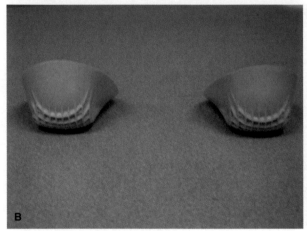

FIGURE A-16 ■ Tuli heel cups.

(Figures A-17 to A-19). In the office setting, there are few things we can do to help arrive at the appropriate shoe prescription. The foot wear pattern reveals three different types: rigid, showing lateral tilt or lateral wear pattern; normal, with no significant tilt and slight lateral wear; and floppy, the pronator with medial wear pattern. Have the patient do a wet test to see their sole imprint. Cushion-curved or semi-curved shoes will offer flexibility to the rigid, underpronating feet. On the other end of the spectrum, motion-control straight shoes are best for the pronators. For those with normal feet, stability shoes are recommended. These are summarized in Figure A-20.[17] Proper shoe care maximizes the shoes' shelf life. It has also been recommended to abandon the old pair after approximately 500 miles. For those not keeping track of their mileage, once the shoe is easily bent with both ends touching each other, then it's time (18).

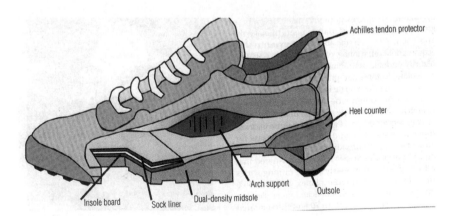

FIGURE A-17 ■ Parts of a shoe.

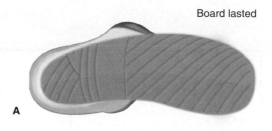

Board lasted

A

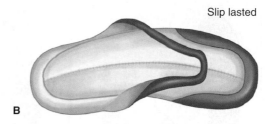

Slip lasted

B

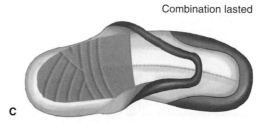

Combination lasted

C

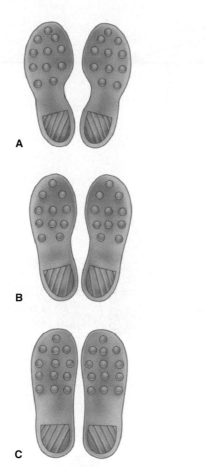

A

B

C

FIGURE A-18 ■ Shoe lasts. Running shoes that have curved lasts (a) provide more support for patients who have high arches. Semi-curved lasts (b) work well for patients with medium arches, and patients who have flat feet or low arches may do best wearing shoes with straight lasts (c).

FIGURE A-19 ■ Shoe lasts. Shoes are constructed by three basic methods. Board-lasted shoes (a) are the most rigid and provide the most motion control for overpronation. Slip-lasted shoes (b) are light and flexible, but they provide much less stability. Runners who have high arches and tend to underpronate may prefer slip-lasted shoes. Because combination-lasted shoes (c) have board only in the heel, they offer hindfoot stability and forefoot flexibility.

Evaluate shoe wear pattern

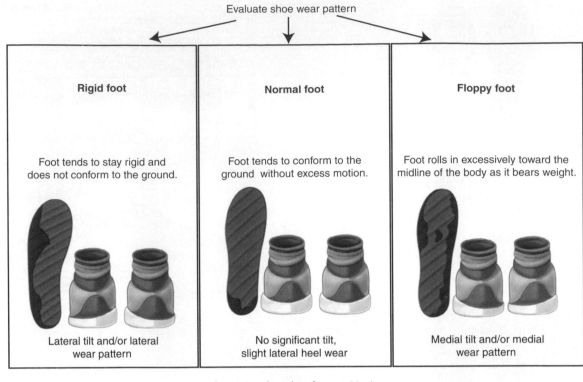

Rigid foot	**Normal foot**	**Floppy foot**
Foot tends to stay rigid and does not conform to the ground.	Foot tends to conform to the ground without excess motion.	Foot rolls in excessively toward the midline of the body as it bears weight.
Lateral tilt and/or lateral wear pattern	No significant tilt, slight lateral heel wear	Medial tilt and/or medial wear pattern

Inspect arch and perform wet test

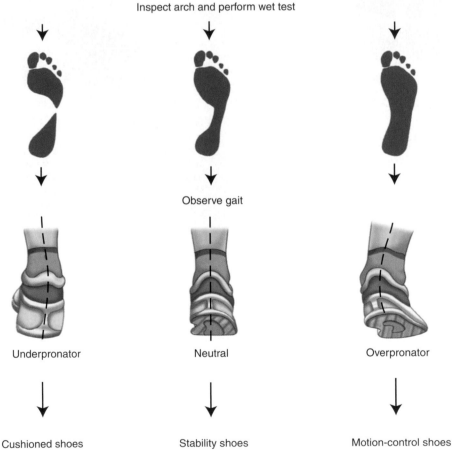

Observe gait

Underpronator   Neutral   Overpronator

Cushioned shoes   Stability shoes   Motion-control shoes

FIGURE A-20 ■ An approach to determine appropriate type of shoes.

REFERENCES

1. Gravlee JR, Van Durme DJ. Braces and splints for musculoskeletal conditions. *Am Family Physician.* 2007;75:343-348.
2. Paluska SA, Mckeag DB. Knee braces: current evidence and clinical recommendations for their use. *Am Family Physician.* 2000;61:411-418.
3. Brown A, Albright JP. The use of knee braces in sports medicine. In: Miller MD, ed. *DeLee and Drez's Orthopedic Sports Medicine.* Philadelphia, PA: Saunders; 2003:2128.
4. American Academy of Pediatrics Committee on Sports Medicine. Technical report: knee brace use in young athletes, 2001;108:503-507.
5. 2006 Donjoy Product Catalog.
6. Boyce SH, Quigley MA, Campbell A. Management of ankle sprains: a randomized controlled trial of treatment of inversion injuries using an elastic support bandage or an Aircast ankle brace. *Br J Sports Med.* 2005;39:91-96.
7. 2006-2007 North Coast Medical Rehabilitation Catalog.
8. Boutis K, Willan AR, et al. A randomized, controlled trial of a removable brace versus casting in children with low-risk ankle fractures. *Pediatrics.* 2007;119:e1256-e1263.
9. Gross MT, Liu HY. The role of ankle bracing for prevention of ankle sprain injuries. *J Orthop Sports Phys Ther.* 2003;33:572-577.
10. Verhagen E, Mechelan W, Vente W. The effect of preventive measures on the incidence of ankle sprains. *Clin J Sports Med.* 2000;10:291-296.
11. Ivins D. Acute ankle sprain: an update. *Am Fam Physician.* 2006;74:1714-1720.
12. Eiff MP, Hatch RL, Calmbach WL. *Radius and Ulna Fractures: Fracture Management for Primary Care.* Philadelphia, PA: Saunders; 2003:128.
13. Plint AC, Perry JJ, et al. A randomized, controlled trial of removable splint versus casting for wrist buckle fractures in children. *Pediatrics.* 2006;117:691-697.
14. Eiff MP, Hatch RL, Calmbach WL. *General Principles of Fracture Care: Fracture Management for Primary Care.* Philadelphia, PA: Saunders; 2003:20.
15. Omey ML, Michelli LJ. Foot and ankle problems in the young athlete. *Med Sci Sports Exerc.* 1999;31:S470-S486.
16. Sanders M, Janisse D. Pads, inserts, and appliances. In: O'Connor PL, Schaller TM, eds. *Footworks II, A Patient's Guide to the Foot and Ankle.* Portage; 2001:66-68.
17. Asplund CA, Brown DL. The running shoe prescription, fit for performance. *Phys Sport Med.* 2005;33(1):17-27.
18. Chew KTL, Lew HL, Date E, et al. Current evidence and clinical applications of therapeutic knee braces. *Am J Phys Med Rehabil.* 2007;86:678-686.
19. http://www.aaos.org/about/ papers/position/1124.asp

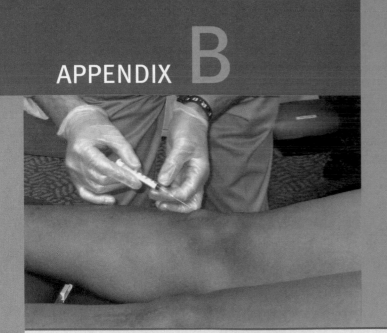

Soft Tissue Injections, Joint Injections, and Aspiration

Eugene Diokno

Evidence-based reviews of injection procedures have not established their efficacy but practice experience supports its effectiveness[1] leading to their vast applications. Diagnostic and therapeutic aspiration of major joints has been an accepted practice in pediatric age group. On the other hand therapeutic injections of joint and soft tissue are rarely indicated or necessary for most sport-related musculoskeletal conditions in children and adolescents. This section provides a short introduction to the topic.

INDICATIONS

General indications for joint and soft tissue injection and aspiration are twofold: diagnostic and therapeutic.[1,2] Aspirating a joint for synovial fluid analysis is a useful diagnostic tool to differentiate an infectious versus an inflammatory etiology. Presence of fat globules in a fresh aspirate may confirm a suspected occult fracture not easily seen on initial plain radiographic studies. Symptomatic relief after injecting a local anesthetic may delineate local from referred pain. A common therapeutic indication is to alleviate the patient's pain and improve range of motion like in a large tense knee effusion. Another indication is to deliver the appropriate pharmacologic agents that usually include a local anesthetic and a form of corticosteroid. Examples of some specific conditions for which these procedures may be called for are listed in Table B-1.

CONTRAINDICATIONS

Any procedure has absolute and relative contraindications.[1,3] Absolute contraindications include joint sepsis,

local cellulitis, fracture, bacteremia, prosthesis, tendinous sites with high risk or rupture, joint prosthesis and allergy for the drugs being used. Relative contraindications are joint instability, coagulopathy, anticoagulation therapy, poor response to previous injections, anatomically inaccessible joints, and uncontrolled diabetes mellitus. All the aforementioned refer to therapeutic injections. An exception is the presence of a septic joint which in itself is an indication for aspiration but a contraindication for therapeutic injection.[1,3]

COMPLICATIONS

These procedures are generally safe and complications are rare.[4] These can be broken into two categories: those attributed to the procedure itself and those from the medication being delivered. Bleeding, infection, and joint injury comprise the first category. A big concern with corticosteroid injection is the risk of tendon rupture. The risk is extremely low but because of the potential adverse

Table B-1.

Indications for Injection

Intra-articular	Nonarticular
Effusion of unknown origin	Bursitis
Rheumatoid arthritis	Tendonitis/tendinosis
Traumatic arthriti	Tenosynovitis
Crystalloid arthropathies	Ganglion
Synovitis	Trigger points
Osteoathritis	Entrapment syndromes
	Fasciitis

outcome, it is one of the important things that need to be included in discussing risks and benefits when obtaining informed consent. Local complications are accelerating a septic joint, subcutaneous fat atrophy, skin depigmentation, steroid flare, cartilage damage, fistulous tract formation, and transient paresis of involved extremity. Facial flushing, gastrointestinal effects, mood alterations, fluid retention, menstrual irregularities, hypothalamic-pituitary axis suppression,[5] and allergic reactions are some of the systemic adverse effects reported.

PRECAUTIONS

Certain general guidelines need to be followed when performing joint aspiration and injection.[4] First and foremost, obtain an informed consent and document. Universal precautions when handling bodily fluids should be practiced. Keeping in mind that the joint space is being invaded, observing sterile technique is paramount. Clinicians should make it a point to thoroughly wash their hands, use sterile gloves, needles, and syringes and wipe the site with an antiseptic solution like povidone-iodine (Betadine®). Sterile draping is optional. For ease of changing syringes either for multiple aspirations or aspiration followed by injection, using a hemostat helps stabilize the hub of the needle already in place. When introducing the needle, the plunger should be drawn back to ensure that it is not in the intravascular space and if so, the needle should be redirected. Injecting into a joint space, bursa, or tendon sheath should be felt with ease. If there is resistance, this may be a sign that the needle tip is within muscle, ligament, or tendon therefore should be readjusted. Patient should be instructed to rest the involved area for the next 24 to 48 hours and be aware of ominous signs to look for that could be related to complications previously discussed.

MATERIALS

As seen in Figure B-1, all the necessary equipment is laid out within reach of the clinician. For non-articular injec-

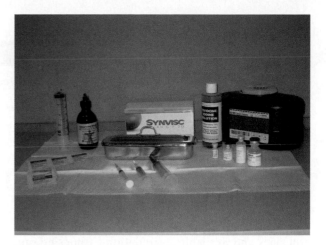

FIGURE B-1 ■ Equipment for injection and aspiration.

tions, alcohol wipes and nonsterile gloves will suffice. For aspirations, an 18- to 20-gauge, 1.5-inch needle and at least 20-mL syringe are preferable. To minimize patient discomfort, a finer 22- to 25-gauge, 1 to 1.5-inch needle can be used for injections. Depending on the involved site, 1- to 10-mL syringe should be available. External local anesthetic like ethyl chloride spray is optional. Application of eutectic lidocaine/prilocaine cream (EMLA®) has not been shown to provide significant analgesic effect with steroid injection into knees of children with juvenile rheumatoid arthritis.[6] The most commonly used local anesthetics are lidocaine, 1% or 2% without epinephrine (Xylocaine®) and bupivacaine, 0.25% or 0.5% (Marcaine®). The latter has a longer onset of action of approximately 30 minutes and duration of action can last up to 8 hours. Prepare sterile tubes or cups for culture studies, kidney basin, hemostat, gauze, adhesive bandage, and compression dressing as necessary.

The exact mechanism of action of corticosteroids is uncertain but is believed to be suppressing inflammation, be it rheumatoid or degenerative in nature, as well as inhibiting the inflammatory damage–repair–damage cycle.[5] It is also postulated that it provides a chondroprotective effect. The more commonly used preparations are listed in Table B-2, which also shows their comparative

Table B-2.

Commonly Used Corticosteroids

Generic	Brand	Potency	Duration	Formulation
Hydrocortisone acetate	Hydrocortone	Low	Short	50 mg/mL
Methylprednisolone acetate	Depo-Medrol	Intermediate	Intermediate	40 & 80 mg/mL
Triamcinolone acetonide	Kenalog Aristocort	Intermediate	Intermediate	40 mg/mL
Dexamethasone sodium phosphate	Decadron	High	Long	4 mg/mL
Betamethasone sodium phosphate/ acetate	Celestone	High	Long	3 & 6mg/mL

Table B-3.

Commonly Injected Sites and Medication Dose Guidelines

Site	Syringe	Needle	1% Lidocaine	Depo-Medrol
Knee	10 cm³	g 22, 1.5 in	2–4 cm³	2 cm³ (80 mg)
Subacromial	10 cm³	g 22, 1.5 in	2–4 cm³	2 cm³ (80 mg)
AC Joint	5 cm³	g 22/25, 1.25 in	1.5 cm³	1.5 cm³ (60 mg)
Lateral epicondyle	5 cm³	g 22/25, 1.25 in	1.5 cm³	1.5 cm³ (60 mg)
Trochanteric bursa	10 cm³	g 22, 1.5 in	2–4 cm³	2 cm³ (80 mg)

potencies and available formulations. Choosing one over another largely depends on the clinician's personal preference that evolved from experience. Some general considerations like duration of action and size of joint space are also taken into account in a case per case basis.

COMMON SITES AND TECHNIQUES

Refer to Table B-3 for common sites and corresponding materials needed for the injection as well as doses of the local anesthetic and corticosteroid.

Knee

The patient is lying supine with the knee extended or a small roll placed in the popliteal side with the knee slightly flexed. Palpate the superior lateral aspect of the patella, and mark one fingerbreadth above and one fin-

gerbreadth lateral to this. Direct the needle to the center of the patella at a 45-degree angle distally. A triangle technique has been described which was claimed to be accurate as well.[7] The patient is seated with the knee flexed at 90 degrees. The inverted triangle borders the patellar edges and the needle is inserted on the lateral side into the space between the patella and femur (Figure B-2).

Subacromial Bursa

The posterolateral approach is commonly used (Figure B-3). Palpate the posterior tip of the acromion. Feel the space between the acromion and the head of the

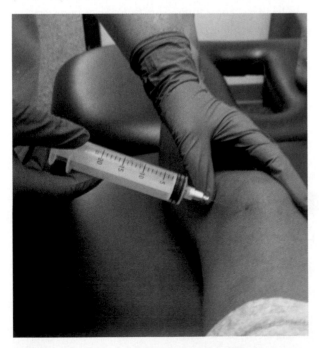

FIGURE B-2 ■ Site for injection and aspiration of the knee.

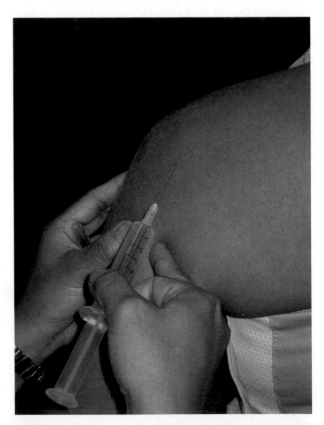

FIGURE B-3 ■ Posterolateral approach for injection of subacromial bursa.

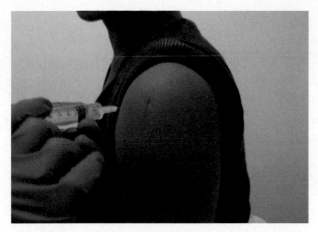

FIGURE B-4 ■ Anterolateral approach for injection of subacromial bursa.

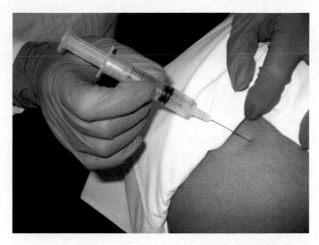

FIGURE B-6 ■ Site for injection or aspiration of trochanteric bursa.

humerus and insert the needle toward the coracoid process. With the anterolateral approach (Figure B-4), the needle is inserted approximately 2 cm lateral to the lateral acromion edge. Neither approach has been shown to be more accurate than the other.[8]

Acromioclavicular Joint

The patient can be supine but the seated position with the arm hanging on the side may slightly separate the AC joint. Palpate the clavicle and walk distally until a depression is felt where the site of the AC joint is. The needle is directed inferiorly and medially at approximately 30 degrees.

Lateral Epicondyle

The most common condition for which this is indicated is lateral epicondylitis or tennis elbow. The patient should lay supine, elbow flexed at 45 degrees and forearm pronated (Figure B-5). Once the lateral epicondlye is palpated, mark and target the point of maximal tenderness. Once the needle is inserted, repeated withdrawal and infiltration using the fanning method can also be done to

cover a broader area. Caution should be exercised that the needle is not inadvertently completely withdrawn prematurely especially that the site is very superficial.

Trochanteric Bursa

Have the patient lie on his side, with the affected side up. Flex the hip and knee to minimize discomfort and to stabilize the hip. Like the tennis elbow, mark the point of maximal tenderness over the bony protrusion of the greater trochanter. The needle is introduced perpendicular to the skin and for individuals of size, a longer needle might be necessary (Figure B-6).[9]

REFERENCES

1. Cardone DA, Tallia AF. Joint and soft tissue injection. *Am Fam Physician*. 2002;66:283-288.
2. Rifat SF, Moeller JL. Basics of joint injection, general techniques and tips for safe, effective use. *Postgrad Med*. 2001;109:157-166.
3. Dooley P, Martin R. Corticosteroid injections and arthocentesis. *Can Fam Physician*. 2002;48:285-292.
4. Rifat SF, Moeller JL. Injection and aspiration techniques for the primary care physician. *Compr Ther*. 2002;28:222-229.
5. Saunders S, Longworth S. The drugs. In: Wolfaard S, ed. *Injection Techniques in Orthopaedics and Sports Medicine*. London: Elsevier; 2006:3-15.
6. Uziel Y, et al. Evaluation of eutectic lidocaine/prilocaine cream (EMLA) for steroid joint injection in children with juvenile rheumatoid arthritis: a double blind, randomized, placebo controlled trial. *J Rheumatol*. 2003;30:594-596.
7. Lockman LE. Practice tips, knee injections and aspirations, the triangle technique. *Can Fam Physician*. 2006;52: 1403-1404.
8. Mathews PV, Glousman RE. Accuracy of subacromial injection: anterolateral versus posterior approach. *J Shoulder Elbow Surg*. 2005;14:145-148.
9. Cardone DA, Tallia AF. Diagnostic and therapeutic injection of the hip and knee. *Am Fam Physician*. 2003;67: 2147-2152.

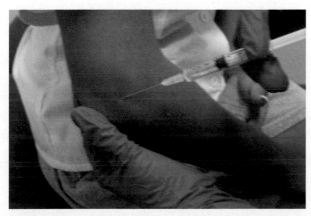

FIGURE B-5 ■ Site for injection of the lateral epicondyle.

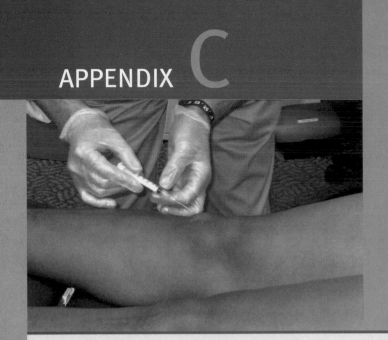

An Illustrated Guide to Some Common Exercises

Eugene Diokno

There are a variety of musculoskeletal conditions and injuries wherein exercises play a vital role in the rehabilitation process. The following instructions are meant for you to disseminate to your patients. Feel free to make them part of your prescription. Individualize the regimen and emphasize proper technique. It is better to demonstrate it while they are in the office with you and have them demonstrate it back. Keep it simple and generally do not exceed three exercises as much as possible keeping in mind they have to do several repetitions for the program to be effective. Like taking medications, the more they have to do, the less adherent they become. Remind them on how they should progress forward depending on their clinical conditions. The stretching exercises should not be painful; otherwise it is time to hold back a little. Give them positive reinforcements on follow-up visits as appropriate. For the healthy ones who are interested in doing home exercises, you can also share these with them. The number of sets and repetitions may vary depending upon the goal of the exercise as well as the stage at which the athlete has progressed in rehabilitation. The number of sets range between 1 and 3 and the repetitions per set range between 8 and 15 (see Ch. 5).

KNEE

See figures C-1 to C-9 with corresponding captions describing the exercises.

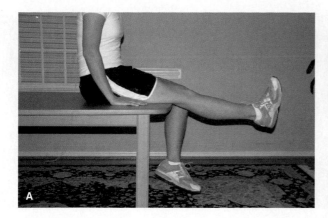

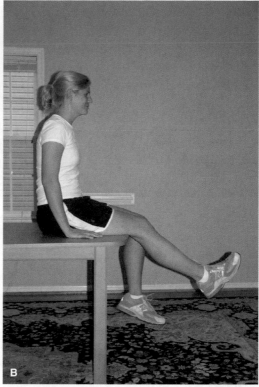

FIGURE C-1 ■ Active extension and flexion (Figure C-1): Sit on a chair. Tighten your front thigh muscle and raise your heel off the floor and straighten your knee. Hold for — seconds. Repeat — sets of —.

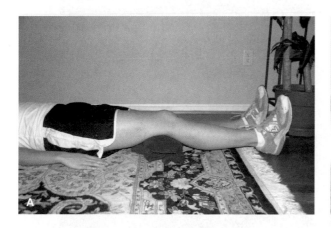

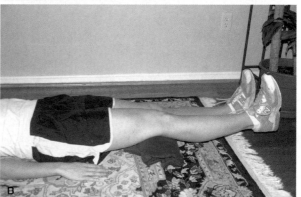

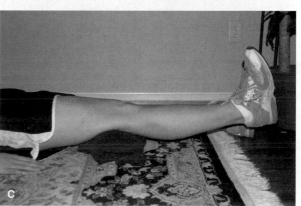

FIGURE C-2 ■ Quadriceps short arcs (Figure C-2): Lie flat and place a towel roll under your knee. Tighten your front thigh muscle and raise your heel off the floor. Hold for — seconds. Repeat — sets of —.

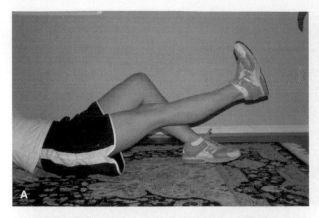

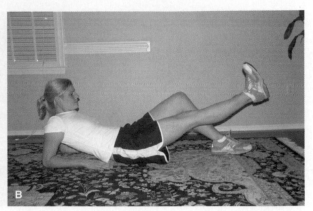

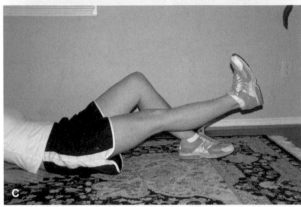

FIGURE C-3 ■ Straight leg raises (Figure C-3): Lie flat on your back. Tighten your front thigh muscle as hard as you can. Slowly raise your leg. Relax and then lower your leg slowly keeping your knee straight throughout. Repeat — sets of —.

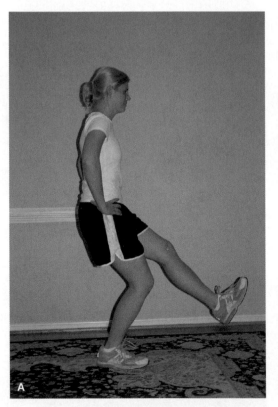

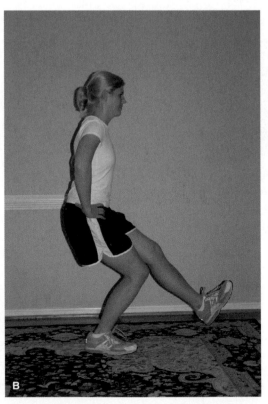

FIGURE C-4 ■ One legged squats (Figure C-4): Stand on one leg with hands on your waist. Slowly bend this leg up to 45 degrees, hold for a few seconds, and then straighten it. Repeat — sets of —.

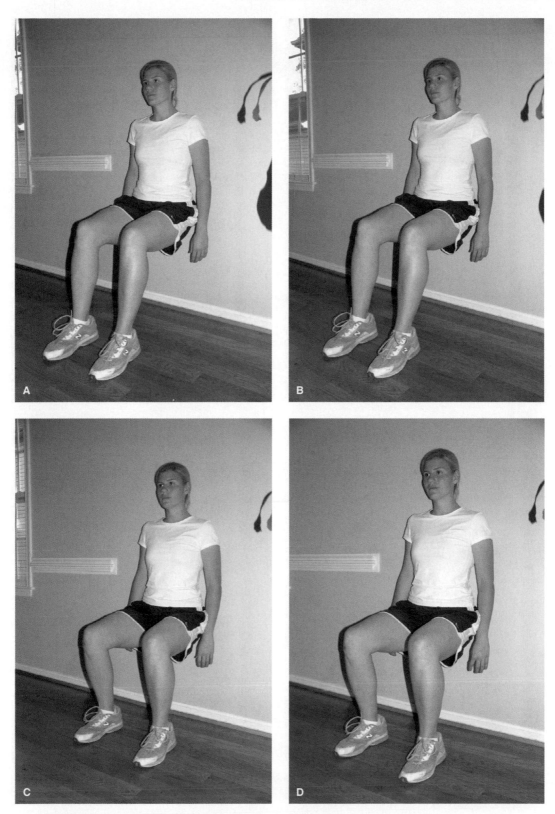

FIGURE C-5 ■ Wall squats (Figure C-5): Stand with your back against a wall with your feet about a foot away. Slowly lower yourself by bending your hips and knees both up to 90 degrees then slowly come up. Repeat — sets of —.

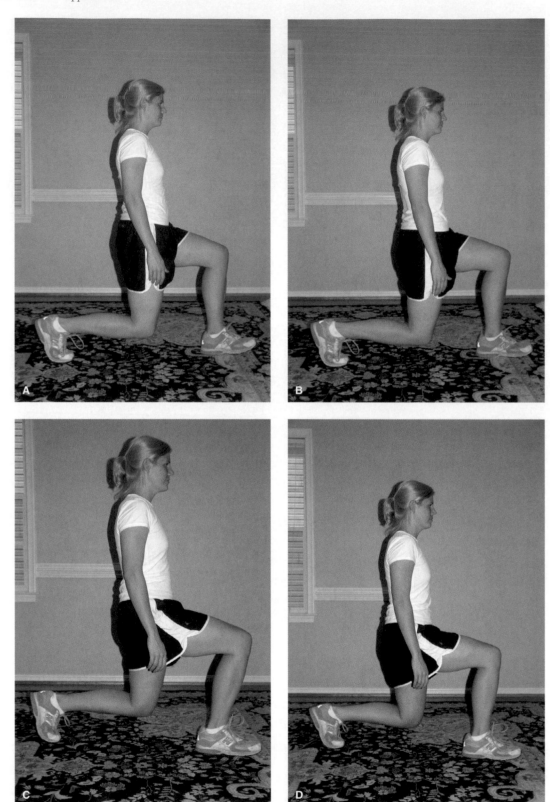

FIGURE C-6 ■ Lunges (Figure C-6): Stand up straight. Lunge forward with one leg, bending your hip and knees to about 90 degrees. Do not let your knees go beyond your toes. Stand back up. Lunge forward with the other leg. Repeat — sets of —.

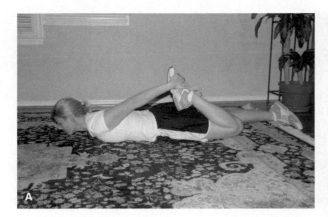

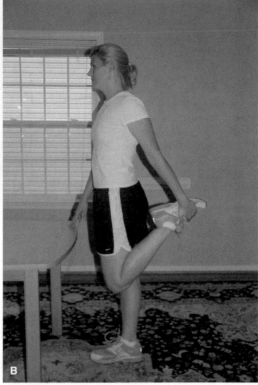

FIGURE C-7 ■ Quadriceps stretch: Lie on your stomach. Grab your foot and pull your heel toward your buttock (Figure C-7A). You can do this standing also (Figure C-7B). You should feel a stretch on your front thigh muscle. Hold the leg for few seconds; repeat — sets of —.

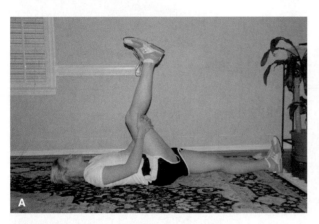

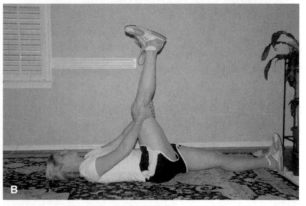

FIGURE C-8 ■ Hamstring stretch (Figure C-8): Lie on your back. With both hands, grab the back of one knee and pull toward you with your foot pointing to the ceiling. Keep the knee straight as far as possible. You should feel a stretch on your back thigh muscle. Hold it for a few seconds. Repeat — sets of —.

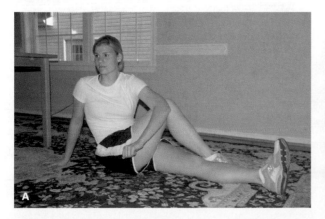

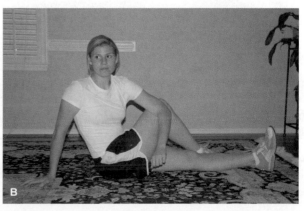

FIGURE C-9 ■ Iliotibial band stretch (Figure C-9): Sit up with one knee bent over the other leg as shown. Twist to the right and push your knee with your left arm. You should feel a stretch on the outer side of your thigh. Hold it for a few seconds. Repeat — sets of —. *(continued)*

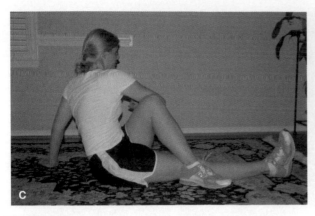
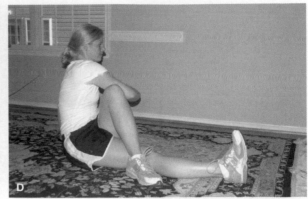

FIGURE C-9 ■ *(Continued).*

ANKLE

See figures C-10 to C-16 with corresponding captions describing the exercises.

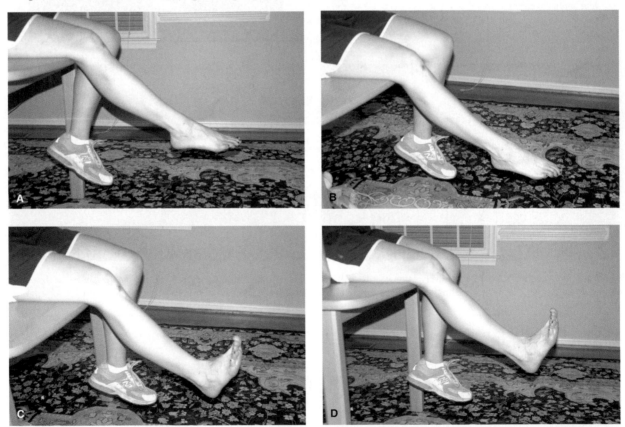

FIGURE C-10 ■ Range of motion: Sit on a chair (Figure C-10). Lift your leg from the floor. Moving only your ankle and foot, draw the alphabet from A to Z in the air. Repeat — sets of the alphabets.

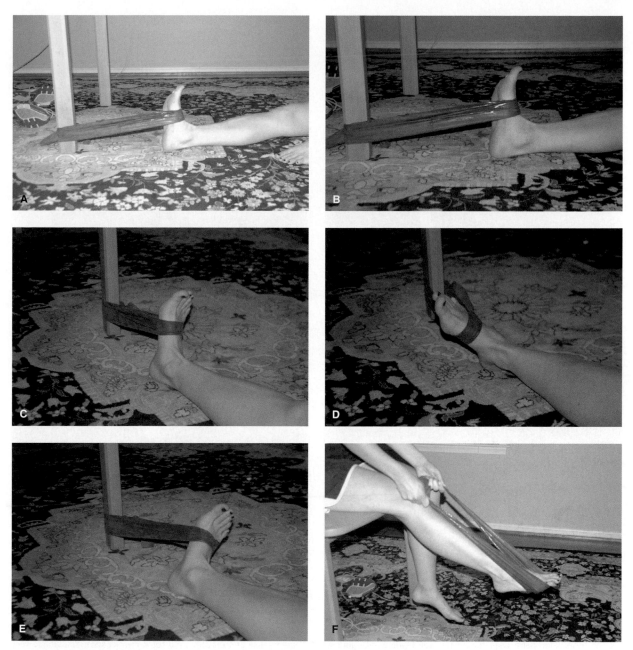

FIGURE C-11 ■ Strengthening: Using an elastic band (that provide various degrees of resistance), loop one end around your foot. Attach the other end to a fixed object. Against the resistance of the elastic band, pull your foot straight up toward you (dorsiflexion) (Figure C-11A to C-11C), pull up and inwards (inversion) (Figure C-11D) and pull up and outwards (eversion) (Figure C-11E). Holding both ends of the band with each hand, loop it around the foot and push your foot downwards against the resistance of the band (plantarflexion) (Figure C-11F). Hold each position for at least 5 seconds, and then return to neutral position. Repeat — sets of.

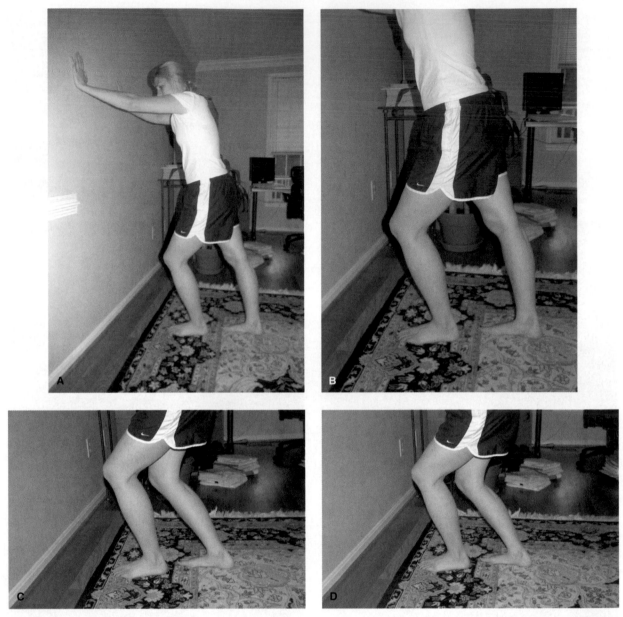

FIGURE C-12 ■ Calf stretching: Stand with palms against a wall with arms straight. Put one leg behind the other. Keep this knee straight and keep the other knee bent. Lean toward the wall leading with your waist (Figure C-12A and C-12B). Hold for a few seconds. You should feel a stretch on your back leg muscle. Repeat the same but this time with the knee bent (Figure C-12C and C-12D). Repeat — sets of —.

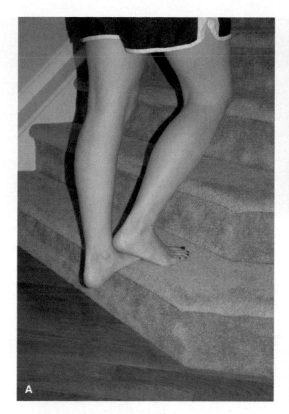

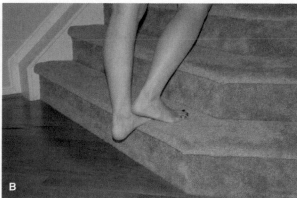

FIGURE C-13 ■ Dorsiflexion and plantarflexion strengthening (Figure C-13): Stand on the edge of the step or a small sturdy stool. Lower your heel below the level of the step. Repeat — sets of —. Repeat with other leg.

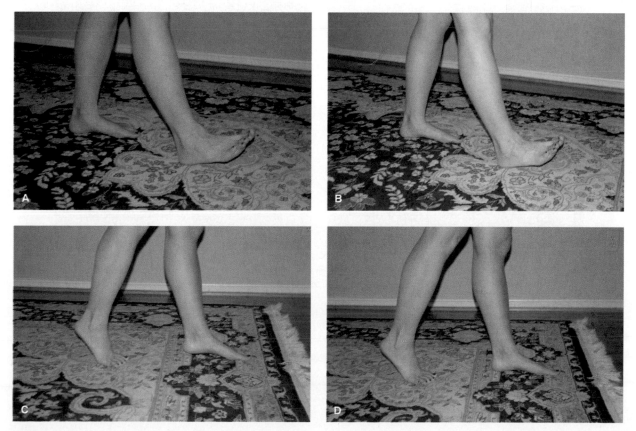

FIGURE C-14 ■ Heel toe walking (Figure C-14): Slowly walk heel to toe raising up fully on toes and then slowly lowering the heels. Do this slowly and repeat for — sets of —.

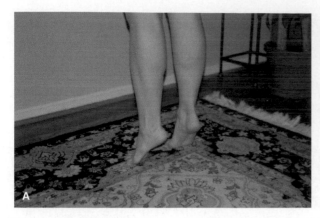 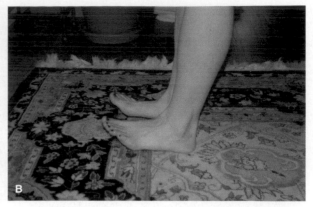

FIGURE C-15 ■ Heel (Figure C-15A) and toe (Figure C-15B) Raises: Raise up on your toes, hold it for a few seconds then go back to standing position. Raise up on your heels, hold for few seconds. Repeat these for — sets of —.

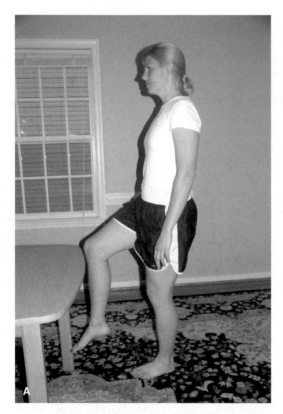 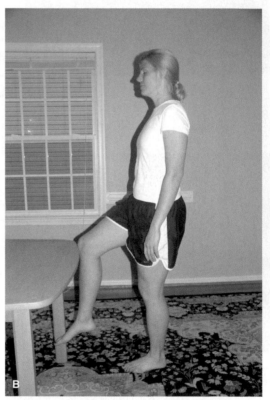

FIGURE C-16 ■ Balance: Stand and balance yourself on one leg for 10 seconds with eyes open (Figure C-16A). You may keep your arms either by your sides or raised up to shoulder level. Repeat with eyes closed (Figure C-16B).

SHOULDER

See figures C-17 to C-19 with corresponding captions describing the exercises.

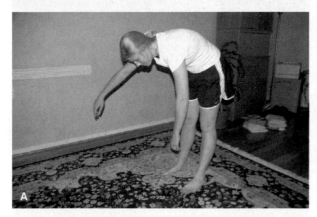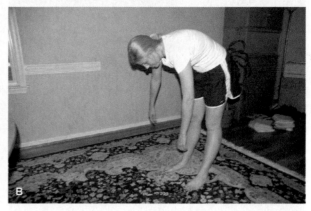

FIGURE C-17 ■ Range of motion (pendulum exercises) (Figure C-17): Lean forward and let your arm hang loose. Gently let your arm move forward, back, and sideways ant then in circles both clockwise and counter clockwise. Repeat — sets of —.

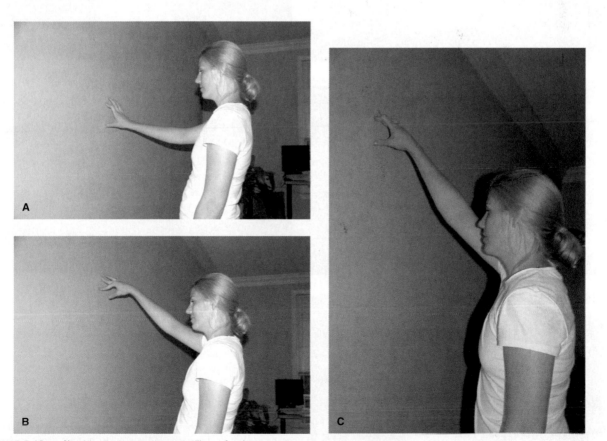

FIGURE C-18 ■ Shoulder flexion (wall crawl) (Figure C-18): Stand near a wall with arm straight touching the wall. Slowly crawl your fingers up until you feel a stretch in the shoulder and then crawl back down. Repeat — sets of —.

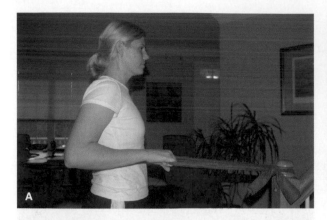

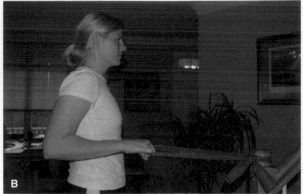

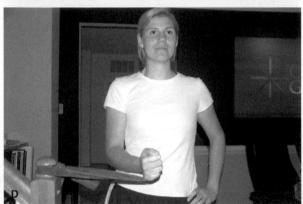

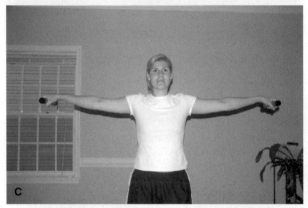

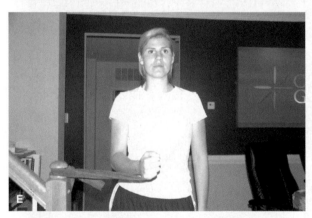

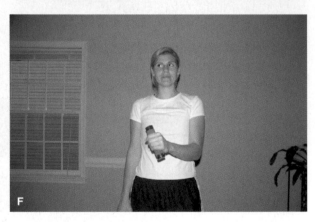

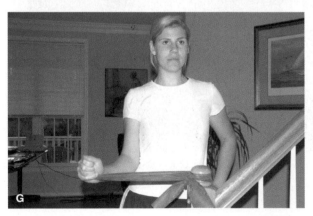

FIGURE C-19 ■ Rotator cuff strengthening: Using an elastic band or holding weight in your hand, do the shoulder motions slowly as shown: flexion, extension (Figure C-19A and C-19B), abduction (Figure C-19C), internal (Figure C-19D to C-19F) and external rotation (Figure C-19G to I). Repeat — sets of —. *(continued)*

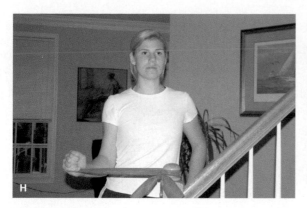
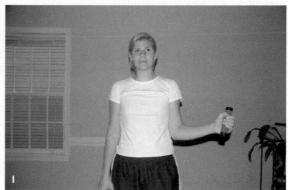

FIGURE C-19 ■ *(Continued)*.

CORE

See figures C-20 to C-26 with corresponding captions describing the exercises.

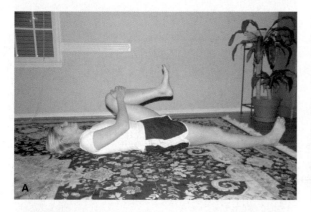
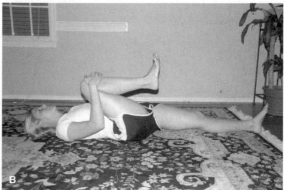

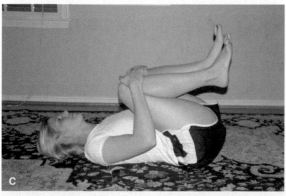

FIGURE C-20 ■ Lumbar flexion (Figure C-20): Lie on your back. Bend one hip, keep back flat, and grab that leg so that your knee touches your chest. Hold for a few seconds. Repeat with both legs at the same time as shown (Figure C-20C). Repeat — sets of —.

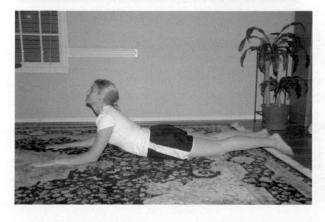

FIGURE C-21 ■ Lumbar extension (Figure C-21): Lie on your stomach. Using your elbows and forearms for support, slowly arch backwards. Do not lift your hips. Hold this position for at least 30 seconds. Return to your starting position. Repeat — sets of —.

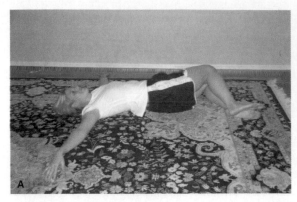
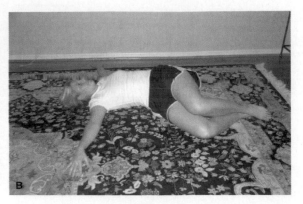

FIGURE C-22 ■ Lumbar rotation (Figure C-22): Lie flat on your back. Stretch your arms out and bend your hips and knees. Keep your shoulders flat on the floor. Roll your knees to one side and hold for a few seconds. Rotate to the other side and hold it for a few seconds. Repeat — sets of —.

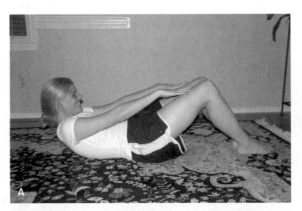
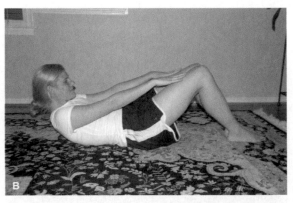

FIGURE C-23 ■ Partial sit-ups (Figure C-23): Lie on your back with the knees bent and arms straight on your thighs. Tuck in your chin and slowly sit up trying to touch your knees. Hold this position for a few seconds and then slowly lay back down. Repeat — sets of —.

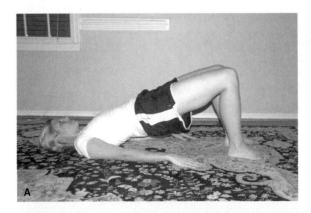
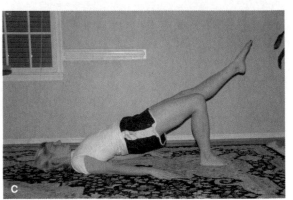

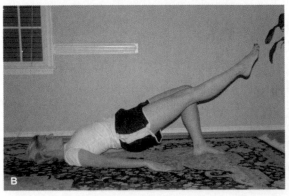

FIGURE C-24 ■ Pelvic lift: Lie on your back with knees bent, feet flat on the floor and arms on your sides. Slowly lift your buttocks up as far up as you can and hold the position for a few seconds (Figure C-24A). Repeat — sets of —. To make it a little harder, straighten one knee with foot pointed up, and then lift your buttocks (Figure C-24B and C-24C).

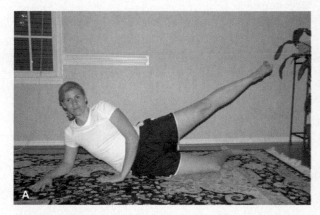
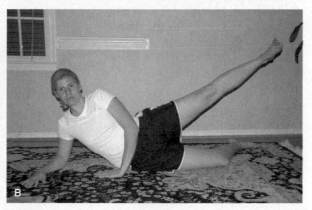

FIGURE C-25 ■ Hip abduction (Figure C-25A and C-25B): Lie on your side. Bend your bottom leg. Support your upper body with your hands. With knee straight and toes pointing, lift your top leg toward the ceiling. Slowly bring it down. Repeat — sets of —.

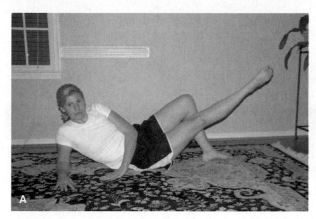
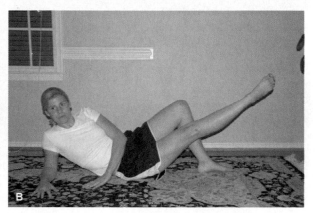

FIGURE C-26 ■ Hip adduction (Figure C-26A and C-26B): Lie on your side. Support your upper body with your arms. With straight knee, slowly lift your bottom leg as high up as you can. Hold it for a few seconds then bring it down. Keep your other leg bent behind it. Repeat — sets of —.

ACKNOWLEDGEMENT

Special thanks to Kelsey Twist for invaluable assistance with preparation of Appendix C.

REFERENCES

1. K Valley Orthopedics Patient Instruction Sheets, Kalamazoo, Michigan, K Valley Orthopedics.

2. Safran M, Stone DA, Zachazewski. *Instructions for Sports Medicine Patients.* Philadelphia, PA: Saunders Elsevier; 2003:40, 42-44, 56, 165-166, 413-415, 505-506.

3. Prentice WE. *Rehabilitation Techniques for Sports Medicine and Athletic Training,* 4th ed. New York, NY: McGraw Hill; 2004:368-691.

APPENDIX D

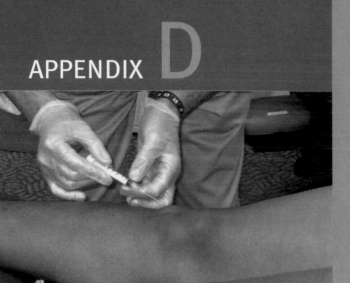

Analgesic and Nonsteroidal Anti-Inflammatory Drugs

Cynthia Feucht

Table D-1.

Anti-Inflammatory Drugs

Generic Name	Brand Name	Adult Dosage	Pediatric Dosage
Non-Steroidal Anti-Inflammatory Drugs			
Diclofenac sodium	Voltaren®	100–200 mg daily (2–4 divided doses) *ER given 1–2 × daily*	2–3 mg/kg/d (2–4 divided doses)
Diclofenac potassium	Cataflam®	100–200 mg daily (2–4 divided doses)	2–3 mg/kg/d (2–4 divided doses)
Diclofenac epolamine	Flector®	180 mg patch every 12 hr	N/A
Etodolac		600–1000 mg daily (2–3 divided doses)	20–30 kg: 400 mg daily 31–45 kg: 600 mg daily 46–60kg: 800 mg daily >60 kg: 1000 mg daily *Age 6–16 y* *Based on ER product*
Fenoprofen calcium	Nalfon®	200–600 mg 3–4 x/d Max 3200 mg/d	N/A
Flurbiprofen	Ansaid®	200–300 mg daily (2–4 divided doses)	N/A
Ibuprofen	Motrin®	1200–3200 mg daily (3–4 divided doses)	4–10 mg/kg/dose 3–4×/d Max 40 mg/kg/d
Indomethacin	Indocin®	50–200 mg daily (2–3 divided doses)	1–2 mg/kg/d (2–4 divided doses) Max 4 mg/kg/d, NTE: 150–200 mg/d *Age >2 y*
Ketoprofen		IR: 150–300 mg daily (3–4 divided doses) ER: 100–200 mg daily	N/A
Ketorolac tromethamine	Toradol®	20 mg initially, 10 mg 4x/d Max 5-d duration	N/A
Meclofenamate sodium		200–400 mg daily (3–4 divided doses)	N/A
Mefenamic acid	Ponstel®	500 mg initially, 250 mg every 6 h as needed (NTE: 1 wk)	N/A

(continued)

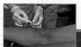

Table D-1. (Continued)

Anti-Inflammatory Drugs

Generic Name	Brand Name	Adult Dosage	Pediatric Dosage
Meloxicam	Mobic®	7.5–15 mg daily	0.125 mg/kg/d Max 7.5 mg daily *Age ≥2 y*
Nabumetone		500–2000 mg daily (1–2 divided doses)	N/A
Naproxen	Naproxen sodium: Anaprox®, Anaprox DS®, Aleve® (OTC) Naproxen: Naprosyn®	Naproxen: 250–500 mg 2×/d Naproxen sodium: 200–500 mg 2×/d Naproxen DR: 375–500 mg 2×/d	*Analgesia: 5–7 mg/kg/ dose every 8–12 h *Inflammatory disease: 10–15 mg/kg/d (2 divided doses) Max 1000 mg/d *Age >2 y*
Oxaprozin	Daypro®	600–1200 mg daily Max 1800 mg daily (in divided doses)	22–31 kg: 600 mg daily 32–54 kg: 900 mg daily ≥55 kg: 1200 mg daily *Age 6–16 y*
Piroxicam	Feldene®	10–20 mg daily	0.2–0.3 mg/kg/d Max 15 mg daily
Sulindac	Clinoril®	150–200 mg 2×/d	2–4 mg/kg/d (2 divided doses) Max 6 mg/kg/d, NTE: 400 mg/d
Tolmetin sodium		600–1800 mg daily (3 divided doses) Max 2000 mg daily	*Analgesia: 5–7 mg/kg/dose every 6–8 h *Inflammatory disease: 15–30 mg/kg/d (3–4 divided doses) NTE: 1800 mg/d *Age ≥2 y*
Celecoxib	Celebrex®	100–400 mg daily (1–2 divided doses)	10–25 kg: 50 mg 2×/d >25 kg: 100 mg 2×/d *Age ≥2 y*

Salicylates

Generic Name	Brand Name	Adult Dosage	Pediatric Dosage
Diflunisal		500–1000 mg daily (2–3 divided doses) Max 1500 mg daily	N/A
Magnesium salicylate	Novosal®, Doan's Extra Strength®	Novosal®: 600 mg 3–4× d, Max 4800 mg daily Doan's®: 934 mg every 6h as needed	N/A
Salsalate	Amigesic®, Salflex®	3000 mg daily (2–4 divided doses)	N/A
Choline magnesium trisalicylate		500–1500 mg 2–3×/d	30–60 mg/kg/d (3–4 divided doses)

IR, immediate-release; ER, extended-release; DR, delayed-release; NTE, not to exceed.
Search monographs [database on the Internet]. Indianapolis (IN); Facts & Comparisons 4.0; 2007 [cited 2007 Jul 23]. Nonsteroidal anti-inflammatory agents; [about 22 screens]. Available from: http://www.online.factsandcomparisons.com/search.aspx?book=DFC&Section=parentMono&search=nsaid.
LexiComp Pediatric Database. http://www.lexi.com. 2007 Jul 23

Table D-2.

Adverse Effects of Anti-Inflammatory Agents

Nausea, vomiting	Photosensitivity
Indigestion, heartburn	Interstitial nephritis
Headache	Acute renal insufficiency
Dizziness	Hyperkalemia
Gastritis	Bronchospasm
GI ulceration/bleeding	Bone marrow suppression
Peptic ulcer	Bruising
Anaphylaxis	Hepatotoxicity
	Increased risk of cardiovascular thrombotic events, myocardial infarction, and stroke
Hypersensitivity reactions	Fluid retention/peripheral edema
Rash	Tinnitus

Search monographs [database on the Internet]. Indianapolis (IN); Facts & Comparisons 4.0; 2007 [cited 2007 Jul 30]. Nonsteroidal anti-inflammatory agents; [about 1 screen]. Available from: http://www.onlinefactsandcomparisons.com/MonoDisp.aspx?book=DIC&monoID=fandc-hp11516&searched=nsaids&#adrs.

Table D-3.

Nonprescription Topical Analgesics

Ingredients	Brand Name
Camphor-based Products	
Camphor 3.1%	JointFlex Cream®
Trolamine Salicylate-based Products	
Trolamine salicylate 10%	Aspercreme Cream®
	Sportscreme Cream®
	Myoflex Cream®
Trolamine salicylate 15%	Myoflex Extra Strength Cream®
Trolamine salicylate 20%	Myoflex Maximum Strength Cream®
Capsaicin-based Products	
Capsaicin 0.025%	Zostrix Arthritis Pain Relief®
	ArthriCare for Women Multi-Action Cream®
Capsaicin 0.035%	Capzasin-P Cream®
Capsaicin 0.075%	Zostrix-HP Arthritis Pain Relief®, Capzasin-HP Cream®
Menthol-based Products	
Menthol 1.27%	Absorbine Jr. Original Liniment®
Menthol 2%	Therapeutic Mineral Ice Gel®
Menthol 4.127%	ActivON Ultra Strength Joint and Muscle®
Menthol 5%	Icy Hot Patch®
	Ultra Strength Ben Gay Relieving Patch®
Menthol 7%	Flexall 454 Gel®
Menthol 12%	Absorbine Jr. Ultra Strength Liquid®
Menthol 16%	Maximum Strength Flexall 454 Gel®

(continued)

Table D-3. (Continued)

Nonprescription Topical Analgesics

Ingredients	Brand Name
Combination Products	
Capsaicin 0.025%, turpentine oil 47%	Sloan's Liniment®
Camphor 3.1%, menthol 16% & methyl salicylate 10%	Flexall Maximum Strength Plus Gel®
Camphor 4%, menthol 10%, methyl salicylate 30%	BenGay Ultra Strength Pain Relieving Cream®
Camphor 4.8%, menthol 2.6%	Vicks VapoRub Ointment®
Camphor 9%, natural menthol 1.3%	Mentholatum Ointment®
Menthol 4.127%, histamine dihydrochloride 0.025%	ActivON Ultra Strength Arthritis®
Menthol 8%, methyl salicylate 30%	Mentholatum Deep Heating Extra Strength Pain Relieving Rub®
	Arthritis Formula Ben Gay Cream®
Menthol 10%, methyl salicylate 30%	Icy Hot Chill Stick®
Menthol 10%, methyl salicylate 15%	Arthritis Hot Pain Relief Creme®

Topical preparations should not be applied more than four times daily. No consensus regarding how long counterirritants should remain in contact with the skin for optimal efficacy.

Wright E. Musculoskeletal injuries and disorders. In: Berardi R, ed. Handbook of Nonprescription Drugs, An Interactive Approach to Self-Care. Washington, DC: American Pharmacists Association; 2006:109-131.

Search monographs [database on the Internet]. Indianapolis (IN): Facts & Comparisons 4.0; 2007 [cited 2007 Jul 23].

Nonprescription drug therapy; rubs and liniments; [about 3 pages]. Available from: http://www.online.factsandcomparisons.com/search.aspx?book=NDT&section=parentMono&Search=rubs/rubs/and/liniments.

Drugstore [homepage on the Internet]. Bellevue: Drugstore.com Inc; c1999-2007 [cited 2007 Jul 23]. Health; rubs and ointments; [about 4 screens]. Available from: http://www.drugstore.com/templates/stdplist/default.asp?catid=9320&trx=GFI-O-EVGR-MCN&trxp1=11&trxp2=9320&trxp3=2&trxp4=ML.

Table D-4.

Topical Analgesic Patient Information

For external use only. Avoid contact with mucous membranes

Apply to affected areas only and avoid contact with irritated skin

Do not use an external source of high heat since irritation and burning may occur

Do not apply tight bandages or wraps over these topical analgesics

Do not apply to broken skin

Re-evaluate therapy if acute pain persists longer than 7–10 d or redness is present

Search monographs [database on the Internet]. Indianapolis (IN): Facts & Comparisons 4.0; 2007 [cited 2007 Jul 23].
Nonprescription drug therapy; rubs and liniments; [about 3 pages]. Available from:
http://www.online.factsandcomparisons.com/search.aspx?book=NDT&section=parentMono&Search=rubs/rubs/and/liniments.

Table D-5.

Sports Drink Comparison Chart

Product	Calories	Carbohydrate (g)	Protein (g)	Sodium (mg)	Potassium (mg)
Accelerade Advanced Sports Drink®	80	15	4	120	15
Gatorade Thirst Quencher®	50	14	None	110	130
Gatorade Endurance Formula®	50	14	None	200	90
PowerAde®	60	17	None	55	30
All Sport Body Quencher®	60	16	None	55	50
Hornet Juice® Powder Packet	60	11	3.7	None	None
SoBe Life Water®	50	13	None	25	None
Vitamin Water Energy®	33.3	8.7	None	None	None
Vitamin Water Power-C®	50	12.7	None	None	None
Vitamin Water Revive®	33.3	8.7	None	None	93.3

Nutritional information based on an 8 ounce serving size.

Sobelifewater.com [homepage on the Internet]. Norwalk: South Beach Beverage Company; c2007 [cited 2007 Jul 26]. Available from: http://www.sobelifewater.com/index_flash.shtml.

Accelerade.com [homepage on the Internet]. New York: Mott's LLP; c2007 [updated 2005 Nov 24; cited 2007 Jul 26]. Available from: http://www.accelerade.com/products/NutritionalInformation.aspx.

Gatorade.com [homepage on the Internet]. Chicago: Quaker Oats Company; c2003-2007 [cited 2007 Jul 26]. Available from: http://www.gatorade.com/products.

Hornetjuice.com [homepage on the Internet]. Auckland, New Zealand: Nature Sport Science Limited; c2007 [cited 2007 Jul 26].
Available from: http://www.hornetjuice.com/image_files/supplements.gif.

Drinkallsport.com [homepage on the Internet]. Austin: All Sport, Inc; c2007 [cited 2007 Jul 26]. Available from: http://www.drinkallsport.com.

Resources for Further Education and Involvement

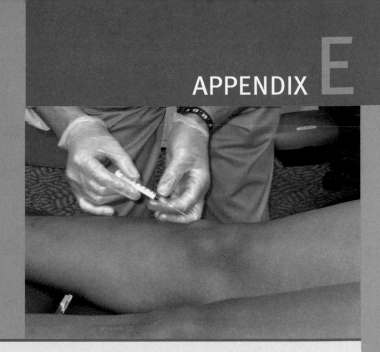

SELECTED SPORTS MEDICINE JOURNALS OF GENERAL INTEREST

American Journal of Sports Medicine
British Journal of Sports Medicine
Clinical Journal of Sports Medicine
Clinics in Sports Medicine
Current Sports Medicine Reports
International Journal of Sports Medicine
Medicine and Science in Sports and Exercise
Scandinavian Journal of Sports Medicine
Sports Medicine

SPORTS MEDICINE ORGANIZATIONS

American College of Sports Medicine, www.acsm.org
American Medical Society for Sports Medicine, www.amssm.org
American Orthopedic Society for Sports Medicine, www.aossm.org
American Osteopathic Academy of Sports Medicine, www.aoasm.org
Canadian Academy of Sports Medicine, www.casm.org
National Athletic Trainers' Association, www.nata.org
National Strength and Conditioning Association, www.nsca.org

North American Society for Pediatric Exercise Medicine, www.naspem.org

LIST OF SELECTED McGRAW-HILL BOOKS

Atlas of Imaging in Sports Medicine (Mark Hargreaves, John Hawley), 2003
Clinical Sports Medicine (Peter Brukner, Karim Khan, with Colleagues), 2007
Current Diagnosis and Treatment in Sports Medicine (Patrick J. McMahon), 2007
Orthopaedic Examination, Evaluation, and Intervention (Mark Dutton), 2004
Therapeutic Modalities for Sports Medicine and Athletic Training (William E. Prentice), 2003
Rehabilitation Techniques in Sports Medicine and Athletic Training (William E. Prentice), 2004
Clinical Sports Nutrition (Louise Burke, Vicki Deakin), 2006
Exercise Physiology (George A. Brooks, Thomas D. Fahey, Kenneth M. Baldwin), 2004
Exercise and Sports Cardiology (Paul D. Thompson), 2002
Preparticipation Physical Evaluation, 2005

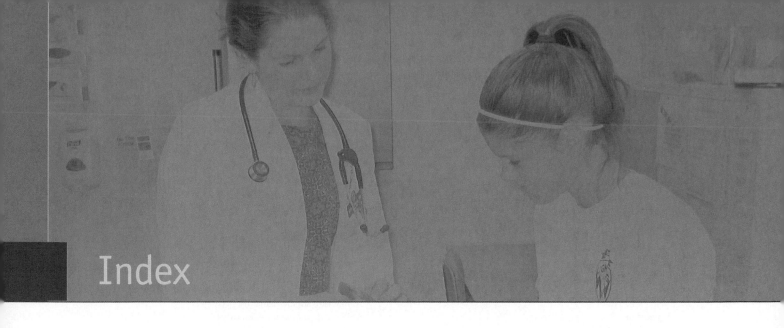

Index